Endocrine Functions and Hypothalamus

Editor: Allan Drake

AMERICAN
MEDICAL PUBLISHERS
www.americanmedicalpublishers.com

AMERICAN
MEDICAL PUBLISHERS
www.americanmedicalpublishers.com

Cataloging-in-Publication Data

Endocrine functions and hypothalamus / edited by Allan Drake.
p. cm.
Includes bibliographical references and index.
ISBN 979-8-88740-094-5
1. Hypothalamic hormones. 2. Hypothalamus--Physiology. 3. Pituitary hormone releasing factors.
4. Hypothalamus--Diseases. 5. Endocrinology. I. Drake, Allan.
QP572.H9 E53 2023
599.014 2--dc23

American Medical Publishers,
41 Flatbush Avenue,
1st Floor, New York,
NY 11217, USA

ISBN 979-8-88740-094-5 (Hardback)

Contents

Preface VII

Chapter 1 ***Nkx2.1* and *Nkx2.4* Genes Function Partially Redundant During Development of the Zebrafish Hypothalamus, Preoptic Region and Pallidum** 1
Martha Manoli and Wolfgang Driever

Chapter 2 **Coexpression Analysis of Nine Neuropeptides in the Neurosecretory Preoptic Area of Larval Zebrafish** 17
Ulrich Herget and Soojin Ryu

Chapter 3 **Characterization of a Mammalian Prosencephalic Functional Plan** 28
Sophie Croizier, Sandrine Chometton, Dominique Fellmann and Pierre-Yves Risold

Chapter 4 **Hypothalamic Glucose Sensing: Making Ends Meet** 41
Vanessa H. Routh, Lihong Hao, Ammy M. Santiago, Zhenyu Sheng and Chunxue Zhou

Chapter 5 **Ontogenesis of Oxytocin Pathways in the Mammalian Brain: Late Maturation and Psychosocial Disorders** 54
Valery Grinevich, Michel G. Desarménien, Bice Chini, Maithé Tauber and Françoise Muscatelli

Chapter 6 **A Unifying Computational Framework for Stability and Flexibility of Arousal** 72
Christin Kosse and Denis Burdakov

Chapter 7 **The Contribution of Hypothalamic Macroglia to the Regulation of Energy Homeostasis** 81
Laura B. Buckman and Kate L. J. Ellacott

Chapter 8 **Notch Signaling and Proneural Genes Work Together to Control the Neural Building Blocks for the Initial Scaffold in the Hypothalamus** 87
Michelle Ware, Houda Hamdi-Rozé and Valérie Dupé

Chapter 9 **Neurons Containing Orexin or Melanin Concentrating Hormone Reciprocally Regulate Wake and Sleep** 99
Roda Rani Konadhode, Dheeraj Pelluru and Priyattam J. Shiromani

Chapter 10 **Thyroid Hormone and the Developing Hypothalamus** 108
Anneke Alkemade

Chapter 11 **Anatomical Organization of MCH Connections with the Pallidum and Dorsal Striatum in the Rat** 117
Sandrine Chometton, Vesna Cvetkovic-Lopes, Christophe Houdayer, Gabrielle Franchi, Amandine Mariot, Fabrice Poncet, Dominique Fellmann and Pierre-Yves Risold

Chapter 12 **Recent Advances in Understanding the Role of the Hypothalamic Circuit During Aggression** 132
Annegret L. Falkner and Dayu Lin

Chapter 13 **Bariatric Surgery in Hypothalamic Obesity** 146
Nathan C. Bingham, Susan R. Rose and Thomas H. Inge

Chapter 14 **Hypothalamic Response to the Chemo-Signal Androstadienone in Gender Dysphoric Children and Adolescents** 155
Sarah M. Burke, Peggy T. Cohen-Kettenis, Dick J. Veltman, Daniel T. Klink and Julie Bakker

Chapter 15 **Role of Estrogen Receptors and G Protein-Coupled Estrogen Receptor in Regulation of Hypothalamus–Pituitary–Testis Axis and Spermatogenesis** 165
Adele Chimento, Rosa Sirianni, Ivan Casaburi and Vincenzo Pezzi

Chapter 16 **Impact of Hypothalamic Reactive Oxygen Species in the Regulation of Energy Metabolism and Food Intake** 173
Anne Drougard, Audren Fournel, Philippe Valet and Claude Knauf

Chapter 17 **Effect of Treatment Modality on the Hypothalamic–Pituitary Function of Patients Treated with Radiation Therapy for Pituitary Adenomas: Hypothalamic Dose and Endocrine Outcomes** 185
Andrew Elson, Joseph Bovi, Kawaljeet Kaur, Diana Maas, Grant Sinson and Chris Schultz

Chapter 18 **The Role of the Lateral Hypothalamus and Orexin in Ingestive Behavior: A Model for the Translation of Past Experience and Sensed Deficits into Motivated Behaviors** 191
Seth W. Hurley and Alan Kim Johnson

Chapter 19 **Hypothalamic Obesity After Craniopharyngioma: Mechanisms, Diagnosis and Treatment** 201
Robert H. Lustig

Chapter 20 **Sweet Taste Signaling Functions as a Hypothalamic Glucose Sensor** 209
Xueying Ren, Ligang Zhou, Rose Terwilliger, Samuel S. Newton and Ivan E. de Araujo

Permissions

List of Contributors

Index

Preface

Every book is initially just a concept; it takes months of research and hard work to give it the final shape in which the readers receive it. In its early stages, this book also went through rigorous reviewing. The notable contributions made by experts from across the globe were first molded into patterned chapters and then arranged in a sensibly sequential manner to bring out the best results.

The hypothalamus is a functionally significant part of the brain. It works as a neural control center for entire endocrine systems, specifically in vertebrates. It maintains the internal balance of the body, which is referred to as homeostasis. Adrenal glands and thyroid gland are the primary endocrine glands in human beings. There are some glands that signal each other in sequence, commonly known as an axis, including hypothalamic-pituitary-adrenal axis. The anterior pituitary regulates several endocrine glands and organs, which is a part of the central neuroendocrine function in hypothalamus. Complex homeostatic mechanisms, several hormonal and behavioral circadian rhythms, crucial behaviors and complicated patterns of neuroendocrine outputs are coordinated through hypothalamus. The extreme lateral part of the ventromedial nucleus of the hypothalamus is liable for controlling food intake. This book contains some path-breaking studies on endocrine functions and hypothalamus. Those in search of information to further their knowledge will be greatly assisted by it.

It has been my immense pleasure to be a part of this project and to contribute my years of learning in such a meaningful form. I would like to take this opportunity to thank all the people who have been associated with the completion of this book at any step.

Editor

nkx2.1 and *nkx2.4* genes function partially redundant during development of the zebrafish hypothalamus, preoptic region and pallidum

Martha Manoli[1] and Wolfgang Driever[1,2]*

[1] Developmental Biology, Faculty of Biology, Institute Biology I, University of Freiburg, Freiburg, Germany
[2] Centre for Biological Signaling Studies (BIOSS), University of Freiburg, Freiburg, Germany

***Correspondence:**
Wolfgang Driever, Institute of Biology 1, Albert-Ludwigs-University Freiburg, Hauptstrasse 1, D-79104 Freiburg, Germany
e-mail: driever@biologie.uni-freiburg.de

During ventral forebrain development, orthologs of the homeodomain transcription factor Nkx2.1 control patterning of hypothalamus, preoptic region, and ventral telencephalon. However, the relative contributions of Nkx2.1 and Nkx2.4 to prosencephalon development are poorly understood. Therefore, we analyzed functions of the previously uncharacterized *nkx2.4*-like *zgc:171531* as well as of the presumed *nkx2.1* orthologs *nkx2.1a* and *nkx2.1b* in zebrafish forebrain development. Our results show that *zgc:171531* and *nkx2.1a* display overlapping expression patterns and a high sequence similarity. Together with a high degree of synteny conservation, these findings indicate that both these genes indeed are paralogs of *nkx2.4*. As a result, we name *zgc:171531* now *nkx2.4a,* and changed the name of *nkx2.1a* to *nkx2.4b*, and of *nkx2.1b* to *nkx2.1*. In *nkx2.1, nkx2.4a,* and *nkx2.4b* triple morpholino knockdown (nkx2TKD) embryos we observed a loss of the rostral part of prosomere 3 and its derivative posterior tubercular and hypothalamic structures. Furthermore, there was a loss of rostral and intermediate hypothalamus, while a residual preoptic region still develops. The reduction of the ventral diencephalon was accompanied by a ventral expansion of the dorsally expressed *pax6,* revealing a dorsalization of the basal hypothalamus. Within the telencephalon we observed a loss of pallidal markers, while striatum and pallium are forming. At the neuronal level, nkx2TKD morphants lacked several neurosecretory neuron types, including avp, *crh*, and *pomc* expressing cells in the hypothalamus, but still form *oxt* neurons in the preoptic region. Our data reveals that, while *nkx2.1, nkx2.4a*, and *nkx2.4b* genes act partially redundant in hypothalamic development, *nkx2.1* is specifically involved in the development of rostral ventral forebrain including the pallidum and preoptic regions, whereas *nkx2.4a* and *nkx2.4b* control the intermediate and caudal hypothalamus.

Keywords: hypothalamus, preoptic region, pallidum, diencephalon, telencephalon, neural patterning, neuroendocrine neurons, zebrafish

INTRODUCTION

Regional specification of the central nervous system (CNS) commences during gastrulation and at neural plate stage, when patterning along the anteroposterior as well as the dorsoventral axes is initiated. The anteroposterior patterning assigns rostrocaudal regional identities (Lumsden and Krumlauf, 1996), and together with the dorsoventral patterning influences cell fate specification and consequently the generation of different neuronal subtypes (Tanabe and Jessell, 1996). Several *Nkx* genes act during patterning of the ventral CNS, and contribute to a molecular code for neuronal differentiation (Shimamura et al., 1995; Ericson et al., 1997; Pabst et al., 1998). Nkx2.1 is a member of the vertebrate Nkx homeobox transcription factor family (Pera and Kessel, 1998; Small et al., 2000; van den Akker et al., 2008). It is also known as thyroid transcription factor 1 (TTF-1) or Thyroid-specific enhancer-binding protein (T/ebp) because of its involvement in thyroid development (Guazzi et al., 1990; Mizuno et al., 1991; Elsalini et al., 2003). Two *nkx2.1* genes in the zebrafish genome have been previously described as paralogs, *nkx2.1a* and *nkx2.1b* (Rohr et al., 2001). Expression of *nkx2.1a* and *b* in the zebrafish CNS was reported to initiate toward the end of gastrulation in a rostrocaudal stripe in the medial anterior neural plate, giving rise to hypothalamus, preoptic region and ventral telencephalon (Rohr et al., 2001). In the medial neural plate and ventral neural tube, expression of mammalian *nkx2.1* has distinct anteroposterior and dorsoventral boundaries (Shimamura et al., 1995; Briscoe et al., 2000; Puelles and Rubenstein, 2003 *nkx2.1a* and *b* expression domains display a common posterior border, which resides in the basal part of prosomere 3 located ventrally to the prethalamus. Both are expressed in the posterior tuberculum and basal hypothalamus. However, the preoptic region, the basal telencephalon around the anterior commissure, and the alar preoptic region exclusively express *nkx2.1b* (Rohr et al., 2001; Lauter et al., 2013). The medial hypothalamus is characterized by *nkx2.1a* expression and low or absent *nkx2.1b* expression.

In mice, development of ventral hypothalamus and telencephalic medial ganglionic eminence depend on NKX2.1. In homozygous *Nkx2.1* knockout mice, ventral forebrain developmental abnormalities start anteriorly in the septal area and extend to the mammillary body of the hypothalamus (Kimura et al., 1996). Loss of NKX2.1 also causes a transformation of medial ganglionic eminence into lateral ganglionic eminence structures (Sussel et al., 1999). In addition, both in mouse and Xenopus embryogenesis removal of *nkx2.1* causes a dorsalization of the basal plate forebrain (Sussel et al., 1999; van den Akker et al., 2008). *Nkx* genes are also involved in neuronal differentiation. In the spinal cord the combinatorial expression of *Nkx* transcription factors (*Nkx6.1, Nkx2.2,* and *Nkx2.9*) specifies ventral identity of neurons (Briscoe et al., 2000; Sander et al., 2000). Less is known about potential involvements of Nkx2 factors in forebrain neuronal differentiation, where Nkx2.1 has been shown to contribute to cortical interneuron subtype specification (Butt et al., 2008).

Here, we report the identification, expression and functional analysis of the zebrafish *nkx2.4a* gene. During embryogenesis *nkx2.4a* is expressed in the hypothalamus in a manner similar to the gene previously reported as *nkx2.1a*. Phylogenetic analysis suggests that *nkx2.4a* resulted from an *nkx2.1* gene duplication event that is not restricted to teleosts (Price, 1993; Small et al., 2000; Wang et al., 2000). In zebrafish, like in mouse (Marín et al., 2002), *nkx2.4a* is expressed in a restricted area of the hypothalamus. In contrast to *nkx2.1*, *nkx2.4a* is not expressed in the telencephalon. Synteny and phylogenetic analysis reveals that the previously reported *nkx2.1a* is in fact a paralog of *nkx2.4*, and not of *nkx2.1*, and thus will be named *nkx2.4b* here in accordance with zebrafish nomenclature. Combined inactivation of *nkx2.1*, *nkx2.4a*, and *nkx2.4b* function by triple Morpholino knockdown (here called nkx2TKD) revealed their contribution to neural patterning and neuronal differentiation. In contrast to single knockdown, the ventral diencephalon of nkx2TKD morphants is dorsalized, revealing that *nkx2.1*, *nkx2.4a*, and *nkx2.4b* act redundantly in hypothalamic patterning. All three genes are required for development of specific subsets of neurosecretory neurons in the hypothalamus.

MATERIALS AND METHODS

ZEBRAFISH HUSBANDRY

Zebrafish breeding and maintenance were carried out under standard conditions at 28.5°C (Westerfield, 2000). We used AB-TL wildtype zebrafish, the enhancer trap *ETvmat2:GFP* (Wen et al., 2008), and smo^{b641} (Barresi et al., 2000), which were identified morphologically. To inhibit pigmentation, embryos were incubated in egg water containing 0.2 mM 1-phenyl-2-thiourea. Embryos were staged according to Kimmel et al. (1995).

INJECTION OF MORPHOLINOS AND RNA

The following morpholinos were used (Gene Tools LLC): *nkx2.4a* TBMO (ATG): 5′-GCTCAGCGACATGGTTCAGCCC GCA-3′, *nkx2.4a* SBMO (e1i1): 5′-TGCATTAGAAGAACTTAC TTGTTGA-3′. The standard control SCMO, p53 ATG (Robu et al., 2007), *nkx2.1* (previously published as *nkx2.1b*) and *nkx2.4b* (published as *nk2.1a-1*) ATG morpholinos have been described (Elsalini et al., 2003). Morpholinos were diluted in H_2O containing 0.05% phenol red or 0.05% rhodamine dextran. *nkx* morpholinos were injected at the one cell stage in different combinations at a total amount of 7.5 ng per embryo, plus an additional 2.5 ng p53 MO. As controls, 7.5 ng standard control morpholino (SCMO) and 2.5 ng p53 MO per embryo were injected.

The efficiency of the *nkx2.4a-e1i1*-SBMO was verified by RT-PCR using cDNA synthesized from 1, 2, and 3 dpf embryos injected with SCMO or *nkx2.4a-e1i1*-SBMO+*nkx2.4b*-MO+*nkx2.1*-MO and *p53*-MO at 2.5 ng each (same conditions as used for all nkx2TKD; **Figure 3B**). The PCR products where sequenced using primers spanning the whole *nkx2.4a* coding region: *nkx2.4a* F: 5′-ATGTCGCTGAGCCCAAAG-3′, *nkx2.4a* R: 5′-CTACCACGTTCTGCCATAAAGC-3′.

To analyse the specificity and efficacy of the translation blocking MOs (TBMOs) directed against the translation start sites of *nkx2.1*, *nkx2.4a*, or *nkx2.4b*, pCS2+-gfp-reporter plasmids were created which each harbor the respective morpholino target sequence, fused in frame to the GFP ORF. *gfp*-reporter mRNAs were generated from plasmids pCS2+-5′UTR-nkx2.4b-gfp, pCS2+-5′UTR-nkx2.1-gfp and pCS2+-5′UTR-nkx2.4a-gfp linearized with NotI, and transcribed using the SP6 mMessage mMachine kit (Ambion). *gfp*-reporter mRNAs were co-injected into one-cell stage embryos in combination with SCMO or the respective specific targeting morpholino. At epiboly stages, embryos were assayed for GFP fluorescence (**Figure 4**). We also attempted to validate the knockdown phenotypes by rescue experiments injecting mRNAs encoding the Nkx2.1 and Nkx2.4, however broad overexpression of Nkx2.1 or Nkx2.4 from injected mRNAs caused severely abnormal development likely because of gain-of-function effects due to ectopic expression (data not shown).

To verify the results obtained with the *nkx2.4a* splice blocking MO, we repeated the nkx2TKD substituting the *nkx2.4a* SBMO with the translation blocking *nkx2.4a* TBMO in the nkx2TKD mix, and analyzed *tyrosine hydroxylase* (*th*), *lhx5*, and *lhx6* expression (**Figure 6**). Both *nkx2.4a* SBMO or TBMO at 2.5 ng per embryo in combination with *nkx2.4b* and *nkx2.1* TBMO generated a similar phenotype.

Synthetic *lefty1* mRNA (mMessage mMachine kit, Ambion) was injected as described (Barth and Wilson, 1995; Thisse and Thisse, 1999).

IN SITU HYBRIDIZATION AND TUNEL STAINING

Whole-mount *in situ* hybridization (WISH) (Lauter et al., 2011) and fluorescent WISH with immunohistochemistry (Filippi et al., 2010) were performed as described. The following digoxigenin-labeled riboprobes were synthesized: *dbx1a* (Fjose et al., 1994), *dlx5a* (Akimenko et al., 1994), *foxa2* (Strähle et al., 1993), *lhx5* and *lhx6* (Toyama et al., 1995), *shha* (Ekker et al., 1995), *otpa* (Del Giacco et al., 2006; Ryu et al., 2007), *pax6* (Krauss et al., 1991b), *pomca* (Herzog et al., 2003), *nkx2.2* (Barth and Wilson, 1995). For generation of *nkx2.4b* (RefSeq NM_131589.1), *nkx2.1(b)* (NM_131776.1), and *nkx2.4a* (NM_001111166.1) probes, the coding sequences were PCR amplified and cloned into the TOPO PCRII vector using the primers *nkx2.4b* F: 5′-ATGTCCTTGA

GCCCCAAAC-3′; *nkx2.4b* R: 5′-TCACCATGTTCTGCCGTACA-3′; *nkx2.1* F: 5′-ATGTCGATGAGCCCTAAGCA-3′; *nkx2.1* R: 5′-TCACCACGTCCTGCCATA-3′ (for *nkx2.4a* see above).

TUNEL assay was performed using the Apoptag *in situ* apoptosis detection kit (Chemicon) (Ryu et al., 2005). Classification of signal: "absent"—no blue stained cell detected in specific brain region; "few cells"—small number of blue stained cell (1–10) dispersed in specific brain region (example telencephalic region in **Figures 3I,J**); "many cells" accumulation of >10 blue stained cells, often clustered, in specific brain region.

MICROSCOPY AND IMAGE ANALYSIS

Transmitted light images were acquired using a Zeiss Axioskop compound microscope. Fluorescently labeled embryos were documented by confocal image stacks using a Zeiss LSM510. Images shown are z-projections of defined sets of consecutive focal planes assembled with the Zeiss Zen 2012 software.

SEQUENCE ALIGNMENTS AND SYNTENY

NKX protein sequences were aligned and analyzed with CLC Genomics Workbench 5 (www.clcbio.com) using the distance based method to generate a phylogenetic tree. The NCBI accession numbers are: NK2.4b [Danio rerio] NP_571664.1, NK2.1(b) [Danio rerio] NP_571851.1, Nkx-2.1 [Mus musculus] NP_001139670.1, Nkx-2.1 isoform 2 [Homo sapiens] NP_003308.1, Nkx-2.1 isoform 1 [Xenopus tropicalis] XP_002935383.1, Nkx-2.4a [Danio rerio] NP_001104636.1, Nkx-2.4 [Mus musculus] NP_075993.1, Nkx-2.4 [Homo sapiens] NP_149416.1, Nkx-2.4 [Xenopus tropicalis] XP_002939478.1, Nkx-2.2 [Homo sapiens] NP_002500.1, Nkx2-2 protein [Mus musculus] AAI38160.1, Nkx-2.2 isoform X1 [Xenopus tropicalis] XP_002939477.1, Nkx-2.2a [Danio rerio] NP_571497.1, Nkx-2.3 [Homo sapiens] NP_660328.2, Nkx2-3 [Mus musculus] CAA72002.1, Nkx-2.3 [Xenopus tropicalis] XP_002937234.1, Nkx2.3 [Danio rerio] AAC05228.1, Nkx-2.5 [Mus musculus] NP_032726.1, Nkx-2.5 isoform 1 [Homo sapiens] NP_004378.1, Nkx2.5 [Danio rerio] AAC05229.1, Nkx2-5 [Xenopus tropicalis] AAI60531.1

Synteny between the mouse and zebrafish *nkx2* genes was visualized using Cinteny (http://cinteny.cchmc.org).

RESULTS

Nkx2.1 AND *Nkx2.4* GENES IN ZEBRAFISH

We systematically searched for zebrafish genes that may interact and be co-expressed with *nkx2.1* transcription factors during ventral diencephalon development, and noticed that the *zgc:171531* gene (ENSDARG00000075107) encodes an NKX2 family member. *zgc:171531* has recently been reported to be expressed in the hypothalamus during late somitogenesis stages (Armant et al., 2013), but its function has not been studied. We analyzed the phylogenetic relationship of Zgc:171531 to other members of the Nkx protein family, and could confirm the suggestion by Armant et al. (2013) that Zgc:171531 is an ortholog of mouse NKX2.4 (**Figure 1**). Phylogenetic tree analysis showed that zebrafish Zgc:171531 is the closest relative of mammalian NKX2.4, and that Zgc:171531and Nkx2.1 are more closely related to each other than to any other Nkx2 transcription factor family member (**Figure 1A**). Therefore, we refer to Zgc:171531 as Nkx2.4a.

To explore the evolutionary history of the *nkx2.1* and *nkx2.4* genes, we searched for synteny conservation. We found that the gene previously reported as zebrafish *nkx2.1b* is located in a microsyntenic chromosomal region related to mouse *Nkx2.1* (**Figure 1B**), thus *nkx2.1b* is indeed the ortholog of mouse *Nkx2.1*. Zebrafish *zgc:171531* resides in a microsyntenic chromosomal region related to mouse *Nkx2.4*. Importantly, also zebrafish *nkx2.4b* (previously named *nkx2.1a*) shares synteny with mouse *Nkx2.4* (**Figure 1C**). Thus, we conclude that *nkx2.4a* and *nkx2.4b* are indeed paralogous NKX2.4 genes derived from the teleost specific genome duplication. In contrast, the previous *nkx2.1a* and *nkx2.1b* are not paralogs, and *zgc:171531* is now named *nkx2.4a*, while *nkx2.1a* is named *nkx2.4b*, and *nkx2.1b* is named *nkx2.1*. This change in nomenclature was approved by the zebrafish gene nomenclature committee (see www.zfin.org).

We analyzed expression of *nkx2.4a* in comparison to *nkx2.1* (**Figure 2**) (Rohr et al., 2001; Tessmar-Raible et al., 2007). At 1 dpf *nkx2.4a* is expressed within the forebrain in basal prosomere 3 including the hypothalamus and the posterior tuberculum, and with decreasing expression levels into the preoptic hypothalamic areas of the basal secondary prosencephalon (**Figure 2E**). In contrast to *nkx2.1* (**Figures 2C,D**), expression of *nkx2.4a* was not detected in the alar hypothalamic region (anterior preoptic region) or the pallidum of the secondary prosencephalon. At 2 dpf *nkx2.4a* expression is downregulated in the basal hypothalamic preoptic area, but continues in the posterior tuberculum and caudal hypothalamus (**Figure 2F**). At 3 dpf *nkx2.4a* expression persists in the posterior tuberculum and hypothalamus (**Figure 2G**), similar to *nkx2.4b* (**Figures 2A,B**). This expression pattern is maintained until 4 dpf (data not shown). Thus, all three *nkx2* genes are expressed in the posterior tuberculum as well as in the basal hypothalamus. However, *nkx2.1* is also expressed in the basal telencephalon around the anterior commissure as well as in the alar hypothalamus preoptic region. *nkx2.4a*, in contrast to *nkx2.4b* (Elsalini et al., 2003), is not expressed in the thyroid gland (**Figure 2H**). Double fluorescent WISH of *nkx2.4a* expression in combination with *nkx2.4b* or *nkx2.1* revealed broad coexpression of *nkx2.4a* and *nkx2.4b* (**Figure 2J**), whereas *nkx2.4a* and *nkx2.1* coexpression is restricted mainly to the intermediate hypothalamus (**Figures 2I,K**).

NODAL AND Shh SIGNALING CONTROL *Nkx2.4a* EXPRESSION

Nodal signaling has been revealed essential for initiation, and Shh for maintenance of *nkx2.1* and *nkx2.4b* expression (Rohr et al., 2001). Smoothened is a key transmembrane effector essential for transmitting Hedgehog signals into the cell (Rohatgi and Scott, 2007). *smoothened homolog* ($smo^{-/-}$) zygotic mutant embryos have severely reduced Shh signaling, although no complete loss occurs due to residual maternal Smo activity (Barresi et al., 2000; Rohr et al., 2001). We detected *nkx2.4a* expression at reduced levels in $smo^{-/-}$ embryos (**Figures 2L,M**), indicating that Hedgehog signaling activity is required to maintain *nkx2.4a* expression. However, Shh is not required for *nkx2.4a* initial induction, similar to what has been shown for *nkx2.4b*.

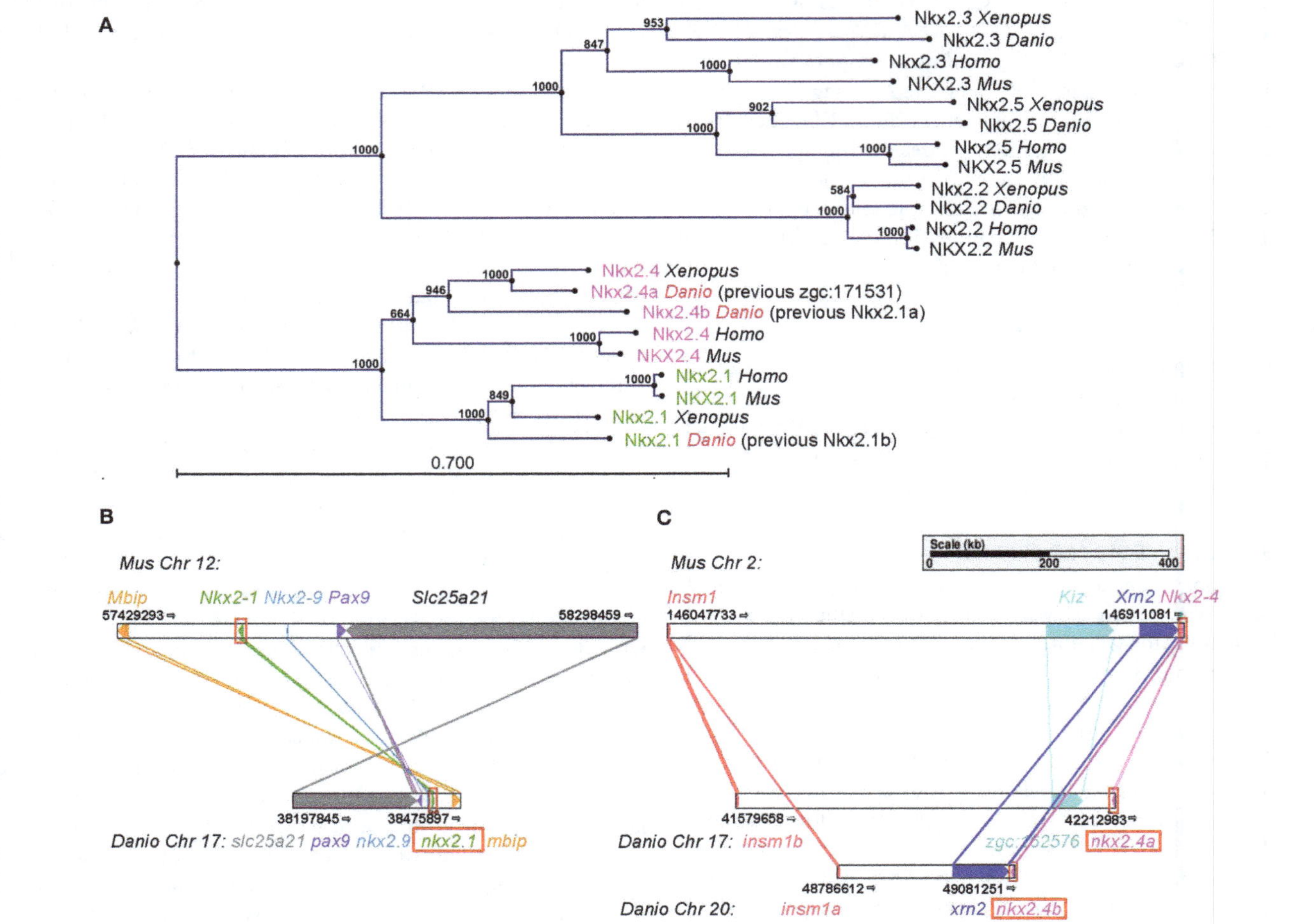

FIGURE 1 | Positioning *nkx2.1* and *nkx2.4* within the *nkx2* homeobox transcription factor family. (A) Phylogenetic tree of five members of the Nkx2 homeobox transcription factor family in zebrafish, Xenopus, mouse, and human. Distance based tree calculations used full-length protein sequences (Materials and Methods). The numbers at the nodes are bootstrap confidence levels from 1000 replicates. The scale bar represents 0.7 substitutions per position. **(B,C)** Genetic synteny at the *nkx2.1* **(B)** and *nkx2.4* **(C)** loci in mouse and zebrafish analyzed using Cinteny (cinteny.cchmc.org). The arrows indicate transcriptional direction.

We then overexpressed *lefty1* mRNA, encoding an inhibitor of Nodal activity, which resulted in complete loss of *nk2.4* expression in >50% of experimental embryos (**Figures 2N,O**). Thus, Nodal is strictly required to induce *nkx2.4a* expression, while Shh contributes to its maintenance.

Nkx2.1 AND *Nkx2.4a/4b* COMBINED KNOCKDOWN SEVERELY AFFECTS THE HYPOTHALAMUS

To examine the role of Nkx2.4a we performed gene knockdown using antisense MOs. The *nkx2.4a* SBMO is complementary to the exon1-intron1 boundary (**Figure 3A**). We have amplified *nkx2.4a* mRNA by RT-PCR from *nkx2.4a* SBMO injected embryos, and found intron1 to be completely retained in the mature mRNA (**Figure 3B**). Sequencing of the splice-blocked mRNA revealed a premature stop codon truncating the Nkx2.4a protein before the homeodomain. To determine the efficiency of the *nkx2.4a* TBMO a *nkx2.4a-gfp* reporter mRNA with the MO binding site at the GFP ATG position was co-injected with the *nkx2.4a* TBMO and shown to completely suppress GFP expression (**Figure 4**). Thus, *nkx2.4a* SBMO and TBMO efficiently inhibit Nkx2.4a expression. Knocking down *nkx2.4a* alone did not result in any detectable morphological phenotype (data not shown).

The similarity in amino acid sequences and the overlapping expression patterns suggest that *nkx2.1, nkx2.4a*, and *nkx2.4b* may act redundantly. Therefore, we aimed at combined knockdown of all three *nkx2* genes. We decided to use Morpholino antisense knockdown to study the combined activity of these three genes, because mutations in none of these genes are available, and even if mutations may become available at some point, the genetic analysis of triple mutations providing the desired phenotype only in one out of 64 embryos is cumbersome. ATG-morpholinos specific to both *nkx2.1* genes have been published (Elsalini et al., 2003). We confirmed their efficacy by knockdown of GFP expression from injected reporter mRNAs (**Figure 4**). *nkx2.4b* TBMO, *nkx2.1* TBMO, and *nkx2.4a* SBMO

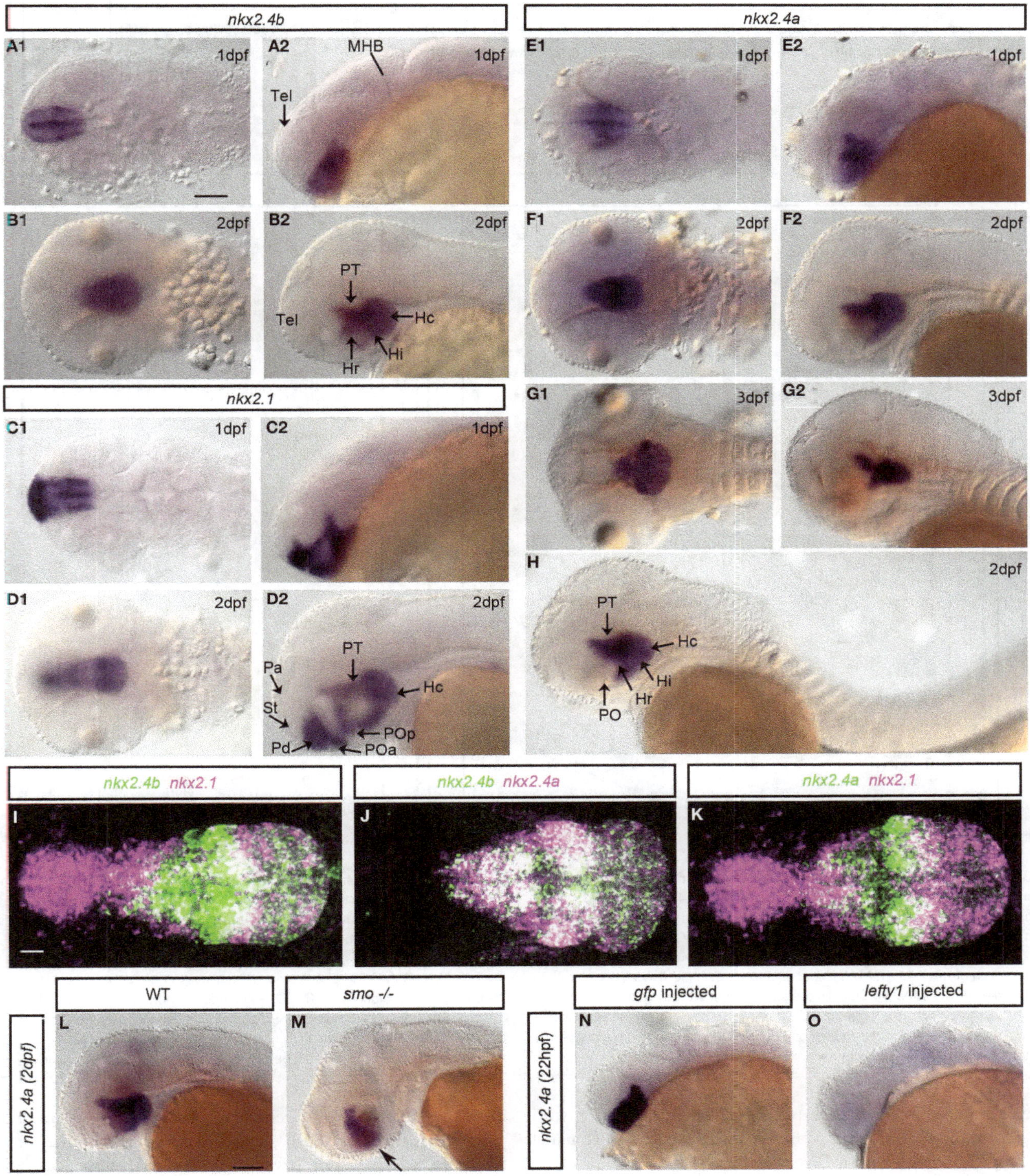

FIGURE 2 | Expression and regulation of *nkx2.1, nkx2.4a,* and *nkx2.4b*. **(A,B)** *nkx2.4b,* **(C,D)** *nkx2.1* and **(E–H)** *nkx2.4a* mRNA expression analyzed by whole mount *in situ* hybridization at indicated stages. **(I–K)** Expression of *nkx2.4a* and *nkx2.4b* and *nkx2.1* were detected by double fluorescent whole mount *in situ* hybridization of 2 dpf embryos, magenta and green channels as indicated in panel headings. Shown are 140–190 μm Z-projections of confocal image stacks. **(L,M)** Expression of *nkx2.4a* in WT and *smo* homozygous mutant embryo. Arrow: residual *nkx2.4a* expressions (**M**, $n = 10$). *nkx2.4a* expression in controls **(N)** and embryos with Nodal signaling inactivated by *lefty1* mRNA injection (**O**: 65% of embryos showed a complete loss, 25% a reduction, 10% normal *nkx2.4a* expression; $n = 25$). **(A1–G1,L-O)** lateral views; **(A2–G2,I–K)** dorsal views. Anterior to left. Scale bar in **A1** = 100 μm (for **A–H**), in **I** = 20 μm (for **I–K**), in **L** = 100 μm (for **L–O**).

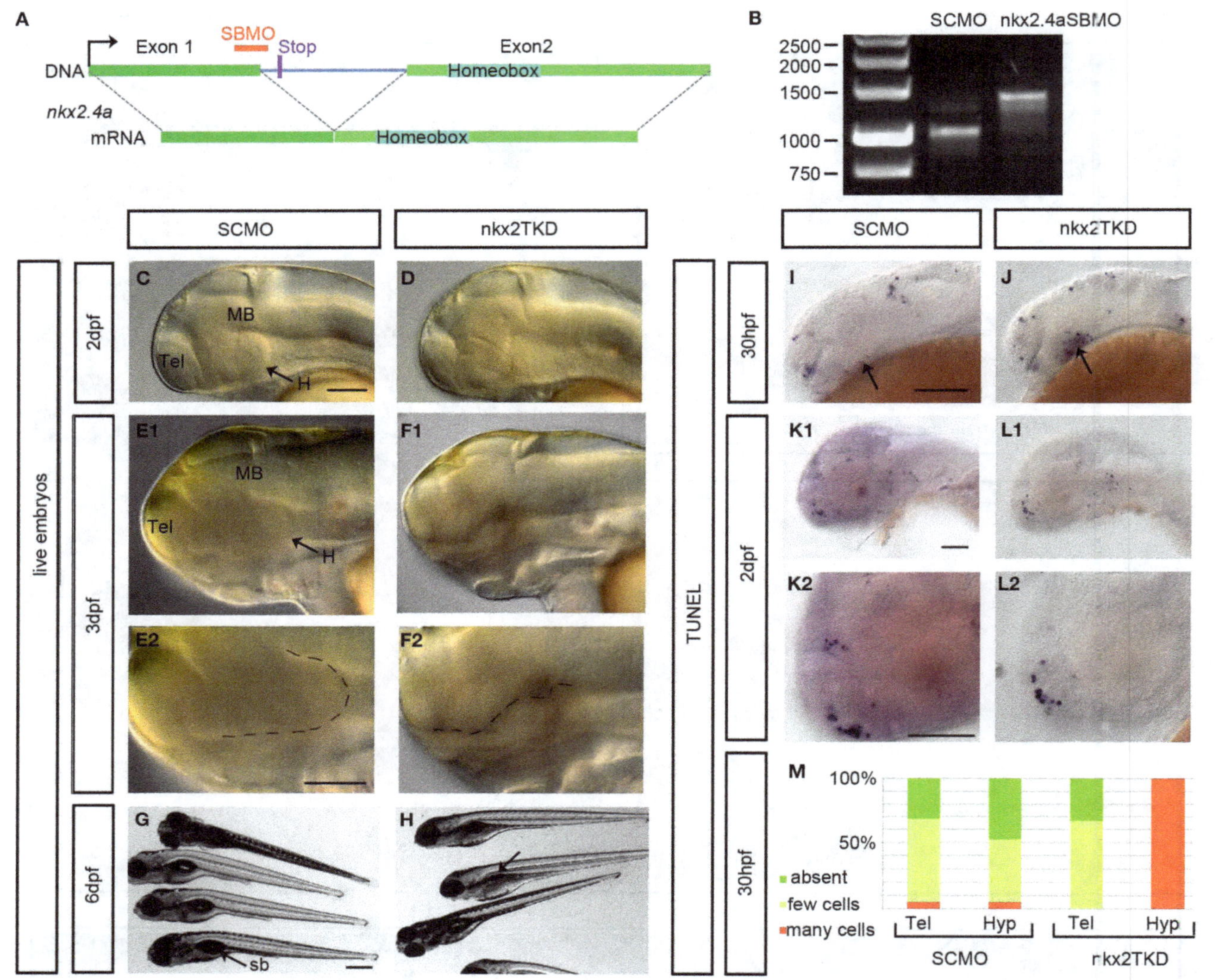

FIGURE 3 | Phenotype of *nkx2.1, nkx2.4a, nkx2.4b* triple (nkx2TKD) morphants. (A) Schematic representation of the *nkx2.4a* gene with the morpholino binding site and the stop codon (12 bases into intron) terminating the protein when intron excision is blocked by the SBMO. **(B)** RT-PCR for *nkx2.4a mRNA* prepared from 3 dpf embryos injected with 7.5 ng SCMO or with 2.5 ng each of *nkx2.4a-e1i1*-MO, *nkx2.4b* and *nkx2.1* ATG MOs. The *nkx2.4a*-e1i1 MO effectively blocks the splice donor site at the exon1-intron1 boundary, giving rise to a longer cDNA. The mature *nkx2.4a* mRNA is nearly completely eliminated under these conditions. **(C–F)** Morphological *in vivo* phenotype of nkxTKD knockdown combined with p53MO knockdown documented using DIC transmitted light microscopy at indicated stages. **(E2–F2)** Close-ups with the ventral border of the diencephalon outlined by dotted lines. **(G,H)** nkxTKD larvae survived at least until 6 dpf (swim bladder is not inflated in fish in **H** indicated by an arrow). **(I–M)** TUNEL staining for apoptotic cells in 30 hpf and 2 dpf SCMO plus p53MO-injected control and nkxTKD plus p53MO morphant embryos (arrows in **I** and **J**: hypothalamus) **(K–L,K2,L2** show close-ups). **(M)** Quantification of number of TUNEL stained apoptotic cells in nkxTKD+p53 ($n = 12$) morphant larvae compared to SCMO+p53MO injected larvae ($n = 19$). Lateral views, anterior at left. Abbreviations see **Table 1**. Scale bars = 100 μm except **G**: scale bar = 400 μm.

were co-injected at 2.5 ng each per embryo in combination with p53 morpholino (for exact amounts used in each figure panel see Supplemental Table 1). Given that some morpholinos cause cell death irrespective of knockdown of specific gene function (Robu et al., 2007), we included p53 MO in our nkx2TKD knockdown mix in all experiments. Live nkx2TKD embryos and larvae were analyzed for morphological abnormalities using transmitted light microscopy (**Figures 3C–H**). At 2 dpf nkx2TKD embryos developed a severe loss of hypothalamic structures, as well as abnormalities in the preoptic region (**Figures 3C,D**). At 3 dpf the massive loss of ventral forebrain tissue became more prominent (**Figures 3E,F**). With the exception of the ventral forebrain, nkx2TKD embryos and larvae developed anatomical structures morphologically similar to control WT embryos, and overall progress of development was not affected. nkx2TKD larvae established blood circulation and survived at least until 6 dpf (**Figures 3G,H**), but frequently did not fully inflate the swim bladder.

To test whether nkx2TKD embryos may develop apoptosis, we performed TUNEL assays. Apoptosis was clearly increased in

Table 1 | Anatomical abbreviations.

1	Basal prosomer 1
2	Basal prosomer 2
3c	Caudal portion of basal prosomer 3 (dbx1+)
3r	Rostral portion of basal prosomer 3 (Pt)
Arc	Arcuate nucleus
H	Hypothalamus
HB	Hindbrain
Hc	Caudal hypothalamus
Hi	Intermediate hypothalamus
Hr	Rostral hypothalamus
MB	Midbrain
OB	Olfactory bulb
P3c	Caudal Prosomere 3
Pa	Pallium
Pd	Pallidum
pit	Pituitary
PO	Preoptic region
POa	Anterior preoptic region
POp	Posterior preoptic region
Pr	Pretectum
PT	Posterior tuberculum
pTh	Prethalamus
sb	Swim bladder
SP	Subpallium
SPV	Supraoptoparaventricular region
St	Striatum
Tel	Telencephalon
Th	Thalamus
zli	Zona limitans intrathalamica

the hypothalamus of morphants compared to SCMO injected embryos at 30 hpf (**Figures 3I,J,M**). However, at 2 dpf apoptosis levels in nkx2TKD morphants were similar to SCMO injected control larvae (**Figures 3K,L**). Thus, nkx2TKD causes increased apoptosis in those brain regions of *nkx2.1/2.4* expression specifically when the hypothalamus forms, but not at later stages.

KNOCKDOWN OF *Nkx2.1/4a/4b* SEVERELY AFFECTS VENTRAL FOREBRAIN PATTERN FORMATION

Shh is a key determinant of ventral pattern formation in the neural plate. Studies have shown that its expression in the basal telencephalon depends on *nkx2.1* function in mice (Sussel et al., 1999). In wild-type zebrafish embryos *shha* (**Figure 5A**) is expressed in floor plate and underlying axial mesoderm, as well as in the zona limitans intrathalamica (ZLI; Scholpp et al., 2006), which is a narrow transverse region between the prethalamus and thalamus (Shimamura et al., 1995; Kiecker and Lumsden, 2004). In *nkx2.1* morphants *shha* expression was mostly normal, with only a minor reduction in the hypothalamus (**Figure 5B**). In *nkx2.4a/4b* double morphants (**Figure 5C**) we detected a more severe reduction of the hypothalamic *shha* expression. In nkx2TKD embryos *shha* expression in the hypothalamus was almost completely eliminated (**Figure 5D**), while in the ZLI and caudal to it *shha* expression appeared normal. Thus, all three *nkx2* genes redundantly regulate *shha* expression in the hypothalamus. Caudal to prosomer 3 *shha* expression was not affected in nkx2TKD morphants. This is consistent with the finding that the expression pattern of *foxa2*, a marker for medial and lateral floor plate caudal to prosomere 2 (Odenthal and Nusslein-Volhard, 1998), appeared unaffected in nkx2TKD morphants with some enlargement of basal prosomeres 1 and 2 (**Figures 5O,P**). With respect to basal prosomere 3, the *nkx2.1* expression extends only into the rostral half of prosomere 3, while *dbx1a* is expressed in the caudal part of basal prosomere 3 (Lauter et al., 2013). *dbx1a* expression was not affected in nkx2TKD morphants, indicating normal development of the caudal portion of prosomer 3 (**Figures 5M,N**). This finding demonstrates that brain regions caudal to the limit of *nkx2.1/4a/4b* expression are not affected upon nkx2TKD.

A target of mouse NKX2.1 in the telencephalon is *Lhx6* (Sussel et al., 1999; Du et al., 2008). In our study, in *nkx2.1* morphants pallidal *lhx6* expression was strongly reduced, but not the diencephalic *lhx6* expression (**Figures 5E,F**). In *nkx2.4a* and *nkx2.4b* double morphants however pallidal *lhx6* expression was maintained, whereas in the diencephalon the caudal posterior tubercular expression was lost (**Figure 5G**). In nkx2TKD morphants, both the pallidal and posterior tubercular *lhx6* expression were severely reduced, while *lhx6* expression in the preoptic supraoptoparaventricular (SPV) region was retained (**Figure 5H**). These results were confirmed by analysing the more broadly expressed *lhx5* (**Figure 5I**). The *lhx5* domains in posterior tuberculum and caudal and rostral hypothalamus were depleted in nkx2TKD morphants, while expression in the alar preoptic region was still detectable (**Figure 5L**). In the telencephalon, the dorsal *lhx5* expression domain expanded ventrally into the pallidal area, from which *lhx5* was absent in wildtype. This ventral expansion of the telencephalic *lhx5* expression was also visible in *nkx2.1* morphants (**Figure 5J**), which otherwise had an unaltered *lhx5* expression pattern. Double *nkx2.4a* and *nkx2.4b* morphants did not develop the telencephalic *lhx5* expansion, but exhibited a reduction of the hypothalamic expression pattern (**Figure 5K**). The nkx2TKD expression changes of *lhx5* and *lhx6* were also validated in triple knockdown embryos using the *nkx2.4a* TBMO (**Figure 6**). The expression of *otpa* in the posterior tuberculum was strongly reduced in nkx2TKD morphants, while expression was still detected in the anterior preoptic area (**Figures 5Q,R**). Analysis of *dlx5a* reveals that the dorsal subpallium (striatum) still forms in nkx2TKD morphants (**Figures 5S,T**). In contrast, the caudal hypothalamic *dlx5a* domain was absent in triple morphants. Similar to what was observed for *lhx6* expression in nkx2TKD morphants, the *dlx5a* expression domain in the alar preoptic region appears expanded ventro-caudally (**Figures 5S,T**). *nkx2.2a* has a rostro-caudal domain extending approximately along the alar-basal boundary of the fore- and midbrain (Puelles and Rubenstein, 1993; Hauptmann and Gerster, 2000). This boundary remained unaffected in the triple morphants. Also, the prethalamic and thalamic as well as preoptic *nkx2.2a* expression domains appeared largely normal, while the caudal hypothalamic expression was reduced (**Figures 5U,V**). Analysing *emx1* expression, we did not observe any effect of nkx2TKD on the pallium (**Figures 5W,X**). In summary, these results show that

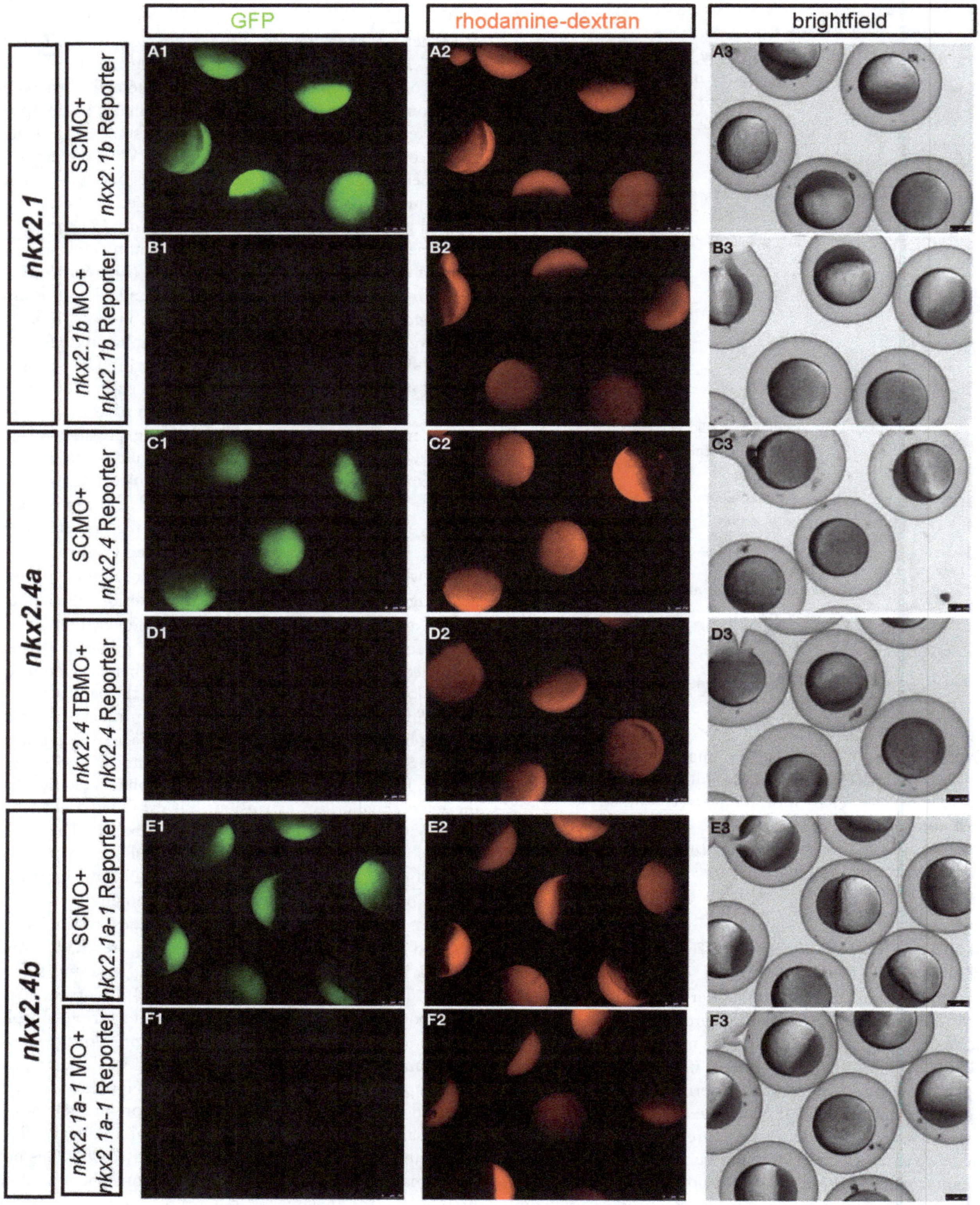

FIGURE 4 | Experimental validation of *in vivo* knockdown efficiency of translation blocking morpholinos used in this study. MO knockdown efficiency was demonstrated by co-injection of GFP reporter mRNAs with the morpholino binding sites engineered at the start ATG of GFP. The following GFP reporter were injected at 100 pg mRNA per embryo: **(A,B)** *5′ UTR-nkx2.1-gfp* mRNA, **(C,D)** *5′ UTR-nkx2.4a-gfp* mRNA, and **(E,F)** *5′ UTR-nkx2.4b-gfp* mRNA. Morpholinos used are indicated in boxes at

(Continued)

FIGURE 4 | Continued
left of each panel and were injected at 5 ng each, controls containing the same amount of SCMO. *nkx2.1* ATG MO and *nkx2.4b* ATG MO morpholinos have been described previously (Elsalini et al., 2003). All embryos were also co-injected with rhodamine-dextran, which was used to sort embryos after 4–5 h. of development for homogenous amounts and distribution of injected material. Knockdown efficiency was then documented between 4 and 5 hpf by pictures taking with the epifluorescence dissecting microscope in the red channel to verify that embryo were injected, in the green channel to control efficiency of GFP knockdown, and in the transmitted light channel to control morphology and viability of embryos. *nkx2.4b* and *nkx2.1* and *nkx2.4a*TBMO morphants were rhodamine-dextran fluorescence levels similar to control-injected embryos but showed no expression of the respective GFP reporters, indicating that these TBMOs effectively bind and block translation of target mRNAs *in vivo*.

loss of *nkx2.1/4a/4b* activity mainly affects three regions of the forebrain. In the caudal diencephalon, there is a loss of the rostral part of basal prosomer 3 and derivative posterior tubercular and hypothalamic structures, while the alar basal boundary appears non-shifted. Further rostrally, there is a loss of rostral and intermediate hypothalamic markers, while a residual preoptic region including the supraoptoparaventricular region develops in nkx2TKD morphants. Within the telencephalon, there is a loss of pallidal markers, while striatum and pallium are forming.

KNOCKDOWN OF *nkx2.1/4a/4b* LEADS TO A DORSALIZATION OF THE VENTRAL DIENCEPHALON

Studies in mice suggested that *Nkx2.1* knockout causes a ventral expansion of dorsal diencephalic marker genes (Kimura et al., 1996). Therefore, we tested whether similar fate shifts occur in nkx2TKD embryos by analysing *pax6a* expression, which is predominantly expressed in dorsal parts of the diencephalon (Krauss et al., 1991a), as well as in cells at the pallial-subpallial boundary (Wullimann and Rink, 2001). In nkx2TKD embryos, *pax6* expression was expanded ventrally in its prethalamic domain, suggesting a loss of basal prosomere 3 (**Figures 5Y–AA**). Together with the data obtained for *dbx1a* expression (**Figures 5M,N**; caudal part of prethalamus and caudal part of basal prosomer 3; Lauter et al., 2013), it appeared that the rostral part of basal prosomere 3 was completely dorsalized, while the caudal *dbx1a* expressing part of prosomere 3 was not affected. Also, it appears that alar *pax6a* expression did not invade into the basal prosomere 1 and 2 regions, which in morphants appeared more pronounced caudal to prosomere 3 (see also 2 dpf *foxa2* expression **Figures 5O,P**). In contrast, when only *nkx2.1* and *nkx2.4b* were knocked down, no obvious ventral expansion of the *pax6a* domain into the hypothalamus was detectable. Thus, *nkx2.4a* can compensate loss of *nkx2.1* and *nkx2.4b* in hypothalamic patterning. In summary these results suggest that the loss of *nkx2.1/4a/4b* activity leads to a dorsalization of the basal prosomer 3 as well as of the pallidum.

Nkx2.1/4a/4b CONTROL EXPRESSION OF *nkx2.1* AND *nkx2.4* GENES

We next analyzed whether Nkx2.1/4a/4b activity is required for continued expression of these genes during embryonic development. Compared to controls, in nkx2TKD morphants the expression domains of all three genes were restricted to more medial forebrain regions, most pronounced for *nkx2.4a* and *nkx2.4b* (**Figure 7**). At 2 dpf, expression of all three genes was maintained in the posterior tubercular portion of the prosomer 3 derived basal hypothalamus in nkx2TKD embryos. In contrast, expression of all three *nkx2* genes was depleted in the intermediate and caudal hypothalamus. *nkx2.1/4a/4b* expression was reduced in the preoptic region. *nkx2.1* expression domains in the alar plate preoptic telencephalon and pallidum were maintained, albeit the size of the domain and the expression level appeared slightly reduced (**Figures 7A,B**). These results suggest that *nkx2.1* and *nkx2.4a/b* activity may be required to maintain their expression in specific domains of the developing forebrain. An alternate explanation may be that some hypothalamic tissue may get lost due to apoptosis (see **Figures 3I,J**).

nkx2TKD AFFECTS HYPOTHALAMIC NEUROSECRETORY POPULATIONS

We next investigated which neuroendocrine systems were affected by loss of *nkx2.1* or *nkx2.4* activity. Expression of *pomca* (Hansen et al., 2003; Lohr and Hammerschmidt, 2011) is lost in the arcuate nucleus as well as the pituitary of nkx2TKD morphants (**Figures 8A,B**). To further characterize differential effects of nkx2TKD on ventral neuroendocrine vs. preoptic hypothalamus, we analyzed expression of the neuroendocrine hormone genes *corticotropin releasing hormone (crh), oxytocin (oxt)*, and *arginine vasopressin (avp)* at 2 and 3 dpf. *crh* expression (Chandrasekar et al., 2007) in the posterior tuberculum and hypothalamus of nkx2TKD morphants was completely absent (**Figures 8C,D**), while *crh* expressing neurons in all other regions developed normally. *oxt* is exclusively expressed in the preoptic region (**Figures 8E,F**), and similar to the preoptic domain of *avp* (**Figures 8E,F**) was not affected in triple morphants. In contrast, *avp* expression in the neuroendocrine ventral hypothalamus was strongly reduced or eliminated in nkx2TKD morphants (**Figures 8G,H**). We also occasionally observed *oxt*-expressing cells at ectopic locations posterior to the domain in the anterior hypothalamus in several nkx2TKD morphants (**Figure 8F**, arrow). In summary, nkx2TKD affects neuroendocrine development selectively in the hypothalamus, but not in the preoptic region.

DISCUSSION

The hypothalamus harbors many highly conserved neuroendocrine and neuromodulatory systems vital for the control of fundamental behavioral patterns and physiology. Hypothalamus organization and major developmental control centers have been well described (Puelles and Rubenstein, 2003; Moreno and Gonzalez, 2011). However, the complex organization and dynamic morphogenesis of the hypothalamus have hindered a more detailed understanding of molecular mechanisms controlling patterning and neuronal differentiation. *Nkx2.1* genes have a crucial role in development of the ventral forebrain, but analysis of mutant mice (Kimura et al., 1996; Sussel et al., 1999; Marín et al., 2002) and knockdown in *Xenopus* (van den Akker et al., 2008) have resulted in phenotypes that differentially affect the alar preoptic region and the basal hypothalamus. Here, we characterize a second *nkx2.1*-related gene in zebrafish, *nkx2.4a*.

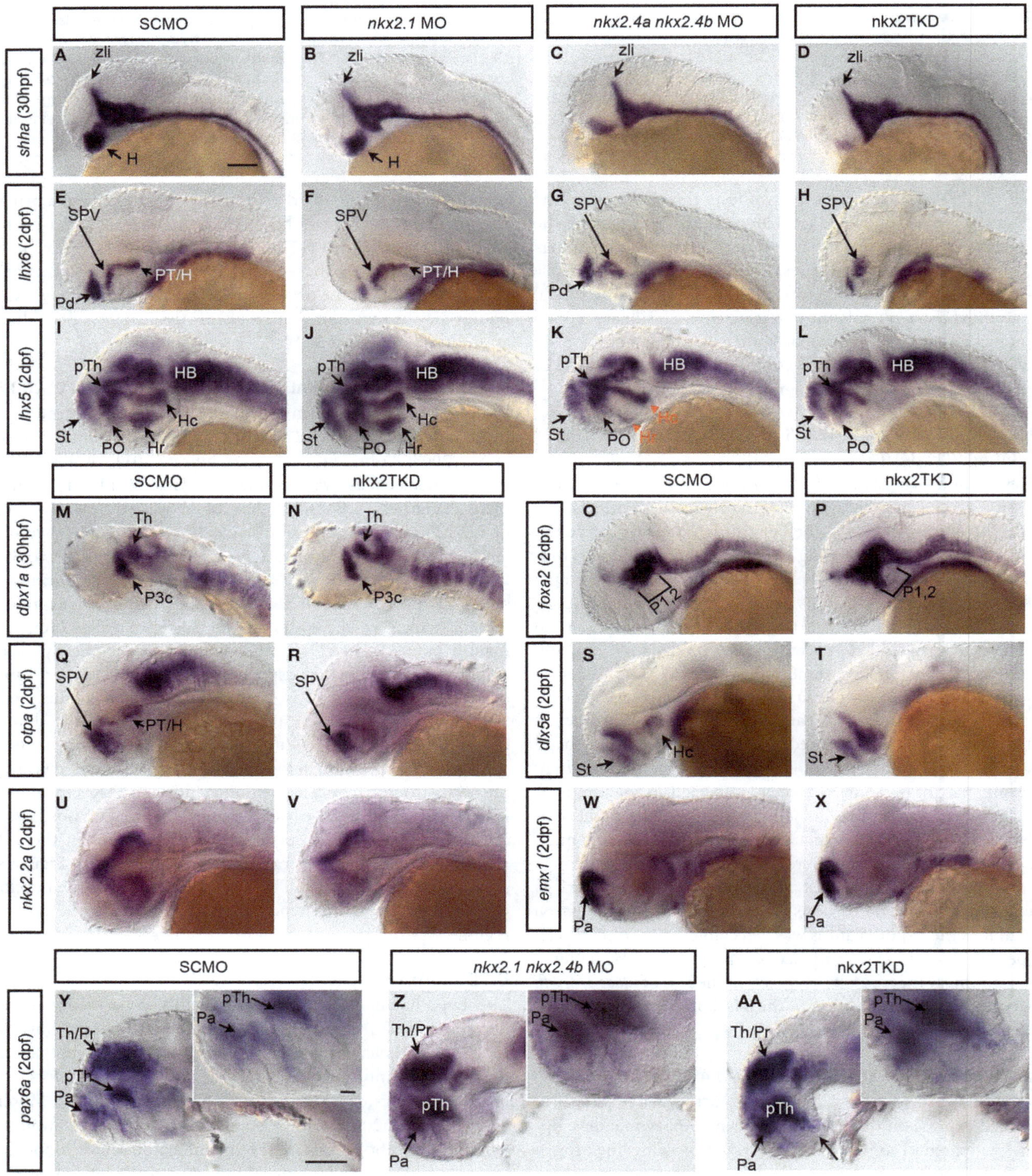

FIGURE 5 | *nkx2.1, nkx2.4a,* and *nkx2.4b* knockdown affects forebrain patterning. Zygotes were injected with single or combinations of Nkx2 gene morpholinos as indicated in boxes above the panels, and incubated until 30 hpf **(A–D,M,N)** or 2 dpf **(E–L,O–AA)**. Expression of patterning genes were analyzed by WISH. **(A–D)** Hypothalamic *shha* expression in **(B)** *nkx2.1* morphants is largely normal, with a minor reduction (n = 10.10); **(C)** *nkx2.4a/4b* double morphants (n = 10.10) is more severely reduced; **(D)** nkx2TKD embryos is severely reduced in the rostral forebrain (n = 29.29). **(E–H)** *lhx6*, and **(I–L)** *lhx5* expression in morphants at 2 dpf (**E**, n = 42.42; **F**, n = 11.11; **G**, n = 4.4; **H**, n = 67.67; **I**, n = 30.30; **J**, n = 7.7; **K**, n = 9.9; **L**, n = 23.23) (red arrowhead in **K** indicates affected area/reduced expression).

(Continued)

FIGURE 5 | Continued
(M,N) *dbx1a* expression was not perturbed by nkx2TKD at 30 hpf. **(O,P)** nkxTKD leads to a slight anterior expansion of *foxa2* expression in basal prosomeres 1 and 2 (**O**, $n = 22.22$; **P**, $n = 11.11$). **(Q,R)** *otpa* and **(S,T)** *dlx5a* expression were affected in the posterior tuberculum and hypothalamus of nkx2TKD morphants at 2 dpf (**Q**, $n = 34.34$; **R**, $n = 60.60$; **S**, $n = 16.16$; **T**, $n = 12.12$). **(U,V)** nkx2TKD affects the expression pattern of *nkx2.2* only in the caudal hypothalamus ($n = 14.14$). **(W,X)** The pallial telencephalic *emx1* expression is not affected in nkx2TKD. **(Y,AA)** In nkx2TKD morphants the prethalamic *pax6* expression domain expands into the ventral hypothalamus (inset in **AA**, $n = 13.13$), while double *nkx2.1* and *nkx2.4b* morphant have a less severe ventral *pax6* expansion (inset in **Z**, $n = 25.25$). Lateral views, anterior is to the left. Abbreviations see **Table 1**. lateral views. Black arrows point at positions of anatomical structures labeled by abbreviation at start of arrow. Scale bar = 100 μm in **(A)** for **(A–X)**, in **(Y)** for **(Y–AA)**.

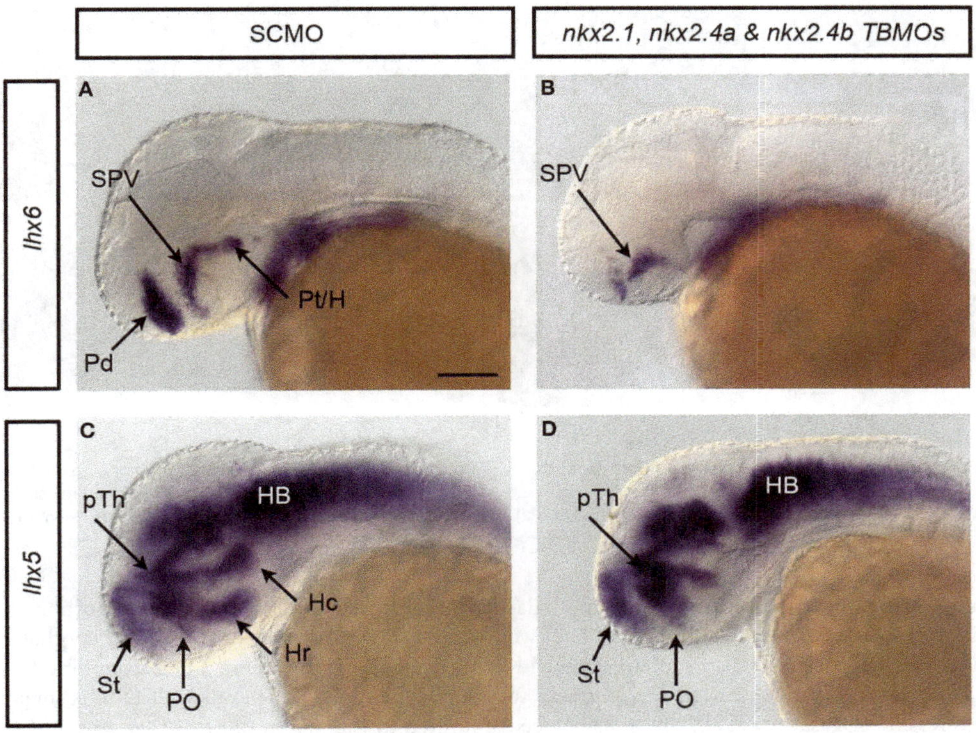

FIGURE 6 | Validation of nkx2TKD phenotype by independent *nkx2.4a* TBMO. By designing a second, non-overlapping MO against *nkx2.4a* (*nkx2.4a* TBMO) concerns with off-target phenotypes can be addressed. The probability of both *nkx2.4a* MOs yielding a similar off-target phenotype is significantly lower compared to a single MO only (Eisen and Smith, 2008). The triple knockdown experiments with the *nkx2.4a* TBMO were analyzed for changes in *lhx6* **(A,B)** and *lhx5* **(C,D)** expression. The observed phenotypes were very similar to the nkx2TKD with the SBMO: the respective expression domains in the pallidum, the posterior tuberculum, the caudal and rostral hypothalamus were depleted in nkx2TKD with the *nkx2.4a* TBMO, while expression in other anatomical domains, including the alar preoptic region, was not significantly affected. Therefore, the analysis of nkx2TKD with the *nkx2.4a* TBMO confirmed the results obtained in our study with the nkx2TKD with the *nkx2.4a* SBMO. Black arrows point at positions of anatomical structures labeled by abbreviation at start of arrow.

Partial redundancies between *nkx2.1* and *nkx2.4a*, which has not been previously knocked out in mice, may explain difficulties in understanding the role of NKX2.1 factors in ventral forebrain development.

zgc:171531 / nkx2.4a encodes a novel zebrafish Nkx2 homeobox transcription factor of high sequence similarity to Nkx2.1 and Nkx2.4. In light of synteny and phylogenetic tree analysis, the previously reported zebrafish *nkx2.1a* is more closely related to *nkx2.4a* than to *nkx2.1*. Recent phylogenetic analysis of rainbow trout Nkx2-4 also suggested zebrafish the previously *nkx2.1a* named gene to be a *nkx2.4* paralog (Uemae et al., 2014). Analysis of *nkx2.4a* expression in relation to the *nkx2.1* genes also reveals a strong similarity to the expression pattern in the brain of the gene previously reported as *nkx2.1a*. *nkx2.4a* is expressed in the posterior tuberculum and hypothalamus. *nkx2.4a* is not expressed in the preoptic region or pallidum, as *nkx2.1* is. For zebrafish, our data indicate that the gene previously named *nkx2.1a* is indeed a paralog of *nkx2.4*, and the two paralogous genes will be named *nkx2.4a* and *nkx2.4b* as orthologs of mammalian *Nkx2.4*, while *nkx2.1* is the only *Nkx2.1* ortholog in zebrafish.

Expression patterns similar to zebrafish have been reported for *nkx2.4* in *Xenopus* (Small et al., 2000; Ermakova et al., 2007). Mouse *Nkx2.4* expression (Price, 1993) is also restricted to the hypothalamus and absent from the preoptic region (Marín et al., 2002). Thus, it appears that the *nkx2.4* expression pattern is conserved throughout evolution, and based on the high sequence

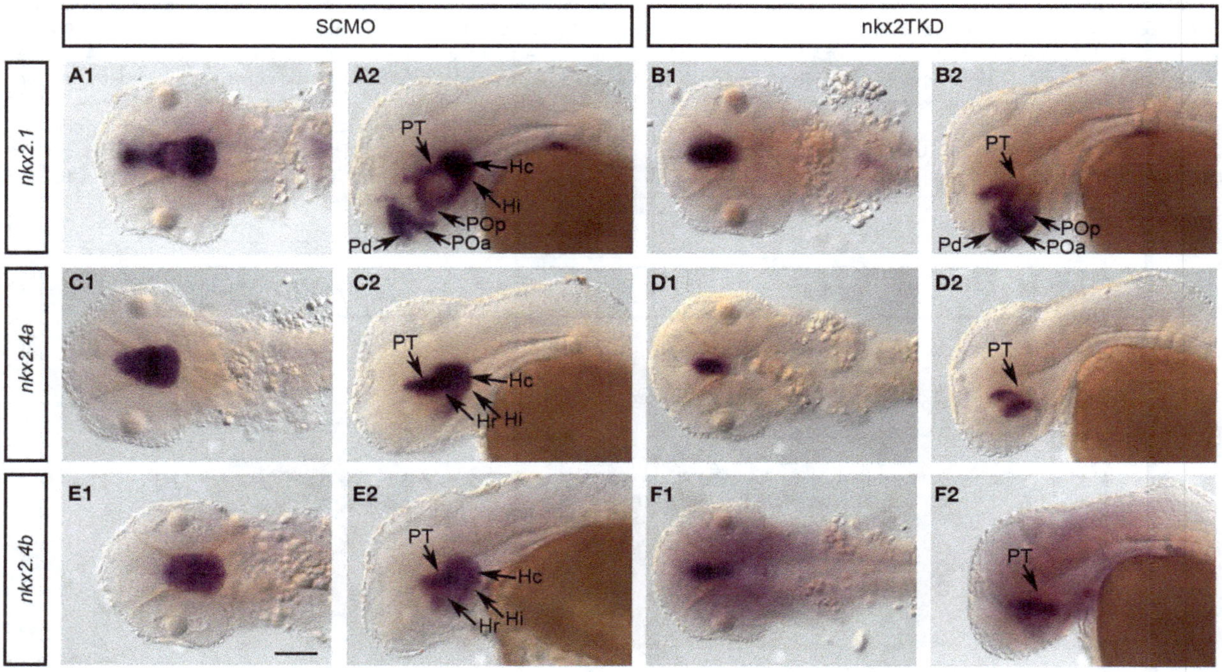

FIGURE 7 | Analysis of *nkx2* gene expression in *nkx2.1*, *nkx2.4a*, and *nkx2.4b* morphants. Expression of *nkx2.1*, *nkx2.4a*, and *nkx2.4b* was analyzed in SCMO **(A,C,E)** and nkx2TKD morphants **(B,D,F)** at 2 dpf. **(A1–F2)** dorsal views, **(A2–F2)** lateral views; anterior is to the left. Abbreviations see **Table 1**. Black arrows point at positions of anatomical structures labeled by abbreviation at start of arrow. Scale bar = 100 μm in **A1** for all panels.

similarity in the homeodomain, may contribute to hypothalamic development in a redundant manner with *nkx2.1*. The two "parallel" *nkx2.1* and *nkx2.4* genes may also explain other riddles, for example *LhjTTF-1/LjNkx2.1* reported for *lampreta* to lack telencephalic expression (Ogasawara et al., 2001) may indeed be a *nkx2.4* ortholog.

Analysis of nkx2TKD embryos revealed that most *nkx2.1/4a/4b* expression in the basal hypothalamus depends on *nkx2.1/4a/4b* activity, except for the posterior tubercular domain. In contrast, it appears that the preoptic and pallidal domain do not strictly depend on *nkx2.1/4a/4b* activity. All three genes are reduced in the medio-lateral extent of their expression in nkx2TKD embryos, which would be in line with a reduced midline-derived activity like Shh required to establish and maintain these domains. Our findings are consistent with reports that *nkx2.1* expression is maintained in a smaller more medial-ventral domain in mice (Sussel et al., 1999), and in *Xenopus* (van den Akker et al., 2008) *nkx2.1* loss-of-function embryos. However, in mouse, expression of *nkx2.4* appears to strictly depend on *nkx2.1* activity (Marín et al., 2002), which would suggest changes in regulatory interactions in evolution.

While morpholino antisense oligonucleotide based knockdown of individual *nkx2.1/4* genes had only subtle effects on hypothalamus development, the combined knockdown of *nkx2.1*, *nkx2.4a* and *nkx2.4b* expression revealed that these genes together control specification and patterning of the basal hypothalamus. **Figure 9** gives an overview of anatomical changes as revealed by marker gene analysis in nkx2TKD morphants. Triple morphant embryos were devoid of the basal hypothalamus including the rostral half of prosomere 3 and extending to the optic commissure. The defects in the nkx2TKD basal hypothalamus are thus limited to the region of *nkx2.1/4a/4b* expression, which extends caudally into the rostral half of basal prosomere 3 (Lauter et al., 2013). In nkx2TKD morphants, the caudal half of prosomer 3 expresses *dbx1a* normally, revealing that the *nkx2.1/4* activity has no effects caudal to its expression limits.

The loss of basal hypothalamic structures upon nkx2TKD is clearly revealed by loss or reduction of the expression domains of *lhx6*, *lhx5*, and *dlx5a* in this region. This basal plate tissue is dorsalized, as the prethalamic expression domain of *pax6a* expands to the ventral edge of the forebrain. However, the ventral expansion of dorsal fates does not reflect a global expansion of alar territories, as the dorsoventral positioning of the *nkx2.2* expression domain, which correlates with the alar-basal boundary, is not shifted. Thus, our data are consistent with the previously published dorsalization of ventral prethalamus in *nkx2.1* mutant mice (Sussel et al., 1999; Marín et al., 2002). They potentially explain discrepancies reported between mouse and *Xenopus* patterning mechanisms. The *xnkx2.1* knockdown has been reported to develop a much weaker basal hypothalamus phenotype (van den Akker et al., 2008) as compared to mice. This could be due to the fact that the *Xenopus nkx2.4* gene (Ermakova et al., 2007) could compensate loss of *nkx2.1*, while in mice *nkx2.4* expression

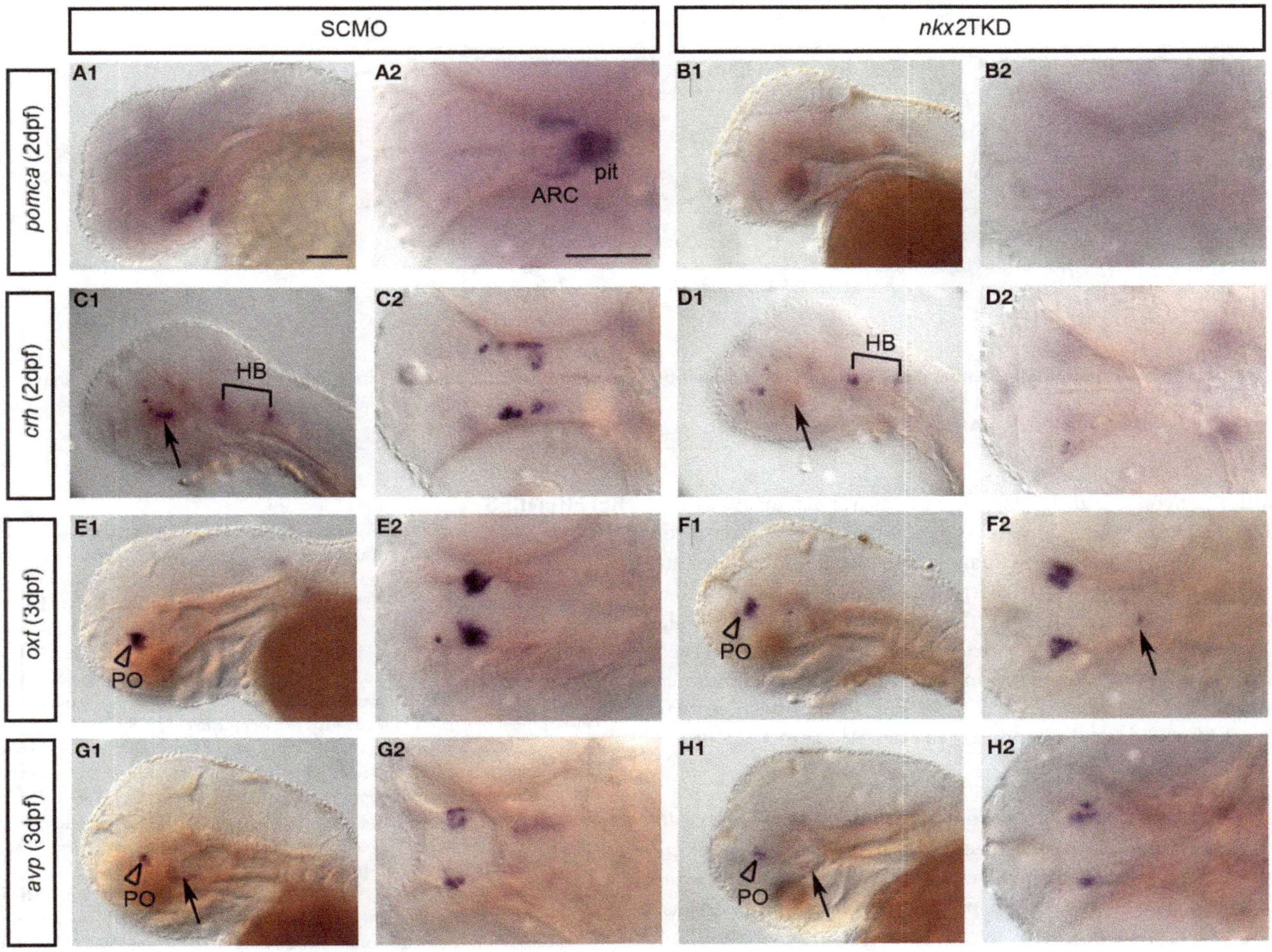

FIGURE 8 | Neuronal differentiation in the hypothalamus of nkx2TKD embryos. Expression of differentiation markers for neuroendocrine neurons analyzed by WISH at 2, 3, and 4 dpf, stages as indicated. **(A,B)** Loss of *pomca* expression in the arcuate nucleus of the hypothalamus (arrowheads) and in the pituitary in nkx2TKD morphants. **(C,D)** *crh* neurons in the posterior tuberculum and hypothalamus (arrows) are reduced in nkx2TKD morphants ($n = 7.7$). **(E,F)** Formation of *oxt*-expressing cells in the PO (arrowheads) is not significantly affected in nkx2TKD morphants. However, in nkx2TKD morphants, *oxt*-expressing cells are detected at ectopic locations within the diencephalon (arrow) ($n = 10.10$). **(G,H)** In nkx2TKD morphants, *avp*-expressing cells in the PC (arrowheads) are still present, but lost in the hypothalamus ($n = 9.9$). **(A1–H1)** lateral views; **(A2–H2)** dorsal views, anterior to the left. The arrows point to the hypothalamus. Abbreviations see **Table 1**. Scale bars = 100 µm in **(A1)** for **(A1–J1)** and in **(A)** for **(A2–J2)**.

depends on *nkx2.1* and thus the *nkx2.1* phenotype is much stronger.

In nkx2TKD morphants the preoptic region is less severely affected, and the SPV appears to develop normally. Both the basal hypothalamus and the preoptic region express *nkx2.1*, except for a small alar plate region of the SPV area characterized by *Orthopedia (otp)* expression (Puelles and Rubenstein, 2003). *otp* is also expressed in the posterior tuberculum and in the arcuate nucleus region. Interestingly, in nkx2TKD morphants the *otpa* expressing domain in the preoptic SPV area was not affected, while the posterior tubercular *otpa* domain was absent. This is consistent with *otpa* in the preoptic SPV not being co-expressed with *nkx2.1/4a/4b*, while in the posterior tuberculum *nkx2.1* is coexpressed (Ryu et al., 2007). The differentiation of neuroendocrine cells in the preoptic region has been studied in detail (Kurrasch et al., 2009; Machluf et al., 2011; Herget et al., 2014) and aids in dissecting the neuroanatomical structures effected in *nkx2.1* mutants. The less severe preoptic phenotype is in line with our finding that neuroendocrine cells develop in the preoptic region of nkx2TKD morphants. In contrast, development of essentially all tested basal hypothalamic neuroendocrine cells depends on *nkx2.1/4a/4b* activity.

The major subdivisions of the larval zebrafish telencephalon, pallium, striatum (dorsal part of area ventralis telencephali, Sdd) and pallidum (ventral part of area ventralis telencephali, Sdv), have been defined by marker gene expression including *lhx6* and *dlx2a* (Mueller et al., 2008; Ganz et al., 2011). Based on loss of *lhx6* expression, triple morphants have a severely reduced pallidum. Mammalian *lhx6* contains a highly conserved Nkx2.1 binding site in its promoter (Du et al., 2008), suggesting a direct and

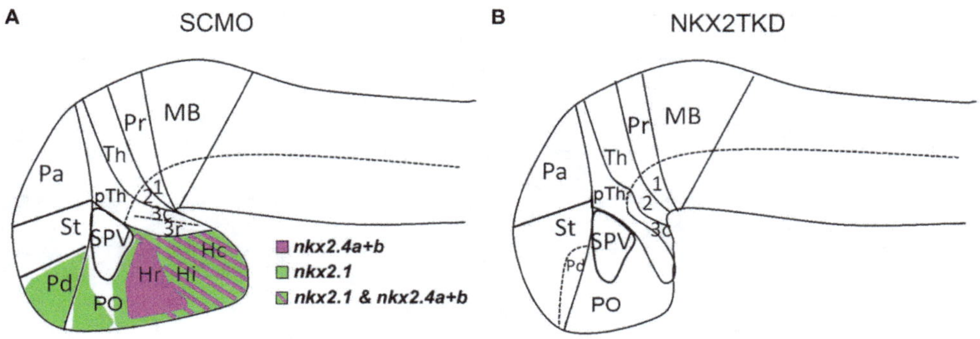

FIGURE 9 | Forebrain patterning abnormalities in nkx2TKD morphants at 2 dpf. (A,B) Schematic sagittal representation of the anatomical domains in the brains of wildtype **(A)** and nkx2TKD morphant **(B)** embryos at 2 dpf. The expression domains of *nkx2.1*, *nkx2.4a*, and *nkx2.4b* are indicated in the wildtype scheme **(A)**, for color code see legend in figure. Abbreviations see **Table 1**.

evolutionary conserved regulation. The ventral expansion of the striatal *lhx5* expression domain suggests that in the absence of *nkx2.1* activity, striatal fate expands into the pallidum, resulting in a dorsalization of the ventral telencephalon similar to that observed in *nkx2.1* mutant mice (Sussel et al., 1999; Marín et al., 2002). When we analyzed *emx* expression, we did not observed an expansion of the pallium, again similar to *nkx2.1* mutant mice (Sussel et al., 1999; Marín et al., 2002), but distinct from reports for *nkx2.1* knockdown in Xenopus (van den Akker et al., 2008).

In summary, our data reveals that *nkx2.1*, *nkx2.4a*, and *nkx2.4b* genes act partially redundant in zebrafish hypothalamic development. *nkx2.1* is specifically involved in the development of rostral ventral forebrain including the pallidum and preoptic regions, but its function in the basal hypothalamus appears redundant with both *nkx2.4* genes. In contrast, *nkx2.4a* and *nkx2.4b* control aspects of basal hypothalamus development including the intermediate and caudal hypothalamus, where loss of *nkx2.4* activity is not fully compensated by *nkx2.1*.

AUTHOR CONTRIBUTIONS

Wolfgang Driever and Martha Manoli designed the study. Martha Manoli performed all experiments and documentation. Martha Manoli and Wolfgang Driever carried out data analysis and wrote and edited the manuscript. Wolfgang Driever obtained funding and supervised the project.

ACKNOWLEDGMENTS

We are grateful to the zebrafish community for plasmids and probes. We thank Thomas Müller, Jörn Schweitzer, Meta Rath, and Alida Filippi for discussion and comments on the manuscript. S. Götter and R. Schlenvogt provided expert care of the fish. This work was supported by the DFG (EXC294-BIOSS), GRK1104 (Martha Manoli), and by the European Commission (FP7, mesDANEURODEV 222999, DOPAMINET 223744, ZFHEALTH 242048) (Wolfgang Driever).

REFERENCES

Akimenko, M. A., Ekker, M., Wegner, J., Lin, W., and Westerfield, M. (1994). Combinatorial expression of three zebrafish genes related to distal-less: part of a homeobox gene code for the head. *J. Neurosci.* 14, 3475–3486.

Armant, O., März, M., Schmidt, R., Ferg, M., Diotel, N., Ertzer, R., et al. (2013). Genome-wide, whole mount *in situ* analysis of transcriptional regulators in zebrafish embryos. *Dev. Biol.* 380, 351–362. doi: 10.1016/j.ydbio.2013.05.006

Barresi, M. J., Stickney, H. L., and Devoto, S. H. (2000). The zebrafish slow-muscle-omitted gene product is required for Hedgehog signal transduction and the development of slow muscle identity. *Development* 127, 2189–2199.

Barth, K. A., and Wilson, S. W. (1995). Expression of zebrafish nk2.2 is influenced by sonic hedgehog/vertebrate hedgehog-1 and demarcates a zone of neuronal differentiation in the embryonic forebrain. *Development* 121, 1755–1768.

Briscoe, J., Pierani, A., Jessell, T. M., and Ericson, J. (2000). A homeodomain protein code specifies progenitor cell identity and neuronal fate in the ventral neural tube. *Cell* 101, 435–445. doi: 10.1016/S0092-8674(00)80853-3

Butt, S. J. B., Sousa, V. H., Fuccillo, M. V., Hjerling-Leffler, J., Miyoshi, G., Kimura, S., et al. (2008). The requirement of Nkx2-1 in the temporal specification of cortical interneuron subtypes. *Neuron* 59, 722–732. doi: 10.1016/j.neuron.2008.07.031

Chandrasekar, G., Lauter, G., and Hauptmann, G. (2007). Distribution of corticotropin-releasing hormone in the developing zebrafish brain. *J. Comp. Neurol.* 505, 337–351. doi: 10.1002/cne.21496

Del Giacco, L., Sordino, P., Pistocchi, A., Andreakis, N., Tarallo, R., Di Benedetto, B., et al. (2006). Differential regulation of the zebrafish orthopedia 1 gene during fate determination of diencephalic neurons. *BMC Dev. Biol.* 6:50. doi: 10.1186/1471-213X-6-50

Du, T., Xu, Q., Ocbina, P. J., and Anderson, S. A. (2008). NKX2.1 specifies cortical interneuron fate by activating Lhx6. *Development* 135, 1559–1567. doi: 10.1242/dev.015123

Eisen, J. S., and Smith, J. C. (2008). Controlling morpholino experiments: don't stop making antisense. *Development* 135, 1735–1743. doi: 10.1242/dev.001115

Ekker, S. C., Ungar, A. R., Greenstein, P., Kessler, D. P. V., Porter, J. A., Moon, R. T., et al. (1995). Patterning activities of vertebrate hedgehog proteins in the developing eye and brain. *Curr. Biol.* 5, 944–955. doi: 10.1016/S0960-9822(95)00185-0

Elsalini, O. A., Gartzen, J., V., Cramer, M., and Rohr, K. B. (2003). Zebrafish hhex, nk2.1a, and pax2.1 regulate thyroid growth and differentiation downstream of Nodal-dependent transcription factors. *Dev. Biol.* 263, 67–80. doi: 10.1016/S0012-1606(03)00436-6

Ericson, J., Rashbass, P., Schedl, A., Brenner-Morton, S., Kawakami, A., van Heyningen, V., et al. (1997). Pax6 controls progenitor cell identity and neuronal fate in response to graded Shh signaling. *Cell* 90, 169–180. doi: 10.1016/S0092-8674(00)80323-2

Ermakova, G. V., Solovieva, E. A., Martynova, N. Y., and Zaraisky, A. G. (2007). The homeodomain factor Xanf represses expression of genes in the presumptive rostral forebrain that specify more caudal brain regions. *Dev. Biol.* 307, 483–497. doi: 10.1016/j.ydbio.2007.03.524

Filippi, A., Mahler, J., Schweitzer, J., and Driever, W. (2010). Expression of the paralogous tyrosine hydroxylase encoding genes th1 and th2 reveals the full complement of dopaminergic and noradrenergic neurons in zebrafish larval and juvenile brain. *J. Comp. Neurol.* 518, 423–438. doi: 10.1002/cne.22213

Fjose, A., Izpisúa-Belmonte, J. C., Fromental-Ramain, C., and Duboule, D. (1994). Expression of the zebrafish gene hlx-1 in the prechordal plate and during CNS development. *Development* 120, 71–81.

Ganz, J., Kaslin, J., Freudenreich, D., Machate, A., Geffarth, M., and Brand, M. (2011). Subdivisions of the adult zebrafish subpallium by molecular marker analysis. *J. Comp. Neurol.* 520, 633–655. doi: 10.1002/cne.22757

Guazzi, S., Price, M., Felice, M., D., Damante, G., Mattei, M. G., and Di Lauro, R. (1990). Thyroid nuclear factor 1 (TTF-1) contains a homeodomain and displays a novel DNA binding specificity. *EMBO J.* 9, 3631–3639.

Hansen, I. A., To, T. T., Wortmann, S., Burmester, T., Winkler, C., Meyer, S. R., et al. (2003). The pro-opiomelanocortin gene of the zebrafish (Danio rerio). *Biochem. Biophys. Res. Commun.* 303, 1121–1128. doi: 10.1016/S0006-291X(03)00475-3

Hauptmann, G., and Gerster, T. (2000). Regulatory gene expression patterns reveal transverse and longitudinal subdivisions of the embryonic zebrafish forebrain. *Mech. Dev.* 91, 105–118. doi: 10.1016/S0925-4773(99)00277-4

Herget, U., Wolf, A., Wullimann, M. F., and Ryu, S. (2014). Molecular neuroanatomy and chemoarchitecture of the neurosecretory preoptic-hypothalamic area in zebrafish larvae. *J. Comp. Neurol.* 522, 1542–1564. doi: 10.1002/cne.23480

Herzog, W., Zeng, X., Lele, Z., Sonntag, C., Ting, J.-W., Chang, C.-Y., et al. (2003). Adenohypophysis formation in the zebrafish and its dependence on sonic hedgehog. *Dev. Biol.* 254, 36–49. doi: 10.1016/S0012-1606(02)00124-0

Kiecker, C., and Lumsden, A. (2004). Hedgehog signaling from the ZLI regulates diencephalic regional identity. *Nat. Neurosci.* 7, 1242–1249. doi: 10.1038/nn1338

Kimmel, C. B., Ballard, W. W., Kimmel, S. R., Ullmann, B., and Schilling, T. F. (1995). Stages of embryonic development of the zebrafish. *Dev. Dyn.* 203, 253–310. doi: 10.1002/aja.1002030302

Kimura, S., Hara, Y., Pineau, T., Fernandez-Salguero, P., Fox, C. H., Ward, J. M., et al. (1996). The T/ebp null mouse: thyroid-specific enhancer-binding protein is essential for the organogenesis of the thyroid, lung, ventral forebrain, and pituitary. *Genes Dev.* 10, 60–69. doi: 10.1101/gad.10.1.60

Krauss, S., Johansen, T., Korzh, V., and Fjose, A. (1991a). Expression pattern of zebrafish pax genes suggests a role in early brain regionalization. *Nature* 353, 267–270. doi: 10.1038/353267a0

Krauss, S., Johansen, T., Korzh, V., Moens, U., Ericson, J. U., and Fjose, A. (1991b). Zebrafish pax[zf-a]: a paired box-containing gene expressed in the neural tube. *EMBO J.* 10, 3609–3619.

Kurrasch, D. M., Nevin, L. M., Wong, J. S., Baier, H., and Ingraham, H. A. (2009). Neuroendocrine transcriptional programs adapt dynamically to the supply and demand for neuropeptides as revealed in NSF mutant zebrafish. *Neural Dev.* 4:22. doi: 10.1186/1749-8104-4-22

Lauter, G., Söll, I., and Hauptmann, G. (2011). Multicolor fluorescent *in situ* hybridization to define abutting and overlapping gene expression in the embryonic zebrafish brain. *Neural Dev.* 6:10. doi: 10.1186/1749-8104-6-10

Lauter, G., Söll, I., and Hauptmann, G. (2013). Molecular characterization of prosomeric and intraprosomeric subdivisions of the embryonic zebrafish diencephalon. *J. Comp. Neurol.* 521, 1093–1118. doi: 10.1002/cne.23221

Lohr, H., and Hammerschmidt, M. (2011). Zebrafish in endocrine systems: recent advances and implications for human disease. *Annu. Rev. Physiol.* 73, 183–211. doi: 10.1146/annurev-physiol-012110-142320

Lumsden, A., and Krumlauf, R. (1996). Patterning the vertebrate neuraxis. *Science* 274, 1109–1115. doi: 10.1126/science.274.5290.1109

Machluf, Y., Gutnick, A., and Levkowitz, G. (2011). Development of the zebrafish hypothalamus. *Ann. N.Y. Acad. Sci.* 1220, 93–105. doi: 10.1111/j.1749-6632.2010.05945.x

Marín, O., Baker, J., Puelles, L., and Rubenstein, J. L. R. (2002). Patterning of the basal telencephalon and hypothalamus is essential for guidance of cortical projections. *Development* 129, 761–773.

Mizuno, K., Gonzalez, F. J., and Kimura, S. (1991). Thyroid-specific enhancer-binding protein (T/EBP): cDNA cloning, functional characterization, and structural identity with thyroid transcription factor TTF-1. *Mol. Cell. Biol.* 11, 4927–4933.

Moreno, N., and Gonzalez, A. (2011). The non-evaginated secondary prosencephalon of vertebrates. *Front. Neuroanat.* 5:12. doi: 10.3389/fnana.2011.00012

Mueller, T., Wullimann, M. F., and Guo, S. (2008). Early teleostean basal ganglia development visualized by Zebrafish Dlx2a, Lhx6, Lhx7, Tbr2 (eomesa), and GAD67 gene expression. *J. Comp. Neurol.* 507, 1245–1257. doi: 10.1002/cne.21604

Odenthal, J., and Nusslein-Volhard, C. (1998). fork head domain genes in zebrafish. *Dev. Genes Evol.* 208, 245–258. doi: 10.1007/s004270050179

Ogasawara, M., Shigetani, Y., Suzuki, S., Kuratani, S., and Satoh, N. (2001). Expression of thyroid transcription factor-1 (TTF-1) gene in the ventral forebrain and endostyle of the agnathan vertebrate, Lampetra japonica. *Genesis* 30, 51–58. doi: 10.1002/gene.1032

Pabst, O., Herbrand, H., and Arnold, H. H. (1998). Nkx2-9 is a novel homeobox transcription factor which demarcates ventral domains in the developing mouse CNS. *Mech. Dev.* 73, 85–93. doi: 10.1016/S0925-4773(98)00035-5

Pera, E. M., and Kessel, M. (1998). Demarcation of ventral territories by the homeobox gene NKX2.1 during early chick development. *Dev. Genes Evol.* 208, 168–171. doi: 10.1007/s004270050170

Price, M. (1993). Members of the Dlx- and Nkx2-gene families are regionally expressed in the developing forebrain. *J. Neurobiol.* 24, 1385–1399. doi: 10.1002/neu.480241010

Puelles, L., and Rubenstein, J. L. (1993). Expression patterns of homeobox and other putative regulatory genes in the embryonic mouse forebrain suggest a neuromeric organization. *Trends Neurosci.* 16, 472–479. doi: 10.1016/0166-2236(93)90080-6

Puelles, L., and Rubenstein, J. L. R. (2003). Forebrain gene expression domains and the evolving prosomeric model. *Trends Neurosci.* 26, 469–476. doi: 10.1016/S0166-2236(03)00234-0

Robu, M. E., Larson, J. D., Nasevicius, A., Beiraghi, S., Brenner, C., Farber, S. A., et al. (2007). p53 activation by knockdown technologies. *PLoS Genet.* 3:e78. doi: 10.1371/journal.pgen.0030078

Rohatgi, R., and Scott, M. P. (2007). Patching the gaps in Hedgehog signalling. *Nat. Cell Biol.* 9, 1005–1009. doi: 10.1038/ncb435

Rohr, K. B., Barth, K. A., Varga, Z. M., and Wilson, S. W. (2001). The nodal pathway acts upstream of hedgehog signaling to specify ventral telencephalic identity. *Neuron* 29, 341–351. doi: 10.1016/S0896-6273(01)00210-0

Ryu, S., Holzschuh, J., Erhardt, S., Ettl, A. K., and Driever, W. (2005). Depletion of minichromosome maintenance protein 5 in the zebrafish retina causes cell-cycle defect and apoptosis. *Proc. Natl. Acad. Sci. U.S.A.* 102, 18467–18472. doi: 10.1073/pnas.0506187102

Ryu, S., Mahler, J., Acampora, D., Holzschuh, J., Erhardt, S., Omodei, D., et al. (2007). Orthopedia homeodomain protein is essential for diencephalic dopaminergic neuron development. *Curr. Biol.* 17, 873–880. doi: 10.1016/j.cub.2007.04.003

Sander, M., Paydar, S., Ericson, J., Briscoe, J., Berber, E., German, M., et al. (2000). Ventral neural patterning by Nkx homeobox genes: Nkx6.1 controls somatic motor neuron and ventral interneuron fates. *Genes Dev.* 14, 2134–2139. doi: 10.1101/gad.820400

Scholpp, S., Wolf, O., Brand, M., and Lumsden, A. (2006). Hedgehog signalling from the zona limitans intrathalamica orchestrates patterning of the zebrafish diencephalon. *Development* 133, 855–864. doi: 10.1242/dev.02248

Shimamura, K., Hartigan, D. J., Martinez, S., Puelles, L., and Rubenstein, J. L. (1995). Longitudinal organization of the anterior neural plate and neural tube. *Development* 121, 3923–3933.

Small, E. M., Vokes, S. A., Garriock, R. J., Li, D., and Krieg, P. A. (2000). Developmental expression of the Xenopus Nkx2-1 and Nkx2-4 genes. *Mech. Dev.* 96, 259–262. doi: 10.1016/S0925-4773(00)00400-7

Strähle, U., Blader, P., Henrique, D., and Ingham, P. W. (1993). Axial, a zebrafish gene expressed along the developing body axis, shows altered expression in cyclops mutant embryos. *Genes Dev.* 7, 1436–1446. doi: 10.1101/gad.7.7b.1436

Sussel, L., Marin, O., Kimura, S., and Rubenstein, J. L. (1999). Loss of Nkx2.1 homeobox gene function results in a ventral to dorsal molecular respecification within the basal telencephalon: evidence for a transformation of the pallidum into the striatum. *Development* 126, 3359–3370.

Tanabe, Y., and Jessell, T. M. (1996). Diversity and pattern in the developing spinal cord. *Science* 274, 1115–1123. doi: 10.1126/science.274.5290.1115

Tessmar-Raible, K., Raible, F., Christodoulou, F., Guy, K., Rembold, M., Hausen, H., et al. (2007). Conserved sensory-neurosecretory cell types in annelid and fish forebrain: insights into hypothalamus evolution. *Cell* 129, 1389–1400. doi: 10.1016/j.cell.2007.04.041

Thisse, C., and Thisse, B. (1999). Antivin, a novel and divergent member of the TGFbeta superfamily, negatively regulates mesoderm induction. *Development* 126, 229–240.

Toyama, R., Curtiss, P. E., Otani, H., Kimura, M., Dawid, I. B., and Taira, M. (1995). The LIM class homeobox gene lim5: implied role in CNS patterning in Xenopus and zebrafish. *Dev. Biol.* 170, 583–593. doi: 10.1006/dbio.1995.1238

Uemae, Y., Sakamoto, J., Hidaka, Y., Hiratsuka, A., Susa, T., Kato, Y., et al. (2014). Gene expression, function, and diversity of Nkx2-4 in the rainbow trout, Oncorhynchus mykiss. *Gen. Comp. Endocrinol.* 206, 193–202. doi: 10.1016/j.ygcen.2014.07.007

van den Akker, W. M. R., Brox, A., Puelles, L., Durston, A. J., and Medina, L. (2008). Comparative functional analysis provides evidence for a crucial role for the homeobox gene Nkx2.1/Titf-1 in forebrain evolution. *J. Comp. Neurol.* 506, 211–223. doi: 10.1002/cne.21542

Wang, C.-C., Brodnicki, T., Copeland, N. G., Jenkins, N. A., and Harvey, R. P. (2000). Conserved linkage of NK-2 homeobox gene pairs Nkx2-2/2-4 and Nkx2-1/2-9 in mammals. *Mamm. Genome* 11, 466–468. doi: 10.1007/s003350010089

Wen, L., Wei, W., Gu, W., Huang, P., Ren, X., Zhang, Z., et al. (2008). Visualization of monoaminergic neurons and neurotoxicity of MPTP in live transgenic zebrafish. *Dev. Biol.* 314, 84–92. doi: 10.1016/j.ydbio.2007.11.012

Westerfield, M. (2000). *The Zebrafish Book: A Guide to the Laboratory Use of Zebrafish (Danio rerio):* Eugene, OR: Univ. of Oregon Press.

Wullimann, M. F., and Rink, E. (2001). Detailed immunohistology of Pax6 protein and tyrosine hydroxylase in the early zebrafish brain suggests role of Pax6 gene in development of dopaminergic diencephalic neurons. *Brain Res. Dev. Brain Res.* 131, 173–191. doi: 10.1016/S0165-3806(01)00270-X

2

Coexpression analysis of nine neuropeptides in the neurosecretory preoptic area of larval zebrafish

Ulrich Herget[1,2] and Soojin Ryu[1]*

[1] Developmental Genetics of the Nervous System, Max Planck Institute for Medical Research, Heidelberg, Germany

[2] The Hartmut Hoffmann-Berling International Graduate School of Molecular and Cellular Biology, University of Heidelberg, Heidelberg, Germany

Correspondence:
Soojin Ryu, Developmental Genetics of the Nervous System, Max Planck Institute for Medical Research, Jahnstr. 29, 69120 Heidelberg, Germany
e-mail. soojin.ryu@mpimf-heidelberg.mpg.de

The paraventricular nucleus (PVN) of the hypothalamus in mammals coordinates neuroendocrine, autonomic and behavioral responses pivotal for homeostasis and the stress response. A large amount of studies in rodents has documented that the PVN contains diverse neuronal cell types which can be identified by the expression of distinct secretory neuropeptides. Interestingly, PVN cell types often coexpress multiple neuropeptides whose relative coexpression levels are subject to environment-induced plasticity. Due to their small size and transparency, zebrafish larvae offer the possibility to comprehensively study the development and plasticity of the PVN in large groups of intact animals, yet important anatomical information about the larval zebrafish PVN-homologous region has been missing. Therefore we recently defined the location and borders of the larval neurosecretory preoptic area (NPO) as the PVN-homologous region in larval zebrafish based on transcription factor expression and cell type clustering. To identify distinct cell types present in the larval NPO, we also generated a comprehensive 3D map of 9 zebrafish homologs of typical neuropeptides found in the mammalian PVN (arginine vasopressin (AVP), corticotropin-releasing hormone (CRH), proenkephalin a (penka)/b (penkb), neurotensin (NTS), oxytocin (OXT), vasoactive intestinal peptide (VIP), cholecystokinin (CCK), and somatostatin (SST)). Here we extend this chemoarchitectural map to include the degrees of coexpression of two neuropeptides in the same cell by performing systematic pairwise comparisons. Our results allowed the subclassification of NPO cell types, and differences in variability of coexpression profiles suggest potential targets of biochemical plasticity. Thus, this work provides an important basis for the analysis of the development, function, and plasticity of the primary neuroendocrine brain region in larval zebrafish.

Keywords: neuroendocrine system, hypothalamus, preoptic region, paraventricular nucleus, zebrafish, coexpression

INTRODUCTION

The vertebrate neuroendocrine system is controlled by specific hypothalamic nuclei. The most extensively studied ones are the paraventricular nucleus (PVN) and supraoptic nucleus (SON) in rodents, which contain neuroendocrine cells expressing secretory neuropeptides. These peptides are transported to the pituitary gland, where they are directly released into the general circulation via the neurohypophysis, or released into the portal system of the adenohypophysis, where they trigger the release of hormones into the general circulation. The two peptides released in the neurohypophsis are arginine vasopressin (AVP), and oxytocin (OXT), and they are produced by distinct magnocellular neurons. Releasing and inhibiting factors acting on adenohypophyseal secretion are instead produced in parvocellular neurons, and include corticotropin-releasing hormone (CRH), thyrotropin-releasing hormone (TRH), methionine or leucine enkephalin (mENK/lENK), neurotensin (NTS), vasoactive intestinal peptide (VIP), cholecystokinin (CCK), and somatostatin (SST) (Swanson and Sawchenko, 1983; Mezey et al., 1985; Simmons and Swanson, 2009).

Coexpression of several of these peptides in the same cell is a common phenomenon in the mammalian PVN. For example, AVP colocalizes with mENK in neurohypophysial terminals in the rat (Martin and Voigt, 1981). Also in rats, CRH can be coexpressed with AVP, OXT, NTS, ENK, VIP, and/or CCK (Burlet et al., 1983; Hökfelt et al., 1983; Roth et al., 1983; Sawchenko et al., 1984a; Mezey et al., 1985; Piekut and Joseph, 1986; Swanson et al., 1986; Sawchenko, 1987; Whitnall and Gainer, 1988; Ceccatelli et al., 1989; Swanson and Simmons, 1989; Arima et al., 2001; Dabrowska et al., 2011). Cells producing OXT were found to also synthesize CRH, CCK, and ENK (Martin and Voigt, 1981; Vanderhaeghen et al., 1981; Rossier et al., 1983; Levin and Sawchenko, 1993). Not all peptide combinations occur, however. The populations of cells producing AVP, OXT, or SST are completely separate in the rat (Swanson and Sawchenko, 1983; Swanson et al., 1986).

The molecular development of the mammalian hypothalamus is largely conserved in zebrafish (Machluf et al., 2011). We have recently defined the location and borders of the larval neurosecretory preoptic area (NPO) as the PVN-homologous region based on transcription factor expression and cell type clustering in larval zebrafish. To identify distinct cell types present in the larval NPO, we also generated a comprehensive 3D map of 9 zebrafish homologs of typical neuropeptides found in the mammalian PVN (*avp*, *crh*, *oxt*, *proenkephalin a* (*penka*), *proenkephalin b* (*penkb*), *nts*, *vip*, *cck*, and *somatostatin* (*sst1.1*); Herget et al., 2014). The larval NPO featured 9 out of 10 peptides also found in the mammalian PVN. One exception was *trh*, which was found to be outside the boundaries of the larval NPO as we defined them. We found a small group of cells producing *cck* at the rostral border of the NPO and cells producing *avp*, *oxt*, *crh*, *penka*, *nts*, or *sst1.1* as dense and intermingled clusters. In contrast, cells producing *penkb* or *vip* appeared to reside in separate subregions of the NPO.

Several of these neuropeptides are coexpressed in the same cells in the mammalian PVN, and extensive coexpression also in the larval NPO seemed likely based on the spatial proximity of cells after 3D registration. We reasoned that definitive classification of distinct cell types cannot be assigned in the larval NPO based on the expression of one neuropeptide alone. Therefore, we analyzed in this study the degree of coexpression of two neuropeptides in the same cell by performing systematic pairwise comparisons of coexpression of *avp*, *crh*, *oxt*, *penka*, *penkb*, *nts*, *cck*, *vip*, and *sst1.1* in the larval zebrafish NPO. Our results show that many of the peptides produced by densely intermingled cells of the larval zebrafish NPO are not coexpressed, while some neuropeptide combinations show occasional, low or moderate levels of coexpression. Interestingly we observed high degrees of coexpression for certain neuropeptide combinations such as *avp* + *crh* and *cck* + *penkb*. These results illustrate that information about coexpressed peptides is essential to identify subclasses of cell types and the classification of cell types should not be based on the expression of one peptide alone within the NPO.

Plastic changes in the coexpression profile of a cell allow it to acquire additional regulatory functions. Indeed, in mammals the coexpression properties of PVN cells are subject to stress-induced plasticity, with different types of stress influencing the expression levels of different neuropeptides (Swanson et al., 1986; Harbuz and Lightman, 1989; Swanson, 1991). The larval zebrafish offers an attractive system to dissect the mechanistic basis of such environment-induced plasticity in the hypothalamus because of the possibility to study the architecture, development, and function of distinct neural circuits in intact and transparent animals. The basal characterization of coexpression profiles is a prerequisite to classify and identify distinct NPO cell types and their plasticity in response to environmental challenges.

MATERIALS AND METHODS

ZEBRAFISH PREPARATION

Zebrafish maintenance and breeding were carried out under standard conditions at 28.5°C (Westerfield, 2000). To avoid pigmentation, embryos were incubated in 0.2 mM 1-phenyl-2-thiourea (Sigma-Aldrich). AB/TL zebrafish larvae were fixed at 5 days post fertilization (dpf) in 4% paraformaldehyde (PFA, Merck; in phosphate buffered saline (PBS), pH 7.2–7.3) overnight. All animals were raised under constant conditions and fixed quickly to avoid chronic environmental or acute handling stress. On the following day, larvae were washed briefly with PBST (phosphate-buffered saline with 0.1% Triton X-100, Merck and Roth), then dehydrated with increasing methanol (Merck) concentrations (25%, 50%, 75%, 100%, in PBST, 5 min steps), and stored in 100% methanol at −20°C. All procedures were performed according to the guidelines of the German animal welfare law and approved by the local government.

WHOLE-MOUNT FLUORESCENT *IN SITU* HYBRIDIZATION

In situ hybridization (ISH) probes for *avp* (Eaton et al., 2008), *oxt* (Unger and Glasgow, 2003), *sst1.1* (Devos et al., 2002), *trh*, *crh* (Löhr et al., 2009), *vip* (Wolf and Ryu, 2013), *cck*, *penka*, *penkb*, and *nts* (Herget et al., 2014) were previously described. Riboprobes were synthesized from linearized plasmids following the instructions provided with the digoxygenin labeling mix (Roche). Fluorescent ISH was performed based on a previously published protocol (Lauter et al., 2011).

MICROSCOPY AND IMAGE PROCESSING

For imaging, larval heads were cleared in 80% glycerol (Gerbu) in PBS for 1 h. Dorsal confocal stacks of larval heads were recorded using a Leica SP5 confocal microscope with a Nikon 20x glycerol objective. Each channel was recorded sequentially, using alternating excitation wavelengths specific for each tyramide, to reduce interfering signals from overlapping emission spectra. Acquisition settings were adjusted for each stack to obtain the optimal image quality of the desired volume. Stacks were evaluated using Amira 5.4 (Visualization Sciences Group) to create maximum intensity projections that were restricted to the volume of interest, excluding signals from planes above or below. Staining signal was analyzed plane by plane within the NPO. Brightness and contrast were adjusted for each channel. Any accumulation of signal with the proper shape and size of a typical cell was included in the analysis and compared to the signal in co-stained channels at the same location. Thus, coexpression was determined by the spatial overlap of cells stained for different peptide markers. Images of single planes and maximum projections were exported from Amira and arranged into figures using Adobe Illustrator. All images show dorsal views of substacks or single planes, with the rostral direction on the left side, unless indicated otherwise.

RESULTS

To comprehensively analyze the degree of coexpression of two peptides in the same cell, we performed cell by cell comparisons of pairwise combinatorial ISH staining of nine peptide markers that we had previously identified to be expressed in the 5 dpf larval NPO. The NPO is defined by the dense clustering of cells expressing these peptides within the transcription factor *orthopedia a* (*otpa*)-positive preoptic area (**Figure 1**). Altogether we examined 36 pairwise combinations of neuropeptides, analyzing a minimum of 5 animals per pair, but the sample size varied and was larger for some peptide combinations. All

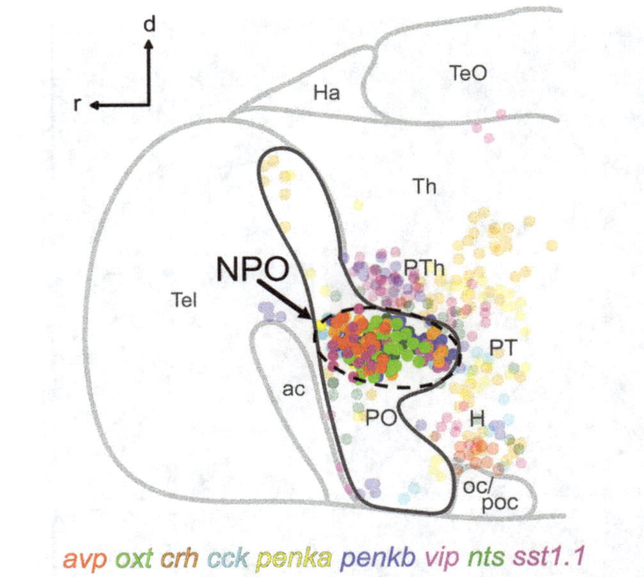

FIGURE 1 | Schematic lateral view of a 5 dpf larval zebrafish brain showing the location of the NPO (dashed line) within the *otpa*-positive part (dark gray line) of the preoptic area, and the spatial distribution of nine cell types expressing the indicated neuropeptides. Cells clustering within the NPO are opaque. For more details, the reader is referred to our previously reported chemoarchitectural map (Herget et al., 2014). Abbreviations: ac, anterior commissure; d, dorsal; H, hypothalamus; Ha, habenula; NPO, neurosecretory preoptic area; oc, optic chiasm; PO, preoptic area; poc, postoptic commissure; PT, posterior tuberculum; PTh, prethalamus; r, rostral; Tel, telencephalon; TeO, optic tectum; Th, thalamus.

data was obtained from 5 dpf larvae, since the original NPO cell type map was generated for that stage. We found broadly three different categories of coexpression extent: (1) Absence of coexpression in all animals; (2) Occurance of coexpression in a single, few or several cells only in some animals analyzed ("variable coexpression"); (3) Coexpression in several cells in all animals analyzed ("consistent coexpression").

NO COEXPRESSION IN ALL ANIMALS

Many of the neuropeptide combinations (16/36) showed no coexpression in the same cell, and often these neuropeptides were expressed in spatially separate clusters. The rostralmost clusters formed by cells expressing *avp*, *crh*, *cck*, or *sst1.1* did not show any overlap with the caudalmost cluster formed by cells expressing *vip* (**Figures 2A–D"**, 5–8 animals analyzed). Among the rostral group, *crh* and *cck* were not coexpressed in the same cells, and *cck* expression was also separate from the large *nts*-positive cluster (**Figures 2E–F"**, 6–7 animals analyzed). The *penka*-expressing cluster extended as far caudally as the small group of *vip*-positive cells, which however occupied a more lateral region (**Figures 2G–G"**, 8 animals analyzed). *oxt*-expressing cells formed a large central cluster, and they did not overlap with the rostrally located *cck*-expressing cells, nor with the caudally located *vip*-expressing group (**Figures 2H–I"**, 6–9 animals analyzed). The *vip*-positive cluster was also separate from cells expressing *penkb* (**Figures 2J–J"**, 7 animals analyzed). The rostral cluster of *cck*-positive cells was close to, but separate from the *avp*-positive and *penka*-positive clusters (**Figures 2K–L"**, 7 animals analyzed). *penkb*-positive cells surrounded the more central *nts*-positive cluster (**Figures 2M–M"**, 5 animals analyzed). Within the center of the NPO, cells expressing *avp* or *oxt* were found intermingled in the same region, but did not overlap (**Figures 2N–O"**, 8 animals analyzed). The central and intermingled clusters of cells expressing *oxt* or *nts* did not show coexpression of these two peptides (**Figures 2P–P"**, 10 animals analyzed). Similar spatial proximity without coexpression was also found for cells expressing *oxt* or *sst1.1* (**Figures 2Q–R"**, 8 animals analyzed).

VARIABLE COEXPRESSION

Occasionally, a single cell was found coexpressing two neuropeptides in a larva, although most of the animals analyzed did not show coexpression. We observed such rarely coexpressing single cells in 10/36 neuropeptide combinations. A single *avp*-positive cell was occasionally found within *nts*-positive cells (**Figure 3A**, 3/11 animals). Similarly, in rare cases, single cells showed coexpression of *crh* and *oxt* (**Figure 3B**, 3/17 animals). The clusters of cells producing *penka* or *penkb* were spatially separate, but in one animal, coexpression could be found in a single cell (**Figure 3C**, 1/16 animals). The intermingled clusters of cells expressing *penka* or *sst1.1* also in rare cases showed one cell with coexpression (**Figure 3D**, 2/14 animals). The *crh*-positive cluster occupied the rostral half of the region covered by both the *penka*-positive and *nts*-positive clusters, and in rarely occuring cells, *crh* was coexpressed with *penka* (**Figure 3E**, 4/14 animals) or *nts* (**Figure 3F**, 1/6 animals). While the *cck*-positive cluster was rostral, occasional coexpression of *sst1.1* was observed (**Figure 3G**, 3/7 animals). The *vip*-producing cluster was caudal and lateral, but a cell that was more rostromedial did in one case coexpress *nts* (**Figure 3H**, 1/9 animals). The central cluster of *penka*-positive cells was intermingled with the clusters of cells expressing *avp* or *oxt*, and occasionally single *penka*-positive cells coexpressed *avp* (**Figure 3I**, 4/21 animals) or *oxt* (**Figure 3J**, 4/33 animals).

The extent of coexpression for other peptide combinations was somewhat higher where more than one cell per animal showed coexpression. In the combination of *crh* and *penkb* staining, many animals showed no coexpression, but in one animal, coexpression was observed in few cells (**Figures 4A–A'"**, 1/12 animals). Similarly few *avp* and *penkb* coexpressing cells were found in some animals analyzed (**Figures 4B–B'"**, 5/15 animals). In those cases in which *crh* and *sst1.1* were coexpressed, we found such coexpression in several cells (**Figures 4C–C'"**, 2/9 animals). Few cells coexpressing *penkb* and *sst1.1* were also found in one animal (**Figures 4D–D'"**, 1/5 animals). Few *avp* and *sst1.1* coexpressing cells were also found in some animals (**Figures 4E–E'"**, 6/25 animals). Some animals showed few *oxt* and *penkb* coexpressing cells (**Figures 4F–F'"**, 4/7 animals). Although in some animals, *penka* and *nts* were not coexpressed, in most animals we found coexpression of these peptides in few cells (**Figures 5A–A'"**, 8/15 animals).

CONSISTENT COEXPRESSION IN ALL ANIMALS

Consistent coexpression in all animals analyzed was found for three peptide combinations. The combination of *nts* and

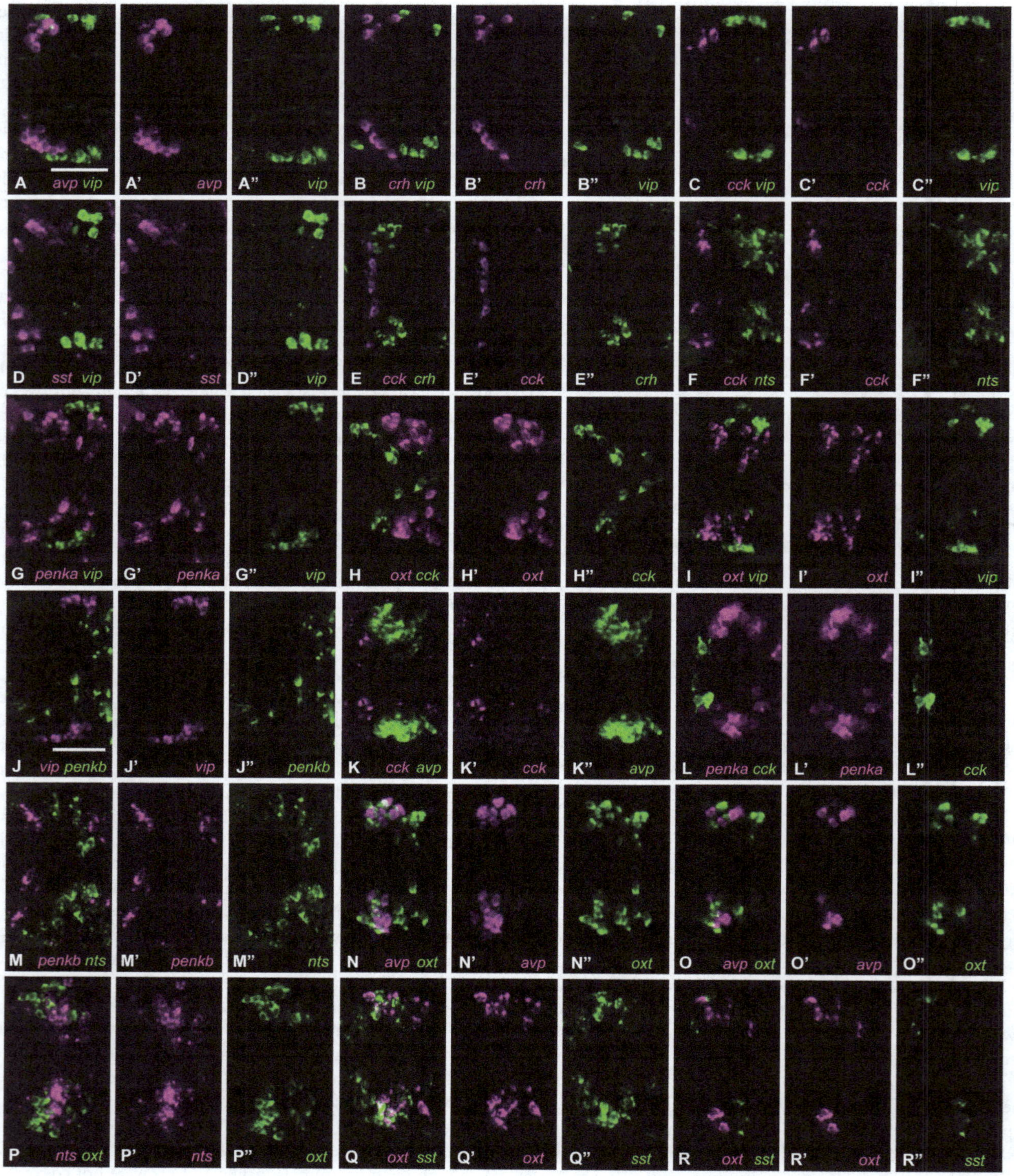

FIGURE 2 | Cell type staining combinations showing no coexpression. **(A)** Cells expressing *avp* **(A')** or *vip* **(A")** form neighboring but separate clusters. **(B)** Cells expressing *crh* **(B')** or *vip* **(B")** are similarly separated. **(C)** Cells expressing *cck* cluster rostrally **(C')**, and are therefore distant from *vip*-positive cells **(C")**. **(D)** Cells expressing *sst1.1* **(D')** also cluster in a separate region from *vip*-positive cells **(D")**. **(E)** *cck*-positive cells **(E')** are rostrally neighboring *crh*-positive cells **(E")**. **(F)** Cells expressing *cck* **(F')** or *nts* **(F")** are separate. **(G)** *penka*-positive cells **(G')** are scattered, but do not overlap with *vip* expression **(G")**. **(H)** *oxt*-positive **(H')** and *cck*-positive cells **(H")** are also separated. **(I)** The clusters formed by cells expressing *oxt* **(I')** or *vip* **(I")** do not show coexpression. **(J)** *vip* **(J')** and *penkb* **(J")** are also not

(*Continued*)

FIGURE 2 | Continued
coexpressed. **(K)** The rostral location of *cck*-positive cells **(K')** is separate from the neighboring *avp*-positive cluster **(K")**. **(L)** *penka*-positive cells **(L')** also are close to the *cck*-positive population **(L")**, but still separate. **(M)** Cells positive for *penkb* **(M')** surround the central *nts*-positive cluster **(M")**. **(N)** Cells expressing *avp* **(N')** or *oxt* **(N")** are intermingled, but the peptides are not coexpressed (single planes: **O–O"**). **(P)** Cells expressing *nts* **(P')** or *oxt* **(P")** have similar locations, but these peptides are not coexpressed. **(Q)** Cells expressing *oxt* **(Q')** or *sst1.1* **(Q")** are also intermingled and do not coexpress these peptides (single planes: **R–R"**). All images show maximum intensity projections, unless indicated otherwise. Scale bar: 50 μm.

sst1.1 showed consistent coexpression in few cells (**Figures 5B–B'''**, 5/5). High degree of coexpression was consistently found for the rostralmost clusters formed by cells producing *penkb* or *cck* (**Figures 5C–C'''**, 13/13 animals). Coexpression was also consistently high for the combination of *avp* and *crh* staining (**Figures 5D–D'''**, 19/19 animals). These results are summarized in **Figure 6**, in which we also indicate the range of coexpression observed (minimum and maximum degrees).

DISCUSSION

Our results show that many of the peptides produced by densely intermingled cells of the larval zebrafish NPO are not coexpressed. Occasional coexpression in one cell can be observed for other peptide staining combinations, and some combinations with low or moderate coexpression appear more frequently. Only three of the 36 combinations show consistent coexpression in all animals analyzed, reaching a high degree only for *avp* + *crh* and *cck* + *penkb*. It should be noted that the presence of RNA does not necessarily mean that the peptide will also be synthesized. For example, there is a distinct cluster of *avp*-expressing cells outside the NPO in the ventral hypothalamus, which can clearly be labeled by ISH, but not by immunohistochemistry (IHC; Eaton et al., 2008; Herget et al., 2014). Still, the information presented here about coexpressed peptide transcripts suggests the existence of subclasses of cell types which can have very different functions.

The large amount of information available on the degree of coexpression of different neuropeptides in the mammalian PVN allows comparisons of our results with those obtained in mammals. Interestingly, many peptide combinations show similar degrees of coexpression both in larval zebrafish and in mammals. The absence of coexpression of *avp* with *oxt* we observed is in line with rat data (Swanson and Sawchenko, 1983). The coexpression of *avp* with *crh* we found to vary between moderate and high levels was also shown to be low or high in the rat (Sawchenko et al., 1984b; Whitnall et al., 1985, 1987; Aubry et al., 1999; Arima et al., 2001; Simmons and Swanson, 2009),

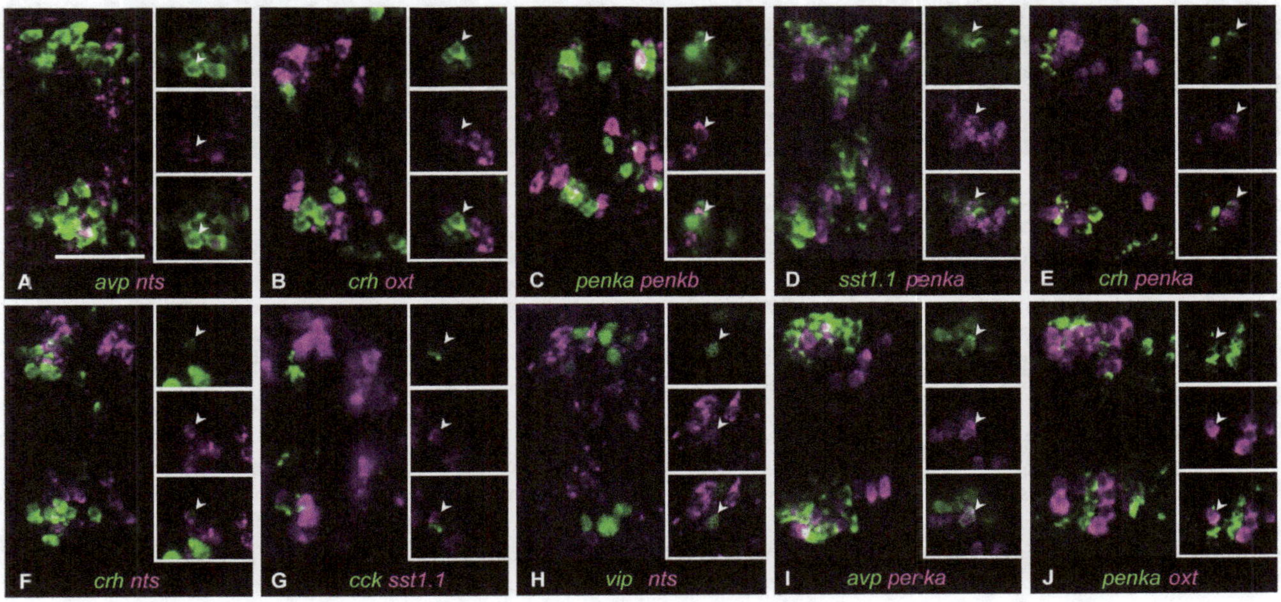

FIGURE 3 | In some cell type staining combinations, occasional and low coexpression can be observed. **(A)** Cells expressing *avp* or *nts* only overlap in rare cases. **(B)** Cells expressing *oxt* or *crh* are usually separate, but occasially these peptides are coexpressed in a single cell. **(C)** Cells expressing *penkb* cells usually surround the *penka*-positive cluster, but in few animals, one cell shows coexpression. **(D)** *penka*-positive cells and *sst1.1*-positive cells are intermingled, and occasionally show low coexpression. **(E)** *crh*-positive cells are intermingled with *penka*-positive cells, but some rare occurences of coexpression were found. **(F)** *crh* can also be coexpressed with *nts* in rare cases. **(G)** *cck*-positive cells appear to faintly coexpress *sst1.1* in few of the animals. **(H)** One isolated cell was sometimes found coexpressing *vip* and *nts*. **(I)** Cells expressing *avp* or *penka* are intermingled and usually these peptides are not coexpressed, but single coexpressing cells do occur. **(J)** Stainings for *oxt* and *penka* often show no coexpressing cells, but sometimes these peptides are coexpressed in few cells. Images show maximum intensity projections, insets show split channels of single confocal planes with coexpressing cells (arrowheads). Scale bar: 50 μm.

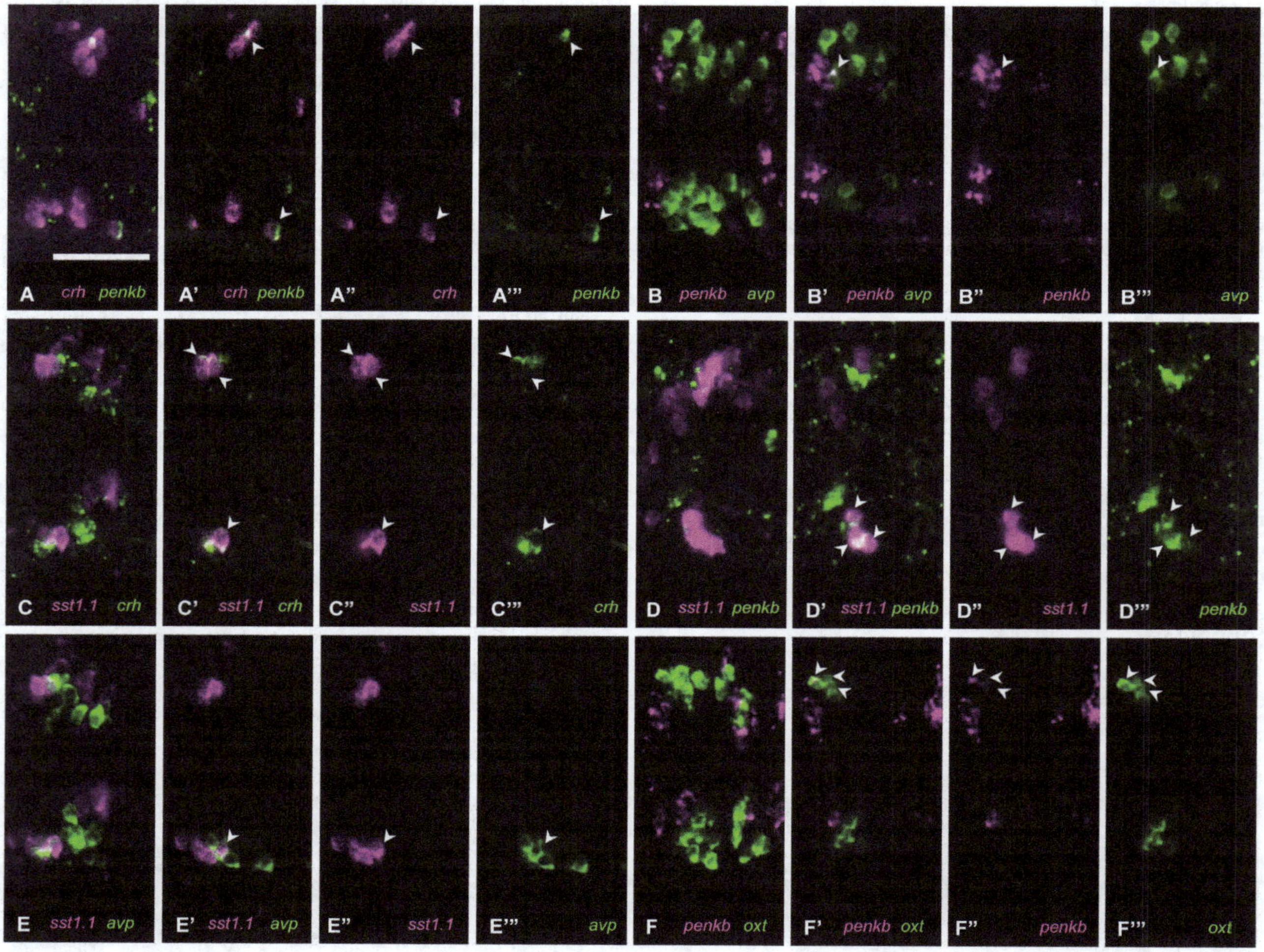

FIGURE 4 | Some peptide combinations show low or moderate coexpression. (A) Coexpression (**(A)** maximum intensity projection; **(A')** single plane) of *crh* **(A'')** and *penkb* **(A''')** rarely occurs, but can be found in more than one cell. **(B)** In some animals, coexpression (**(B)** maximum intensity projection; **(B')** single plane) of *penkb* **(B'')** and *avp* **(B''')** can be found. **(C)** Moderate coexpression (**(C)** maximum intensity projection; **(C')** single plane) of *sst1.1* **(C'')** and *crh* **(C''')** can be observed in some animals. **(D)** Few cells also show coexpression (**(D)** maximum intensity projection; **(D')** single plane) of *sst1.1* **(D'')** and *penkb* **(D''')**. **(E)** Coexpression is found in few cells (**(E)** maximum intensity projection; **(E')** single plane) labeled for *sst1.1* **(E'')** and *avp* **(E''')**. **(F)** In some animals, moderate coexpression (**(F)** maximum intensity projection; **(F')** single plane) of *penkb* **(F'')** and *oxt* **(F''')** can be found. Arrowheads mark coexpressing cells. Scale bar: 50 μm.

and was low in the mouse or sheep (Rivalland et al., 2005; Biag et al., 2012). Recently, it was found that only magnocellular CRH-positive cells coexpress AVP in the rat (Dabrowska et al., 2013). Coexpression of CRH and AVP was also found in other teleosts (Yulis and Lederis, 1987; Olivereau et al., 1988; Fryer, 1989). We found rare coexpression of *oxt* with *penka*, and low coexpression of *oxt* with *penkb*, and coexpression of OXT with ENK was also seen in the rat (Martin and Voigt, 1981; Rossier et al., 1983). OXT and SST do not overlap in the rat (Swanson and Sawchenko, 1983), and we saw the same absence of coexpression in the fish. We observed rare coexpression of *crh* with *penka*, and low coexpression of *crh* with *penkb*, while ENK coexpression with CRH seems to be higher in rats (Hökfelt et al., 1983; Ceccatelli et al., 1989; Pretel and Piekut, 1990), or sheep (Rivalland et al., 2005). However, one more recent study also found only low coexpression of ENK in CRH-producing cells in the rat (Dabrowska et al., 2013), which is more in line with our results. NTS and ENK are coexpressed in low degrees in the rat (Ceccatelli et al., 1989), and we also saw consistent coexpression of *nts* with *penka*, but not with *penkb*. It was reported that very few NTS cells coexpress VIP in the rat (Ceccatelli et al., 1989), and the coexpression of *nts* and *vip* was also rare here.

Other peptide coexpression profiles we observed in larval zebrafish deviate from previously established mammalian data. AVP and ENK are thought to be coexpressed in the rat (Martin and Voigt, 1981), and moderately coexpressed in the sheep (Rivalland et al., 2005), but *penka* was only rarely coexpressed with *avp*, and *penkb* showed only low coexpression with *avp* in our case. We did not find coexpression of *avp* with *cck*,

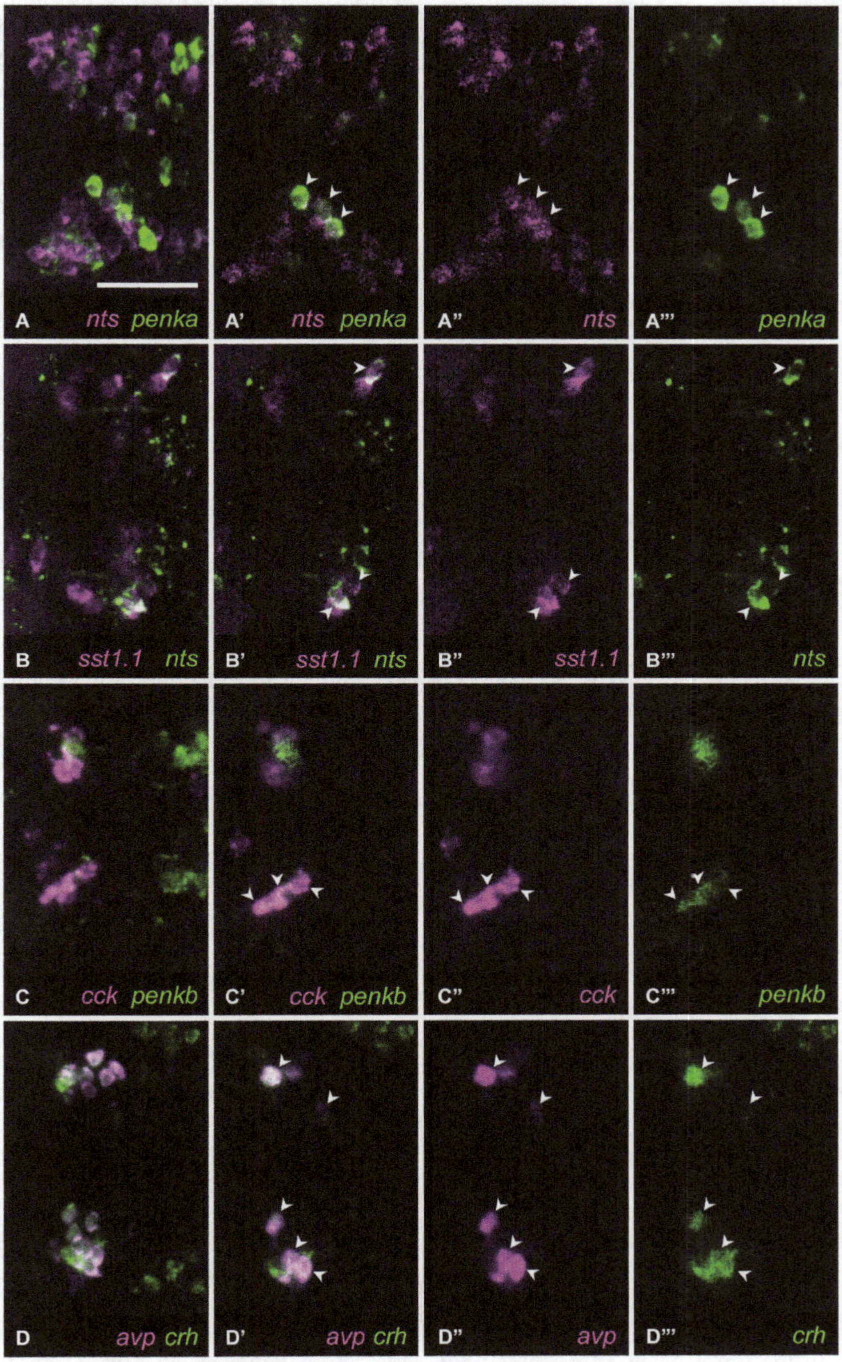

FIGURE 5 | Four combinations of neuropeptides show higher coexpression. **(A)** In most animals, several cells show coexpression (**(A)** maximum intensity projection; **(A')** single plane) of *nts* **(A'')** with *penka* **(A''')**. **(B)** In all animals, few cells show coexpression (**(B)** maximum intensity projection; **(B')** single plane) of *sst1.1* **(B'')** and *nts* **(B''')**. **(C)** High coexpression can be found (**(C)** maximum intensity projection; **(C')** single plane) in the rostral clusters of cells expressing *cck* **(C'')** or *penkb* **(C''')**. **(D)** Consistently high coexpression (**(D)** maximum intensity projection; **(D')** single plane) can be observed for the intermingled *avp*-positive **(D'')** and *crh*-positive clusters **(D''')**. Arrowheads mark coexpressing cells. Scale bar: 50 μm.

but there are many such cells in the rat (Mezey et al., 1986). Our observation showed low coexpression of *avp* with *sst1.1*, but those are non-overlapping cell types in the rat (Swanson and Sawchenko, 1983). *oxt* coexpression with *crh* was rare here, but variably low or high in the rat (Sawchenko et al., 1984a; Dabrowska et al., 2013), and low in the mouse (Biag et al., 2012).

avp							
oxt	crh	penka	penkb	nts	cck	vip	sst1.1
-	+/+++	-/+	-/++	-/+	-	-	-/++
oxt							
avp	crh	penka	penkb	nts	cck	vip	sst1.1
-	-/+	-/+	-/++	-	-	-	-
crh							
avp	oxt	penka	penkb	nts	cck	vip	sst1.1
++/+++	-/+	-/+	-/++	-/+	-	-	-/+
penka							
avp	oxt	crh	penkb	nts	cck	vip	sst1.1
-/+	-/+	-/+	-/+	-/++	-	-	-/+
penkb							
avp	oxt	crh	penka	nts	cck	vip	sst1.1
-/++	-/++	-/++	-/+	-	++/+++	-	-/+
nts							
avp	oxt	crh	penka	penkb	cck	vip	sst1.1
-/+	-	-/+	-/++	-	-	-/+	+
cck							
avp	oxt	crh	penka	penkb	nts	vip	sst1.1
-	-	-	-	++/+++	-	-	-/++
vip							
avp	oxt	crh	penka	penkb	nts	cck	sst1.1
-	-	-	-	-	-/+	-	-
sst1.1							
avp	oxt	crh	penka	penkb	nts	cck	vip
-/++	-	-/+	-/+	-/+	+	-/+	-

FIGURE 6 | Overview of coexpression profiles of cells expressing *avp*, *oxt*, *crh*, *penka*, *penkb*, *nts*, *cck*, *vip*, or *sst1.1*. Coexpression degrees indicate complete absence (−), rare occurrence (+), low coexpression (++), or high coexpression (+++). In many combinations, coexpression was variable, and the minimum and maximum degrees are indicated (min/max). Differences between the coexpression of one peptide in one cell type and vice versa are caused by differences in cell cluster sizes.

In the zebrafish, one study reported colocalization of *oxt* and *crh* in the preoptic area (Chandrasekar et al., 2007), but with our increased resolution, we can clarify that those cells only reside in the same region, and are in fact intermingled. OXT and CCK are coexpressed in the rat (Vanderhaeghen et al., 1981; Bondy et al., 1989; Levin and Sawchenko, 1993), but we saw no such coexpression in the zebrafish. CRH coexpression with NTS was reported to be low (Sawchenko et al., 1984a) or moderate in the rat (Ceccatelli et al., 1989), but according to our results coexpression only occurs rarely. CRH and CCK are coexpressed in some cells in the rat (Mezey et al., 1986; Ceccatelli et al., 1989), but not at all in our data. CRH and VIP were reported to be coexpressed in low levels in the rat (Ceccatelli et al., 1989), but they are not coexpressed here. ENK and VIP are coexpressed in the rat (Hökfelt et al., 1987), but neither *penka* nor *penkb* overlap with *vip* in our results. NTS and CCK show very low coexpression in the rat (Ceccatelli et al., 1989), but no coexpression in our results. All observed differences can originate from differences in both species and age, since we compare larval zebrafish data with adult mammalian results. Changes in coexpression levels during continued development from the larval stage detailed here into adulthood can also be expected.

To our knowledge, several peptide combinations were never addressed as far as coexpression is concerned. *avp* coexpression with *nts* was not discussed before, and rarely occurs here. Also, *crh* coexpression with *sst1.1* was not addressed before, and is rare here. We found that *penka* is not coexpressed with *cck*, which was not addressed before. Coexpression of *penkb* with *cck* was high, and is reported here for the first time. Similarly, coexpression of *penka* or *penkb* with *sst1.1* was not reported before, and we found rare or low coexpression. Also the coexpression of *sst1.1* and *nts* is shown here for the first time. Coexpression of *cck* and *vip* was never addressed before, and we found that they do not coexpress. We also report rare coexpression of *cck* with *sst1.1* for the first time. Lastly, we also show that the expression of *vip* does not overlap with that of *oxt* or *sst1.1*.

The rarely observed coexpression in only few cells or few animals is a deviation from the otherwise complete absence of coexpression seen in most cells or animals for these combinations of stainings. Potential causes of such rare coexpression could be transitional stages in the development of these cells, mismapping due to lack of resolution, or stochastic variation. The confocal microscopy used allowed sufficient depth resolution to spatially separate cells in all three dimensions and therefore mismapping is unlikely.

The high degree of coexpression of *avp* and *crh* observed has immediate functional implications. Similar to CRH, AVP stimulates adrenocorticotropic hormone (ACTH) secretion (Gillies and Lowry, 1979; Rivier and Vale, 1983). A wide range of coexpression levels was reported in different fish species. Coexpression of *avp* and *crh* was very high, reported as 100%, in *Catostomus*, but absent in *Anguilla* (Yulis and Lederis, 1987; Olivereau and Olivereau, 1990). In humans, AVP/CRH coexpression increases with age, and a connection with stress has been implied (Raadsheer et al., 1993). In addition to CRH and AVP, CCK can also stimulate ACTH release, and CCK acting in concert with AVP has a similar ACTH-releasing potency as CRH alone (Mezey et al., 1986). We saw no coexpression of *cck* with *avp* or *crh*. In contrast to CRH, AVP, and CCK, OXT generally inhibits stress responses, while local, endogenous OXT potentiates hypothalamo-pituitary-adrenal (HPA) axis activity, suggesting a dual mechanism of OXT released within the PVN (Neumann, 2002). In our results, coexpression of *oxt* and *crh* was very rare, and only present in single cells when it occurred. The spatial proximity of the densely intermingled cells positive for *oxt* or *crh* suggests that local release of Oxt could have immediate effects on *crh*-producing cells. ENK, CRH, and AVP were found to be colocalized within the same secretory vesicles (Hisano et al., 1987), suggesting that coexpressed peptides are packaged into common vesicles and coreleased at the synapse. We found that either *penka* or *penkb* can be coexpressed in both *crh*-positive and *avp*-positive cells. The concerted action of coreleased CRH and ENK is thought to fine-tune stress regulation (Pretel and Piekut, 1990).

In the rat, CRH-positive innervation of the neurohypophysis was suggested by observations of CRH in neurohypophyseal terminals (Bloom et al., 1982). The coexpression of CRH in magnocellular cells innervating the neurohypophysis could allow direct CRH release to the general circulation. The stress axis is also affected by VIP (Westendorf et al., 1983; Tilders et al., 1984), and NTS (Gudelsky et al., 1989). In the parvocellular PVN, coexpression of NTS and CRH was found, and the fractions of CRH-positive cells that coexpress AVP or NTS form different discrete subsets (Sawchenko et al., 1984a). The reported segregation of cells expressing AVP or CRH in rats cannot be found in larval zebrafish, and *vip* is not coexpressed with *crh* here, but we did find coexpression of *nts* and *crh*.

The CRH-producing cells coexpressing AVP were reported to be stress-responsive, while the AVP-negative CRH-producing cells do not respond to stress (Whitnall, 1993). Under osmotic stress, ENK and CRH levels are increased, but restraint and swimming stress only elevated CRH, not ENK (Harbuz and Lightman, 1989). Such findings demonstrate the functional implications of coexpression differences. For a cell, switching on the coexpression of another peptide is an elegant strategy to change its function without the need for major structural rearrangement of input or target projections, which could impose much stronger metabolic demands. Neurochemical switching in response to alterations in environmental conditions has been suggested as a relevant biological phenomenon in PVN neurons (Kiss, 1988; Swanson, 1991). Dynamic adaptation of neuroendocrine transcription to altered supply or demand for neuropeptides has also been suggested in zebrafish larvae (Kurrasch et al., 2009). With the coexpression profiles established here for the larval zebrafish under basal conditions, alterations triggered by environmental challenges can be studied in a model organism that has important advantages for the analysis of neural structure and function in intact and genetically tractable animals.

ACKNOWLEDGMENTS

We are grateful for helpful comments and critical discussion of the data by Rodrigo De Marco, Jose Arturo Gutierrez-Triana, and Colette vom Berg. We appreciate the suggestions and critical reading of the manuscript by Mario Wullimann. We also thank Regina Singer for technical assistance, Gabi Shoeman, Christiane Brandel and Angelika Schoell for fish care, and Mona Friedrich for additional staining and imaging.

REFERENCES

Arima, H., House, S. B., Gainer, H., and Aguilera, G. (2001). Direct stimulation of arginine vasopressin gene transcription by cAMP in parvocellular neurons of the paraventricular nucleus in organotypic cultures. *Endocrinology* 142, 5027–5030. doi: 10.1210/endo.142.11.8595

Aubry, J. M., Bartanusz, V., Jezova, D., Belin, D., and Kiss, J. Z. (1999). Single stress induces long-lasting elevations in vasopressin mRNA levels in CRF hypophysiotrophic neurones, but repeated stress is required to modify AVP immunoreactivity. *J. Neuroendocrinol.* 11, 377–384. doi: 10.1046/j.1365-2826.1999.00338.x

Biag, J., Huang, Y., Gou, L., Hintiryan, H., Askarinam, A., Hahn, J. D., et al. (2012). Cyto- and chemoarchitecture of the hypothalamic paraventricular nucleus in the C57BL/6J male mouse: a study of immunostaining and multiple fluorescent tract tracing. *J. Comp. Neurol.* 520, 6–33. doi: 10.1002/cne.22698

Bloom, F. E., Battenberg, E. L., Rivier, J., and Vale, W. (1982). Corticotropin releasing factor (CRF): immunoreactive neurones and fibers in rat hypothalamus. *Regul. Pept.* 4, 43–48. doi: 10.1016/0167-0115(82)90107-0

Bondy, C. A., Whitnall, M. H., Brady, L. S., and Gainer, H. (1989). Coexisting peptides in hypothalamic neuroendocrine systems: some functional implications. *Cell Mol. Neurobiol.* 9, 427–446. doi: 10.1007/bf00712791

Burlet, A., Tonon, M. C., Tankosic, P., Coy, D., and Vaudry, H. (1983). Comparative immunocytochemical localization of corticotropin releasing factor (CRF-41) and neurohypophysial peptides in the brain of Brattleboro and Long-Evans rats. *Neuroendocrinology* 37, 64–72. doi: 10.1159/000123517

Ceccatelli, S., Eriksson, M., and Hökfelt, T. (1989). Distribution and coexistence of corticotropin-releasing factor-, neurotensin-, enkephalin-, cholecystokinin-, galanin- and vasoactive intestinal polypeptide/peptide histidine isoleucine-like peptides in the parvocellular part of the paraventricular nucleus. *Neuroendocrinology* 49, 309–323. doi: 10.1159/000125133

Chandrasekar, G., Lauter, G., and Hauptmann, G. (2007). Distribution of corticotropin-releasing hormone in the developing zebrafish brain. *J. Comp. Neurol.* 505, 337–351. doi: 10.1002/cne.21496

Dabrowska, J., Hazra, R., Ahern, T. H., Guo, J. D., McDonald, A. J., Mascagni, F., et al. (2011). Neuroanatomical evidence for reciprocal regulation of the corticotrophin-releasing factor and oxytocin systems in the hypothalamus and the bed nucleus of the stria terminalis of the rat: Implications for balancing stress and affect. *Psychoneuroendocrinology* 36, 1312–1326. doi: 10.1016/j.psyneuen.2011.03.003

Dabrowska, J., Hazra, R., Guo, J. D., Dewitt, S., and Rainnie, D. G. (2013). Central CRF neurons are not created equal: phenotypic differences in CRF-containing neurons of the rat paraventricular hypothalamus and the bed nucleus of the stria terminalis. *Front. Neurosci.* 7:156. doi: 10.3389/fnins.2013.00156

Devos, N., Deflorian, G., Biemar, F., Bortolussi, M., Martial, J. A., Peers, B., et al. (2002). Differential expression of two somatostatin genes during zebrafish embryonic development. *Mech. Dev.* 115, 133–137. doi: 10.1016/s0925-4773(02)00082-5

Eaton, J. L., Holmqvist, B., and Glasgow, E. (2008). Ontogeny of vasotocin-expressing cells in zebrafish: selective requirement for the transcriptional regulators orthopedia and single-minded 1 in the preoptic area. *Dev. Dyn.* 237, 995–1005. doi: 10.1002/dvdy.21503

Fryer, J. N. (1989). Neuropeptides regulating the activity of goldfish corticotropes and melanotropes. *Fish Physiol. Biochem.* 7, 21–27. doi: 10.1007/bf00004686

Gillies, G., and Lowry, P. (1979). Corticotrophin releasing factor may be modulated vasopressin. *Nature* 278, 463–464. doi: 10.1038/278463a0

Gudelsky, G. A., Berry, S. A., and Meltzer, H. Y. (1989). Neurotensin activates tuberoinfundibular dopamine neurons and increases serum corticosterone concentrations in the rat. *Neuroendocrinology* 49, 604–609. doi: 10.1159/000125176

Harbuz, M. S., and Lightman, S. L. (1989). Responses of hypothalamic and pituitary mRNA to physical and psychological stress in the rat. *J. Endocrinol.* 122, 705–711. doi: 10.1677/joe.0.1220705

Herget, U., Wolf, A., Wullimann, M. F., and Ryu, S. (2014). Molecular neuroanatomy and chemoarchitecture of the neurosecretory preoptic-hypothalamic area in zebrafish larvae. *J. Comp. Neurol.* 522, 1542–1564. doi: 10.1002/cne.23480

Hisano, S., Tsuruo, Y., Katoh, S., Daikoku, S., Yanaihara, N., and Shibasaki, T. (1987). Intragranular colocalization of arginine vasopressin and methionine-enkephalin-octapeptide in CRF-axons in the rat median eminence. *Cell Tissue Res.* 249, 497–507. doi: 10.1007/bf00217321

Hökfelt, T., Fahrenkrug, J., Ju, G., Ceccatelli, S., Tsuruo, Y., Meister, B., et al. (1987). Analysis of peptide histidine-isoleucine/vasoactive intestinal polypeptide-immunoreactive neurons in the central nervous system with special reference to their relation to corticotropin releasing factor- and enkephalin-like immunoreactivities in the paraventricular hypothalamic nucleus. *Neuroscience* 23, 827–857. doi: 10.1016/0306-4522(87)90162-X

Hökfelt, T., Fahrenkrug, J., Tatemoto, K., Mutt, V., Werner, S., Hulting, A. L., et al. (1983). The PHI (PHI-27)/corticotropin-releasing factor/enkephalin immunoreactive hypothalamic neuron: possible morphological basis for integrated control of prolactin, corticotropin, and growth hormone secretion. *Proc. Natl. Acad. Sci. U S A* 80, 895–898. doi: 10.1073/pnas.80.3.895

Kiss, J. Z. (1988). Dynamism of chemoarchitecture in the hypothalamic paraventricular nucleus. *Brain Res. Bull.* 20, 699–708. doi: 10.1016/0361-9230(88)90080-9

Kurrasch, D. M., Nevin, L. M., Wong, J. S., Baier, H., and Ingraham, H. A. (2009). Neuroendocrine transcriptional programs adapt dynamically to the supply and demand for neuropeptides as revealed in *NSF* mutant zebrafish. *Neural Dev.* 4:22. doi: 10.1186/1749-8104-4-22

Lauter, G., Söll, I., and Hauptmann, G. (2011). Multicolor fluorescent in situ hybridization to define abutting and overlapping gene expression in the embryonic zebrafish brain. *Neural Dev.* 6:10. doi: 10.1186/1749-8104-6-10

Levin, M. C., and Sawchenko, P. E. (1993). Neuropeptide co-expression in the magnocellular neurosecretory system of the female rat: evidence for differential modulation by estrogen. *Neuroscience* 54, 1001–1018. doi: 10.1016/0306-4522(93)90591-3

Löhr, H., Ryu, S., and Driever, W. (2009). Zebrafish diencephalic A11-related dopaminergic neurons share a conserved transcriptional network with neuroendocrine cell lineages. *Development* 136, 1007–1017. doi: 10.1242/dev.033878

Machluf, Y., Gutnick, A., and Levkowitz, G. (2011). Development of the zebrafish hypothalamus. *Ann. N Y Acad. Sci.* 1220, 93–105. doi: 10.1111/j.1749-6632.2010.05945.x

Martin, R., and Voigt, K. H. (1981). Enkephalins co-exist with oxytocin and vasopressin in nerve terminals of rat neurohypophysis. *Nature* 289, 502–504. doi: 10.1038/289502a0

Mezey, E., Reisine, T. D., Skirboll, L., Beinfeld, M., and Kiss, J. Z. (1985). Cholecystokinin in the medial parvocellular subdivision of the paraventricular nucleus. Co-existence with corticotropin-releasing hormone. *Ann. N Y Acad. Sci.* 448, 152–156. doi: 10.1111/j.1749-6632.1985.tb29915.x

Mezey, E., Reisine, T. D., Skirboll, L., Beinfeld, M., and Kiss, J. Z. (1986). Role of cholecystokinin in corticotropin release: coexistence with vasopressin and corticotropin-releasing factor in cells of the rat hypothalamic paraventricular nucleus. *Proc. Natl. Acad. Sci. U S A* 83, 3510–3512. doi: 10.1073/pnas.83.10.3510

Neumann, I. D. (2002). Involvement of the brain oxytocin system in stress coping: interactions with the hypothalamo-pituitary-adrenal axis. *Prog. Brain Res.* 139, 147–162. doi: 10.1016/s0079-6123(02)39014-9

Olivereau, M., Moons, L., Olivereau, J., and Vandesande, F. (1988). Coexistence of corticotropin-releasing factor-like immunoreactivity and vasotocin in perikarya of the preoptic nucleus in the eel. *Gen. Comp. Endocrinol.* 70, 41–48. doi: 10.1016/0016-6480(88)90092-5

Olivereau, M., and Olivereau, J. (1990). Effect of pharmacological adrenalectomy on corticotropin-releasing factor-like and arginine vasotocin immunoreactivities in the brain and pituitary of the eel: immunocytochemical study. *Gen. Comp. Endocrinol.* 80, 199–215. doi: 10.1016/0016-6480(90)90165-i

Piekut, D. T., and Joseph, S. A. (1986). Co-existence of CRF and vasopressin immunoreactivity in parvocellular paraventricular neurons of rat hypothalamus. *Peptides* 7, 891–898. doi: 10.1016/0196-9781(86)90111-7

Pretel, S., and Piekut, D. (1990). Coexistence of corticotropin-releasing factor and enkephalin in the paraventricular nucleus of the rat. *J. Comp. Neurol.* 294, 192–201. doi: 10.1002/cne.902940204

Raadsheer, F. C., Sluiter, A. A., Ravid, R., Tilders, F. J., and Swaab, D. F. (1993). Localization of corticotropin-releasing hormone (CRH) neurons in the paraventricular nucleus of the human hypothalamus; age-dependent colocalization with vasopressin. *Brain Res.* 615, 50–62. doi: 10.1016/0006-8993(93)91113-7

Rivalland, E. T., Iqbal, J., Clarke, I. J., Turner, A. I., and Tilbrook, A. J. (2005). Co-localization and distribution of corticotrophin-releasing hormone, arginine vasopressin and enkephalin in the paraventricular nucleus of sheep: a sex comparison. *Neuroscience* 132, 755–766. doi: 10.1016/j.neuroscience.2005.01.045

Rivier, C., and Vale, W. (1983). Interaction of corticotropin-releasing factor and arginine vasopressin on adrenocorticotropin secretion in vivo. *Endocrinology* 113, 939–942. doi: 10.1210/endo-113-3-939

Rossier, J., Liston, D., Patey, G., Chaminade, M., Foutz, A. S., Cupo, A., et al. (1983). The enkephalinergic neuron: implications of a polyenkephalin precursor. *Cold Spring Harb. Symp. Quant. Biol.* 48(Pt. 1), 393–404. doi: 10.1101/sqb.1983.048.01.043

Roth, K. A., Weber, E., Barchas, J. D., Chang, D., and Chang, J. K. (1983). Immunoreactive dynorphin-(1–8) and corticotropin-releasing factor in subpopulation of hypothalamic neurons. *Science* 219, 189–191. doi: 10.1126/science.6129700

Sawchenko, P. E. (1987). Evidence for differential regulation of corticotropin-releasing factor and vasopressin immunoreactivities in parvocellular neurosecretory and autonomic-related projections of the paraventricular nucleus. *Brain Res.* 437, 253–263. doi: 10.1016/0006-8993(87)91641-6

Sawchenko, P. E., Swanson, L. W., and Vale, W. W. (1984a). Corticotropin-releasing factor: co-expression within distinct subsets of oxytocin-, vasopressin- and neurotensin-immunoreactive neurons in the hypothalamus of the male rat. *J. Neurosci.* 4, 1118–1129.

Sawchenko, P. E., Swanson, L. W., and Vale, W. W. (1984b). Co-expression of corticotropin-releasing factor and vasopressin immunoreactivity in parvocellular neurosecretory neurons of the adrenalectomized rat. *Proc. Natl. Acad. Sci. U S A* 81, 1883–1887. doi: 10.1073/pnas.81.6.1883

Simmons, D. M., and Swanson, L. W. (2009). Comparison of the spatial distribution of seven types of neuroendocrine neurons in the rat paraventricular nucleus: toward a global 3D model. *J. Comp. Neurol.* 516, 423–441. doi: 10.1002/cne.22126

Swanson, L. W. (1991). Biochemical switching in hypothalamic circuits mediating responses to stress. *Prog. Brain Res.* 87, 181–200. doi: 10.1016/S0079-6123(08)63052-6

Swanson, L. W., and Sawchenko, P. E. (1983). Hypothalamic integration: organization of the paraventricular and supraoptic nuclei. *Annu. Rev. Neurosci.* 6, 269–324. doi: 10.1146/annurev.ne.06.030183.001413

Swanson, L. W., Sawchenko, P. E., and Lind, R. W. (1986). Regulation of multiple peptides in CRF parvocellular neurosecretory neurons: implications for the stress response. *Prog. Brain Res.* 68, 169–190. doi: 10.1016/s0079-6123(08)60238-1

Swanson, L. W., and Simmons, D. M. (1989). Differential steroid hormone and neural influences on peptide mRNA levels in CRH cells of the paraventricular nucleus: a hybridization histochemical study in the rat. *J. Comp. Neurol.* 285, 413–435. doi: 10.1002/cne.902850402

Tilders, F., Tatemoto, K., and Berkenbosch, F. (1984). The intestinal peptide PHI-27 potentiates the action of corticotropin-releasing factor on ACTH release from rat pituitary fragments in vitro. *Endocrinology* 115, 1633–1635. doi: 10.1210/endo-115-4-1633

Unger, J. L., and Glasgow, E. (2003). Expression of isotocin-neurophysin mRNA in developing zebrafish. *Gene Expr. Patterns* 3, 105–108. doi: 10.1016/S1567-133X(02)00064-9

Vanderhaeghen, J. J., Lotstra, F., Vandesande, F., and Dierickx, K. (1981). Coexistence of cholecystokinin and oxytocin-neurophysin in some magnocellular hypothalamo-hypophyseal neurons. *Cell Tissue Res.* 221, 227–231. doi: 10.1007/bf00216585

Westendorf, J. M., Phillips, M. A., and Schonbrunn, A. (1983). Vasoactive intestinal peptide stimulates hormone release from corticotropic cells in culture. *Endocrinology* 112, 550–557. doi: 10.1210/endo-112-2-550

Westerfield, M. (2000). *The Zebrafish Book. A Guide for the Laboratory Use of Zebrafish (Danio rerio)*. 4th Edn. Eugene: University of Oregon Press.

Whitnall, M. H. (1993). Regulation of the hypothalamic corticotropin-releasing hormone neurosecretory system. *Prog. Neurobiol.* 40, 573–629. doi: 10.1016/0301-0082(93)90035-Q

Whitnall, M. H., and Gainer, H. (1988). Major pro-vasopressin-expressing and pro-vasopressin-deficient subpopulations of corticotropin-releasing hormone neurons in normal rats. Differential distributions within the paraventricular nucleus. *Neuroendocrinology* 47, 176–180. doi: 10.1159/000124910

Whitnall, M. H., Mezey, E., and Gainer, H. (1985). Co-localization of corticotropin-releasing factor and vasopressin in median eminence neurosecretory vesicles. *Nature* 317, 248–250. doi: 10.1038/317248a0

Whitnall, M. H., Smyth, D., and Gainer, H. (1987). Vasopressin coexists in half of the corticotropin-releasing factor axons present in the external zone of the median eminence in normal rats. *Neuroendocrinology* 45, 420–424. doi: 10.1159/000124768

Wolf, A., and Ryu, S. (2013). Specification of posterior hypothalamic neurons requires coordinated activities of Fezf2, Otp, Sim1a and Foxb1.2. *Development* 140, 1762–1773. doi: 10.1242/dev.085357

Yulis, C. R., and Lederis, K. (1987). Co-localization of the immunoreactivities of corticotropin-releasing factor and arginine vasotocin in the brain and pituitary system of the teleost Catostomus commersoni. *Cell Tissue Res.* 247, 267–273. doi: 10.1007/BF00218308

3

Characterization of a mammalian prosencephalic functional plan

Sophie Croizier[†], Sandrine Chometton, Dominique Fellmann and Pierre-Yves Risold*

EA 3922, SFR FED 4234, UFR Sciences Médicales et Pharmaceutiques, Université de Franche-Comté, Besançon, France

Correspondence:
Pierre-Yves Risold, EA 3922, SFR FED 4234, UFR Sciences Médicales et Pharmaceutiques, Université de Franche-Comté, 19 rue Ambroise Paré, 25030 Besançon cedex, France
e-mail: pierre-yves.risold@univ-fcomte.fr

[†]Present address:
Sophie Croizier, The Saban Research Institute, Neuroscience Program, Children's Hospital Los Angeles, University of Southern California, Los Angeles, California 90027, USA

Hypothalamic organizational concepts have greatly evolved as the primary hypothalamic pathways have been systematically investigated. In the present review, we describe how the hypothalamus arises from a molecularly heterogeneous region of the embryonic neural tube but is first differentiated as a primary neuronal cell cord (earliest mantle layer). This structure defines two axes that align onto two fundamental components: a longitudinal tractus postopticus(tpoc)/retinian component and a transverse supraoptic tract(sot)/olfactory component. We then discuss how these two axonal tracts guide the formation of all major tracts that connect the telencephalon with the hypothalamus/ventral midbrain, highlighting the existence of an early basic plan in the functional organization of the prosencephalic connectome.

Keywords: melanin concentrating hormone, cell cord, pioneer tracts, lateral hypothalamic area, medial forebrain bundle

INTRODUCTION

As a whole, the hypothalamus is involved in an extremely large range of functions, including neuroendocrine and visceral responses, thermogenesis, circadian or seasonal cycles, sleep or general arousal, the expression of specific instinctive behaviors, the control of rhythmic cortical (hippocampal) neuron firing, emotion and reward. Therefore, the hypothalamus is a complex structure composed of dozens of cell groups or nuclei that are often involved in several of these responses. Classically, the hypothalamus has been divided into four anteroposterior regions (preoptic, anterior, tuberal and posterior regions) and three longitudinal zones (periventricular, medial and lateral zones) (Swanson, 1987). This organizational scheme has been widely accepted by anatomists and physiologists during the past decades but is not satisfactory, as most of the borders are not clear and are often arbitrarily drawn. In light of anatomical findings acquired during the late 1980s and early 1990s, the organization of the hypothalamus has been revised around the concept of a behavioral control column that is composed of the medial zone nuclei (**Figure 1A**; Swanson, 2000, 2005). Following this new concept, each medial zone nucleus is involved in pathways that include the tectum, thalamus and telencephalon, referencing the classical circuit described by Papez in 1937 (Papez, 1995). This new view of the hypothalamic organization is interesting as it suggests that this region is fully integrated within the complex prosencephalic networks that control behavioral expression. Therefore, the hypothalamus is capable of influencing telencephalic centers, including the cerebral cortex, as well as being influenced by descending projections (Risold and Swanson, 1996, 1997; Risold et al., 1997). Conspicuous convergences have appeared between the organization of these connections and those of the classical striato-nigral and mesotelencephalic circuits, and a revision of the telencephalic organization has been proposed (**Figure 1B**; Risold et al., 1997; Swanson, 2000, 2003; Risold, 2004).

Although interesting, this concept primarily involves the medial zone nuclei at hypothalamic levels but ignores large sections of this structure, especially the entire hypothalamic lateral zone (lateral hypothalamic area, LHA) (**Figure 1A**). The LHA is a poorly differentiated region that has always been viewed as a rostral extension of the brainstem reticular formation or a bed nucleus of the medial forebrain bundle (mfb). The mfb is the major fiber tract of the basal prosencephalon that passes through the LHA and bidirectionally connects more than fifty cell groups in the brainstem and telencephalon (Nieuwenhuys et al., 1982; Swanson, 1987). The mfb is a specific attribute of the LHA

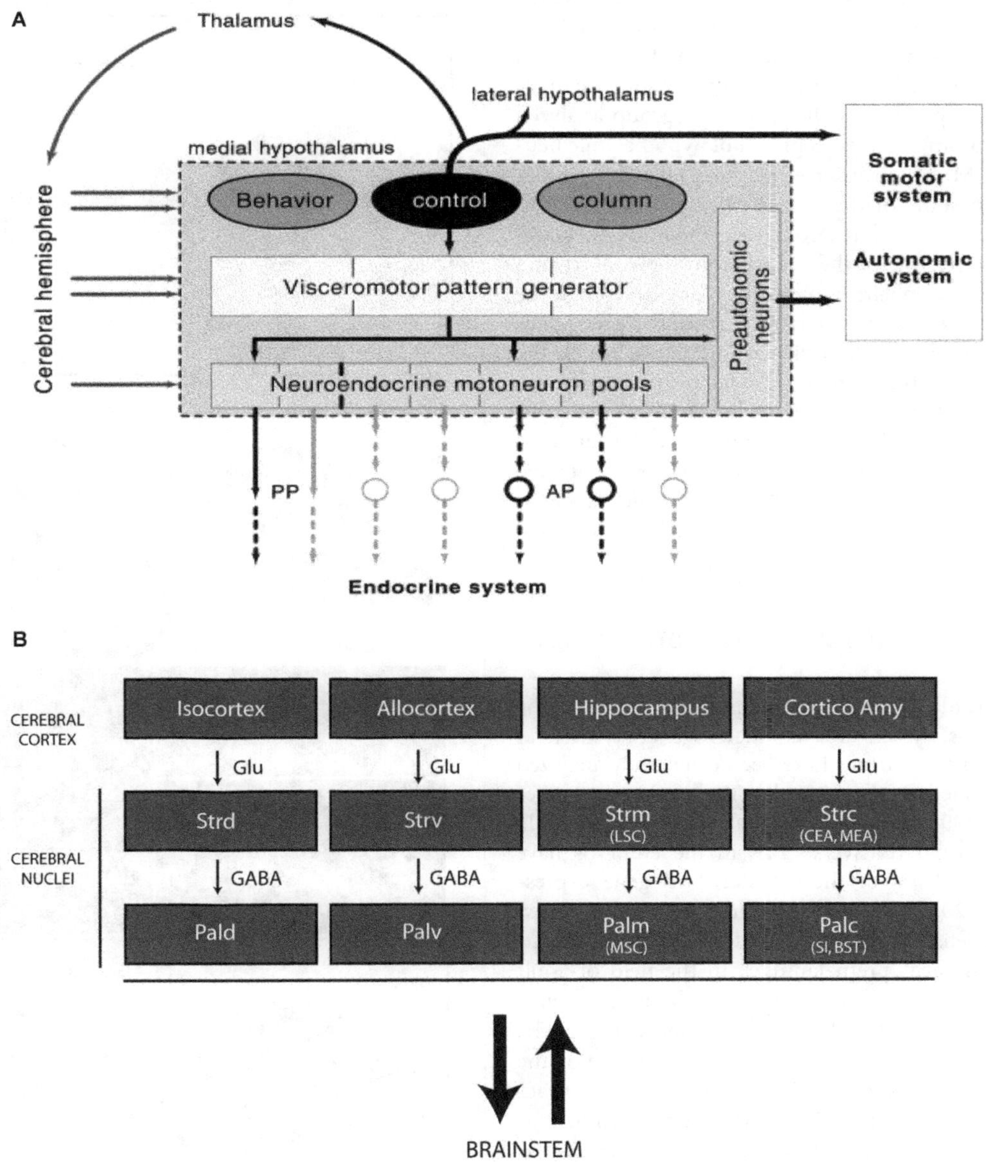

FIGURE 1 | (A) Diagram illustrating the recent concept of the morphofunctional organization of the hypothalamus. Hypothalamic periventricular structures form a visceromotor pattern generator (VMPG) network that controls neuroendocrine and visceral responses. This VMPG is influenced by medial zone nuclei. These nuclei form a behavioral control column and are involved in the expression of goal oriented behaviors. They control somatic motor responses through projections in the tectum (periaqueductal gray), but they are also involved in closed loop circuits with the telencephalon, in particular through projections to the thalamus. Reproduced with permission from Thompson and Swanson, 2003. **(B)** Schematic representation of the organization of the telencephalon (adapted from Risold, 2004). The cerebral cortex as a whole, including the cortico-amygdaloid nuclei, topographically projects onto the striatum (dorsal, ventral, medial, and posterior divisions), which is connected with the pallidum (similarly parceled into dorsal, ventral, medial and posterior divisions). While projections from the cortex are glutamatergic, the striatum and pallidum are massively GABAergic and are bidirectionally connected with the brainstem. Abbreviations: AP: anterior pituitary; BST: bed nuclei of the stria terminalis; CEA: central nucleus amygdala; Cortico Amy: cortical nuclei amygdala; GABA: gamma aminobutyric acid; Glu: glutamate; LSC: lateral septal complex; MEA: medial nucleus amygdala; MSC: medial septal complex; Pal d-v-m-c: dorsal, ventral, medial and caudal divisions of the pallidum; PP: posterior pituitary; SI: substantia inominata; Str d-v-m-c: dorsal, ventral, medial and caudal divisions of the striatum.

throughout its entire alar-basal extent. However, the LHA is not homogeneous. The basal portion of the LHA contains abundant cell populations that are characterized by the expression of specific peptides, such as melanin-concentrating hormone (MCH) and hypocretins/orexins, and widespread projections from the cerebral cortex to the spinal cord.

Tremendous progress in expanding the general knowledge of the forebrain embryonic development has been made over the last twenty years. Recent studies, alongside anatomical data, have led to a better understanding of the organization of the vertebrate forebrain, which has allowed for a better comprehension of its evolution (Puelles, 2001; Aboitiz, 2011). To understand the organization of the basal portion of the LHA, our group analyzed the comparative anatomy and development of hypothalamic neurons that produce MCH (Croizier et al., 2013). In the present analysis, we revised some of these observations from past and recent developmental studies regarding the forebrain to better understand the relative role of the LHA within the context of a putative general prosencephalic framework. We observed that the whole ventral prosencephalon is organized around a precocious structure, previously named the cell cord and from which the LHA differentiates, in a timely manner. This primary structure defines two axes that align onto two fundamental components: a tractus postopticus (tpoc)/retinian component and a supraoptic tract (sot)/olfactory component. These two axes determine the path of the mfb and provide what can be described as a basic structural framework for a prosencephalic "functional plan".

DEVELOPMENTAL GENE PATTERNS AND HYPOTHALAMIC SUBDIVISIONS

Very complex molecular interactions occur at the origin of the hypothalamic regions, which are very heterogeneous, even at the earliest stages. These patterns have been extensively analyzed in many more detailed works to which the reader may refer (Shimamura et al., 1995; Nieuwenhuys et al., 1998; Puelles et al., 2012). Longitudinal and transverse axes in the embryos have been revised on the basis of these patterns of gene expression (Puelles et al., 2012). Although the terminology proposed by Puelles and Rubenstein is widely used in the developmental field (see for instance "prethalamus"), in the field of adult neuroanatomy the traditional axes and nomenclature are maintained. Since we strive to be clear for all interested readers, "adult" or "developmental", we often hesitate to use one or the other name for a structure or spatial relation. For this practical reason, and in particular to respect the main information flows in the adult brain, we have used sometimes similar rostrocaudal and dorsoventral axes in the embryonic brain as are used in the adult brain (for example see in **Figure 3**). We also use the terminology prethalamus-ventral thalamus, in this way adding "prethalamus", as is often done in developmental studies, for the presumptive regions of the zona incerta and the ventral lateral geniculate nuclei. The preoptic region (POA) (actually a part of the telencephalon, see below), the anterior region (or alar hypothalamus) that is supraoptic and regions that are posterior (basal) or postoptic represent no problem (**Figure 2**).

From the general literature in this field one important observation retained our attention: very early in development, these gene expression patterns bear resemblances to and are contiguous with those in structures adjacent to the hypothalamus, which suggests that some hypothalamic boundaries are not sharply delineated (**Figure 2A**). Consider the following examples.

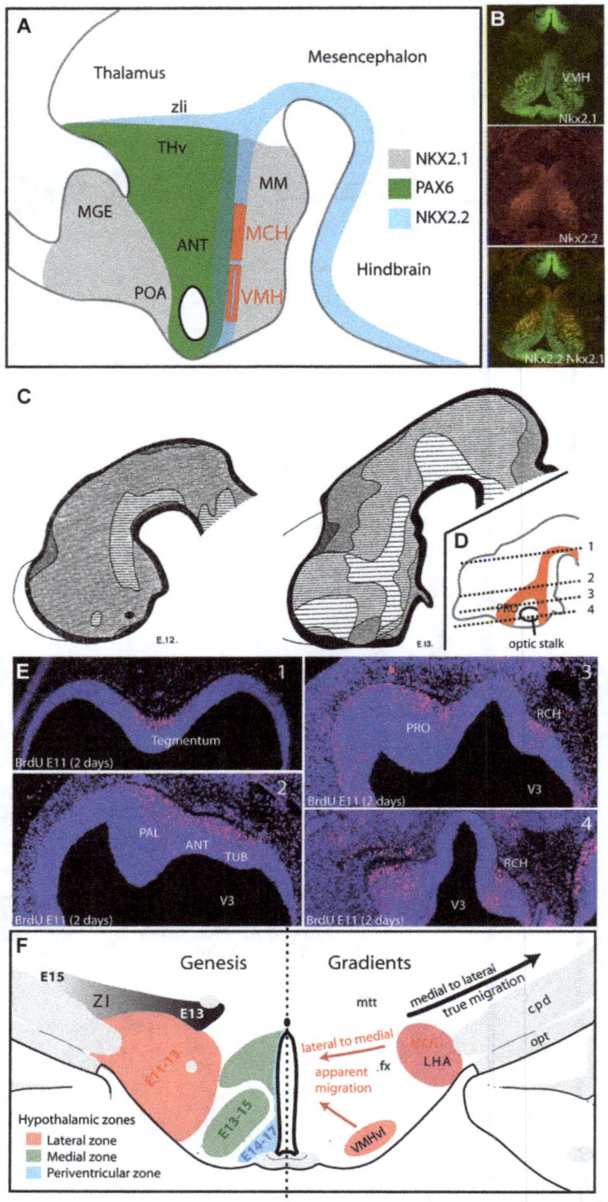

FIGURE 2 | (A) The distribution patterns of transcription factors agree well with the alar-basal divisions of the hypothalamus into preoptic, anterior and posterior/postoptic regions. However, these patterns extend outside the borders of the hypothalamus, involving the ventral telencephalon, prethalamus-ventral thalamus and ventral midbrain. MCH neurons and neurons of the VMH are generated from Nkx2.1/Nkx2.2 expressing neuroepithelial zones in the postoptic region. **(B)** Based on immunohistochemical analysis of a horizontal section of an E15 rat embryonic hypothalamus, the VMH clearly express both Nkx2.1 and Nkx2.2. **(C)** Figures from Keyser (1972) illustrating the differentiation of the early neurogenic zone in E12 and E13 Chinese hamster embryos: the first appearance of a longitudinal zone in the ventral mesencephalon and dorsal hypothalamus correspond to the cell cord **(A)**. At E13, neurogenesis involved larger regions in the preoptic/ventral telencephalon; in other figure from Keyser that is not shown here, this author observed these regions forming one single continuum (as in **D**). This continuum takes the shape of

(Continued)

FIGURE 2 | Continued
an inverted Y. **(D,E)** Figure adapted from Croizier et al., 2011 illustrating the distribution of neurons generated at E11 on an E13 rat embryo. BrdU was injected into the pregnant dam at E11, and embryos were taken 2 days later at E13. BrdU was detected by immunohistochemistry on horizontal sections. The distribution pattern of these nuclei is schematized on a sagittal section in **(D)**. BrdU-labeled nuclei follow an inverted Y pattern. In **(E)** pictures are arranged from dorsal (1) to ventral (4). **(F)** Gradients of neurogenesis in the ventral diencephalon. Left side: Schematic representation of the neurogenic gradients in the hypothalamus and prethalamus-ventral thalamus, as described by Altman and Bayer (1986). The LHA is generated between E11and E13, the medial hypothalamus from E13 to E15 and the periventricular zone from E14 to E17. Note the medial to lateral gradient in the prethalamus-ventral thalamus (generated from E13 to E15). Right side: Drawing summarizing the gradients in the ventral diencephalon: lateral to medial gradients (red arrows) in the hypothalamus suggest the apparent or passive migrations of neurons in lateral territories (LHA or VMHvl), but the prethalamus-ventral thalamus requires the effective migration of cells away from the ventricular surface (black arrow). Abbreviations: ANT: anterior hypothalamic area; cpd: cerebral peduncle; fx: fornix; LHA: lateral hypothalamic area; MCH: melano-concentrating hormone expressing neurons; MGE: medial ganglionic eminence; MM: mammillary body; mtt: mammillothalamic tract; opt: optic tract; PAL: pallidum; POA: preoptic area; PRO: presumptive preoptic area; RCH: retrochiasmatic region; THv: prethalamus or ventral thalamus; TUB: presumptive tuberal hypothalamic region; VMH: ventromedial hypothalamic nucleus; VMHvl: ventrolateral part of the VMH; ZI: zona incerta; zli: zona limitans intrathalamica; V3: third ventricle.

THE HYPOTHALAMIC/TELENCEPHALIC BORDER

The POA shares many characteristics and developmental expression patterns with the pallidum, and has been considered a telencephalic structure (Moreno and González, 2011; Puelles et al., 2012). The preoptic anlage expresses the telencephalic marker Foxg1, distinguishing it from hypothalamic structures. Shh and Nkx2.1 are co-distributed in the POA, but their expression patterns extend into the pallidal anlage. Although the POA expresses Shh, it does not express Nkx2.2, whereas the hypothalamic regions do express Nkx2.2. Defining the telencephalo-hypothalamic limit has always been problematic, despite functional and connectional studies in adult animals that have been interpreted in favor of including the POA as part of the hypothalamus (Swanson, 1987; Risold et al., 1997). Earlier authors often viewed this region to be a medial and unevaginated section of the telencephalon or telencephalon impar (His, 1893; Herrick, 1910; Kuhlenbeck, 1929). These early claims have been strengthened by recent studies of gene expression patterns (Moreno and González, 2011). This definition is further reinforced by recent findings that, similar to the lateral and medial ganglionic eminences (LGE and MGE, respectively), the POA produces GABAergic (gamma aminobutyric acid) interneurons that tangentially migrate into the cerebral cortex (Brown et al., 2011; Gelman et al., 2011; Vitalis and Rossier, 2011). In addition, migrating cells from the olfactory epithelium colonize the medial septal and preoptic areas. Many of these cells express GnRH (gonadotropin-releasing hormone) and are neuroendocrine neurons, including in the septal region. Neuroendocrine functions are a hallmark of the hypothalamus, but a putative neuroendocrine zone extends beyond the actual rostral border of the hypothalamus. *Therefore, a putative hypothalamo/telencephalic limit at the septal/preoptic border is not delineated by the distribution pattern of neuroendocrine GnRH neurons, the origin of GABAergic interneurons migrating into the pallium, or developmental gene expression patterns.*

ANTERIOR HYPOTHALAMUS/PRETHALAMUS-VENTRAL THALAMUS

At early embryonic stages, Pax6 is expressed in a continuum that includes the presumptive prethalamus-ventral thalamus and extends into the optic vesicle (Stoykova et al., 1996; Puelles et al., 2013). In the hypothalamus, this pattern involves a strip of tissue between the optic stalk and the prethalamus-ventral thalamus (**Figure 2A**). The *Pax6* expression pattern (encompassing the alar hypothalamus and prethalamic eminence) clearly suggests an elongation of the primary embryonic brain (see the interesting paper of (Suzuki et al., 2014) about the rise of the eyes in chordates). As previously noted, Pax family members are involved in the formation of the retina and are also involved in the guidance of retinal projections and the differentiation of retinorecipient structures into the suprachiasmatic nucleus (SCN). In vertebrates, such as lampreys or batrachians, the SCN is adjacent to the prethalamus. In the anuran, Dominguez confirmed this close and continuous positioning of the anterior hypothalamus and prethalamus (Dominguez et al., 2013). In some species, projections from the prethalamus and from the tectum reach the retina through the optic tract. In mammals, the ventral geniculate body has retained a strong retinal afferent, and the intergeniculate leaflet, a small structure of prethalamic-ventral thalamic origin, has strong bidirectional connections with the SCN, reminiscent of the adjacent positions of the SCN and the prethalamus in non-amniote vertebrates (see the recent work of Suzuki et al., 2014 as well). *Therefore, early Pax6 expression patterns prefigure optic related pathways that in the alar hypothalamus and in the prethalamus-ventral thalamus.*

THE HYPOTHALAMUS AS A ROSTRAL STRUCTURE

Also of particular interest for the development of the hypothalamus are the longitudinal expression patterns of Shh and Nkx2.2, which label a band of hypothalamic neuroepithelial tissue that rostrally extends from a similar band in the ventral mesencephalon (Shimamura et al., 1995; Alvarez-Bolado et al., 2012). When the anterior neuropore closure occurs, the initial expression patterns of Shh and Nkx2.2 involve the differentiating zona limitans intrathalamica (zli), at the junction between the prethalamus and thalamus. At roughly the same stage, corresponding to the beginning of neurogenesis, Shh expression (but not Nkx2.2) appears in a telencephalic region. The domain of Nkx2.2 overlaps partially with both Pax6 and Nkx2.1 expression domains (Croizier et al., 2011). The Pax6/Nkx2.2-rich region gives rise to anterior hypothalamic structures whose composition in the adult are not yet completely clear. However, the Nkx2.1/Nkx2.2 regions give rise to vast portions of the basal hypothalamus. We have clearly shown (Croizier et al., 2011) that neurons that produce MCH are generated and differentiate under the control of Shh (Szabó et al., 2009; Alvarez-Bolado et al., 2012) in this sector of the embryonic wall. In the model of Puelles, this is the RTu-I portion of the basal hypothalamus (Puelles et al.,

2012); in this way, the MCH cells would represent a precocious peduncular superficial derivative of the dorsal retrotuberal basal domain.

The ventromedial hypothalamic nucleus is produced by a more rostral portion of the Nkx2.1/Nkx2.2 region (**Figure 2B**, and see (Altman and Bayer, 1986) for the origin of this nucleus). Shimogori identified this region as the "intrahypothalamic diagonal", on the basis of multiple gene expression patterns ("diagonal", that is, neither columnar nor prosomeric, but somewhat in the middle of both, rather confusingly) (Shimogori et al., 2010). The Nkx2.2 and Shh expression patterns extend into the brainstem and are known to be involved in the genesis of other very early defined neurons, including serotonergic neurons, which have diffuse projection patterns similar to MCH neurons (Ye et al., 1998). Somewhat later, Shh is also involved in the differentiation of dopaminergic ventral midbrain neurons (Riddle and Pollock, 2003; Perez-Balaguer et al., 2009). *Therefore, the co-expression of two primary markers of the basal neural tube extends into the postoptic (i.e., basal) hypothalamus*, and we observe the early production of specific neuron populations with diffuse projection patterns as MCH and serotonergic neurons in corresponding hypothalamic regions and hindbrain.

The mammillary nuclei and regions of the very ventromedial hypothalamus (VMH, arcuate nucleus) are generated by an Nkx2.1 expressing neuroepithelial zone (Puelles and Rubenstein, 2003). This appears to be the only pattern that does not show any sign of extension outside of the hypothalamic borders (although, see Puelles et al., 2013).

From all these observations we can conclude that the hypothalamus has diverse origins. Patterns of gene expressions are very complex, and precise combinations of gene expression are associated with specific cell groups or nuclei. However, at the very early stages, the patterns of Shh, Pax6, Nkx2.2 and Nkx2.1 expression indicate that the POA is a part of the telencephalon (Puelles et al., 2012) and the anterior (alar hypothalamus) and postoptic regions (basal hypothalamus) share some gene expression patterns with the prethalamus and the ventral (basal) brainstem.

EARLY NEUROGENESIS IN THE HYPOTHALAMUS—EVIDENCE OF A PRIMARY STRUCTURE

In the embryonic neural tube, neurogenesis (neuron production and therefore the formation of a postmitotic "mantle layer") begins in the ventral hindbrain, behind the cephalic flexure. This neurogenic zone extends both caudally and rostrally. In more rostral regions, Keyser very precisely depicted the patterns of morphologic modifications that occur in the hypothalamic periventricular and mantle layers of the Chinese hamster (Keyser, 1972), describing the development of a "matrix" that can be translated into a very dynamic view of the pattern of neurogenesis in the diencephalon (**Figure 2C**, right and left diagrams). These observations by Keyser can easily be correlated with neurogenesis studies using tritiated nucleotides or BrdU. Keyser showed that the early pattern of neuron production is not uniform throughout the hypothalamus. Neurogenesis begins in a column of cells that was named the "cell cord" by Gilbert in 1935 in the human embryo (cited in Keyser, 1972), and it was more recently observed again in the mouse embryo by Croizier (Croizier et al., 2011; **Figures 2D,E**). The position of the cell cord on the model of Puelles is probably basal, immediately under the alar-basal boundary (Puelles et al., 2012). This column of early neurogenesis gives rise to the first generated hypothalamic neurons that ultimately form the postchiasmatic lateral hypothalamus, and extends into the ventral midbrain. MCH expressing neurons are among the first generated cells in this region, and we showed their early differentiation within this cell cord (Croizier et al., 2011). From this original sector, neurogenesis involves more rostral territories (presumptive entopeduncular nucleus (Altman and Bayer, 1986)). Therefore, the early mantle layer forms the shape of an inverted Y in the hypothalamic primordium (**Figures 2C,D**). The vertical (postoptic) limb and stem of the Y are longitudinal and correspond with the Shh/Nkx2.2/Pax6 expression patterns. The supraoptic arm, however, does not respect these longitudinal patterns and is transversally oriented (longitudinal and transverse here in the sense of the model by Puelles et al., 2012). A chronological correlation could be made between the development of this supraoptic arm and the differentiation of the zli (another transverse feature), the differentiation of the telencephalic vesicle or the telencephalic expression of Shh. However, causal links have not yet been demonstrated.

Keyser also observed that the development of the mantle layer extends from these hypothalamic initial regions, in both the ventral (hypothalamic) and dorsal (ventral thalamic/prethalamic) directions (Keyser, 1972). Altman and Bayer described a lateral to medial gradient of neurogenesis in the hypothalamus (lateral to periventricular) that is clearly in agreement with the observations of Keyser (**Figure 2F**; Altman and Bayer, 1986). A similar gradient was also clearly demonstrated for MCH expressing neurons (Brischoux et al., 2001; Croizier et al., 2010). On the contrary, both Altman and Bayer (1986) in the rat, and Keyser (1972) in the Chinese hamster, described a medial to lateral gradient of neurogenesis in the prethalamus that generates the zona incerta (adult ventral thalamus). This gradient is opposite to the hypothalamic gradient, although both structures are generated during the same period (between E11 and E16 in the rat). Therefore, these two opposing gradients involving two adjacent structures, lateral to medial for the hypothalamus and medial to lateral for the zona incerta, clearly designate a unique sector of origin, and the region giving rise to the cell cord is a good candidate. The opposite (lateral-medial and medial-lateral) gradients of genesis in the hypothalamus and prethalamus-ventral thalamus suggest distinct strategies of cell migration; the lateral to medial hypothalamic gradient suggests a dominant passive migration, as was shown for MCH expressing neurons in the dorsal hypothalamus and is also evident for the VMH. However, the medial to lateral gradient of the zona incerta indicates that lateral neurons must actively migrate far from the ventricular surface (**Figure 2F**; Keyser, 1972; Altman and Bayer, 1986).

Therefore, the initial neurogenesis in the hypothalamus produces a primary inverted Y-shaped structure named here the cell cord (although this structure is slightly different but encompasses the original cell cord). The prethalamus-ventral thalamus and medial hypothalamus are then produced through inverted gradients that are dorsal and ventromedial to this initial cell cord, respectively.

THE STRUCTURAL WIRING OF THE HYPOTHALAMUS AND THE CHRONOTOPIC DIFFERENTIATION OF THE WHOLE PROSENCEPHALON

Gene expression patterns indicate that the development of the hypothalamus is a multifactorial process, but gradients of neurogenesis show that time is a key parameter. The study by Altman and Bayer (1986) emphasized this point when these authors described three waves of genesis to form the three longitudinal zones of the hypothalamus, even if "three waves" might not to be literally considered (Alvarez-Bolado et al., 2012). Time is also a critical parameter according the description of the "matrix" (mantle layer) and cell cord by Keyser (1972). Relying on the development of MCH expressing neurons, we have more recently illustrated the importance of chronology in the organization of this conspicuous neuron population in the posterior hypothalamus in both rat and mouse (Croizier et al., 2010, 2011). Therefore, an analysis of the hypothalamic wiring is inseparable from the timely and sequential events that lead to the morphofunctional organization of the whole prosencephalon.

Tract formation in the hypothalamus immediately follows neurogenesis and accompanies the differentiation of hypothalamic regions. The main axonal bundles of the prosencephalon, transverse and longitudinal, have been illustrated on the prosomeric model by Puelles et al. (see their Figure 8.34) (Puelles et al., 2012). Pioneer tracts have been well described in a series of papers (Herrick, 1910; Easter et al., 1993; Mastick and Easter, 1996). Pioneer tract organization is very well conserved in the young embryo of all vertebrates, from fishes to mammals. The tpoc is the first prosencephalic tract. It is composed of commissural axons (postoptic commissure) and axons running toward the ventral midbrain, parallel to the Nkx2.2 expression domain. This tract joins the medial longitudinal fasciculus (mlf) in the midbrain. The sot and the stria medullaris are formed in the preoptic/entopeduncular primordium. The sot joins the tpoc by passing over the optic stalk (Anderson and Key, 1996), while the stria medullaris runs toward the dorsal diencephalon. The long projections of the hypothalamus subsequently organize along these pioneer tracts, and several stages can be recognized. *Each stage is correlated with a different degree of organization in the embryonic brain and is reflected in the structure of the adult hypothalamus.*

- The first stage is concerned with the initial formation of the pioneer tracts. Guidance cues, such as Slit/ROBO family members, and transcription factors, such as Pax6, play important roles in constraining the paths of pioneer tracts (Mastick et al., 1997; Nural and Mastick, 2004; Ricaño-Cornejo et al., 2011). Both tpoc and sot clearly recall the early neurogenic pattern and travel along the inverted Y-shaped cell cord.

  Initially, these tracts are composed of descending axons. The first MCH expressing neurons and the first neurons in the ventrolateral VMH are generated during this preliminary stage (**Figure 3A**). MCH and SF-1 are expressed in neurons within the dorsal and ventral cell cords, respectively, and their axons have been traced in the tpoc running toward the mesencephalon (Croizier et al., 2011; Cheung et al., 2013). In the adult hypothalamus, this first stage is represented by spinally projecting MCH neurons (Brischoux et al., 2001; Croizier et al., 2010, 2011) that are located very laterally in the rat LHA (**Figure 3E**). Neurons in the lateral region of the adult VMH, where the first SF1-labeled cells settle, send abundant projections through the supraoptic commissures (Canteras et al., 1994), and this pattern is also clearly reminiscent of descending SF-1 projections in the tpoc.
- The second stage is characterized by the growth of ascending projections along the tpoc and sot. This growth is particularly well illustrated by the differentiation of ascending projecting MCH expressing neurons (**Figure 3A**). During this stage, large bundles of ascending axons containing neurotransmitters, such as serotonin and dopamine, develop from the brainstem. The projections from hindbrain serotonergic or ventral midbrain dopaminergic neurons are initially longitudinal as they follow the tpoc, changing course in the basal hypothalamus and becoming transversally oriented in order to migrate towards the telencephalon (**Figures 3B–D**). MCH expressing neurons settle in the hypothalamic region, where these axons change direction. Moreover, in the rat, the phenotype of MCH expressing neurons change drastically as the mesotelencephalic dopaminergic pathway develops. As mentioned above, the first MCH expressing neurons send descending axons to the spinal cord. However, MCH expressing neurons produced during the second stage, as the dopaminergic mesotelencephalic axons progress in the mfb, project axons toward the telencephalon but not the spinal cord in the adult rat (Brischoux et al., 2002; Croizier et al., 2010, 2011; **Figure 3E**).

The mechanisms responsible for the change in the axial organization of the MCH population appear to be related to the differentiation of the telencephalic vesicles (Croizier et al., 2011). The growth and differentiation of telencephalic vesicles involves complex interactions between morphogenic molecular actors, such as Fgf8 and Wnts (Rubenstein et al., 1998; Aboitiz, 2011). These proteins are produced by organizing centers and may diffuse and act far from their production sites. Croizier also detected a sharp increase in the production of the chemoattractant Netrin1 in the telencephalon following the onset of neurogenesis (Croizier et al., 2011). Therefore, the telencephalon exerts a strong influence on the developing rostral brainstem as it differentiates. This influence likely increases as the rostral brainstem becomes involved in very active neurogenesis (**Figure 4A**). Although not fully understood, the telencephalic organizing centers, such as the ventral and cortical hems, and the diencephalic organizing centers, such as the zli, interact through the production of morphogenic protein gradients (Marín et al., 2002; Pottin et al., 2011; Rash and Grove, 2011). These processes are important for the coordinated growth of the cortex and thalamus and for the establishment

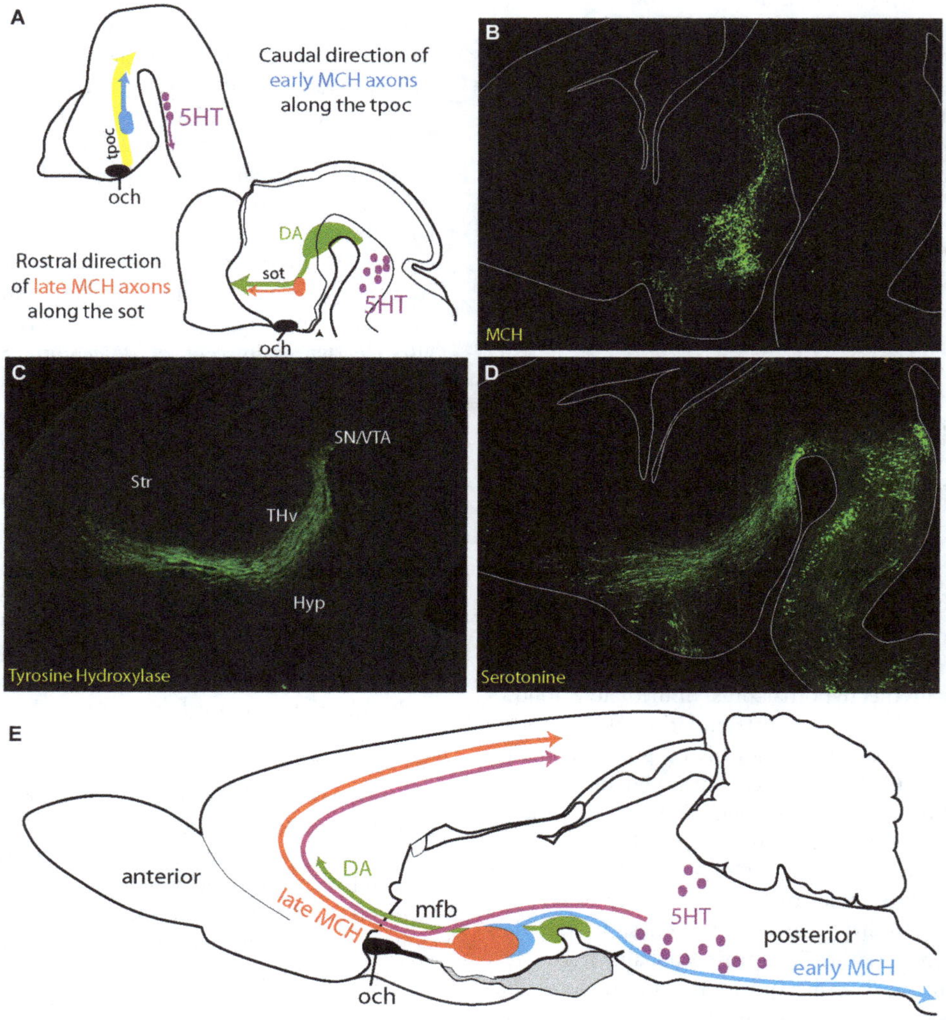

FIGURE 3 | (A) Initial projections of MCH expressing neurons follow pioneer tracts, but their direction changes as the embryo matures. Axons of first generated MCH expressing neurons follow the tpoc toward the midbrain. Axons from late generated MCH expressing neurons follow the sot toward the telencephalon, along DA and 5HT axons (see Croizier et al., 2011). **(B–D)** Distribution of serotonin, MCH (MCH-GFP, revealed with an anti-GFP antibody; see Croizier et al., 2011) and tyrosine hydroxylase (dopamine) in three adjacent sections cut in the parasagittal plane and passing through the mfb of an E14 mouse embryonic brain. Serotonergic and dopaminergic axons from respectively the hindbrain and midbrain travel along the tpoc and arch rostrally at the level of the posterior hypothalamus, where MCH expressing cells are found. Note the pattern of serotonergic axons that closely follows the inverted Y pattern of the sot/tpoc. **(E)** Schematic illustration of the ascending serotonergic and dopaminergic pathways to the telencephalon through the mfb and the distribution patterns of early and late MCH projections in the adult rat central nervous system. Abbreviations: DA: dopaminergic neurons; Hyp: hypothalamus; MCH: melano-concentrating hormone containing neurons; mfb: medial forebrain bundle; och: optic chiasm (or presumptive position of the optic tract in **A**); SN: substantia nigra; sot: supraoptic tract; Str: presumptive striatal region; THv: ventral thalamic region; tpoc: tractus postopticus; VTA: ventral tegmental area (presumptive); 5HT: serotonergic neurons.

of corticothalamic and thalamocortical connections. However, the second stage also corresponds to an outburst of neurogenesis throughout the hypothalamus and the ventral mesencephalon. The dopaminergic neurons of the substantia nigra and ventral tegmental area are representative of this second stage. Their soma migrate through pre-existing premotor or motor midbrain structures, such as the Edinger-Westfall or oculomotor nuclei, to settle in the ventral midbrain. Their ascending projections through the lateral mfb to the striatum define them anatomically. The outburst of neurogenesis in the hypothalamus includes cortically projecting MCH expressing neurons and most of the hypothalamic medial zone that is generated between E13 and E15 in the rat (Altman and Bayer, 1986). During the same stage, Cheung reported ascending SF-1 expressing axons from the VMH in the mfb (Cheung et al., 2013).

Therefore, the second stage in the development of the hypothalamus is characterized by the differentiation of most of the hypothalamic lateral and medial cell groups and is concomitant with the differentiation of the dopaminergic ventral midbrain.

- The third stage corresponds with the differentiation of the thin periventricular hypothalamic zone and neuroendocrine pathways, as neurogenesis reaches exhaustion in the hypothalamic anlage. Most of the late produced periventricular structures are regions of the visceromotor pattern generator (VMPG) that was described by Thompson and Swanson (Thompson and Swanson, 2003). These structures are often perichiasmatic or involve dorsal hypothalamic cell groups (dorsomedial nucleus, dorsomedial capsule of the VMH). The last generated MCH expressing neurons in the rat are periventricular and project to the arcuate nucleus (Croizier et al., 2010), and some others can be characterized as neuroendocrine in nature (Cvetkovic et al., 2003). These last produced MCH expressing neurons can be viewed as part of the VMPG. Therefore, most of the VMPG and LHA could have a common origin in the periventricular dorsal hypothalamus but be generated at different periods.
- Finally, perinatal processes that are not further evocated here and that are associated with the functional organization of the hypothalamus might constitute a fourth stage. For example, the morphological modifications induced by hormones, such as sexual steroids or leptin, are now well described during the perinatal period (Bouret et al., 2004; Simerly, 2005; Ciofi et al., 2007).

HYPOTHALAMIC TRACT TOPOGRAPHIC ORGANIZATION

The anatomical dispositions of all the major tracts crossing or bounding the hypothalamus of the adult animal are summarized in **Figure 4B** and supplementary information. From this, it appears that all of the major tracts that originate in the dorsal or ventral telencephalon or in the retina converge in the anterior hypothalamic region (alar hypothalamus). However, upon reaching the caudal hypothalamus, they all follow adjacent pathways. This topographical organization closely follows the initial scaffolding provided by the tpoc in the caudal hypothalamus, as well as that provided by the sot for descending tracts from the telencephalon. The more ventral of these tracts (fornix, stria terminalis, ventral lateral hypothalamic tract, neuroendocrine tracts) end in the neurohypophysis and caudal hypothalamus, while the others (mfb, cerebral peduncle) take divergent routes at the mesencephalic limit. The relative path of these tracts can be illustrated on a schematic sagittal view of the embryonic brain (**Figure 4C**). We therefore observed that the descending tracts from the telencephalon traveled along a transverse path related to the sot, but as they joined the optic tract at the level of the posterior hypothalamus, their course became longitudinal, coincident with that of the tpoc and optic tract. Only the stria medullaris escaped from this general scheme.

STRUCTURAL ORGANIZATION OF THE HYPOTHALAMUS AND THE PROSENCEPHALIC FUNCTIONAL PLAN

The development of the hypothalamus and the adjacent "prethalamus-ventral thalamus" involves several stages. The first stage includes the differentiation of the cell cord. The inverted Y-shaped arrangement is the first differentiated structure of the prosencephalon and guides the first pioneer tracts, including the tpoc and sot. Following the differentiation of the cell cord, neurogenesis becomes generalized in the prosencephalon, preceding the formation of all of the major fiber tracts that connect the telencephalon with the hypothalamus and mesencephalon. Therefore, as new neurons settle medially or dorsally to the cell cord, fiber tracts topographically organize dorsally or medially to the early mfb. The tpoc also guides the optic tract and the supraoptic commissures. Therefore, while the supraoptic arm of the initial inverted Y-shaped pattern appears to guide the olfactory projections in the hypothalamus, the postoptic guides tracts parallel to retinal projections (**Figure 5A**).

These first and second stages in the forebrain differentiation leave traces that are found in the adult anatomical organization of the hypothalamus. In the adult brain, neurons that were initially derived from the cell cord form a large part of the reticularly organized hypothalamus, including the LHA. This structure can be considered, at a functional level, a rostral extension of the primary medial mantle layer that originates in the hindbrain and from which serotonergic neurons are produced. The concept of a deep structure in the brain with a reticular like appearance that is involved in general arousal in all vertebrates and that forms a reticular core is quite ancient. For example, this reticular core was termed the isodentritic core by Ramon-Moliner and Nauta and was also compared to the deep ancient brain described by McLean (Ramón-Moliner and Nauta, 1966; Nieuwenhuys et al., 1998; Swanson, 2003). Pfaff recently argued that primitive mechanisms involving the reticular formation of all vertebrates are important for initiating the activation of behaviors (Pfaff et al., 2012). The hypothalamic cell cord along with a more caudal cell cord are reminiscent of such primitive structures. In the adult brain, structures along the cell cord serve synchronizing and patterning functions; MCH and the cognate hypocretin expressing neurons play roles in the sleep/wake cycle. MCH knockout mice have modified locomotor activities, and in humans, the absence of hypocretin in the dorsal hypothalamus is associated with narcolepsy (Peyron et al., 2000; Verret et al., 2003). This cell cord could also have important functions during all stages of brain development. Serotonergic neurons, which are among the very first generated cells in the hindbrain, act as pacemakers to synchronize the electrical activity of local motoneurons (Moruzzi et al., 2009). Later, the sot and tpoc are the precocious frames for the mfb. The early mfb contains dopamine and serotonin projections, and both neurotransmitters play key roles in the development of telencephalic structures. Dopamine modulates the cell cycle and proliferation in the ganglionic eminences and influences the maturation of the local circuitry (Diaz et al., 1997; Goffin et al., 2010). Serotonin has well recognized developmental effects. Alterations of early serotonergic or dopaminergic pathways lead to pathological conditions, such as autism or schizophrenia (Herlenius and Lagercrantz, 2001; Kinast et al., 2013). MCH is also suspected to have trophic actions (Cotta-Grand et al., 2009).

However, the second stage of forebrain development is more specifically associated with the differentiation of the hypothalamic medial regions and structures belonging to the

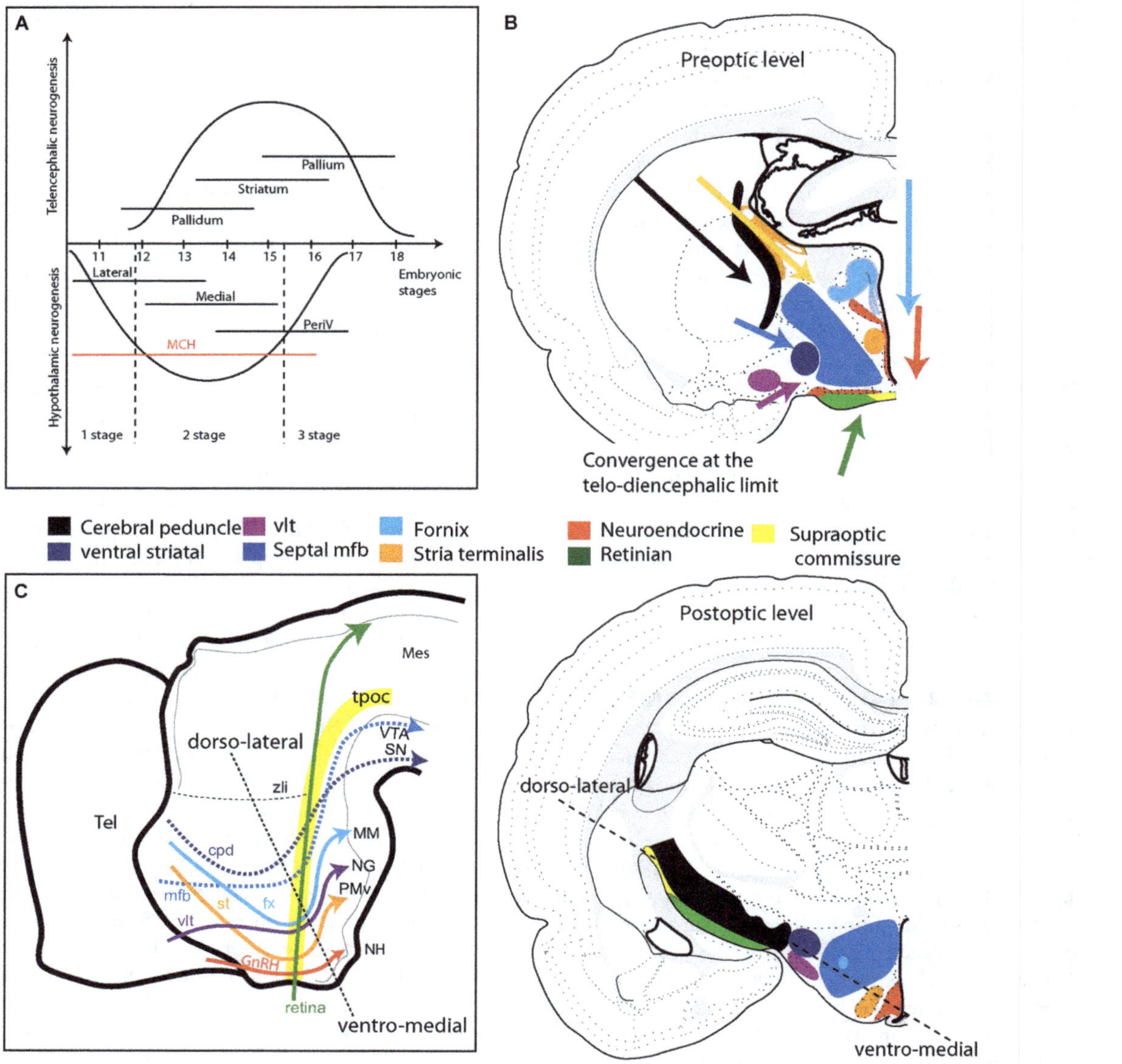

FIGURE 4 | (A) Schematic comparison of neurogenesis in the hypothalamus and telencephalon in the rat (see text for details). Neurogenesis in the hypothalamus is described as involving three stages: an early stage that produces only the lateral zone; a second that is concomitant to neurogenesis in the telencephalon and produces neurons in all hypothalamic longitudinal zones, but mostly the medial; a late third stage that concerns mainly periventricular zone neurons. Note that MCH neurons are produced during all three stages. **(B)** Illustration of the primary fiber tracts in the hypothalamus; these tracts originate in the telencephalon or retina and converge at the diencephalon-telencephalon limit at preoptic level (top drawing). In the postoptic hypothalamus (bottom drawing), these tracts are all aligned according to an axis determined by the dashed line. See text and supplementary information for details. **(C)** Schematic representation of the primary descending tracts in the ventral prosencephalon on a sagittal view of the embryonic brain. The tracts are topographically organized. Descending pathways from the telencephalon end in more posterior regions as they are distributed more dorsally in the hypothalamus. The dashed line recalls the ventro-medial/dorso-lateral axis, as in **(B)**. Abbreviations: cpd: cerebral peduncle; fx: fornix; GnRH: gonadotropin-releasing hormone; MCH: melano-concentrating hormone; mes: mesencephalon; mfb: medial forebrain bundle; MM: mammillary body; NG: nucleus Gemini; NH: neurohypophysis; periV: periventricular; PMv: ventral premmamillary nucleus; SN: substantia nigra; st: stria terminalis; tel: telencephalon; tpoc: tractus postopticus; vlt: ventrolateral hypothalamic tract; VTA: ventral tegmental area; zli: zona limitans intrathalamica.

classical striato-nigral pathways. These structures share genetic, topographic and chronotopic characteristics during development. This developmental stage coincides with the concept of a convergence in the anatomical organization of circuits involving these regions in the adult. It therefore becomes very attractive to describe the circuits connecting the pallium, striatum, pallidum and rostral brainstem as a series of parallel interacting loops (**Figures 5B,C**). Alexander described several putative circuits

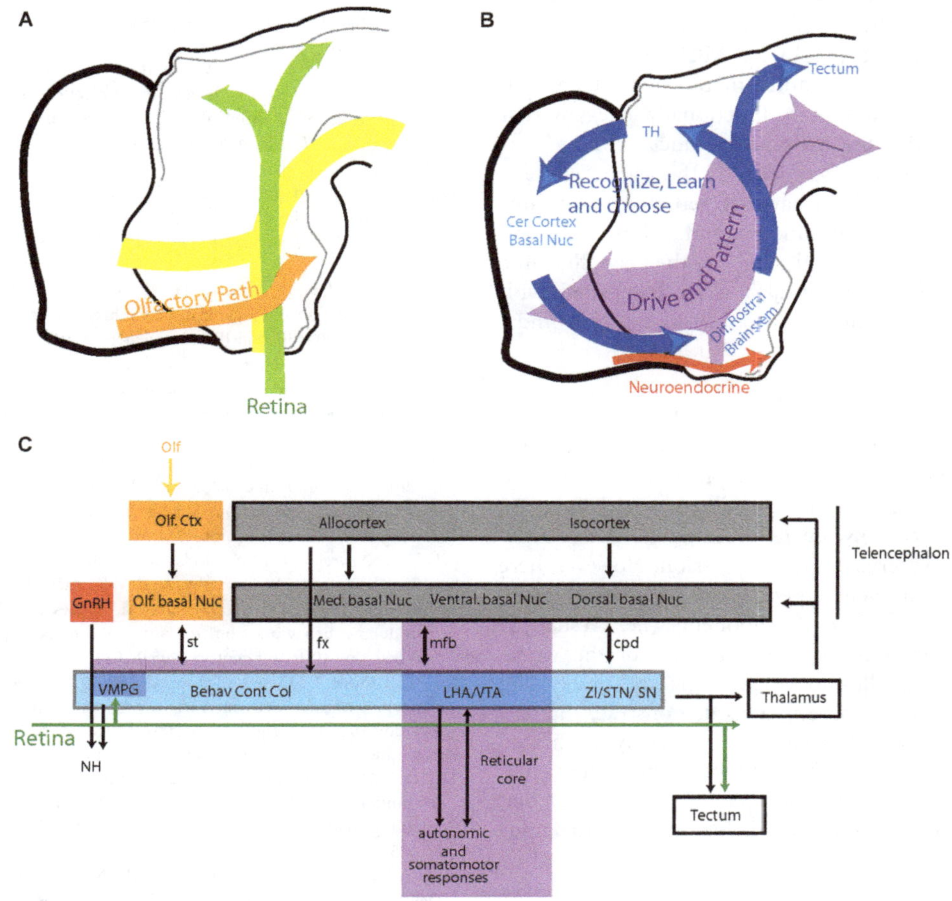

FIGURE 5 | (A) Schematic organization of olfactory and optic pathways in the hypothalamus compared to the cell cord. **(B,C)** Organization of the prosencephalic connectivity. The hypothalamus and ventral midbrain are engaged in circuit loops (blue in **B**) that involve topographically organized descending inputs from the telencephalon and topographically organized outputs to the thalamus and tectum. These circuits play roles in behavioral expressions, voluntary motor responses and learning/memory. They are superimposed on a reticular core (including the VMPG), which is rostrally contiguous to the reticular brainstem, recalling the scaffold of the original cell cord, and are mostly involved with driving and patterning brain activities. See text for details. Abbreviations: Behav Cont Col: behavioral control column (medial zone nuclei of the hypothalamus); cer: cerebral; cpd: cerebral peduncle; ctx: cortex; fx: fornix; GnRH: gonadotropin-releasing hormone; LHA: lateral hypothalamic area; med: medial; mfb: medial forebrain bundle; NH: neurohypophysis; nuc: nucleus; olf: olfactory; SN: substantia nigra; st: stria terminalis; STN: subthalamic nucleus; TH: thalamus; VMPG: visceromotor pattern generator; VTA: ventral tegmental area; ZI: zona incerta.

involving dorsal and ventral striatal components (Alexander et al., 1990). The Swanson group described several other circuits, involving medial and posterior striatal/pallidal structures and hypothalamic medial zone nuclei, suggesting the existence of a basic organizational plan (see Section Introduction; Swanson, 2003; Thompson and Swanson, 2010). We believe that we can now hypothesize that these sets of circuits are developmentally linked and can identify this as to be basic mammalian forebrain functional plan. Each of these circuits shows specific cytoarchitectonic characteristics and are either reticularly or nuclearly organized, likely under the control of the specific expression and localization of adherence molecules (CAM, cadherins) along the corresponding pathways (for example, for the nuclearly organized amygdala and medial hypothalamic nuclei connected through the stria terminalis). Some may even be characterized by the expression of specific transcription factors (again, as illustrated for the amygdala and hypothalamus, concerning reproductive and defensive pathways—Choi et al., 2005).

"Classic" authors have already suggested that well differentiated structures of highly organized brains must have emerged during evolution from primordial reticularly organized forms. Ramon-Moliner and Nauta used of the term "phylogenetic segregation" to characterize these evolutionary processes (Ramón-Moliner and Nauta, 1966). Pre- and postoptic hypothalamic structures have been observed in amphibians, as has a dopamine rich posterior tuberculum; however, laterally organized structures cannot be found in these species. Obviously, lateral and medial hypothalamic structures are phylogenetically recent but made of neurons that derivate from phylogenetically ancient populations (see in Croizier et al., 2013 for MCH and the dorsal hypothalamus), as are the substantia nigra/ventral tegmental area in the ventral midbrain. It is functionally relevant that these structures, including the mammillary nuclei (which contain head direction cells and are part of the Papez circuit), evolved in parallel. A larger behavioral repertory in mammals, especially related to reproductive and agonistic behaviors, is related to the differentiation of the hypothalamic medial and lateral zones, but is also likely associated with increased voluntary motor controls allowed by the extrapyramidal pathways.

To conclude, it has become obvious that the classical hypothalamus with its four regions does not constitute one single neurological entity, at least from the developmental point of view. The divergence in the origins of the collection of nuclei and areas that are usually gathered between its arbitrary borders can be traced to the earliest patterns of gene expression. However, here we contend that early neurogenesis gives rise to a first mantle layer, with longitudinal and transverse components (i.e., Y-shaped) that serves as a foundation for the formation of the whole forebrain connectivity, guiding most ascending and descending tracts appearing later. These observations demonstrate that the structures of the hypothalamic region are intimately implicated within complex networks along the extrapyramidal pathway and act together for the expression of behaviors. They also suggest that these circuits that involve the telencephalon and hypothalamus share a basic organizational plan.

ACKNOWLEDGMENTS

The authors are particularly grateful to Dr Gonzalo Alvarez-Bolado (Anatomisches Institut, Universität Heidelberg, Germany) and Philippe Ciofi (Institut Magendie, Bordeaux, France) for helpful discussions and careful reading of the manuscript.

REFERENCES

Aboitiz, F. (2011). Genetic and developmental homology in amniote brains. Toward conciliating radical views of brain evolution. *Brain Res. Bull.* 84, 125–136. doi: 10.1016/j.brainresbull.2010.12.003

Alexander, G. E., Crutcher, M. D., and Delong, M. R. (1990). Basal ganglia-thalamocortical circuits: parallel substrates for motor, oculomotor, "prefrontal" and "limbic" functions. *Prog. Brain Res.* 85, 119–146. doi: 10.1016/s0079-6123(08)62678-3

Altman, J., and Bayer, S. A. (1986). The development of the rat hypothalamus. *Adv. Anat. Embryol. Cell Biol.* 100, 1–178.

Alvarez-Bolado, G., Paul, F. A., and Blaess, S. (2012). Sonic hedgehog lineage in the mouse hypothalamus: from progenitor domains to hypothalamic regions. *Neural Dev.* 7:4. doi: 10.1186/1749-8104-7-4

Anderson, R. B., and Key, B. (1996). Expression of a novel N-CAM glycoform (NOC-1) on axon tracts in embryonic Xenopus brain. *Dev. Dyn.* 207, 263–269. doi: 10.1002/(sici)1097-0177(199611)207:3<263::aid-aja3>3.0.co;2-f

Bouret, S. G., Draper, S. J., and Simerly, R. B. (2004). Trophic action of leptin on hypothalamic neurons that regulate feeding. *Science* 304, 108–110. doi: 10.1126/science.1095004

Brischoux, F., Cvetkovic, V., Griffond, B., Fellmann, D., and Risold, P. Y. (2002). Time of genesis determines projection and neurokinin-3 expression patterns of diencephalic neurons containing melanin-concentrating hormone. *Eur. J. Neurosci.* 16, 1672–1680. doi: 10.1046/j.1460-9568.2002.02229.x

Brischoux, F., Fellmann, D., and Risold, P. Y. (2001). Ontogenetic development of the diencephalic MCH neurons: a hypothalamic 'MCH area' hypothesis. *Eur. J. Neurosci.* 13, 1733–1744. doi: 10.1046/j.0953-816x.2001.01552.x

Brown, K. N., Chen, S., Han, Z., Lu, C. H., Tan, X., Zhang, X. J., et al. (2011). Clonal production and organization of inhibitory interneurons in the neocortex. *Science* 334, 480–486. doi: 10.1126/science.1208884

Canteras, N. S., Simerly, R. B., and Swanson, L. W. (1994). Organization of projections from the ventromedial nucleus of the hypothalamus: a Phaseolus vulgaris-leucoagglutinin study in the rat. *J. Comp. Neurol.* 348, 41–79. doi: 10.1002/cne.903480103

Cheung, C. C., Kurrasch, D. M., Liang, J. K., and Ingraham, H. A. (2013). Genetic labeling of steroidogenic factor-1 (SF-1) neurons in mice reveals ventromedial nucleus of the hypothalamus (VMH) circuitry beginning at neurogenesis and development of a separate non-SF-1 neuronal cluster in the ventrolateral VMH. *J. Comp. Neurol.* 521, 1268–1288. doi: 10.1002/cne.23226

Choi, G. B., Dong, H. W., Murphy, A. J., Valenzuela, D. M., Yancopoulos, G. D., Swanson, L. W., et al. (2005). Lhx6 delineates a pathway mediating innate reproductive behaviors from the amygdala to the hypothalamus. *Neuron* 46, 647–660. doi: 10.1016/j.neuron.2005.04.011

Ciofi, P., Lapirot, O. C., and Tramu, G. (2007). An androgen-dependent sexual dimorphism visible at puberty in the rat hypothalamus. *Neuroscience* 146, 630–642. doi: 10.1016/j.neuroscience.2007.02.028

Cotta-Grand, N., Rovère, C., Guyon, A., Cervantes, A., Brau, F., and Nahon, J. L. (2009). Melanin-concentrating hormone induces neurite outgrowth in human neuroblastoma SH-SY5Y cells through p53 and MAPKinase signaling pathways. *Peptides* 30, 2014–2024. doi: 10.1016/j.peptides.2009.06.015

Croizier, S., Amiot, C., Chen, X., Presse, F., Nahon, J. L., Wu, J. Y., et al. (2011). Development of posterior hypothalamic neurons enlightens a switch in the prosencephalic basic plan. *PLoS One* 6:e28574. doi: 10.1371/journal.pone 00 28574

Croizier, S., Cardot, J., Brischoux, F., Fellmann, D., Griffond, B., and Risold, P. Y. (2013). The vertebrate diencephalic MCH system: a versatile neuronal population in an evolving brain. *Front. Neuroendocrinol.* 34, 65–87. doi: 10.1016/j.yfrne.2012.10.001

Croizier, S., Franchi-Bernard, G., Colard, C., Poncet, F., La Roche, A., and Risold, P. Y. (2010). A comparative analysis shows morphofunctional differences between the rat and mouse melanin-concentrating hormone systems. *PLoS One* 5:e15471. doi: 10.1371/journal.pone.0015471

Cvetkovic, V., Brischoux, F., Griffond, B., Bernard, G., Jacquemard, C., Fellmann, D., et al. (2003). Evidence of melanin-concentrating hormone-containing neurons supplying both cortical and neuroendocrine projections. *Neuroscience* 116, 31–35. doi: 10.1016/s0306-4522(02)00557-2

Diaz, J., Ridray, S., Mignon, V., Griffon, N., Schwartz, J. C., and Sokoloff, P. (1997). Selective expression of dopamine D3 receptor mRNA in proliferative zones during embryonic development of the rat brain. *J. Neurosci.* 17, 4282–4292.

Dominguez, L., Morona, R., González, A., and Moreno, N. (2013). Characterization of the hypothalamus of Xenopus laevis during development. I. The alar regions. *J. Comp. Neurol.* 521, 725–759. doi: 10.1002/cne.23222

Easter, S. S. Jr., Ross, L. S., and Frankfurter, A. (1993). Initial tract formation in the mouse brain. *J. Neurosci.* 13, 285–299.

Gelman, D., Griveau, A., Dehorter, N., Teissier, A., Varela, C., Pla, R., et al. (2011). A wide diversity of cortical GABAergic interneurons derives from the embryonic preoptic area. *J. Neurosci.* 31, 16570–16580. doi: 10.1523/jneurosci.4068-11.2011

Goffin, D., Ali, A. B., Rampersaud, N., Harkavyi, A., Fuchs, C., Whitton, P. S., et al. (2010). Dopamine-dependent tuning of striatal inhibitory synaptogenesis. *J. Neurosci.* 30, 2935–2950. doi: 10.1523/jneurosci.4411-09.2010

Herlenius, E., and Lagercrantz, H. (2001). Neurotransmitters and neuromodulators during early human development. *Early Hum. Dev.* 65, 21–37. doi: 10.1016/s0378-3782(01)00189-x

Herrick, C. J. (1910). The morphology of the forebrain in amphibian and reptilian. *J. Comp. Neurol.* 20, 413–547.

His, W. (1893). Vorschläge zur eintheilung des gehirns. *Arch. Anat. Entwickel* 3/4, 173–179.

Keyser, A. (1972). The development of the diencephalon of the Chinese hamster. An investigation of the validity of the criteria of subdivision of the brain. *Acta Anat. Suppl. (Basel)* 59, 1–178.

Kinast, K., Peeters, D., Kolk, S. M., Schubert, D., and Homberg, J. R. (2013). Genetic and pharmacological manipulations of the serotonergic system in early life: neurodevelopmental underpinnings of autism-related behavior. *Front. Cell. Neurosci.* 7:72. doi: 10.3389/fncel.2013.00072

Kuhlenbeck, H. (1929). Die grundbestandteile des enddhirns im lichte der bauplanlehre. *Anat. Anzig* 67, 1–51.

Marín, O., Baker, J., Puelles, L., and Rubenstein, J. L. (2002). Patterning of the basal telencephalon and hypothalamus is essential for guidance of cortical projections. *Development* 129, 761–773.

Mastick, G. S., and Easter, S. S., Jr. (1996). Initial organization of neurons and tracts in the embryonic mouse fore- and midbrain. *Dev. Biol.* 173, 79–94. doi: 10.1006/dbio.1996.0008

Mastick, G. S., Davis, N. M., Andrew, G. L., and Easter, S. S. Jr. (1997). Pax-6 functions in boundary formation and axon guidance in the embryonic mouse forebrain. *Development* 124, 1985–1997.

Moreno, N., and González, A. (2011). The non-evaginated secondary prosencephalon of vertebrates. *Front. Neuroanat.* 5:12. doi: 10.3389/fnana.2011.00012

Moruzzi, A. M., Abedini, N. C., Hansen, M. A., Olson, J. E., and Bosma, M. M. (2009). Differential expression of membrane conductances underlies spontaneous event initiation by rostral midline neurons in the embryonic mouse hindbrain. *J. Physiol.* 587, 5081–5093. doi: 10.1113/jphysiol.2009.180091

Nieuwenhuys, R., Geeraedts, L. M., and Veening, J. G. (1982). The medial forebrain bundle of the rat. I. General introduction. *J. Comp. Neurol.* 206, 49–81. doi: 10.1002/cne.902060106

Nieuwenhuys, R., Ten Donkelaar, H. J., and Nicholson, C. (1998). *The Central Nervous System of Vertebrates.* Berlin: Springer-Verlag.

Nural, H. F., and Mastick, G. S. (2004). Pax6 guides a relay of pioneer longitudinal axons in the embryonic mouse forebrain. *J. Comp. Neurol.* 479, 399–409. doi: 10.1002/cne.20317

Papez, J. W. (1995). A proposed mechanism of emotion. 1937. *J. Neuropsychiatry Clin. Neurosci.* 7, 103–112.

Perez-Balaguer, A., Puelles, E., Wurst, W., and Martinez, S. (2009). Shh dependent and independent maintenance of basal midbrain. *Mech. Dev.* 126, 301–313. doi: 10.1016/j.mod.2009.03.001

Peyron, C., Faraco, J., Rogers, W., Ripley, B., Overeem, S., Charnay, Y., et al. (2000). A mutation in a case of early onset narcolepsy and a generalized absence of hypocretin peptides in human narcoleptic brains. *Nat. Med.* 6, 991–997. doi: 10.1038/79690

Pfaff, D. W., Martin, E. M., and Faber, D. (2012). Origins of arousal: roles for medullary reticular neurons. *Trends Neurosci.* 35, 468–476. doi: 10.1016/j.tins.2012.04.008

Pottin, K., Hinaux, H., and Rétaux, S. (2011). Restoring eye size in Astyanax mexicanus blind cavefish embryos through modulation of the Shh and Fgf8 forebrain organising centres. *Development* 138, 2467–2476. doi: 10.1242/dev.054106

Puelles, L. (2001). Thoughts on the development, structure and evolution of the mammalian and avian telencephalic pallium. *Philos. Trans. R. Soc. Lond. B Biol. Sci.* 356, 1583–1598. doi: 10.1098/rstb.2001.0973

Puelles, L., Harrison, M., Paxinos, G., and Watson, C. (2013). A developmental ontology for the mammalian brain based on the prosomeric model. *Trends Neurosci.* 36, 570–578. doi: 10.1016/j.tins.2013.06.004

Puelles, L., Martinez-De-La-Torre, M., Bardet, S., and Rubenstein, J. L. R. (2012). "Hypothalamus," in *The Mouse Nervous System*, eds C. Watson, G. Paxinos and L. Puelles (London: Elsevier), 221–312.

Puelles, L., and Rubenstein, J. L. (2003). Forebrain gene expression domains and the evolving prosomeric model. *Trends Neurosci.* 26, 469–476. doi: 10.1016/s0166-2236(03)00234-0

Ramón-Moliner, E., and Nauta, W. J. (1966). The isodendritic core of the brain stem. *J. Comp. Neurol.* 126, 311–335. doi: 10.1002/cne.901260301

Rash, B. G., and Grove, E. A. (2011). Shh and Gli3 regulate formation of the telencephalic-diencephalic junction and suppress an isthmus-like signaling source in the forebrain. *Dev. Biol.* 359, 242–250. doi: 10.1016/j.ydbio.2011.08.026

Ricaño-Cornejo, I., Altick, A. L., García-Peña, C. M., Nural, H. F., Echevarría, D., Miquelajáuregui, A., et al. (2011). Slit-Robo signals regulate pioneer axon pathfinding of the tract of the postoptic commissure in the mammalian forebrain. *J. Neurosci. Res.* 89, 1531–1541. doi: 10.1002/jnr.22684

Riddle, R., and Pollock, J. D. (2003). Making connections: the development of mesencephalic dopaminergic neurons. *Brain Res. Dev. Brain Res.* 147, 3–21. doi: 10.1016/j.devbrainres.2003.09.010

Risold, P. Y. (2004). "The septal region," in *The Rat Nervous System*, ed G. Paxinos (Amsterdam: Elsevier), 605–632.

Risold, P. Y., and Swanson, L. W. (1996). Structural evidence for functional domains in the rat hippocampus. *Science* 272, 1484–1486. doi: 10.1126/science.272.5267.1484

Risold, P. Y., and Swanson, L. W. (1997). Connections of the rat lateral septal complex. *Brain Res. Brain Res. Rev.* 24, 115–195. doi: 10.1016/s0165-0173(97)00009-x

Risold, P. Y., Thompson, R. H., and Swanson, L. W. (1997). The structural organization of connections between hypothalamus and cerebral cortex. *Brain Res. Brain Res. Rev.* 24, 197–254. doi: 10.1016/s0165-0173(97)00007-6

Rubenstein, J. L., Shimamura, K., Martinez, S., and Puelles, L. (1998). Regionalization of the prosencephalic neural plate. *Annu. Rev. Neurosci.* 21, 445–477. doi: 10.1146/annurev.neuro.21.1.445

Shimamura, K., Hartigan, D. J., Martinez, S., Puelles, L., and Rubenstein, J. L. (1995). Longitudinal organization of the anterior neural plate and neural tube. *Development* 121, 3923–3933.

Shimogori, T., Lee, D. A., Miranda-Angulo, A., Yang, Y., Wang, H., Jiang, L., et al. (2010). A genomic atlas of mouse hypothalamic development. *Nat. Neurosci.* 13, 767–775. doi: 10.1038/nn.2545

Simerly, R. B. (2005). Wired on hormones: endocrine regulation of hypothalamic development. *Curr. Opin. Neurobiol.* 15, 81–85. doi: 10.1016/j.conb.2005.01.013

Stoykova, A., Fritsch, R., Walther, C., and Gruss, P. (1996). Forebrain patterning defects in Small eye mutant mice. *Development* 122, 3453–3465.

Suzuki, D. G., Murakami, Y., Escriva, H., and Wada, H. (2014). A comparative examination of neural circuit and brain patterning between the lamprey and amphioxus reveals the evolutionary origin of the vertebrate visual center. *J. Comp. Neurol.* 523, 251–261. doi: 10.1002/cne.23679

Swanson, L. W. (1987). "The hypothalamus," in *Handbook of Chemical Neuroanatomy, Integrated Systems of the CNS, Part I*, eds T. H. A. Björklund and L. W. Swanson (Amsterdam: Elsevier), 1–124.

Swanson, L. W. (2000). Cerebral hemisphere regulation of motivated behavior. *Brain Res.* 886, 113–164. doi: 10.1016/s0006-8993(00)02905-x

Swanson, L. W. (2003). *Brain Architecture, Understanding The Basic Plan.* New York: Oxford University Press.

Swanson, L. W. (2005). Anatomy of the soul as reflected in the cerebral hemispheres: neural circuits underlying voluntary control of basic motivated behaviors. *J. Comp. Neurol.* 493, 122–131. doi: 10.1002/cne.20733

Szabó, N. E., Zhao, T., Cankaya, M., Theil, T., Zhou, X., and Alvarez-Bolado, G. (2009). Role of neuroepithelial Sonic hedgehog in hypothalamic patterning. *J. Neurosci.* 29, 6989–7002. doi: 10.1523/jneurosci.1089-09.2009

Thompson, R. H., and Swanson, L. W. (2003). Structural characterization of a hypothalamic visceromotor pattern generator network. *Brain Res. Brain Res. Rev.* 41, 153–202. doi: 10.1016/s0165-0173(02)00232-1

Thompson, R. H., and Swanson, L. W. (2010). Hypothesis-driven structural connectivity analysis supports network over hierarchical model of brain architecture. *Proc. Natl. Acad. Sci. U S A* 107, 15235–15239. doi: 10.1073/pnas.1009112107

Verret, L., Goutagny, R., Fort, P., Cagnon, L., Salvert, D., Léger, L., et al. (2003). A role of melanin-concentrating hormone producing neurons in the central regulation of paradoxical sleep. *BMC Neurosci.* 4:19. doi: 10.1186/1471-2202-4-19

Vitalis, T., and Rossier, J. (2011). New insights into cortical interneurons development and classification: contribution of developmental studies. *Dev. Neurobiol.* 71, 34–44. doi: 10.1002/dneu.20810

Ye, W., Shimamura, K., Rubenstein, J. L., Hynes, M. A., and Rosenthal, A. (1998). FGF and Shh signals control dopaminergic and serotonergic cell fate in the anterior neural plate. *Cell* 93, 755–766. doi: 10.1016/s0092-8674(00)81437-3

4

Hypothalamic glucose sensing: making ends meet

Vanessa H. Routh[1]*, Lihong Hao[1,2], Ammy M. Santiago[1,2], Zhenyu Sheng[1] and Chunxue Zhou[1,2]

[1] Department of Pharmacology and Physiology, New Jersey Medical School, Rutgers University, Newark, NJ, USA

[2] Department of Pharmacology and Physiology and Graduate School of the Biomedical Sciences, New Jersey Medical School, Rutgers University, Newark, NJ, USA

***Correspondence:**
Vanessa H. Routh, Department of Pharmacology and Physiology, New Jersey Medical School, Rutgers University, Medical Science Building, 185 S. Orange Ave., Newark, NJ 07103, USA
e-mail: routhvh@njms.rutgers.edu

The neuroendocrine system governs essential survival and homeostatic functions. For example, growth is needed for development, thermoregulation maintains optimal core temperature in a changing environment, and reproduction ensures species survival. Stress and immune responses enable an organism to overcome external and internal threats while the circadian system regulates arousal and sleep such that vegetative and active functions do not overlap. All of these functions require a significant portion of the body's energy. As the integrator of the neuroendocrine system, the hypothalamus carefully assesses the energy status of the body in order to appropriately partition resources to provide for each system without compromising the others. While doing so the hypothalamus must ensure that adequate glucose levels are preserved for brain function since glucose is the primary fuel of the brain. To this end, the hypothalamus contains specialized glucose sensing neurons which are scattered throughout the nuclei controlling distinct neuroendocrine functions. We hypothesize that these neurons play a key role in enabling the hypothalamus to partition energy to meet these peripheral survival needs without endangering the brain's glucose supply. This review will first describe the varied mechanisms underlying glucose sensing in neurons within discrete hypothalamic nuclei. We will then evaluate the way in which peripheral energy status regulates glucose sensitivity. For example, during energy deficit such as fasting specific hypothalamic glucose sensing neurons become sensitized to decreased glucose. This increases the gain of the information relay when glucose availability is a greater concern for the brain. Finally, changes in glucose sensitivity under pathological conditions (e.g., recurrent insulin-hypoglycemia, diabetes) will be addressed. The overall goal of this review is to place glucose sensing neurons within the context of hypothalamic control of neuroendocrine function.

Keywords: glucose-excited neurons, glucose-inhibited neurons, hypoglycemia, starvation, glucose homeostasis, orexin, agouti-related peptide, nitric oxide

INTRODUCTION

Our neuroendocrine systems maintain homeostasis against changing internal and external stressors. In order to do this, it is necessary to carefully partition fuel to each system which requires energy without compromising a constant brain glucose supply. The primary responsibility for this fuel partitioning falls upon the hypothalamus. The hypothalamus integrates autonomic responses and endocrine function with behaviors, especially those concerned with the homeostatic requirements of everyday life. There are five basic physiological needs which are governed by the hypothalamus. These are the regulation of blood pressure and electrolyte composition, body temperature, energy metabolism, reproduction, and the emergency response to stress. In order to do this, the hypothalamus receives sensory information from the entire body. This input includes visceral sensory afferents as well as circulating hormones. The hypothalamus possesses internal sensory neurons which detect changes in local temperature, osmolality, electrolytes and nutrients such as glucose and free fatty acids. The hypothalamus then compares the information from this input with biological set points and adjusts an array of autonomic, endocrine and behavioral responses in order to maintain homeostasis (Oomura et al., 1969; Steffens et al., 1972, 1988; Sawchenko, 1998; Beverly et al., 2001; Lindberg et al., 2013; Valassi et al., 2014). This review will focus on the mechanisms underlying hypothalamic glucose sensing and the role of this system in glucose homeostasis.

Glucose is the primary fuel of the brain, thus it is essential to maintain adequate levels for brain function at all times. Hypothalamic glucose sensing neurons were discovered in the 1960s, and there is evidence that they play a role in maintaining cerebral glucose levels (Anand et al., 1964; Oomura et al., 1964; Levin et al., 2004; Fioramonti et al., 2010b). The hypothalamus also receives and integrates input from other central and peripheral glucose sensors (Routh et al., 2013). Interestingly, glucose sensing neurons make up subpopulations of hypothalamic nuclei involved in varied aspects of neuroendocrine function (Fioramonti et al., 2007; Gonzalez et al., 2008; Melnick et al., 2011; Roland and Moenter, 2011; Stanley et al., 2013). This suggests that glucose sensing neurons may contribute to the coordination of nutrient partitioning amongst neuroendocrine systems.

However, given the need of the brain for glucose, we hypothesize that the main function of hypothalamic glucose sensing neurons is to ensure that brain needs are prioritized above those of other neuroendocrine or bodily functions.

GLUCOSE ENTRY INTO THE BRAIN

When considering the physiological significance of brain glucose sensing, it is important to consider the regulation of glucose entry into the brain. The saturable glucose transporter isoform-1 is the primary glucose transporter at the blood brain barrier (Cardoso et al., 2010). However, the regulation of blood glucose entry is clearly more complicated than simple transport, and suggests the evidence of distinct diffusion barriers as will be discussed below (Mullier et al., 2009; Langlet et al., 2013). As a result, glucose concentrations in the brain are lower than that of the periphery. A landmark study by Silver and Erecinska in the 1990s showed that ventromedial hypothalamic (VMH) glucose levels in anesthetized rats were ~2.5 mM at baseline (~7.6 mM blood glucose due to the hyperglycemic effects of anesthesia) and 0.16 mM during hypoglycemia (~2.8 mM blood glucose). In this study, VMH glucose levels never exceeded 4.5 mM even when blood glucose was raised to 20 mM (Silver and Erecinska, 1994). Later microdialysis studies using the zero net flux technique in awake animals indicated that brain glucose levels at peripheral euglycemia (~5.5 mM) were ~1.5–2 mM, not only in the hypothalamus but the hippocampus and striatum as well (McNay and Gold, 1999; McNay et al., 2000, 2001; De Vries et al., 2003). Brain glucose varies with blood glucose, declining to ~0.7 mM after an overnight fast. During peripheral hypoglycemia, hypothalamic glucose fell to ~0.3 mM (Dunn-Meynell et al., 2009). These studies indicate that hypothalamic glucose levels range from ~0.2 to 4.5 mM as blood glucose levels vary from pathological hypoglycemia to hyperglycemia. Physiological hypothalamic glucose levels vary from ~0.7 to 2.5 mM between the fasted and fed state. This issue is important because although glucose concentration in the hypothalamus was first measured nearly 20 years ago, until fairly recently the majority of *in vitro* studies of glucose sensing neurons still used standard extracellular solutions containing 10–20 mM glucose. These glucose concentrations would even be considered analogous to diabetes when occurring in the blood. Thus, experimental conditions need to be considered when evaluating the relevance of the results obtained from studies of glucose sensing neurons.

There are several likely reasons for the resistance to studies of neurons *in vitro* using physiologically relevant glucose concentrations. One technical reason is that lower glucose concentrations were thought to be damaging to neurons *in vitro* or to cause neuronal silencing (Mobbs et al., 2001). This was reflected by the fact that until recently it was impossible to purchase stock neuronal culture media containing less than 20 mM glucose (media is now available without glucose to allow investigator control). However, for over 15 years our laboratory and others have routinely studied hypothalamic neurons in brain slices or after dissociation using ~2 mM glucose in the bathing medium with no evidence of neuronal damage or silencing (Levin et al., 1993; Routh et al., 1997; Song et al., 2001; Kang et al., 2004; Wang et al., 2004; Song and Routh, 2005, 2006; Burdakov et al., 2006; Canabal et al., 2007b; Fioramonti et al., 2007; Gonzalez et al., 2008; Cotero and Routh, 2009; Cotero et al., 2009; Murphy et al., 2009a,b; Melnick et al., 2011; Medeiros et al., 2012; Karnani et al., 2013; Vazirani et al., 2013). In fact, we find that glucose concentrations of 5 mM and higher obscure glucose sensing in some subtypes of glucose sensing neurons (Canabal et al., 2007a).

A more compelling argument for the use of higher glucose concentrations relates to brain regions near circumventricular organs. One important example is the arcuate nucleus (ARC) within the VMH which surrounds the median eminence. VMH glucose levels discussed above are often taken to reflect those within the larger ventromedial nucleus (VMN), which lies dorsal to the ARC. In contrast, since the median eminence possesses a fenestrated endothelium it was assumed that ARC glucose levels would be more similar to that of the blood than to the VMN. However, Dunn-Meynell et al., showed that ARC and VMN glucose levels do not differ (Dunn-Meynell et al., 2009). In this regard, the work of Vincent Prevot and colleagues also deserves careful consideration (Mullier et al., 2009). This group has convincingly demonstrated that differential organization and expression of the tight junction proteins within the ependymal cells which line the third ventricle and the median eminence leads to distinct patterns of diffusion from blood and cerebrospinal fluid. When blue Evans dye was injected into the blood, staining was restricted to the median eminence and did not diffuse into the ARC. In contrast, when the dye was injected into the third ventricle, staining was present in the ARC but not in the adjacent VMN. These data suggest that distinct diffusion barriers exist between the cerebrospinal fluid, circumventricular organs (e.g., median eminence) and the brain (even between adjacent brain regions). However, the physiological significance of diffusion from cerebrospinal fluid to the ARC is unclear given that the cerebrospinal fluid is thought predominantly to drain the brain. An even more intriguing observation from these investigators is that these barriers are not constant under all physiological conditions. For example, during fasting and glucoprivation the structural components of these hypothalamic diffusion barriers were altered such that ARC glucose levels significantly exceeded those in the VMN, although they did not reach blood levels. Furthermore, blood glucose levels appear to play a key role in driving these structural changes in the blood- and cerebrospinal fluid-brain barriers (Langlet et al., 2013). Together, these data indicate that while brain glucose levels are clearly lower than those of the blood, there exist privileged routes for glucose diffusion to distinct brain regions (e.g., from cerebrospinal fluid to ARC but not VMN) which are regulated by nutritional status. These observations also underscore the putative role of central glucose sensing in modulating glucose levels in order to meet the needs of the brain.

CELLULAR MECHANISMS OF GLUCOSE SENSING

The existence of glucose sensing neurons was suggested by 2 independent groups in 1964, one using cats and the other dogs (Anand et al., 1964; Oomura et al., 1964). In these studies, reciprocal changes in single unit activity were measured in the VMH and lateral hypothalamus (regions formerly called the "satiety" and "feeding" centers, respectively) during intravenous glucose or insulin injections. Glucose increased neuronal activity in the VMH while the converse occurred in the lateral hypothalamus. Later work from Oomura's laboratory demonstrated that hypothalamic neurons were directly regulated by glucose *in vitro*. This group coined the terms *glucose responsive* for neurons that increased their activity with increased glucose and *glucose sensitive* for those that decreased their activity as glucose increased (Oomura et al., 1964). Today, these subtypes of glucose sensing neurons are more commonly referred to respectively as *glucose-excited* (GE) or *glucose-inhibited* (GI) neurons based on their response to physiological changes in extracellular glucose (Song et al., 2001; Kang et al., 2004; Wang et al., 2004; Burdakov et al., 2005; Melnick et al., 2011). The following discussion of glucose sensing mechanism will focus primarily on studies using physiological glucose concentrations unless this information is not available. These data are summarized in **Table 1**. We are defining physiological glucose concentration as being below 5 mM in order to account for variability in blood or cerebrospinal fluid to brain glucose ratio under differing physiological conditions. Data from studies which used tissue or cellular preparations which do not discriminate between the ARC and VMN will be referred to as "VMH," whereas studies in which neuronal location was verified

Table 1 | Putative role of glucose-inhibited and glucose-excited neurons in substrate partitioning during energy deficit.

Nuclei/Peptide phenotype	Glucose Sensing phenotype	Mechanism of glucose sensing	Putative effect on brain fuel supply during energy deficit	Mechanism by which brain fuel may be altered	Representative references
ARC NPY	Inhibited	nNOS independent	Increase	Increase food intake Decrease energy expenditure Initiate ketogenesis	Murphy et al., 2009b; Joly-Amado et al., 2012; Leshan et al., 2012; Warne et al., 2013; Wang et al., 2014
ARC GHRH	Inhibited	Unknown	Increase	Caloric mobilization	Stanley et al., 2013
VMN nNOS	Inhibited	NO/AMPK/Cl^- channel	Increase	Glucagon, epinephrine secretion	Song et al., 2001; Song and Routh, 2006; Murphy et al., 2009a; Fioramonti et al., 2010a, 2013
LH orexin	Inhibited	Metabolism independent K^+ channel	Increase	Reward feeding Arousal	Antunes et al., 2001; Burdakov et al., 2005; Harris et al., 2005; Gonzalez et al., 2008; Williams et al., 2008; Sheng et al., 2014
LH NPY	Inhibited	K^+ channel	?		Marston et al., 2011
LH GABA	Inhibited	Metabolism independent Mixed ionic conductance	?	?	Karnani et al., 2013
PVN pre-autonomic	Inhibited	Unknown	?	?	Melnick et al., 2011
LH MCH	Excited	K^+ channel	Decrease	Anabolic (increase fat mass)*	Burdakov et al., 2005; Naufahu et al., 2013
PO/AHA GnRH	Excited	AMPK Non–selective cation channel	Decrease	Divert fuels to reproductive axis	Roland and Moenter, 2011; Beall et al., 2012
VMN unknown	Excited	KATP channel	?	?	Ashford et al., 1990a; Song et al., 2001
PVN pre-autonomic	Excited	KATP independent Non–selective cation channel	?	?	Melnick et al., 2011

The overall hypothesis presented here is that during energy deficit the glucose-sensing function of these neurons reinforces the mechanisms which provide brain-specific fuels while reducing the drive for other fuel consuming neuroendocrine systems. The predictions regarding the putative effect on brain fuel supply and underlying mechanisms are based on net positive input to downstream circuitry and would be reversed if their net effect was inhibitory.

**While MCH neurons increase food intake, they are associated with anabolic processes which could divert fuel away from the brain.*

visually or via microdissection as being from one region or the other will be referred to as such.

GLUCOSE-EXCITED (GE) NEURONS

GE neurons are found in many hypothalamic regions including the ARC, VMN, anterior hypothalamus, paraventricular nucleus, and the lateral hypothalamus (Oomura et al., 1964; Ashford et al., 1990a,b; Shian and Lin, 1991; Burdakov et al., 2005; Melnick et al., 2011; Roland and Moenter, 2011). The neurotransmitter phenotype of VMN GE neurons is largely unknown and there are conflicting reports regarding whether ARC POMC neurons are GE neurons (Wang et al., 2004; Claret et al., 2007; Fioramonti et al., 2007; Parton et al., 2007). In contrast, GE neurons have been found among the gonadotropin releasing hormone neurons (GnRH) of the anterior hypothalamus (Roland and Moenter, 2011; Beall et al., 2012), the preautonomic neurons in the paraventricular nucleus (Melnick et al., 2011), and the melanin concentrating hormone neurons of the lateral hypothalamus (Burdakov et al., 2005). The mechanism underlying glucose sensing by VMH GE neurons has been the most extensively characterized. Michael Ashford was the first to show that the majority of these GE neurons utilize a glucose sensing mechanism similar to that of the pancreatic β- cell (Ashford et al., 1990a). That is, like the β-cell, increased glucose metabolism raises the ATP/ADP ratio and closes the ATP sensitive potassium channel (KATP) leading to depolarization. Despite the fact that Ashford's original studies were performed using non-physiological glucose concentrations, his findings have stood the test of time (and glucose concentration) (Song et al., 2001). Barry Levin's laboratory demonstrated a second important similarity between many VMH GE neurons and the pancreatic β-cell: the initial phosphorylation of glucose to glucose-6-phosphate is catalyzed by the pancreatic form of hexokinase IV, glucokinase (Dunn-Meynell et al., 2002; Kang et al., 2006). In addition to a lower affinity for glucose than other hexokinases, glucokinase is not subject to end-product inhibition. This allows for activity at a rate proportional to glucose concentration (Magnuson, 1990). Thus, the presence of glucokinase is often used to predict glucose sensing in neuronal populations (Navarro et al., 1996; Yang et al., 1999; Lynch et al., 2000; Maekawa et al., 2000; Mobbs et al., 2001; Dunn-Meynell et al., 2002; Levin, 2002; Penicaud et al., 2002; Ramonet et al., 2004; Balfour et al., 2006; Kang et al., 2006; Zhou et al., 2010; Beall et al., 2012).

In addition to the ubiquitous glucose transporter 3 (GLUT3), subpopulations of VMH GE neurons also express GLUT2 and the insulin-sensitive GLUT4. Interestingly, a fairly large percentage of GE neurons express both GLUT4 and the insulin receptor (Kang et al., 2004). About 25% of VMH GE neurons possess the sodium glucose co-transporter (SGLT) which could couple glucose uptake with membrane depolarization (Kang et al., 2004). The cellular fuel sensor AMP activated protein kinase (AMPK) may mediate glucose sensing in some GE neurons. For example AMPK dependent glucose sensing has been reported for POMC neurons, as well as for the GnRH neurons in the anterior hypothalamus (Claret et al., 2007; Roland and Moenter, 2011; Beall et al., 2012). Finally, the KATP channel does not mediate glucose sensing in all GE neurons. GnRH neurons and PVN GE neurons use a non-selective cation channel, while the melanin-concentrating hormone neurons use an unidentified K channel (Burdakov et al., 2005; Melnick et al., 2011; Roland and Moenter, 2011). Thus, while many GE neurons could be considered the brain's "pancreatic β-cell," there is clearly a high degree of heterogeneity within this category of glucose sensing neurons.

GLUCOSE-INHIBITED (GI) NEURONS

GI neurons are also widely dispersed throughout the hypothalamus, including the VMN, ARC, paraventricular nucleus, dorsomedial nucleus, and the lateral hypothalamus (Song et al., 2001; Burdakov et al., 2005; Song and Routh, 2006; Fioramonti et al., 2007; Williams et al., 2008; Marston et al., 2011; Melnick et al., 2011). There are two broad categories of GI neurons, those whose activity is regulated by glucose metabolism (e.g., by changes in ATP) and those that respond to the glucose molecule itself. The *metabolism dependent* GI neurons most likely utilize GK since, like GE neurons, the majority of GI neurons express GK (Dunn-Meynell et al., 2002; Kang et al., 2006). Moreover, like GE neurons, subpopulations of metabolism dependent GI neurons also express GLUT2, GLUT4, SGLT2, and/or the insulin receptor (Kang et al., 2004). The most studied of the metabolism dependent GI neurons are located in the VMH. These GI neurons are activated in low glucose via an interaction between AMPK and the gaseous messenger nitric oxide (NO) which leads to chloride channel closure, membrane depolarization, and increased action potential frequency (Song et al., 2001; Song and Routh, 2005; Murphy et al., 2009a; Fioramonti et al., 2010a). VMH NO production by the neuronal NO synthase (nNOS) and NO signaling through its receptor, soluble guanylyl cyclase (sGC) are critical for both glucose sensing by GI neurons and the *in vivo* counterregulatory response (CRR) to hypoglycemia suggesting a role for these GI neurons in hypoglycemia detection (Murphy et al., 2009a; Fioramonti et al., 2010a, 2013). There is also a very significant overlap between VMH NO producing neurons and GI neurons (Canabal et al., 2007b). Thus, while the peptide neurotransmitter phenotype of these GI neurons remains unclear, it is reasonable to refer to them as nNOS-GI neurons based on their gaseous transmitter phenotype.

The above studies provided consistent results using either electrophysiological recordings of VMN GI neurons in brain slices or membrane potential dye imaging in freshly isolated VMH neurons. The electrophysiological experiments were performed on visually identified VMN neurons; whereas studies using isolated VMH neurons did not allow discrimination between VMN and ARC neurons. It is likely that mechanistic data concerning AMPK-NO signaling obtained from imaging isolated VMH neurons reflect VMN vs. ARC GI neurons for several reasons. Technically, VMN neurons vastly outnumber ARC neurons in this preparation and thus the significant majority of GI neurons analyzed would be VMN- vs. ARC-GI neurons. Moreover, the ARC neuropeptide Y (NPY)/agouti-related peptide (AgRP) co-expressing neurons, half of which are GI neurons, do not express nNOS nor do changes in intracellular AMPK appear to affect their activity (Sternson et al., 2005; Fioramonti et al., 2007; Leshan et al., 2012). Thus, together these data suggest distinct glucose sensing mechanisms for VMN nNOS-GI and ARC

NPY/AgRP-GI neurons. The exact cellular mechanism underlying glucose sensing in the ARC NPY/AgRP-GI neurons is not known. However, it could still be argued that regardless of what the mechanism is ultimately determined to be, the NPY/AgRP-GI neurons are metabolism-dependent since they are clearly regulated by changes in AMPK activity in presynaptic terminals synapsing onto NPY/AgRP neurons (Yang et al., 2011).

Denis Burdakov's laboratory has extensively characterized the *metabolism-independent,* orexin expressing GI neurons, which are only found in the lateral, perifornical and dorsomedial hypothalamus (Burdakov et al., 2005; Gonzalez et al., 2008; Williams et al., 2008). Orexin neurons are equally inhibited by glucose and by the non-metabolizable glucose analog, 2-deoxyglucose. Thus, they respond to the glucose molecule itself rather than downstream metabolites (Gonzalez et al., 2008; Sheng et al., 2014). Glucose clearly activates a leak tandem-pore potassium (K2P) channel in these neurons (Burdakov et al., 2006; González et al., 2009). Moreover, Twik-related acid-sensitive potassium-like (TASK) 1/3 channels, which belong to the K2P ion channel family, regulate high frequency firing in orexin neurons. However, TASK 1/3 channels do not appear to be critical for glucose sensing (González et al., 2009). Thus, at the present time the precise ion channel which mediates glucose inhibition in metabolism-independent GI neurons remains to be determined. Interestingly, there are two different glucose responses for metabolism-independent GI neurons. A non-adapting response is characterized by sustained glucose inhibition, while "adapting" GI neurons are transiently inhibited when glucose concentration rises but resume firing action potentials after several minutes in high glucose (Williams et al., 2008). The adaptive response appears to be due to a spontaneous decrease in inhibitory K^+ currents (Williams et al., 2008). In addition to the orexin neurons, GI neurons also exist within the NPY and gamma-aminobutyric acid (GABA) neurons of the lateral hypothalamus (Marston et al., 2011; Karnani et al., 2013). The GABA-GI neurons are also metabolism independent. However, they are distinct from the orexin-GI neurons in that the glucose sensitive conductance appears to be carried by a mixture of ion channels (Marston et al., 2011). It is not known whether the lateral hypothalamic NPY-GI neurons are metabolism dependent or independent (Karnani et al., 2013). The paraventricular nucleus GI neurons may also be metabolism independent because they do not appear to express GK (Stanley et al., 2013).

GLUCOSE SENSING GLIAL CELLS

Neurons are not the only glucose sensitive cells within the brain. An increasing body of knowledge suggests that glucose sensing by hypothalamic glial cells may play an important role in glucose and energy homeostasis. For example, the data discussed above indicates that the cells composing the blood brain barrier are responsive to changes in glucose (Langlet et al., 2013). Specialized ependymal cells known as tanycytes which line the third ventricle express GK, GLUT2 and KATP channels, suggesting that they are capable of sensing glucose (Garcia et al., 2003). In support of this, glucose increases intracellular calcium levels within cultured tanycytes (Orellana et al., 2012). Hypothalamic GK inhibition by alloxan *in vivo* reduces food intake, impairs the hyperglycemic response to a glucoprivic challenge and destroys tanycytes; all of which reverse 2 weeks after alloxan injection. These data suggest that hypothalamic tanycytes play a role in the physiological response to hypoglycemia (Sanders et al., 2004). Astrocytes also play a role in glucose sensing. Numerous studies suggest that the glucose transporter 2 (GLUT2) plays a role in hypothalamic glucose sensing (Garcia et al., 2003; Guillod-Maximin et al., 2004; Marty et al., 2005; Bady et al., 2006; Stolarczyk et al., 2010). Interestingly, hypothalamic GLUT2 is primarily expressed in astrocytes (Guillod-Maximin et al., 2004). Thus, it is clear that hypothalamic glucose sensing is a complex system involving coordination between a wide variety of neuronal and glial populations.

REGULATION OF GLUCOSE SENSING BY SIGNALS OF PERIPHERAL ENERGY HOMEOSTASIS

HORMONAL SIGNALS OF ENERGY HOMEOSTASIS

Hypothalamic glucose sensing is modulated by the hormonal milieu which reflects peripheral energy homeostasis. Insulin and the adipose derived hormone leptin, both of which are considered "satiety" hormones, inhibit VMH GE neurons in the presence of high extracellular glucose by opening the KATP channel (Spanswick et al., 1997, 2000). The effect of insulin persisted in physiological glucose concentrations (Cotero and Routh, 2009); however leptin had no effect on VMH GE neurons in 2.5 mM glucose (Wang et al., 2004). Insulin also prevents inhibition of VMH GE neurons when glucose is lowered (Cotero and Routh, 2009; Cotero et al., 2009). Interestingly, hypothalamic insulin infusion suppresses hepatic glucose production *in vivo* (Rojas and Schwartz, 2014). A role for VMH GE neurons in altered glucose homeostasis is also suggested by the observation that VMH GE neurons from *db/db* mice and *fa/fa* Zucker rats with peripheral insulin resistance are also insulin resistant (Spanswick et al., 2000; Cotero et al., 2009). Interestingly, ghrelin, which is released from the stomach during hunger, indirectly inhibits ARC POMC (GE?) neurons (Cowley et al., 2003; Ibrahim et al., 2003). Similar effects of ghrelin and leptin on GE neurons is counterintuitive. However, it is well established that leptin activates POMC neurons (Cowley et al., 2001). Moreover, the effect of ghrelin on glucose sensitivity of POMC neurons has not yet been evaluated nor is there agreement as to whether POMC neurons are truly GE neurons (Wang et al., 2004; Fioramonti et al., 2007).

Metabolically relevant hormones also regulate both the activity and the glucose sensitivity of GI neurons. Leptin inhibits ARC NPY/AgRP neurons (50% of which are GI neurons) as well as lateral hypothalamic orexin-GI neurons (Shiraishi et al., 2000; Yamanaka et al., 2003; Kohno et al., 2007; Louis et al., 2010; Baver et al., 2014). Leptin also blunts the activation of both VMH- and lateral hypothalamic orexin-GI neurons by decreased glucose (Murphy et al., 2009b; Sheng et al., 2014). In contrast, activation of VMN GI neurons by decreased glucose is blunted in the neuronal insulin-receptor knockout (NIRKO) mouse (Diggs-Andrews et al., 2010) and insulin stimulates NO production by VMH GI neurons in decreased glucose (Canabal et al., 2007b). These observations are consistent with insulin-induced potentiation of the response to low glucose in these neurons. The effect of insulin on lateral hypothalamus orexin-GI neurons is not clear. These neurons are clearly activated by insulin-induced hypoglycemia; however whether this is simply because they are GI neurons or whether insulin is having an independent effect is not known (Griffond et al., 1999; Moriguchi et al., 1999; Cai et al., 2001; Zhao et al., 2005). As predicted given the inhibitory effect of leptin, ghrelin activates both NPY-GI and orexin-GI neurons (Kohno et al., 2003; Yamanaka et al., 2003). Ghrelin also increases the activation of orexin-GI neurons in low glucose (Sheng et al., 2014).

NUTRIENTS OTHER THAN GLUCOSE

Hypothalamic glucose sensing neurons also respond to other nutrient-related signals in addition to glucose. Within the VMH, there is overlap between GE and GI neurons and neurons whose activity is altered by free fatty acids and ketones (Wang et al., 2005; Le Foll et al., 2013, 2014). Neuronal fatty acid sensing is consistent with data showing that central fatty acid infusion modulates glucose-induced insulin secretion and peripheral insulin sensitivity (Cruciani-Guglielmacci et al., 2004; Migrenne et al., 2006; Marsollier et al., 2009; Le Foll et al., 2013). In contrast to glucose and fatty acids, direct evidence of amino acid sensing neurons has been elusive. Administration of the branched chain amino acid L-leucine, but not valine, into the third ventricle decreases food intake; an effect which appears to be mediated by the hypothalamic mammalian target of rapamycin (mTOR) (Cota et al., 2006). The mTOR inhibitor rapamycin restores NO production by VMH GI neurons during hyperglycemia suggesting potential overlap in glucose and amino acid sensing pathways in these neurons (Canabal et al., 2007a). Moreover, Blouet et al. demonstrated that direct application of leucine increased the action potential frequency of POMC neurons (Blouet et al., 2009). Taken together these data support the hypothesis that hypothalamic glucose sensing neurons integrate multiple nutrient signals; however this has yet to be definitely shown for amino acids.

PHYSIOLOGICAL ROLE OF GLUCOSE SENSING NEURONS

While the existence of glucose sensing neurons has been known for half a century (Anand et al., 1964; Oomura et al., 1964), their exact physiological functions remain elusive. In the following discussion, we have attempted to relate what is known about the different subpopulations of glucose sensing neurons with the function of the region or peptide phenotype in which they are found. **Table 1** summarizes these data. Our overall hypothesis is that glucose sensitivity within multiple populations of neurons involved in metabolic control enables the brain to broadly reinforce the neurocircuitry which compensates for energy deficit when glucose levels fall. This would be beneficial in order to ensure an adequate neuronal fuel supply (glucose, ketones) at all times.

HYPOGLYCEMIA DETECTION

When considering a physiological role for glucose sensing neurons, hypoglycemia detection seems an obvious choice, especially since the majority of glucose sensing neurons are most sensitive to a decline in extracellular glucose levels below that which would be seen during normal fed conditions (Song et al., 2001; Wang et al., 2004; Song and Routh, 2005; Murphy et al., 2009b). This hypothesis is also attractive when considering that glucose is the primary fuel of the brain and that hypoglycemia clearly has deleterious central effects (Languren et al., 2013). Insulin-induced hypoglycemia increases *cfos* activation in a number of hypothalamic nuclei, including the ARC, the paraventricular and dorsomedial nuclei and the lateral hypothalamus (Niimi et al., 1995; Diggs-Andrews et al., 2010; Fergani et al., 2014). Moreover, hypoglycemia or central glucoprivation induces *cfos* expression in several known hypothalamic glucose sensing populations including the lateral hypothalamic orexin neurons as well as NPY neurons in the ARC, dorsomedial nucleus and lateral hypothalamus (Cai et al., 2001; Ferenczi et al., 2010; Marston et al., 2011). Interestingly, although the VMN contains GI neurons and plays a role in hypoglycemia detection, *cfos* activation was not detected in this brain region following insulin-induced hypoglycemia or glucoprivation (Niimi et al., 1995; Borg et al., 1997; Diggs-Andrews et al., 2010; Zhu et al., 2010; Szepietowska et al., 2011; Stanley et al., 2013). One reason for this apparent discrepancy may be because activation of VMN nNOS-GI neurons by decreased glucose requires the NO-sGC pathway, which may not be represented by *cfos* activation.

Although VMN *cfos* does not increase after hypoglycemia, functional studies support a key role for VMN GI neurons in the CRR. For example, repetitive hypoglycemic episodes shift the glycemic threshold for initiation of the CRR to lower glucose levels (Dagogo-Jack et al., 1993; Cryer, 2013; Moheet et al., 2014). Similarly, after recurrent hypoglycemia VMN GE and GI neurons show blunted inhibition or activation, respectively, as glucose levels decline (Song and Routh, 2006; Kang et al., 2008; Fioramonti et al., 2010b). Moreover, VMH lactate infusion *in vivo* blunts the CRR while lactate perfusion *in vitro* blunts activation of VMN GI neurons by decreased glucose (Song and Routh, 2005). VMH NO signaling is critical for glucose sensing by VMN nNOS-GI neurons as well as for the full CRR. That is, nNOS inhibition prevents activation of VMN nNOS-GI neurons by decreased glucose and neurons which are activated by decreased glucose are not detectable in brain sections from nNOS knockout mice (Fioramonti et al., 2010a). Similarly, the CRR is significantly impaired in nNOS knockout mice, after VMH NOS or sGC inhibition, or when NO-sGC signaling is disrupted by a post-translational modification of sGC known as S-nitrosation which renders it NO resistant (Fioramonti et al., 2010a, 2013). Interestingly, when S-nitrosation during recurrent hypoglycemia is prevented both glucose sensing by VMH GI neurons as well as the CRR are preserved. Taken together, these data suggest a clear role for GI, and in particular VMN nNOS-GI, neurons in detecting hypoglycemia and initiating the CRR.

FASTING AND STARVATION

In addition to hypoglycemia detection, another potential role for glucose sensing neurons is to maintain the brain's energy supply during starvation. In fact, since insulin-induced hypoglycemia is an iatrogenic consequence of treating Type 1 and advanced Type 2 Diabetes Mellitus in the modern world, glucose sensing neurons probably evolved as a defense against starvation. During starvation, the hypothalamic-pituitary-adrenal axis and the sympathetic nervous system play a key role in energy mobilization (Straub et al., 2010). The energetic needs of the body and the brain are first supplied by mobilization of liver glycogen stores for gluconeogenesis. After several hours adipocyte lipolysis provides fatty acids, which then fuel most organ systems. However, the brain cannot utilize fatty acids as fuel. Thus, preserving adequate blood glucose for the brain during starvation is one of the most important actions of the neuroendocrine system. When liver glycogen is depleted, muscle catabolism is initially necessary to provide amino acids as substrates for gluconeogenesis. Muscle catabolism is clearly detrimental in the long term and after several days of starvation, increased conversion of fatty acids to ketones in the liver provides fuel to the brain and spares lean body mass (Straub et al., 2010). It seems likely that glucose sensing neurons, particularly GI neurons, are important for informing the brain of the potential magnitude of a threat to the brain energy supply during starvation and aiding in energy mobilization.

In support of this, in general the hormonal changes which occur during fasting (e.g., reduced leptin and increased ghrelin) activate GI neurons and/or enhance their activation by decreased glucose (Cai et al., 1999; López et al., 2000; Diano et al., 2003; Kohno et al., 2003, 2008; Yamanaka et al., 2003; Murphy et al., 2009b; Sheng et al., 2014). A role for ARC NPY/AgRP-GI neurons in defending the brains energy supply during starvation stands out in particular. Fasting increases NPY gene expression as well as *cfos* expression and action potential frequency in ARC NPY/AgRP-GI neurons (Mizuno et al., 1999; Takahashi and Cone, 2005; Becskei et al., 2009; Murphy et al., 2009b). Fasting also increases hypothalamic NPY release and the activation of NPY/AgRP-GI neurons in response to decreased glucose (Murphy et al., 2009b). These data are consistent with the overall role of hypothalamic NPY/AgRP neurons to stimulate food intake (Billington and Levine, 1992; White, 1993). NPY expressing neurons are found in several brain regions which regulate energy homeostasis including the ARC and brainstem. However, AgRP expression is restricted to the ARC where it is found in 95% of the NPY neurons (Broberger et al., 1998). AgRP is an endogenous inhibitor of the melanocortin receptor. Thus, NPY/AgRP neurons oppose the effects of the anorexigenic POMC neurons at their targets. These targets include the hypothalamic paraventricular nucleus; a key site for regulating metabolism and food intake. The corticotrophin releasing hormone neurons which drive the hypothalamic-pituitary-adrenal axis as well as pre-autonomic neurons which activate the sympathetic nervous system reside in the paraventricular nucleus (Steffens et al., 1972, 1988; van Dijk et al., 1994; Ahima et al., 2000; Elmquist, 2001; Watts and Sanchez-Watts, 2002). In addition to opposing POMC neurons, NPY/AgRP neurons regulate energy partitioning and substrate utilization in a melanocortin-independent fashion (Joly-Amado et al., 2012). Importantly, AgRP deficiency impairs ketone body release from the liver during starvation (Warne et al., 2013). AgRP also mediates the gluconeogenic effects of ghrelin (Wang et al., 2014). Thus, increased AgRP release, especially in response to low glucose during starvation, may play a role in enhancing gluconeogenesis as well as triggering increased ketone production to fuel the brain. Similarly, increased activation of VMN nNOS-GI neurons during low glucose is consistent with enhanced gluconeogenesis (Fioramonti et al., 2010a). Orexin is associated with enhanced reward-based feeding behavior as well as increased sympathetic activity. Increased activity in low glucose, especially during fasting, is consistent with this line of reasoning (Antunes et al., 2001; Harris et al., 2005; Kelley et al., 2005; Zheng et al., 2007; Choi et al., 2010; Perello et al., 2010; Sheng et al., 2014). Moreover, we have recently shown that low glucose enhances excitatory glutamate neurotransmission onto ventral tegmental area dopamine neurons in an orexin dependent manner (Sheng et al., 2014). This observation strongly supports a role for orexin-GI neurons in reinforcing feeding behavior when glucose levels decline. Finally, since growth hormone is also released during hypoglycemia, it makes sense that growth hormone releasing hormone neurons are also GI neurons (Stanley et al., 2013). Together these data are consistent with an overall role for hypothalamic GI neurons in providing the brain with fuel during energy deficit. An important caveat to the above discussion is that the neurocircuitry which controls autonomic and neuroendocrine systems is extremely complex and its activation should never be considered in "all or none" terms. Rather, the above is a generalization in order to propose a physiological role for glucose sensing neurons and form a framework for designing experiments which test these hypotheses.

LINK NEUROENDOCRINE SYSTEMS WITH GLUCOSE STATUS

Another putative function for hypothalamic glucose sensing neurons is to prevent activation of neuroendocrine systems which use rather than provide fuel during energy deficit or conversely to allow energy to be diverted to these systems when it will not threaten the brain. For example, this may explain why subpopulations GnRH neurons are glucose sensing (Roland and Moenter, 2011). In contrast to the GI neurons described above, GnRH neurons are excited by glucose. Thus, when glucose levels are sufficient reproductive function is supported. Conversely, during times when food is scarce and glucose levels are low, the glucose sensing function of these neurons would contribute to inhibition of the reproductive axis. Moreover, while melanocortin concentrating hormone neurons stimulate food intake, they are also associated with anabolic processes (increased fat mass, reproduction) which could divert fuel away from the brain (Naufahu et al., 2013). Thus, reduced activity of melanocortin concentration hormone-GE neurons in low glucose is consistent with our overall hypothesis. However, one must use caution when trying to apply this reasoning to all GE or GI neurons because the relationship between the direction of glucose sensing (i.e., excited or inhibited by glucose) will depend on whether that particular glucose sensing neuron is inhibitory or stimulatory to the system in question. This is further evidenced by the observation that both GE and GI neurons are often found in the same hypothalamic nuclei. As mentioned above, the homeostatic mechanisms regulated by the hypothalamus are diverse and extremely complex. Thus, extreme caution is warranted when attempting to generalize the function of hypothalamic GE and GI neurons. Moreover, it is important to realize that there will be numerous exceptions to any rule for these systems.

WHAT ABOUT ENERGY SURPLUS?

The preceding discussion of hypothalamic glucose sensing neurons has focused on their role in sensing energy deficit. The main reasons for this bias are as follows. Although glucose concentration-response curves have only been published for VMH GE and GI neurons, these data suggest that glucose sensing neurons are primarily responsive to decreases in glucose below brain glucose concentrations associated with peripheral euglycemia (Wang et al., 2004; Song and Routh, 2005; Kang et al., 2006; Murphy et al., 2009b). In addition, their glucose sensitivity is altered under conditions associated with a need to sense energy deficit. That is, fasting reduces the inhibitory effect of glucose on VMH GI neurons leading to increased activation in response to smaller declines in glucose (Murphy et al., 2009b). Moreover, the glucose sensitivity of both VMH GE and GI neurons shifts in parallel with the ability of the brain to sense and respond to insulin-induced hypoglycemia (Song and Routh, 2005, 2006; Kang et al., 2008; Diggs-Andrews et al., 2010; Fioramonti et al., 2010a,b, 2013). In contrast, there is less known about glucose sensing neurons during hyperglycemia. We found that acute hyperglycemia prevents VMH GI neurons from producing NO and depolarizing in response to decreased glucose as a result of mTOR inhibition of AMPK (Canabal et al., 2007a). Conversely, while inhibition of VMH GE neurons from diabetic *db/db* mice to a maximal glucose decrease to 0.1 mM was identical to that of non-diabetic controls, the inhibition in response to a mid-range decrease (0.5 mM) was significantly enhanced in the diabetic mice (Cotero et al., 2009). Spanswick and colleagues found no difference in glucose sensitivity of VMH GE neurons in Zucker obese *fa/fa* rats compared to lean *Fa/Fa* rats; however they only evaluated the response of these neurons to a glucose decrease from 10 to 0 mM (Spanswick et al., 2000). Finally, 2 additional subtypes of ARC glucose sensing neurons have been identified which respond to changes in extracellular glucose above 5 mM: the high-GE (HGE) and high-GI (HGI) neurons (Fioramonti et al., 2004). As mentioned above, brain glucose concentrations above 5 mM have never been observed. However, since the permeability of the blood brain barrier changes with nutrient status it is possible that these glucose sensing neurons may play a role in glucose detection under some situations (Langlet et al., 2013). Such a role is consistent with data from Luc Penicaud's group showing that centrally restricted glucose infusion via the carotid artery increased *cfos* expression in ARC and paraventricular nucleus neurons and astrocytes which was associated with transient peripheral insulin secretion (Guillod-Maximin et al., 2004). Based on the above findings, it is tempting to speculate that the brain has a mechanism for sensing hyperglycemia and modulating peripheral metabolism in response. Furthermore, disrupted glucose sensing in diabetes suggests that glucose sensing neurons may play a role in the pathology of metabolic syndrome. In fact, an enhanced response to glucose deficit during conditions of energy sufficiency or even surplus (e.g., obesity/diabetes) could potentially lead to similar compensatory mechanisms as in response to fasting or starvation. Such changes could further enhance the obese state. However, due to a lack of data such comments are purely speculative at this time.

INTERACTION WITH NON-HYPOTHALAMIC GLUCOSE SENSORS

While the focus of this review is on hypothalamic glucose sensing neurons, glucose sensing neurons are also found in many other brain regions including the amygdala (Nakano and Oomura, 1986; Zhou et al., 2010), nucleus solitarius (Adachi et al., 1984) and midbrain (Levin, 2000). Moreover, although glucose sensing neurons *per se* have not been identified in the hindbrain, neurons within this region clearly respond to glucoprivation (Ritter et al., 1998, 2011; Routh et al., 2013). There are also glucose sensors located in numerous peripheral sites including the carotid bodies (Alvarez-Buylla and de Alvarez-Buylla, 1998; Pardal and Lopez-Barneo, 2002; Lopez-Barneo, 2003), portal-mesenteric vein (Donovan et al., 1994; Hevener et al., 1997; Matveyenko and Donovan, 2006) and intestine (Sayegh et al., 2004; Raybould, 2007; Ackroff et al., 2010). The regulation of glucose homeostasis clearly involves integration of information from multiple glucose sensing regions. For example, the hypothalamus, hindbrain and portal-mesenteric vein glucose sensors are all critical for hypoglycemia detection and full initiation of the CRR (Routh et al., 2013). Unraveling the physiological function of the many glucose sensing brain regions and how they work together is an evolving field which requires a great deal more work in order to understand.

CONCLUSION: THE SELFISH BRAIN

In conclusion, the hypothalamus is the primary site of integration for the neuroendocrine and autonomic responses which maintain energy and glucose homeostasis. Within the hypothalamus sensory neurons respond to circulating nutrients and hormones in order to inform the brain regarding peripheral metabolic homeostasis. The presence of glucose sensing neurons within the hypothalamus suggests a sensitive mechanism for maintaining a constant glucose supply to the brain. There is evidence for a role of glucose sensing neurons in hypoglycemia detection and initiation of the CRR during modern iatrogenic hypoglycemia (Song and Routh, 2006; Fioramonti et al., 2010a,b, 2013; Routh et al., 2013). However, it is likely that glucose sensing neurons actually evolved to protect the brain during intermittent starvation. For example, fasting increases the activation of NPY/AgRP-GI and orexin-GI neurons by decreased glucose (Murphy et al., 2009b). This could provide glucose for the brain in several ways; including increased food intake, initiating gluconeogenesis and mediating the shift to ketogenesis should the threat be sufficient (Beck, 2000; Joly-Amado et al., 2012; Warne et al., 2013; Sheng et al., 2014; Wang et al., 2014). Should similar fasting-induced changes in the glucose sensitivity of VMN nNOS- and growth hormone releasing hormone-GI neurons occur, this could also contribute to ensuring adequate fuel to the brain (Cai et al., 1999; Fioramonti et al., 2010a; Stanley et al., 2013). In contrast, other subtypes of glucose sensing neurons may divert energy away from competing systems (e.g., reproductive axis Roland and Moenter, 2011) when glucose levels are low. On the other hand, when the energy needs of the brain are met, the response of glucose sensing neurons to low glucose may be "deactivated" as seen for the effect of leptin and insulin on VMH GI and GE neurons, respectively (Cotero and Routh, 2009; Murphy et al., 2009b). Thus, we hypothesize that during energy deficit glucose sensing neurons are enlisted in order to enable the brain to prioritize its own energy needs at the expense of other energy requiring systems. However, clearly much work remains to determine the viability of our hypothesis.

AUTHOR CONTRIBUTIONS

VHR provided the original intellectual conception for the work and drafted and revised the manuscript. Lihong Hao, Ammy M. Santiago, Zhenyu Sheng and Chunxue Zhou provided intellectual discussion during conception and provided critical revision of the draft. All authors provide final approval and agree to be accountable for all aspects of the work in ensuring that questions related to the accuracy or integrity of any part of the work are appropriately investigated and resolved.

ACKNOWLEDGMENTS

Supported in part by NIDDK RO1 DK81538, the American Heart Association Grant in Aid 14GRNT20380639, and the NJ Health Foundation.

REFERENCES

Ackroff, K., Yiin, Y.-M., and Sclafani, A. (2010). Post-oral infusion sites that support glucose-conditioned flavor preferences in rats. *Physiol. Behav.* 99, 402–411. doi: 10.1016/j.physbeh.2009.12.012

Adachi, A., Shimizu, N., Oomura, Y., and Kobashi, M. (1984).Convergence of hepatoportal glucose-sensitive afferent signals to glucose-sensitive units within the nucleus of the solitary tract. *Neurosci. Lett.* 46, 215–218. doi: 10.1016/0304-3940(84)90444-0

Ahima, R. S., Saper, C. B., Flier, J. S., and Elmquist, J. K. (2000). Leptin regulation of neuroendocrine systems. *Front. Neuroendocrinol.* 21:197. doi: 10.1006/frne.2000.0197

Alvarez-Buylla, R., and de Alvarez-Buylla, E. R. (1998). Carotid sinus receptors participate in glucose homeostasis. *Respir. Physiol.* 72, 347–360. doi: 10.1016/0034-5687(88)90093-X

Anand, B. K., China, G. S., Sharma, K. N., Dua, S., and Singh, B. (1964). Activity of single neurons in the hypothalamus feeding centers: effect of glucose. *Am. J. Physiol.* 2207, 1146–1154.

Antunes, V. R., Brailoiu, G. C., Kwok, E. H., Scruggs, P., and Dun, N. J. (2001). Orexins/hypocretins excite rat sympathetic preganglionic neurons *in vivo* and *in vitro*. *Am. J. Physiol. Regul. Integr. Comp. Physiol.* 281, R1801–R1807.

Ashford, M. L. J., Boden, P. R., and Treherne, J. M. (1990a). Glucose-induced excitation of hypothalamic neurones is mediated by ATP-sensitive K^+ channels. *Pfugers Arch.* 415, 479–483.

Ashford, M. L. J., Boden, P. R., and Treherne, J. M. (1990b). Tolbutamide excites rat glucoreceptive ventromedial hypothalamic neurones by indirect inhibition of ATP-sensitive K^+ channels. *Br. J. Pharmacol.* 101, 531–540. doi: 10.1111/j.1476-5381.1990.tb14116.x

Bady, I., Marty, N., Dallaporta, M., Emery, M., Gyger, J., Tarussio, D., et al. (2006). Evidence from Glut2-Null mice that glucose is a critical physiological regulator of feeding. *Diabetes* 55, 988–995. doi: 10.2337/diabetes.55.04.06.db05-1386

Balfour, R. H., Hansen, A. M. K., and Trapp, S. (2006). Neuronal responses to transient hypoglycaemia in the dorsal vagal complex of the rat brainstem. *J. Physiol.* 570, 469–484. doi: 10.1113/jphysiol.2005.098822

Baver, S. B., Hope, K., Guyot, S., Bjørbaek, C., Kaczorowski, C., and O'Connell, K. M. S. (2014). Leptin Modulates the intrinsic excitability of AgRP/NPY neurons in the arcuate nucleus of the hypothalamus. *J. Neurosci.* 34, 5486–5496. doi: 10.1523/JNEUROSCI.4861-12.2014

Beall, C., Hamilton, D., Gallagher, J., Logie, L., Wright, K., Soutar, M., et al. (2012). Mouse hypothalamic GT1-7 cells demonstrate AMPK-dependent intrinsic glucose-sensing behaviour. *Diabetologia* 55, 2432–2444. doi: 10.1007/s00125-012-2617-y

Beck, B. (2000). Neuropeptides and obesity. [Review] [170 refs]. *Nutrition* 16, 916–923. doi: 10.1016/S0899-9007(00)00410-X

Becskei, C., Lutz, T. A., and Riediger, T. (2009). Blunted fasting-induced hypothalamic activation and refeeding hyperphagia in late-onset obesity. *Neuroendocrinology* 90, 371–382. doi: 10.1159/000251723

Beverly, J. L., De Vries, M. G., Bouman, S. D., and Arseneau, L. M. (2001). Noradrenergic and GABAergic systems in the medial hypothalamus are activated during hypoglycemia. *Am. J. Physiol.* 280, R563–R569.

Billington, C. J., and Levine, A. S. (1992). Hypothalamic neuropeptide Y regulation of feeding and energy metabolism. *Curr. Opin. Neurobiol.* 2, 847–851. doi: 10.1016/0959-4388(92)90144-A

Blouet, C., Jo, Y.-H., Li, X., and Schwartz, G. J. (2009). Mediobasal Hypothalamic leucine sensing regulates food intake through activation of a hypothalamus–brainstem circuit. *J. Neurosci.* 29, 8302–8311. doi: 10.1523/JNEUROSCI.1668-09.2009

Borg, M. A., Sherwin, R. S., Borg, W. P., Tamborlane, W. V., and Shulman, G. I. (1997). Local ventromedial hypothalamus glucose perfusion blocks counterregulation during systemic hypoglycemia in awake rats. *J. Clin. Invest.* 99, 361–365. doi: 10.1172/JCI119165

Broberger, C., Johansen, J., Johansson, C., Schalling, M., and Hokfelt, T. (1998). The neuropeptide Y/agouti gene-related protein (AGRP) brain circuitry in normal, anorectic, and monosodium glutamate-treated mice. *Proc. Natl. Acad. Sci. U.S.A.* 95, 15043–15048. doi: 10.1073/pnas.95.25.15043

Burdakov, D., Gerasimenko, O., and Verkhratsky, A. (2005). Physiological Changes in glucose differentially modulate the excitability of hypothalamic melanin-concentrating hormone and orexin neurons *in situ*. *J. Neurosci.* 25, 2429–2433. doi: 10.1523/JNEUROSCI.4925-04.2005

Burdakov, D., Jensen, L. T., Alexopoulos, H., Williams, R. H., Fearon, I. M., O'Kelly, I., et al. (2006). Tandem-Pore K^+ channels mediate inhibition of orexin neurons by glucose. *Neuron* 50, 711–722. doi: 10.1016/j.neuron.2006.04.032

Cai, X. J., Evans, M. L., Lister, C. A., Leslie, R. A., Arch, J. R., Wilson, S., et al. (2001). Hypoglycemia activates orexin neurons and selectively increases hypothalamic orexin-B levels: responses inhibited by feeding and possibly mediated by the nucleus of the solitary tract. *Diabetes* 50, 105–112. doi: 10.2337/diabetes.50.1.105

Cai, X. J., Widdowson, P. S., Harrold, J., Wilson, S., Buckingham, R. E., Arch, J. R., et al. (1999). Hypothalamic orexin expression: modulation by blood glucose and feeding. *Diabetes* 48, 2132–2137. doi: 10.2337/diabetes.48.11.2132

Canabal, D. D., Potian, J. G., Duran, R. G., McArdle, J. J., and Routh, V. H. (2007a). Hyperglycemia impairs glucose and insulin regulation of nitric oxide production in glucose-inhibited neurons in the ventromedial hypothalamus. *Am. J. Physiol. Regul. Integr. Comp. Physiol.* 293, R592–R600. doi: 10.1152/ajpregu.00207.2007

Canabal, D. D., Song, Z., Potian, J. G., Beuve, A., McArdle, J. J., and Routh, V. H. (2007b). Glucose, insulin and leptin signaling pathways modulate nitric oxide (NO) synthesis in glucose-inhibited (GI) neurons in the ventromedial hypothalamus (VMH). *J. Physiol. Regul. Integr. Comp. Physiol.* 292, R1418–R1428. doi: 10.1152/ajpregu.00216.2006

Cardoso, F. L., Brites, D., and Brito, M. A. (2010). Looking at the blood–brain barrier: molecular anatomy and possible investigation approaches. *Brain Res. Rev.* 64, 328–363. doi: 10.1016/j.brainresrev.2010.05.003

Choi, D. L., Davis, J. F., Fitzgerald, M. E., and Benoit, S. C. (2010). The role of orexin-A in food motivation, reward-based feeding behavior and food-induced neuronal activation in rats. *Neuroscience* 167, 11–20. doi: 10.1016/j.neuroscience.2010.02.002

Claret, M., Smith, M. A., Batterham, R. L., Selman, C., Choudury, A. I., Fryer, L. G., et al. (2007). AMPK is essential for energy homeostasis regulation and glucose sensing by POMC and AgRP neurons. *J. Clin. Invest.* 117, 2325–2336. doi: 10.1172/JCI31516

Cota, D., Proulx, K., Smith, K. A. B., Kozma, S. C., Thomas, G., Woods, S. C., et al. (2006). Hypothalamic mTOR signaling regulates food intake. *Science* 312, 927–930. doi: 10.1126/science.1124147

Cotero, V. E., and Routh, V. H. (2009). Insulin blunts the response of glucose-excited (GE) neurons in the ventrolateral-ventromedial hypothalamic nucleus (VL-VMN) to decreased glucose. *Am. J. Physiol. Endocrinol. Metab.* 296, E1101–E1109. doi: 10.1152/ajpendo.90932.2008

Cotero, V. E., Zhang, B. B., and Routh, V. H. (2009). The response of glucose-excited neurones in the ventromedial hypothalamus to decreased glucose is enhanced in a murine model of type 2 diabetes mellitus. *J. Neuroendocrinol.* 22, 65–74. doi: 10.1111/j.1365-2826.2009.01938.x

Cowley, M. A., Smart, J. L., Rubinstein, M., Cerdan, M. G., Diano, S., Horvath, T. L., et al. (2001). Leptin activates anorexigenic POMC neurons through a neural network in the arcuate nucleus. *Nature* 411, 480–484. doi: 10.1038/35078085

Cowley, M. A., Smith, R. G., Diano, S., Tschop, M., Pronchuk, N., Grove, K. L., et al. (2003). The distribution and mechanism of action of ghrelin in the cns demonstrates a novel hypothalamic circuit regulating energy homeostasis. *Neuron* 37, 649–661. doi: 10.1016/S0896-6273(03)00063-1

Cruciani-Guglielmacci, C., Hervalet, A., Douared, L., Sanders, N. M., Levin, B. E., Ktorza, A., et al. (2004). Beta oxidation in the brain is required for the effects of non-esterified fatty acids on glucose-induced insulin secretion in rats. *Diabetologia* 47, 2032–2038. doi: 10.1007/s00125-004-1569-2

Cryer, P. E. (2013). Mechanisms of hypoglycemia-associated autonomic failure in diabetes. *N. Eng. J. Med.* 369, 362–372. doi: 10.1056/NEJMra1215228

Dagogo-Jack, S. E., Craft, S., and Cryer, P. E. (1993). Hypoglycemia-associated autonomic failure in insulin-dependent diabetes mellitus. Recent antecedent hypoglycemia reduces autonomic responses to, symptoms of, and defense against subsequent hypoglycemia. *J. Clin. Invest.* 91, 819–828. doi: 10.1172/JCI116302

De Vries, M. G., Arseneau, L. M., Lawson, M. E., and Beverly, J. L. (2003). Extracellular glucose in rat ventromedial hypothalamus during acute and recurrent hypoglycemia. *Diabetes* 52, 2767–2773. doi: 10.2337/diabetes.52.11.2767

Diano, S., Horvath, B., Urbanski, H. F., Sotonyi, P., and Horvath, T. L. (2003). Fasting activates the nonhuman primate hypocretin (orexin) system and its postsynaptic targets. *Endocrinology* 144, 3774–3778. doi: 10.1210/en.2003-0274

Diggs-Andrews, K. A., Zhang, X., Song, Z., Daphna-Iken, D., Routh, V. H., and Fisher, S. J. (2010). Brain insulin action regulates hypothalamic glucose sensing and the counterregulatory response to hypoglycemia. *Diabetes* 59, 2271–2280. doi: 10.2337/db10-0401

Donovan, C. M., Hamilton-Wessler, M., Halter, J. B., and Bergman, R. N. (1994). Primacy of liver glucosensors in the sympathetic response to progressive hypoglycemia. *Proc. Natl. Acad. Sci. U.S.A.* 91, 2863–2867. doi: 10.1073/pnas.91.7.2863

Dunn-Meynell, A. A., Routh, V. H., Kang, L., Gaspers, L., and Levin, B. E. (2002). Glucokinase is the likely mediator of glucosensing in both glucose-excited and glucose-inhibited central neurons. *Diabetes* 51, 2056–2065. doi: 10.2337/diabetes.51.7.2056

Dunn-Meynell, A. A., Sanders, N. M., Compton, D., Becker, T. C., Eiki, J. I, Zhang, B. B., et al. (2009). Relationship among brain and blood glucose levels and spontaneous and glucoprivic feeding. *J. Neurosci.* 29, 7015–7022. doi: 10.1523/JNEUROSCI.0334-09.2009

Elmquist, J. K. (2001). Hypothalamic pathways underlying the endocrine, autonomic, and behavioral effects of leptin. *Physiol. Behavior.* 74, 703–708. doi: 10.1016/S0031-9384(01)00613-8

Ferenczi, S., Zelei, E., Pintér, B., Szoke, Z., and Kovács, K. J. (2010). Differential regulation of hypothalamic neuropeptide Y hnRNA and mRNA during psychological stress and insulin-induced hypoglycemia. *Mol. Cell. Endocrinol.* 321, 138–145. doi: 10.1016/j.mce.2010.02.036

Fergani, C., Routly, J. E., Jones, D. N., Pickavance, L. C., Smith, R. F., and Dobson, H. (2014). Kisspeptin, c-Fos and CRFR Type 2 Co-expression in the hypothalamus after insulin-induced hypoglycaemia. *Reprod. Domest. Anim.* 49, 433–440. doi: 10.1111/rda.12293

Fioramonti, X., Contie, S., Song, Z., Routh, V. H., Lorsignol, A., and Penicaud, L. (2007). Characterization of glucosensing neuron subpopulations in the arcuate nucleus: integration in NPY and POMC networks? *Diabetes* 56, 1219–1227. doi: 10.2337/db06-0567

Fioramonti, X., Deak, A., Deshpande, S., Carneiro, L., Zhou, C., Sayed, N., et al. (2013). Hypothalamic S-nitrosylation contributes to the counter-regulatory response impairment following recurrent hypoglycemia. *PLoS ONE* 8:e68709. doi: 10.1371/journal.pone.0068709

Fioramonti, X., Lorsignol, A., Taupignon, A., and Penicaud, L. (2004). A New ATP-Sensitive K^+ channel-independent mechanism is involved in glucose-excited neurons of mouse arcuate nucleus. *Diabetes* 53, 2767–2775. doi: 10.2337/diabetes.53.11.2767

Fioramonti, X., Marsollier, N., Song, Z., Fakira, K. A., Patel, R. M., Brown, S., et al. (2010a). Ventromedial hypothalamic nitric oxide production is necessary for hypoglycemia detection and counterregulation. *Diabetes* 59, 519–528. doi: 10.2337/db09-0421

Fioramonti, X., Song, Z., Vazirani, R. P., Beuve, A., and Routh, V. H. (2010b). Hypothalamic nitric oxide in hypoglycemia detection and counterregulation: a two two edged sword. *Antioxid. Redox Signal.* 14, 505–517. doi: 10.1089/ars.2010.3331

Garcia, M., Millan, C., Balmaceda-Aguilera, C., Castro, T., Pastor, P., Montecinos, H., et al. (2003). Hypothalamic ependymal-glial cells express the glucose transporter GLUT2, a protein involved in glucose sensing. *J. Neurochem.* 86, 709–724. doi: 10.1046/j.1471-4159.2003.01892.x

González, J. A., Jensen, L. T., Doyle, S. E., Miranda-Anaya, M., Menaker, M., Fugger, L., et al. (2009). Deletion of TASK1 and TASK3 channels disrupts intrinsic excitability but does not abolish glucose or pH responses of orexin/hypocretin neurons. *Eur. J. Neurosci.* 30, 57–64. doi: 10.1111/j.1460-9568.2009.06789.x

Gonzalez, J. A., Jensen, L. T., Fugger, L., and Burdakov, D. (2008). Metabolism-Independent sugar sensing in central orexin neurons. *Diabetes* 57, 2569–2576. doi: 10.2337/db08-0548

Griffond, B., Risold, P.-Y., Jacquemard, C., Colard, C., and Fellmann, D. (1999). Insulin-induced hypoglycemia increases preprohypocretin (orexin) mRNA in the rat lateral hypothalamic area. *Neurosci. Lett.* 262, 77–80. doi: 10.1016/S0304-3940(98)00976-8

Guillod-Maximin, E., Lorsignol, A., Alquier, T., and Penicaud, L. (2004). Acute intracarotid glucose injection towards the brain induces specific c-fos activation in hypothalamic nuclei: involvement of astrocytes in cerebral glucose-sensing in rats. *J. Neuroendocrinol.* 16, 464–471. doi: 10.1111/j.1365-2826.2004.01185.x

Harris, G. C., Wimmer, M., and Aston-Jones, G. (2005). A role for lateral hypothalamic orexin neurons in reward seeking. *Nature* 437, 556–559. doi: 10.1038/nature04071

Hevener, A. L., Bergman, R. N., and Donovan, C. M. (1997). Novel glucosensor for hypoglycemic detection localized to the portal vein. *Diabetes* 46, 1521–1525. doi: 10.2337/diab.46.9.1521

Ibrahim, N., Bosch, M. A., Smart, J. L., Qiu, J., Rubinstein, M., Ronnekleiv, O. K., et al. (2003). Hypothalamic proopiomelanocortin neurons are glucose responsive and express K(ATP) channels. *Endocrinol* 144, 1331–1340. doi 10.1210/en.2002-221033

Joly-Amado, A., Denis, R. G. P., Castel, J., Lacombe, A., Cansell, C., Rouch, C., et al. (2012). Hypothalamic AgRP-neurons control peripheral substrate utilization and nutrient partitioning. *EMBO J.* 31, 4276–4288. doi: 10.1038/emboj.2012.250

Kang, L., Dunn-Meynell, A. A., Routh, V. H., Gaspers, L. D., Nagata, Y., Nishimura, T., et al. (2006). Glucokinase is a critical regulator of ventromedial hypothalamic neuronal glucosensing. *Diabetes* 55, 412–420. doi: 10.2337/diabetes.55.02.06.db05-1229

Kang, L., Routh, V. H., Kuzhikandathil, E. V., Gaspers, L., and Levin, B. E. (2004). Physiological and molecular properties of rat hypothalamic ventromedial nucleus glucosensing neurons. *Diabetes* 53, 559. doi: 10.2337/diabetes.53.3.549

Kang, L., Sanders, N. M., Dunn-Meynell, A. A., Gaspers, L. D., Routh, V. H., Thomas, A. P., et al. (2008). Prior hypoglycemia enhances glucose responsiveness in some ventromedial hypothalamic glucosensing neurons. *Am. J.Physiol. Regul. Integr. Comp. Physiol.* 294, R784–R792. doi: 10.1152/ajpregu.00645.2007

Karnani, M. M., Szabó G., Erdélyi, F., and Burdakov, D. (2013). Lateral hypothalamic GAD65 neurons are spontaneously firing and distinct from orexin-and melanin-concentrating hormone neurons. *J. Physiol.* 591, 933–953. doi: 10.1113/jphysiol.2012.243493

Kelley, A. E., Baldo, B. A., and Pratt, W. E. (2005). A proposed hypothalamic–thalamic–striatal axis for the integration of energy balance, arousal, and food reward. *J. Comp. Neurol.* 493, 72–85. doi: 10.1002/cne.20769

Kohno, D., Gao, H. Z., Muroya, S., Kikuyama, S., and Yada, T. (2003). Ghrelin directly interacts with neuropeptide-Y-Containing neurons in the rat arcuate nucleus: Ca^{2+} signaling via protein kinase a and N-Type channel-dependent mechanisms and cross-talk with leptin and orexin. *Diabetes* 52, 948–956. doi: 10.2337/diabetes.52.4.948

Kohno, D., Nakata, M., Maekawa, F., Fujiwara, K., Maejima, Y., Kuramochi, M., et al. (2007). Leptin suppresses ghrelin-induced activation of neuropeptide y neurons in the arcuate nucleus via phosphatidylinositol 3-kinase- and phosphodiesterase 3-mediated pathway. *Endocrinology* 148, 2251–2263. doi: 10.1210/en.2006-1240

Kohno, D., Sone, H., Minokoshi, Y., and Yada, T. (2008). Ghrelin raises $[Ca^{2+}]$i via AMPK in hypothalamic arcuate nucleus NPY neurons. *Biochem. Biophys. Res. Commun.* 366, 388–392. doi: 10.1016/j.bbrc.2007.11.166

Langlet, F., Levin Barry, E., Luquet, S., Mazzone, M., Messina, A., Dunn-Meynell Ambrose, A., et al. (2013). Tanycytic VEGF-A boosts blood-hypothalamus barrier plasticity and access of metabolic signals to the arcuate nucleus in response to fasting. *Cell Metab.* 17, 607–617. doi: 10.1016/j.cmet.2013.03.004

Languren, G., Montiel, T., Julio-Amilpas, A., and Massieu, L. (2013). Neuronal damage and cognitive impairment associated with hypoglycemia: an integrated view. *Neurochem. Int.* 63, 331–343. doi: 10.1016/j.neuint.2013.06.018

Le Foll, C., Dunn-Meynell, A. A., Miziorko, H. M., and Levin, B. E. (2014). Regulation of hypothalamic neuronal sensing and food intake by ketone bodies and fatty acids. *Diabetes* 63, 1259–1269. doi: 10.2337/db13-1090

Le Foll, C., Dunn-Meynell, A., Musatov, S., Magnan, C., and Levin, B. E. (2013). FAT/CD36: a major regulator of neuronal fatty acid sensing and energy homeostasis in rats and mice. *Diabetes* 62, 2709–2716. doi: 10.2337/db12-1689

Leshan, R. L., Greenwald-Yarnell, M., Patterson, C. M., Gonzalez, I. E., and Myers, M. G. (2012). Leptin action through hypothalamic nitric oxide synthase-1-expressing neurons controls energy balance. *Nat. Med.* 18, 820–823. doi: 10.1038/nm.2724

Levin, B. E. (2000). Glucose-regulated dopamine release from substantia nigra neurons. *Brain Res.* 874, 158–164. doi: 10.1016/S0006-8993(00)02573-7

Levin, B. E. (2002). Metabolic sensors. Viewing glucosensing neurons from a broader perspective. *Physiol. Behavior.* 76, 397–401. doi: 10.1016/S0031-9384(02)00763-1

Levin, B. E., Planas, B., Routh, V. H., Hamilton, J., Stern, J. S., and Horwitz, B. A. (1993). Altered alpha 1-adrenoceptor binding in intact and adrenalectomized obese Zucker rats (fa/fa). *Brain Res.* 614, 146–154. doi: 10.1016/0006-8993(93)91028-Q

Levin, B. E., Routh, V. H., Kang, L., Sanders, N. M., and Dunn-Meynell, A. A. (2004). Neuronal glucosensing: what do we know after 50 years? *Diabetes* 53, 2521–2528. doi: 10.2337/diabetes.53.10.2521

Lindberg, D., Chen, P., and Li, C. (2013). Conditional viral tracing reveals that steroidogenic factor 1-positive neurons of the dorsomedial subdivision of the ventromedial hypothalamus project to autonomic centers of the hypothalamus and hindbrain. *J. Comp. Neurol.* 521, 3167–3190. doi: 10.1002/cne.23338

Lopez-Barneo, J. (2003). Oxygen and glucose sensing by carotid body glomus cells. *Curr. Opin. Neurobiol.* 13, 493–499. doi: 10.1016/S0959-4388(03)00093-X

López, M., Seoane, L., del Carmen García, M., Lago, F., Casanueva, F. F., Señarís, R., et al. (2000). Leptin regulation of prepro-orexin and orexin receptor mRNA levels in the hypothalamus. *Biochem. Biophys. Res. Commun.* 269, 41–45. doi: 10.1006/bbrc.2000.2245

Louis, G. W., Leinninger, G. M., Rhodes, C. J., and Myers, M. G. Jr. (2010). Direct innervation and modulation of orexin neurons by lateral hypothalamic LepRb neurons. *J. Neurosci.* 30, 11278–11287. doi: 10.1523/JNEUROSCI.1340-10.2010

Lynch, R. M., Tompkins, L. S., Brooks, H. L., Dunn-Meynell, A. A., and Levin, B. E. (2000). Localization of glucokinase gene expression in the rat brain. *Diabetes* 49, 693–700. doi: 10.2337/diabetes.49.5.693

Maekawa, F., Toyoda, Y., Torii, N., Miwa, I., Thompson, R. C., Foster, D. L., et al. (2000). Localization of glucokinase-like immunoreactivity in the rat lower brain stem: for possible location of brain glucose-sensing mechanisms. *Endocrinology* 141, 375–384. doi: 10.1210/endo.141.1.7234

Magnuson, M. A. (1990). Glucokinase gene structure. Functional implications of molecular genetic studies. [Review] [31 refs]. *Diabetes* 39, 523–527. doi: 10.2337/diab.39.5.523

Marsollier, N., Kassis, N., Mezghenna, K., Soty, M., Fioramonti, X., Lacombe, A., et al. (2009). Deregulation of hepatic insulin sensitivity induced by central lipid infusion in rats is mediated by nitric oxide. *PLoS ONE* 4:e6649. doi: 10.1371/journal.pone.0006649

Marston, O. J., Hurst, P., Evans, M. L., Burdakov, D. I., and Heisler, L. K. (2011). Neuropeptide Y cells represent a distinct glucose-sensing population in the lateral hypothalamus. *Endocrinology* 152, 4046–4052. doi: 10.1210/en.2011-1307

Marty, N., Dallaporta, M., Foretz, M., Emery, M., Tarussio, D., Bady, I., et al. (2005). Regulation of glucagon secretion by glucose transporter type 2 (glut2) and astrocyte-dependent glucose sensors. *J. Clin. Invest.* 115, 3545–3553. doi: 10.1172/JCI26309

Matveyenko, A. V., and Donovan, C. M. (2006). Metabolic sensors mediate hypoglycemic detection at the portal vein. *Diabetes* 55, 1276–1282. doi: 10.2337/db05-1665

McNay, E. C., Fries, T. M., and Gold, P. E. (2000). Decreases in rat extracellular hippocampal glucose concentration associated with cognitive demand during a spatial task. *Proc. Natl. Acad. Sci. U.S.A.* 97, 2881–2885. doi: 10.1073/pnas.050583697

McNay, E. C., and Gold, P. E. (1999). Extracellular glucose concentrations in the rat hippocampus measured by zero-net-flux: effects of microdialysis flow rate, strain, and age. *J Neurochem.* 72, 785–790. doi: 10.1046/j.1471-4159.1999.720785.x

McNay, E. C., McCarty, R. C., and Gold, P. E. (2001). Fluctuations in brain glucose concentration during behavioral testing: dissociations between brain areas and between brain and blood. *Neurobiol. Learn. Mem.* 75, 325–337. doi: 10.1006/nlme.2000.3976

Medeiros, N., Dai, L., and Ferguson, A. V. (2012). Glucose-responsive neurons in the subfornical organ of the rat—a novel site for direct CNS monitoring of circulating glucose. *Neuroscience* 201, 157–165. doi: 10.1016/j.neuroscience.2011.11.028

Melnick, I. V., Price, C. J., and Colmers, W. F. (2011). Glucosensing in parvocellular neurons of the rat hypothalamic paraventricular nucleus. *Eur. J. Neurosci.* 34, 272–282. doi: 10.1111/j.1460-9568.2011.07742.x

Migrenne, S., Cruciani-Guglielmacci, C., Kang, L., Wang, R., Rouch, C., Lefevre, A. L., et al. (2006). Fatty acid signaling in the hypothalamus and the neural control of insulin secretion. *Diabetes* 55, S139–S144. doi: 10.2337/db06-S017

Mizuno, T. M., Makimura, H., Silverstein, J., Roberts, J. L., Lopingco, T., and Mobbs, C. V. (1999). Fasting regulates hypothalamic neuropeptide, Y., agouti-related peptide, and proopiomelanocortin in diabetic mice independent of changes in leptin or insulin. *Endocrinology* 140, 4551–4557.

Mobbs, C. V., Kow, L. M., and Yang, X. J. (2001). Brain glucose-sensing mechanisms: ubiquitous silencing by aglycemia vs. hypothalamic neuroendocrine responses. *Am. J. Physiol.* 281, E649–E654.

Moheet, A., Kumar, A., Eberly, L. E., Kim, J., Roberts, R., and Seaquist, E. R. (2014). Hypoglycemia-Associated autonomic failure in healthy humans: comparison of two vs three periods of hypoglycemia on hypoglycemia-induced counterregulatory and symptom response 5 days later. *J. Clin. Endocrinol. Metab.* 99, 664–670. doi: 10.1210/jc.2013-3493

Moriguchi, T. S. T., Nambu, T., Yanagisawa, M., and Goto, K. (1999). Neurons containing orexin in the lateral hypothalamic area of the adult rat brain are activated by insulin-induced acute hypoglycemia. *Neurosci. Lett.* 264, 101–104. doi: 10.1016/S0304-3940(99)00177-9

Mullier, A., Bouret, S. G., Prevot, V., and Dehouck, B. (2009). Differential distribution of tight junction proteins suggests a role for tanycytes in blood-hypothalamus barrier regulation in the adult mouse brain. *J. Comp. Neurol.* 518, 943–962. doi: 10.1002/cne.22273

Murphy, B. A., Fakira, K. A., Song, Z., Beuve, A., and Routh, V. H. (2009a). AMP-activated Protein Kinase (AMPK) and Nitric Oxide (NO) regulate the glucose sensitivity of ventromedial hypothalamic (VMH) glucose-inhibited (GI) neurons. *Am. J. Physiol. Cell Physiol.* 297, C750–C758. doi: 10.1152/ajpcell.00127.2009

Murphy, B. A., Fioramonti, X., Jochnowitz, N., Fakira, K., Gagen, K., Contie, S., et al. (2009b). Fasting enhances the response of arcuate neuropeptide Y (NPY)-glucose-inhibited (GI) neurons to decreased extracellular glucose. *Am. J. Physiol. Cell Physiol.* 296, 746–756. doi: 10.1152/ajpcell.00641.2008

Nakano, Y., and Oomura, Y. (1986). Feeding-related activity of glucose- and morphine-sensitive neurons in the monkey amygdala. *Brain Res.* 399, 167–172. doi: 10.1016/0006-8993(86)90613-X

Naufahu, J., Cunliffe, A. D., and Murray, J. F. (2013). The roles of melanin-concentrating hormone in energy balance and reproductive function: are they connected? *Reproduction* 145, R141–R150. doi: 10.1530/REP-12-0385

Navarro, M., Rodriquez de Fonseca, F., Alvarez, E., Chowen, J. A., Zueco, J. A., Gomez, R., et al. (1996). Colocalization of glucagon-like peptide-1 (GLP-1) receptors, glucose transporter GLUT-2, and glucokinase mRNAs in rat hypothalamic cells: evidence for a role of GLP-1 receptor agonists as an inhibitory signal for food and water intake. *J. Neurochem.* 67, 1982–1991. doi: 10.1046/j.1471-4159.1996.67051982.x

Niimi, M., Sato, M., Tamaki, M., Wada, Y., Takahara, J., and Kawanishi, K. (1995). Induction of fos protein in the rat hypothalamus elicited by insulin-induced hypoglycemia. *Neurosci. Res.* 23, 361–364. doi: 10.1016/0168-0102(95)00965-V

Oomura, Y., Kimura, K., Ooyama, H., Maeo, T., Iki, M., and Kuniyoshi, N. (1964). Reciprocal activities of the ventromedial and lateral hypothalamic area of cats. *Science* 143, 484–485. doi: 10.1126/science.143.3605.484

Oomura, Y., Ono, H., Ooyama, H., and Wayner, M. J. (1969). Glucose and osmosensitive neurons of the rat hypothalamus. *Nature* 222, 282–284. doi: 10.1038/222282a0

Orellana, J. A., Sáez, P. J., Cortés-campos, C., Elizondo, R. J., Shoji, K. F., Contreras-Duarte, S., et al. (2012). Glucose increases intracellular free $Ca2^{+}$ in tanycytes via ATP released through connexin 43 hemichannels. *Glia* 60, 53–68. doi: 10.1002/glia.21246

Pardal, R., and Lopez-Barneo, J. (2002). Low glucose-sensing cells in the carotid body. *Nat. Neurosci.* 5, 197–198. doi: 10.1038/nn812

Parton, L. E., Ye, C. P., Coppari, R., Enriori, P. J., Choi, B., Zhang, C. Y., et al. (2007). Glucose sensing by POMC neurons regulates glucose homeostasis and is impaired in obesity. *Nature* 449, 228–232. doi: 10.1038/nature 06098

Penicaud, L., Leloup, C., Lorsignol, A., Alquier, T., and Guillod, E. (2002). Brain glucose sensing mechanism and glucose homeostasis. *Curr. Opin. Clin. Nutr. Metab. Care* 5, 539–543. doi: 10.1097/00075197-200209000-00013

Perello, M., Sakata, I., Birnbaum, S., Chuang, J.-C., Osborne-Lawrence, S., Rovinsky, S. A., et al. (2010). Ghrelin increases the rewarding value of high-fat diet in an orexin-dependent manner. *Biol. Psychiatry* 67, 880–886. doi: 10.1016/j.biopsych.2009.10.030

Ramonet, D., Rodriguez, M. J., Pugliese, M., and Mahy, N. (2004). Putative glucosensing property in rat and human activated microglia. *Neurobiology Disease* 17, 1–9. doi: 10.1016/j.nbd.2003.11.019

Raybould, H. E. (2007). Sensing of glucose in the gastrointestinal tract. *Auton. Neurosci.* 133, 86–90. doi: 10.1016/j.autneu.2007.01.006

Ritter, S., Li, A.-J., Wang, Q., and Dinh, T. T. (2011). Minireview: the value of looking backward: the essential role of the hindbrain in counterregulatory responses to glucose deficit. *Endocrinology* 152, 4019–4032. doi: 10.1210/en. 2010-1458

Ritter, S., Llewellyn-Smith, I., and Dinh, T. T. (1998). Subgroups of hindbrain catecholamine neurons are selectively activated by 2-deoxy-D-glucose induced metabolic challenge. *Brain Res.* 805, 41–54. doi: 10.1016/S0006-8993(98) 00655-6

Rojas, J. M., and Schwartz, M. W. (2014). Control of hepatic glucose metabolism by islet and brain. *Diabetes, Obes. Metab.* 16, 33–40. doi: 10.1111/dom.12332

Roland, A. V., and Moenter, S. M. (2011). Glucosensing by GnRH Neurons: inhibition by androgens and involvement of AMP-Activated protein kinase. *Mol. Endocrinol.* 25, 847–858. doi: 10.1210/me.2010-0508

Routh, V. H., Donovan. C. M., and Ritter, S. (2013). Hypoglycemia Detection. *Transl. Endocrinol. Metab.* 3, 47–87. doi: 10.1210/TEAM.9781936704200.ch2

Routh, V. H., McArdle, J. J., and Levin, B. E. (1997). Phosphorylation modulates the activity of the ATP-sensitive K^{+} channel in the ventromedial hypothalamic nucleus. *Brain Res.* 778, 107–119. doi: 10.1016/S0006-8993(97)01043-3

Sanders, N. M., Dunn-Meynell, A. A., and Levin, B. E. (2004). Third ventricular alloxan reversibly impairs glucose counterregulatory responses. *Diabetes* 53, 1230–1236. doi: 10.2337/diabetes.53.5.1230

Sawchenko, P. E. (1998). Toward a new neurobiology of energy balance, appetite, and obesity: the anatomists weigh in. *J. Comp. Neurol.* 402, 435–441.

Sayegh, A. I., Covasa, M., and Ritter, R. C. (2004). Intestinal infusions of oleate and glucose activate distinct enteric neurons in the rat. *Auton. Neurosci.* 115, 54–63. doi: 10.1016/j.autneu.2004.08.006

Sheng, Z., Santiago, A. M., Thomas, M. P., and Routh, V. H. (2014). Metabolic regulation of lateral hypothalamic glucose-inhibited orexin neurons may influence midbrain reward neurocircuitry. *Mol. Cell. Neurosci.* 62, 30–41. doi: 10.1016/j.mcn.2014.08.001

Shian, L. R., and Lin, M. T. (1991). Insulin acts on the hypothalamic glucose-facilitated neurons to induce hyperglycemia and hyperinsulinemia in the rat. *Experientia* 47, 942–944. doi: 10.1007/BF01929887

Shiraishi, T., Oomura, Y., Sasaki, K., and Wayner, M. J. (2000). Effects of leptin and orexin-A on food intake and feeding related hypothalamic neurons. *Physiol. Behav.* 71, 251–261. doi: 10.1016/S0031-9384(00)00341-3

Silver, I. A., and Erecinska, M. (1994). Extracellular glucose concentration in mammalian brain: continuous monitoring of changes during increased neuronal activity and upon limitation in oxygen supply in normo-, hypo-, and hyperglycemic animals. *J. Neurosci.* 14, 5068–5076.

Song, Z., Levin, B. E., McArdle, J. J., Bakhos, N., and Routh, V. H. (2001). Convergence of pre- and postsynaptic influences on glucosensing neurons in the ventromedial hypothalamic nucleus. *Diabetes* 50, 2673–2681. doi: 10.2337/diabetes.50.12.2673

Song, Z., and Routh, V. H. (2005). Differential effects of glucose and lactate on glucosensing neurons in the ventromedial hypothalamic nucleus. *Diabetes* 54, 15–22. doi: 10.2337/diabetes.54.1.15

Song, Z., and Routh, V. H. (2006). Recurrent hypoglycemia reduces the glucose sensitivity of glucose-inhibited neurons in the ventromedial hypothalamus nucleus (VMN). *Am. J. Physiol. Regul. Integr. Comp. Physiol.* 291, R1283–R1287. doi: 10.1152/ajpregu.00148.2006

Spanswick, D., Smith, M. A., Groppi, V. E., Logan, S. D., and Ashford, M. L. J. (1997). Leptin inhibits hypothalamic neurons by activation of ATP-sensitive potassium channels. *Nature* 390, 521–525. doi: 10.1038/37379

Spanswick, D., Smith, M. A., Mirshamsi, S., Routh, V. H., and Ashford, M. L. J. (2000). Insulin activates ATP-sensitive K^{+} channels in hypothalamic neurons of lean, but not obese rats. *Nat. Neurosci.* 3, 757–758. doi: 10.1038/77660

Stanley, S., Domingos Ana, I., Kelly, L., Garfield, A., Damanpour, S., Heisler, L., et al. (2013). Profiling of glucose-sensing neurons reveals that GHRH neurons are activated by hypoglycemia. *Cell Metab.* 18, 596–607. doi: 10.1016/j.cmet.2013.09.002

Steffens, A. B., Mogenson, G. J., and Stevenson, J. A. (1972). Blood glucose, insulin, and free fatty acids after stimulation and lesions of the hypothalamus. *Am. J. Physiol.* 222, 1446–1452.

Steffens, A. B., Scheurink, A. J., Luiten, P. G., and Bohus, B. (1988). Hypothalamic food intake regulating areas are involved in the homeostasis of blood glucose and plasma FFA levels. *Physiol. Behav.* 44, 581–589. doi: 10.1016/0031-9384(88)90322-8

Sternson, S. M., Shepherd, G. M. G., and Friedman, J. M. (2005). Topographic mapping of VMH [rarr] arcuate nucleus microcircuits and their reorganization by fasting. *Nat. Neurosci.* 8, 1356–1363. doi: 10.1038/nn1550

Stolarczyk, E., Guissard, C., Michau, A., Even, P. C., Grosfeld, A., Serradas, P., et al. (2010). Detection of extracellular glucose by GLUT2 contributes to hypothalamic control of food intake. *Am. J. Physiol. Endocrinol. Metab.* 298, E1078–E1087. doi: 10.1152/ajpendo.00737.2009

Straub, R. H., Cutolo, M., Buttgereit, F., and Pongratz, G. (2010). Energy regulation and neuroendocrine–immune control in chronic inflammatory diseases. *J. Intern. Med.* 267, 543–560. doi: 10.1111/j.1365-2796.2010.02218.x

Szepietowska, B., Zhu, W., Chan, O., Horblitt, A., Dziura, J., and Sherwin, R. S. (2011). Modulation of β-Adrenergic receptors in the ventromedial hypothalamus influences counterregulatory responses to hypoglycemia. *Diabetes* 60, 3154–3158. doi: 10.2337/db11-0432

Takahashi, K. A., and Cone, R. D. (2005). Fasting induces a large, leptin-dependent increase in the intrinsic action potential frequency of orexigenic arcuate nucleus neuropeptide Y/Agouti-Related protein neurons. *Endocrinology* 146, 1043–1047. doi: 10.1210/en.2004-1397

Valassi, E., Scacchi, M., and Cavagnini, F. (2014). Neuroendocrine control of food intake. *Nutr. Metab. Cardiovasc. Dis.* 18, 158–168. doi: 10.1016/j.numecd.2007.06.004

van Dijk, G., Bottone, A. E., Strubbe, J. H., and Steffens, A. B. (1994). Hormonal and metabolic effects of paraventricular hypothalamic administration of neuropeptide Y during rest and feeding. *Brain Res.* 660, 96–103. doi: 10.1016/0006-8993(94)90843-5

Vazirani, R. P., Fioramonti, X., and Routh, V. H. (2013). Membrane potential dye imaging of ventromedial hypothalamus neurons from adult mice to study glucose sensing. *J. Vis. Exp.* 81:e50861. doi: 10.3791/50861

Wang, Q., Liu, C., Uchida, A., Chuang, J.-C., Walker, A., Liu, T., et al. (2014). Arcuate AgRP neurons mediate orexigenic and glucoregulatory actions of ghrelin. *Mol. Metab.* 3, 64–72. doi: 10.1016/j.molmet.2013.10.001

Wang, R., Cruciani-Guglielmacci, C., Migrenne, S., Magnan, C., Cotero, V. E., and Routh, V. H. (2005). The effects of oleic-acid (OA) on distinct populations of neurons in the hypothalamic arcuate nucleus (ARC) are dependent on extracellular glucose levels. *J. Neurophysiol.* 55, 1491–1498. doi: 10.1152/jn.00697.2005

Wang, R., Liu, X., Hentges, S. T., Dunn-Meynell, A. A., Levin, B. E., Wang, W., et al. (2004). The regulation of glucose-excited neurons in the hypothalamic arcuate nucleus by glucose and feeding-relevant peptides. *Diabetes* 53, 1959–1965. doi: 10.2337/diabetes.53.8.1959

Warne, J. P., Varonin, J. M., Nielsen, S. S., Olofsson, L. E., Kaelin, C. B., Chua, S., et al. (2013). Coordinated regulation of hepatic energy stores by leptin and hypothalamic agouti-related protein. *J. Neurosci.* 33, 11972–11985. doi: 10.1523/JNEUROSCI.0830-13.2013

Watts, A. G., and Sanchez-Watts, G. (2002). Interactions between heterotypic stressors and corticosterone reveal integrative mechanisms for controlling corticotropin-releasing hormone gene expression in the rat paraventricular nucleus. *J. Neurosci.* 22, 6282–6289.

White, J. D. (1993). Neuropeptide Y: a central regulator of energy homeostasis. *Reg. Pept.* 49, 93–107.

Williams, R. H., Alexopoulos, H., Jensen, L. T., Fugger, L., and Burdakov, D. (2008). Adaptive sugar sensors in hypothalamic feeding circuits. *Proc. Natl. Acad. Sci. U.S.A.* 105, 11975–11980. doi: 10.1073/pnas.0802687105

Yamanaka, A., Beuckmann, C. T., Willie, J. T., Hara, J., Tsujino, N., Mieda, M., et al. (2003). Hypothalamic orexin neurons regulate arousal according to energy balance in mice. *Neuron* 38, 701–713. doi: 10.1016/S0896-6273(03)00331-3

Yang, X. J., Kow, L. M., Funabashi, T., and Mobbs, C. V. (1999). Hypothalamic glucose sensor: similarities to and differences from pancreatic beta-cell mechanisms. *Diabetes* 48, 1763–1772. doi: 10.2337/diabetes.48.9.1763

Yang, Y., Atasoy, D., Su Helen, H., and Sternson Scott, M. (2011). Hunger states switch a flip-flop memory circuit via a synaptic AMPK-dependent positive feedback loop. *Cell* 146, 992–1003. doi: 10.1016/j.cell.2011.07.039

Zhao, Y. Y., Guo, L., Du, J., and Liu, G. L. (2005). Effects of acute hypoglycemia on the orexin system in rat. *Chin. Med. Sci. J.* 20, 55–58.

Zheng, H., Patterson, L. M., and Berthoud, H.-R. (2007). Orexin signaling in the ventral tegmental area is required for high-fat appetite induced by opioid stimulation of the nucleus accumbens. *J. Neurosci.* 27, 11075–11082. doi: 10.1523/JNEUROSCI.3542-07.2007

Zhou, L., Podolsky, N., Sang, Z., Ding, Y., Fan, X., Tong, Q., et al. (2010). The medial amygdalar nucleus: a novel glucose-sensing region that modulates the counterregulatory response to hypoglycemia. *Diabetes* 59, 2646–2652. doi: 10.2337/db09-0995

Zhu, W., Czyzyk, D., Paranjape, S. A., Zhou, L., Horblitt, A., Szabó, G., et al. (2010). Glucose prevents the fall in ventromedial hypothalamic GABA that is required for full activation of glucose counterregulatory responses during hypoglycemia. *Am. J. Physiol. Endocrinol. Metab.* 298, E971–E977. doi: 10.1152/ajpendo.00749.2009

5

Ontogenesis of oxytocin pathways in the mammalian brain: late maturation and psychosocial disorders

***Valery Grinevich*[1*†], *Michel G. Desarménien*[2†], *Bice Chini*[3†], *Maithé Tauber*[4,5†] and *Françoise Muscatelli*[6,7*†]**

[1] *Schaller Research Group on Neuropeptides, German Cancer Research Center and CellNetwork Cluster of Excellence of the University of Heidelberg, Heidelberg, Germany*
[2] *Institute of Functional Genomics, Centre National de la Recherche Scientifique, Institut National de la Santé et de la Recherche Médicale, Université Montpellier 1, Université Montpellier 2, Montpellier, France*
[3] *Consiglio Nazionale delle Ricerche Institute of Neuroscience, Milan, Italy*
[4] *Reference Centre for Prader-Willi Syndrome – Department of Pediatric Endocrinology, Hôpital des Enfants Centre Hospitalier Universitaire de Toulouse 330, Toulouse, France*
[5] *Institut National de la Santé et de la Recherche Médicale Unité Mixe de Recherche 1043, Paul Sabatier University Toulouse III, Toulouse, France*
[6] *Institut de Neurobiologie de la Méditerranée Unité Mixe de Recherche U901, Institut National de la Santé et de la Recherche Médicale, Parc Scientifique de Luminy, Marseille, France*
[7] *Aix-Marseille Université, Institut de Neurobiologie de la Méditerranée Unité Mixe de Recherche 901, Marseille, France*

Correspondence:
Valery Grinevich, Schaller Research Group on Neuropeptides (V078), German Cancer Research Center, CellNetwork Cluster of Excellence, University of Heidelberg, Im Neuenheimer Feld 581 (TP4), Office 3.301, D-69120 Heidelberg, Germany
e-mail: v.grinevich@dkfz-heidelberg.de; Valery.Grinevich@mpimf-heidelberg.mpg.de;
Françoise Muscatelli, Institut de Neurobiologie de la Méditerranée, INMED UMR U901, INSERM, Parc Scientifique de Luminy, Aix-Marseille Université, INMED UMR 901, 13273 Marseille, France
e-mail: francoise.muscatelli@inserm.fr

† These authors have contributed equally to this work.

Oxytocin (OT), the main neuropeptide of sociality, is expressed in neurons exclusively localized in the hypothalamus. During the last decade, a plethora of neuroendocrine, metabolic, autonomic and behavioral effects of OT has been reported. In the urgency to find treatments to syndromes as invalidating as autism, many clinical trials have been launched in which OT is administered to patients, including adolescents and children. However, the impact of OT on the developing brain and in particular on the embryonic and early postnatal maturation of OT neurons, has been only poorly investigated. In the present review we summarize available (although limited) literature on general features of ontogenetic transformation of the OT system, including determination, migration and differentiation of OT neurons. Next, we discuss trajectories of OT receptors (OTR) in the perinatal period. Furthermore, we provide evidence that early alterations, from birth, in the central OT system lead to severe neurodevelopmental diseases such as feeding deficit in infancy and severe defects in social behavior in adulthood, as described in Prader-Willi syndrome (PWS). Our review intends to propose a hypothesis about developmental dynamics of central OT pathways, which are essential for survival right after birth and for the acquisition of social skills later on. A better understanding of the embryonic and early postnatal maturation of the OT system may lead to better OT-based treatments in PWS or autism.

Keywords: oxytocin, oxytocin receptor, ontogenesis, somatodendritic release, axonal release, autisn, Prader-Willi syndrome

INTRODUCTION

Oxytocin (OT) is a neuropeptide which is synthesized in defined nuclei of the hypothalamus, paraventricular (PVN), supraoptic (SON), and accessory (AN) nuclei and secreted both in the blood circulation as a hormone and in the brain as a neuromodulator. During the last decade, hundreds of original reports and reviews have been published, clearly showing that the OT system is a key regulator of all the aspects of social behavior, including those involved in reproduction and care of the offspring (Lee et al., 2009). Notably, in humans, OT facilitates the processing of social information and improves cognitive emphatic abilities, representing a potential new approach for the treatment of autism spectrum disorders, as extensively reviewed elsewhere (Meyer-Lindenberg et al., 2011). Even if OT is currently regarded as a "prosocial" drug, this does not implicate *per se* a "positive" connotation. OT has been found to increase trust and generosity (Kosfeld et al., 2005), but also gloating and envy (Shamay-Tsoory et al., 2009), which are also manifestations of complex "social" behaviors. Similarly, OT increases in-group but not out-group cooperation, an ethnocentric behavior that can promote prejudice, xenophobia, and intergroup violence (De Dreu et al., 2011). Furthermore, OT has been found to induce adverse behavior in borderline-personality disorders (Bartz et al., 2011). These results suggest that the selection of patients will play a crucial role in determining the outcome of the symptomatic treatment with this neuropeptide, the use of which should be restricted to those individuals who could benefit from it. An understanding of the OT-mediated cellular and molecular mechanisms on neuronal networks underlying social and feeding behavior is needed for a successful employment of this peptide in neuropsychiatric and genetic disorders. However, despite the large body of knowledge about physiology and central pathways of OT (see reviews from Landgraf and Neumann, 2004; Ross and Young, 2009; Lee et al., 2009; Knobloch and Grinevich, 2014), the developmental aspect of the OT system remains the *"locus minoris"* of neuroscience and neuroendocrinology. Here, we collected virtually all of the available information, including our personal ongoing research, and provide some general conclusions regarding the dynamics of central OT pathways in prenatal and early postnatal ontogenesis. Furthermore, we clearly demonstrate, by investigating a mouse model for the Prader-Willi syndrome (PWS), that changes in the developmental maturation of the OT system cause metabolic and social alterations. These can be significantly improved or even fully compensated by OT treatment in the first days after birth, opening the door for a powerful pharmacological therapy for PWS in early infancy.

THE BIRTH OF OT-ERGIC NUCLEI

In many species (rodent, human, zebrafish, chicken), all oxytocin (OT) neurons are generated from the proliferative ("convoluted") neuroepithelium of the diamond shaped third ventricle (**Table 1** and **Figure 1**). Birth-dating studies revealed that these hypothalamic neurons are generated in the second half of the gestational period in rodents, within the first quarter of the gestational period (E30-43; length of pregnancy ~165 days) in macaques (Markakis, 2002) and at the middle of pregnancy in humans (Swaab, 1995).

In rodents, the SON and PVN appear very early. At embryonic day (E) 12.5 dpc (days post-coîtum), two groups of cells are identified in the mouse: one near the third ventricle and the other moved lateral to the surface pial to give rise to the SON (Dongen and Nieuwenhuys, 1989). At E14.5 dpc, the PVN and the SON are settled (Nakai et al., 1995), while AN are recognized later (probably due to their small size and relatively small number of cells; Altman and Bayer, 1978a,b,c). At this stage, an antibody recognizing the Neurophysin-I (the carrier protein for OT) reveals a positive immunosignal (**Figure 1B**), consistent with the expression of the OT-prohormone, not yet detected at E12.5 dpc. Furthermore, an antibody recognizing the intermediate forms of OT (VA10) reveals a positive immunosignal of the OT-intermediate forms at E16.5 dpc (**Figure 1C**), but not at E14.5 dpc. Importantly, the mature, amidated form of OT is detected at birth (see **Table 1**) and co-exists with immature forms of OT during the entire postnatal life (**Figure 1D**). The role of an earlier production of the non-mature forms of OT has not been studied, although a functional role of these forms during the embryonic development has been suggested (Tribollet et al., 1988).

In humans, the SON and PVN are completely formed at 25 weeks of gestation (Dörner and Staudt, 1972) and OT-immunoreactivity is first detected at the age of 26 weeks (Wierda et al., 1991). At that age, the number of stained OT neurons is relatively similar in the fetal and adult hypothalamus (Van der Woude et al., 1995), while the morphological analysis of individual magnocellular neurons suggests that these cells are still immature, as can be seen by the gradual increase of their nuclear volume (Rinne et al., 1962; was also observed in the rat by Crespo et al., 1988).

GENETIC HIERARCHY OF OT NEURON FORMATION

The signaling molecules and transcription factors that are involved in the determination and differentiation of OT neurons are not well known, only a few mouse studies reported factors

Table 1 | Birth of OT neurons and OT synthesis.

Biosynthesis	Mouse	Rat	Primates/Human
Birth of OT neurons	E10.5-12.5: postmitotic neurons giving rise to the PVN, SON, AN (Caqueret et al., 2006) E13.5-E15.5: terminal differentiation of PVN and SON neurons (Caqueret et al., 2006)	E13-E15 for the PVN E13-E14 for the SON (Altman and Bayer, 1978a,b,c)	In macaques: E30-E38 for the PVN E40-E43 for the SON (van Eerdenburg and Rakic, 1994)
Initial OT gene expression (based on *in situ* hybridization)	E15.5 E15.5 (presumptive PVN) and E18.5 (SON) (Allan Brain Atlas, Jing et al., 1998)	E16-E17 (SON, PVN) (Laurent et al., 1989; Trembleau et al., 1995)	15 Weeks of human gestation (Allan Brain Atlas)
Initial synthesis of pre-proOT (based on immunohistochemistry)	E14.5 PVN, SON, AN (**Figure 1** of this review)	E16 (PVN, SON) (Whitnall et al., 1985; Altstein and Gainer, 1988)	ND
Initial production of mature form of OT	P0 (birth) in PVN, SON, AN (Schaller et al., 2010)	E21-P0 (SON, PVN, AN) (Boer et al., 1980; Buijs et al., 1980; Sinding et al., 1980; Whitnall et al., 1985; Altstein and Gainer, 1988)	14 Weeks of gestation (Schubert et al., 1981; Goudsmit et al., 1992; Swaab et al., 1995)

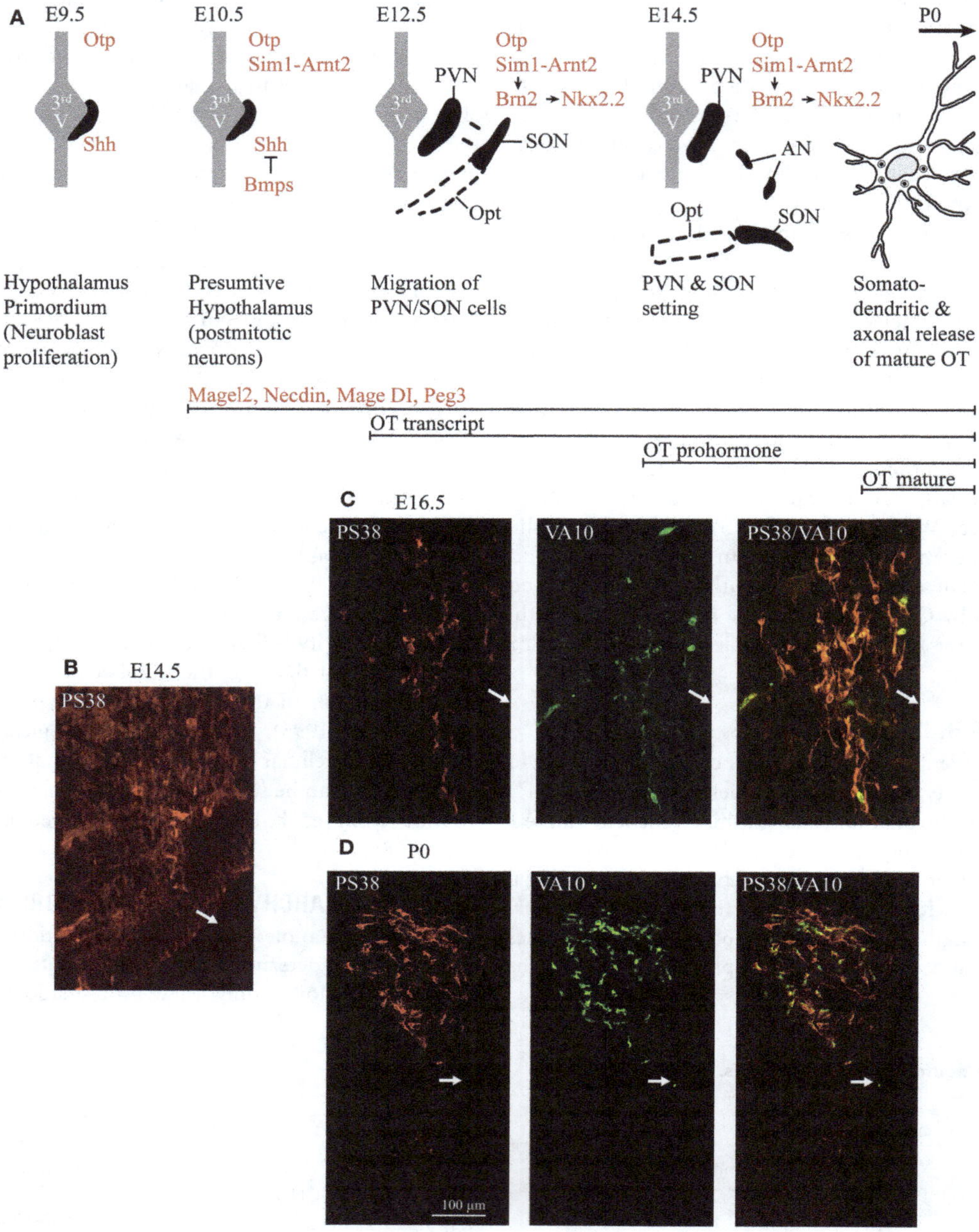

FIGURE 1 | Ontogenesis of the OT neurons during mouse embryonic development. (A) The developmental stages and transcription factors (in red in the drawings) known to be involved in the setting of the PVN, SON, and AN. Below are indicated several genes known to be expressed in OT neurons and the inactivation of each of these genes alters OT neurons. The developmental stages from which an expression of *OT* transcript, OT prohormone and OT-mature form are detected are also indicated (in black). **(B)** Immunohistochemical detection of the OT-neurophysin I (associated with OT prohormone) using the PS38 antibody (in red) and of the OT-intermediate forms using the VA10 antibody (in green). At E12.5 pcd, we did not detect any signal (not shown). At E14.5 pcd we first detect few cells expressing the OT-neurophysin I **(B)**, probably the OT-prohormone, but not OT intermediate forms. **(C)** At E16.5 pcd we detect both OT-neurophysin I and the OT intermediate forms. **(D)** At the day of birth virtually all OT neurons of the PVN co-express both OT-neurophysin I and immature forms of OT. White arrows indicate the location of the third ventricle.

involved in the early stages of development of the hypothalamic-neurohypophyseal system (Carrel and Allen, 2000; Caqueret et al., 2006; Szarek et al., 2010).

The early patterning of hypothalamus has been shown to depend on a cascade of transcription factors (**Figure 1A**): firstly the sonic hedgehog (SHH) is necessary to establish the hypothalamus primordium (E9.5 dpc in mouse) (Mathieu et al., 2002; see also Blaess et al. (2014) in this Research Topic of Frontiers in Neuroanatomy); the local production of the bone morphogenetic proteins (BMPs) is then required to down-regulate SHH and establish region specific transcription profiles (Ohyama et al., 2003). The bHLH-PAS (basic helix-loop-helix PER-ART-SIM) transcription factor SIM1 is expressed in the incipient PVN, SON and AN from E10.5 dpc (Caqueret et al., 2006) where it dimerises with ARNT2 (Michaud et al., 2000; Hosoya et al., 2001). A key downstream target of SIM1/ARNT2 is Brn2, a POU domain transcription factor required for OT (as well as for two other types of neuroendocrine neurons, expressing arginine-vasopressin (AVP) and corticotropin releasing hormone neurons of the PVN/SON/AN and expressed from E11.5 dpc, Nakai et al., 1995; Schoneman et al., 1995). In a parallel or convergent SIM1/ARNT2 pathway, the homeobox orthopedia (OTP) factor is also necessary for Brn2 expression (Caqueret et al., 2006), which is still expressed at E15.5 dpc, with Nkx2.2. All of these factors are required to define at E12.5 dpc the prospective PVN domain, however, from this stage on, the factors that will specify the parvocellular[1] and magnocellular OT neurons have not been identified. The ablation of Brn2 results in a loss of all neurons of the PVN, SON and presumably of the AN (Nakai et al., 1995; Schoneman et al., 1995). Importantly the lack of axonal projections of magnocellular OT and AVP neurons in the Brn2 knock-out mice to the pituitary (Schoneman et al., 1995), as also observed in the Arnt2-knockout mice (Hosoya et al., 2001), leads to progressive loss of pituicytes (pituitary astrocyte-like glial cells). All together, these results suggest a role of OT and/or AVP in the formation of the neurohypophysis. Indeed, in the absence of OT, the neurovascular interface in the neurohypophysis does not form in zebra fish (Gutnick et al., 2011).

One approach to identify such factors involved in the determination and differentiation of OT cells is the analysis of the OT promoter and its upstream and downstream sequences. Interestingly, genomic DNA constructs, including more than 500 base pairs (bp) upstream and 3.6 kb downstream of the OT gene, enabled an expression of OT or EGFP-reporter in OT-neurons only (Young et al., 1990; Belenky et al., 1992) in adult transgenic rodents. Later, a genomic analysis of the OT-promoter (500 bp) defined a minimal promoter sufficient for expression in OT-neurons (magnocellular neurons) of adult rodents (Fields et al., 2012; Gainer, 2012). Several binding sites for transcription factors (ERE, COUP-TF, SF1) have been identified in this sequence, but not the ones for the transcription factors described above (**Figure 1A**), suggesting that the DNA sequence required for the development of OT cells is not present in these 500 bp.

In conclusion, from the E12.5 dpc stage, the transcriptional factors that will specify the parvocellular and magnocellular OT neurons have not yet been characterized.

Several other genes such as *fibroblast growth factor 8* (Brooks et al., 2010), the *Mage-D1*, *Necdin* and *Magel2* genes, *CD38*, *Peg3* (**Figure 1** and **Table 3**), are known to be expressed in mouse hypothalamus during development. Their knock-out (KO) alters the number and/or function of OT-neurons, but their role in OT-neurons is not clarified yet.

[1] Parvocellular OT neurons belong to a relatively small population of PVN cells, which project to the brainstem and spinal cord (Sawchenko and Swanson, 1982) and control appetite, nociception and autonomic functions. The development of these particular neurons has not been studied.

THE BIOSYNTHESIS OF OT IN ONTOGENESIS

In the rat and mouse, the OT can be detected by several techniques (such as radioimmunoassay, enzyme immunoassay, immunohistochemistry) from the beginning of the second gestational week (**Table 1**). However, all of these techniques are based on the use of OT antibodies. The specificity of these antibodies, in particular against the different forms of OT, is not always established. The most reliable and relevant studies have been performed with the use of antibodies characterized by Harold Gainer's laboratory or using Mass Spectrometry Ànalysis, which, unfortunately, has not been used in developmental studies. Based on the tools used for OT detection, the OT prohormone is found in embryos just after the appearance of the OT mRNA, while the mature OT peptide is only released from birth on (**Table 1** and **Figure 1**). The OT gene encodes for the Pre-Pro-OT-Neurophysin I (pre-pro-hormone), which is cleaved by different enzymes to give rise to different OT intermediate forms and to the Neurophysin I, and finally to the mature amidated form that is released (**Figure 2**). It has been shown that the steady state of the mature OT form can be controlled by an oxytocinase (P-LAP) that is produced in periphery and centrally by the OT-magnocellular neurons. Noticeably, P-LAP is also expressed in parvocellular OT neurons and in other brain structures (Tobin et al., 2014).

Before birth, there is a delay in OT prohormone processing with an accumulation of the OT intermediate forms in OT neurons until birth. This delay was not observed for AVP processing as the amidated AVP form is detected as early as E16.5 dpc (Whitnall et al., 1985; Altstein and Gainer, 1988). Furthermore, morphological and electrophysiological properties of the magnocellular OT neurons are not mature at birth; their morphological and electrophysiological properties develop progressively during the first two postnatal weeks (see below, as well as Swaab, 1995, 1997a,b). Thus, although functional at birth, the OT-ergic system undergoes a progressive maturation during early postnatal life and is not mature before weaning in rodents and, most likely, in human infants as well. However, a comparison of immature and mature forms of OT in human development has never been studied.

ELECTRICAL PROPERTIES OF OT NEURONS AFTER BIRTH

To our knowledge, no electrophysiological studies have been performed on embryonic OT neurons. However, the groups of Francoise Moos and Michel G. Desarmenien systematically analyzed electrical activity of magnocellular neurons (although without distinction between OT and AVP) in the SON of rats during early postnatal life. Three main features arise from these studies: the importance of the second postnatal week (PW2), the role of autocontrol by OT, presumably released from soma and dendrites, and the determinant role of the development of electrophysiological features on the morphological maturation of the neurons. At birth and during PW1, the membrane potential is unstable and cells fire small and large erratic action potentials. During PW2, the membrane potential stabilizes to a more

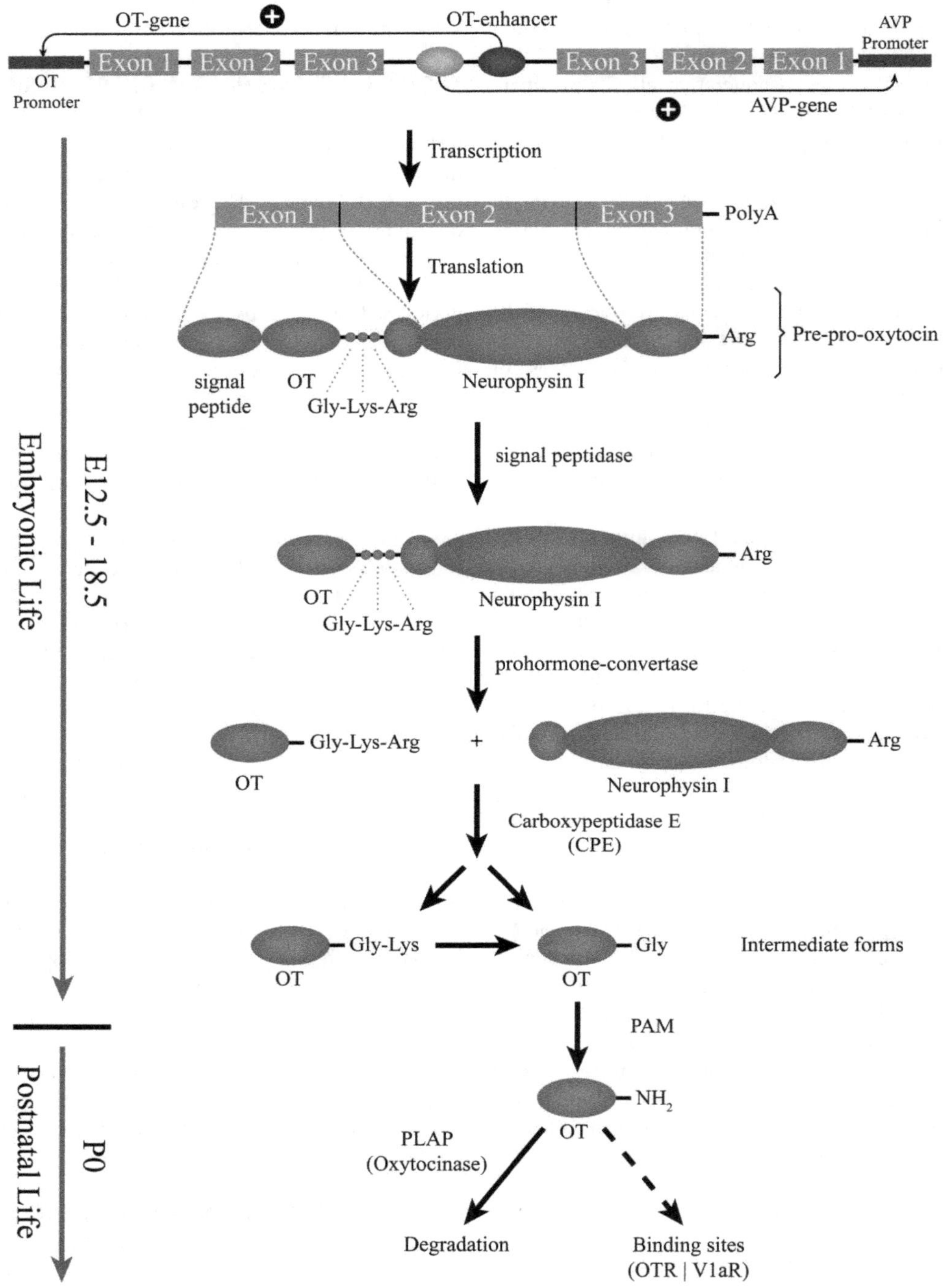

FIGURE 2 | Starting from the gene: the biosynthesis of the different forms of OT. This scheme represents the genomic structure of the OT gene, which is contiguous to the AVP-gene; regulatory elements might be shared. The transcription and translation steps of the *OT* gene are then indicated. First, OT preprohormone is produced, that will be cleaved and matured by successive enzymes. The OT intermediate forms are produced from E16.5 (see above) but the mature amidated OT form is detected only from birth. The released mature form is then degraded by an oxytocinase (PLAP) or binds to OT binding sites (OTR or V1a-receptors). PAM, alpha-amidating monooxygenase; PLAP, placental leucine aminopeptidase.

hyperpolarized value, the spontaneous activity becomes organized and the action potential progressively increases in size and decreases in duration, leading to a decrease in action potential-evoked calcium entry (Widmer et al., 1997; Chevaleyre et al., 2000). At the end of PW2 and during PW3, a switch in regulation of intracellular free calcium from extrusion to sequestration into the reticulum also occurs (Lee et al., 2007a). These two modifications of calcium entry and regulation may have important consequences on peptide secretion. The PW2 is also the period during which the chloride equilibrium potential becomes hyperpolarized, GABA becomes inhibitory and glutamatergic activity appears (Chevaleyre et al., 2001), together with an increase in NMDA receptor expression (Hussy et al., 1997). Most interestingly, this period of action potential and synaptic activity maturation is concomitant with the appearance of a major feature of SON neurons: autocontrol (**Figure 3**).

OTR has been shown to play an important role in autoregulation of magnocellular neuronal activity (Richard et al., 1997) and it is well established that OTRs are expressed in adult PVN (van Leeuwen et al., 1985; Freund-Mercier et al., 1987; Tribollet et al., 1988; Yoshimura et al., 1993; Adan et al., 1995). During ontogenesis, cells expressing OTR mRNA have been observed in SON and PVN starting from P1 (Yoshimura et al., 1996), a finding consistent with the faint and diffuse expression of OTR present throughout the hypothalamus at this stage (Tribollet et al., 1989). An increase in OTR mRNA expression is detected from P7 and is then maintained fairly stably to adulthood (Yoshimura et al., 1996).

Consistently with changes in OTR expression during PW2, OT and its related analog are most efficient in increasing electrical activity on one-third of SON neurons (supposed to be OT-ergic neurons since they were insensitive to AVP) and somatodendritic release of native OT (Chevaleyre et al., 2000).

The somatodendritic release of OT not only activates action potential firing, it is also determinant for the maturation of glutamatergic synaptic activity and of the neuronal morphology. Indeed at birth, supraoptic neurons display an oblong soma from which 2-3 dendrites with few proximal branches arise (Chevaleyre et al., 2001). However, during PW2, the interplay between incoming glutamatergic inputs and autocontrol induces an intense sprouting of dendritic branches (Chevaleyre et al., 2002), as if neurons were exploring the environment to establish new connections. This sprouting is transient and the neurons acquire their mature morphology (Randle et al., 1986) by the end of PW2. Although partial and concerning only SON OT neurons, these data point to a determinant role of autocontrol of OT neurons during PW2 in rats. This information should be taken into account in our understanding of how OT treatments during infancy can have lifelong consequences on OT-related social diseases (see the chapter below).

ESTABLISHMENT OF OT CIRCUITRY

Since neuroendocrinology was established as a new discipline, it has been clearly demonstrated that magnocellular (both OT and AVP) neurons of adult vertebrate species, including mammals, are primarily projecting to the posterior pituitary lobe to release these hormones into the systemic blood stream (Knobloch and Grinevich, 2014 and references therein). However, embryogenesis of pituitary OT projections remains unexplored. In fact, only two studies demonstrate such projection in rats without discrimination between OT and AVP components. The first study by the Ann-Judith Silverman group (Silverman et al., 1980) showed the existence of neurophysin-positive (i.e. without

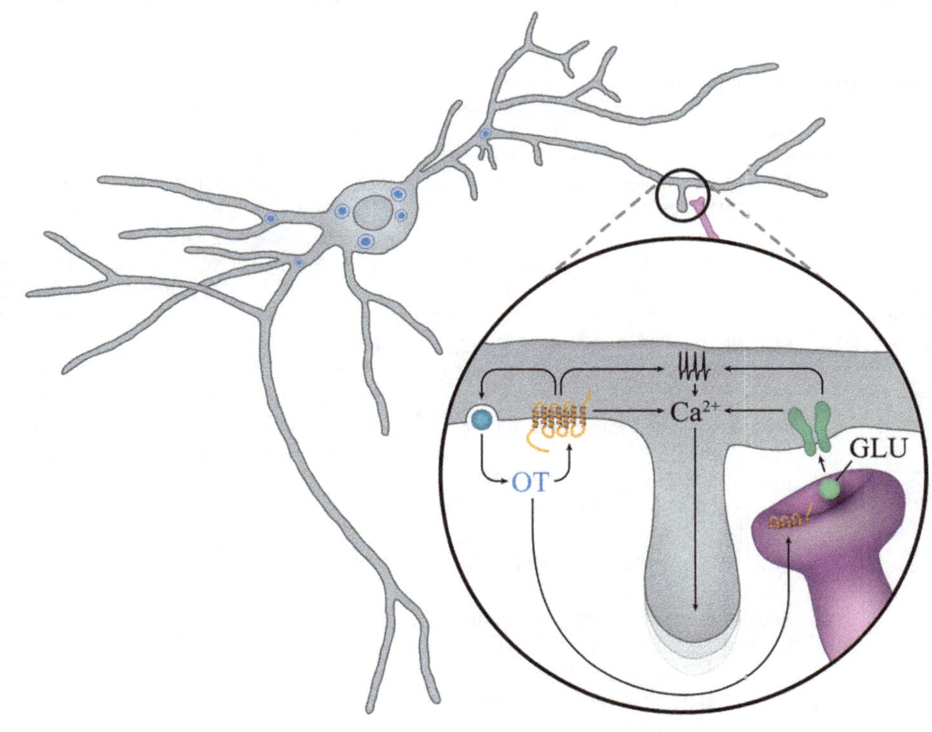

FIGURE 3 | "Auto-control" of OT neurons in early postnatal ontogenesis. In the rat SON during the second PN week, locally released OT promotes calcium mobilization and OT release, and favors the maturation of glutamatergic inputs. Activation of NMDA and OTR increases electrical activity and mobilization of calcium from intracellular stores and promotes growth of new dendritic branches.

discrimination between OT and AVP) fibers in the posterior pituitary. Another study by the Michael Ugrumov and André Calas groups (Makarenko et al., 2000, 2002), employing DiI-based retrograde tracing in fixed brains, showed certain dynamics of these projections: first connections between the main part of the SON and pituitary are established earlier (detected at E15—earliest time point of the experiment), while the PVN and retrochiasmatic parts of the SON project to the pituitary later—at E17 (Makarenko et al., 2000). Intriguingly, the AN, composed mostly of OT neurons, projects to the pituitary only after birth (Makarenko et al., 2002).

Remarkable work on zebra fish larvae showed that OT is essential for the formation of an effective neurovascular interface (i.e., contacts of axonal OT terminals with fenestrated capillaries in the posterior pituitary; Gutnick et al., 2011). Unfortunately, such observation has not been extended to mice lacking OT or OTR, in which the analysis of the pituitary structure has not been reported.

Although central projections of OT neurons in adult rodents (mice, rats, and voles) have been significantly explored during last years (Ross et al., 2009; Knobloch et al., 2012; Dölen et al., 2013), the literature lacks reports on embryogenesis and early postnatal development of OT projections. This concerns both ascending projections of magnocellular OT neurons to the forebrain and descending projections of parvocellular OT neurons terminating in the brain stem and spinal cord.

The major inputs carrying visceral sensory information to the SON and PVN are relayed by catecholaminergic and non-catecholaminergic (glucagon-like peptide 1) neurons whose soma are located in the nucleus of the solitary tract and ventrolateral medulla. Both direct and indirect arguments indicate that these afferents are not functional at birth and develop during the first postnatal week (see review by Rinaman, 2007). Similarly, although no anatomical studies on the dynamics of innervation of OT neurons by glutamate and GABA have been performed, electrophysiological data summarized above suggest long-term postnatal maturation of synaptic inputs.

THE DEVELOPMENTAL TRAJECTORIES OF OT RECEPTOR EXPRESSION

The developmental trajectories of OT receptor (OTR) expression in the nervous system have been investigated in mice, rats, voles and humans by different experimental approaches such as autoradiography, *in situ* hybridization and transcriptomic analysis, which provide complementary information. While autoradiography maps high affinity OTR at subcellular sites, which grossly correspond to receptor site(s) of activity on neuronal cell bodies and processes, *in situ* hybridization maps the neuronal bodies in which OTR mRNA accumulates. Transcriptomic analysis provides clues on brain regions actively synthesizing OTR mRNA without giving details on the cell types and subpopulations involved (see **Table 2** for the available literature).

Among mammalian species, the rat has been by far the most extensively investigated. In this animal, the three aforementioned techniques resulted in highly comparable and consistent results, which made it possible to trace a developmental trajectory of OTR ontogenesis. This has been schematically summarized in **Table 3** and **Figure 4** (Shapiro and Insel, 1989; Snijdewint et al., 1989;

Table 2 | Studies of OTR trajectories in development.

Mice	Rats	Voles	Human
Method: autoradiography (^{125}I-OTA) Age: E18.5, P0, PN7, PN14, PN21, PN35, PN60 Subject: all embryos and brain (Hammock and Levitt, 2013) Method: transcriptomic analysis Age: PN4, PN6, PN8, PN10, PN14, P180 Subject: primary somatosensory cortex (Fertuzinhos et al., 2014; http://hbatlas.org/mouseNCXtranscriptome/)	Method: autoradiography (^{125}I-OTA) Age: PN1, PN5, PN10, PN14, PN18, PN24, PN60 Subject: brain (Shapiro and Insel, 1989) Method: autoradiography (^{125}I-OTA) Age: E12, E14, E16, E18, E20, PN1, PN3, PN5, PN10, PN13, PN16, PN19, PN22, PN25, PN30, PN35, PN40, PN45, PN60, PN90 Subject: brain and spinal cord (Tribollet et al., 1989) Method: autoradiography (^{125}I-OTA) Age: E12, E14, E16, E18, E20, PN1, PN3, PN5, PN10, PN13, PN16, PN19, PN22, PN25, PN30, PN35, PN40, PN45, PN60, PN90 Subject: forebrain (Lukas et al., 2010) Method: autoradiography (^{3}H-OT) Age: E20, PN1, PN5, PN15 Subject: brain (Snijdewint et al., 1989) Method: *In situ* hybridization Age: E9, E13, E14, E15, E17, E20, PN1, PN3, PN7, PN13, PN14, PN22, PN50 Subject: brain and spinal cord (Yoshimura et al., 1996)	Method: autoradiography (^{125}I-OTA) Age: PN1, 1 week, 2 weeks, 3 weeks, 3 months Subject: lateral septum (Wang and Young, 1997) Method: autoradiography (^{125}I-OTA) Age: PN6, PN9, PN12, PN15, PN18, PN21, PN60 Subject: forebrain (Prounis and Ophir, 2013)	Method: transcriptomic analysis Age: 15 different periods of life from early embryonic (10-13PCW) to late adulthood (60Y+) Subject: Cerebellar cortex, mediodorsal nucleus of the thalamus, striatum, amygdala, hippocampus and 11 areas of neocortex (Kang et al., 2011)

Table 3 | Brain structures expressing OTR in different periods of prenatal and early postnatal life in rats.

Expression pattern	Structure
Appearance in prenatal and/or early postnatal life and permanence to adult life	Dorsal nucleus of the vagus nerve Anterior olfactory nucleus Amygdaloid complex Nucleus accumbens° Dorsal peduncular cortex Lateral septum CA1 subfield of the hippocampus Ventral tegmental area Bed nucleus of the stria terminalis* Hypothalamic ventromedial nucleus* Ventral subiculum
Transient expression in prenatal and/or early postnatal life	Parietal cortex Cingulate cortex Retrosplenial cerebral cortex Mammillary complex Dorsal subiculum Caudate putamen Anterior and paraventricular thalamic nuclei Reticular nucleus Substantia gelatinosa of the V nerve Nucleus of the hypoglossus
Expression in late postnatal life	Olfactory tuberculum (Calleja islands) Ventral pallidum

° In the adult, binding in the accumbens has been reported to almost completely disappear (Tribollet et al., 1989) or to be greatly reduced as compared to its pick at PN20 (Shapiro and Insel, 1989).

**The appearance of OTR in the hypothalamic ventromedial nucleus has been reported to appear at PN1 (Tribollet et al., 1989) or to emerge only in the adult brain (Shapiro and Insel, 1989).*

Tribollet et al., 1989; Yoshimura et al., 1996; Lukas et al., 2010; Workman et al., 2013). Throughout the embryonic development and the first post-natal days, OTR progressively appears in several brain regions, reaching a well-defined "infant" pattern of distribution around PN10. After PN13, an abrupt decline of OTR density is observed in several areas, accompanied by expression in novel brain regions; this phase has been referred to as the first transition to the adult pattern and is basically completed at PN18. Around and after weaning, a second transition occurs, characterized by a novel reshaping of OTR expression, which slowly disappears from some areas and increases in others. Finally, the adult pattern of OTR expression is achieved at P60-90. Brain structures expressing OTR in different periods of prenatal and early postnatal life in rats (according to Shapiro and Insel, 1989; Tribollet et al., 1989; Lukas et al., 2010) are reported in **Table 3**.

OTR appears as early as E14 pcd is the posterior portion of the neuronal tube that will become the vagal motor nucleus. Even though the mature OT is not detected until much later in development (see above), immature C-terminal extended forms of OT have been visualized much earlier (E16 pcd, see above). It is thus tempting to speculate that some immature OT forms may have an unrecognized role during early development in the vagal subregion. Mechanistically, the delivery of immature OT to the vagal nucleus can be achieved either via the neuropeptide diffusion through the brain tissue after somatodendritic release or via the transventricular pathway (Knobloch and Grinevich, 2014).

Strongly labeled areas of the "infant pattern" around PN10, schematically reported in **Figure 4B**, include the anterior olfactory nucleus, caudate putamen, accumbens, cingulate cortex, bed nucleus of the stria terminalis, some septal, thalamic and amygdaloid nuclei and the dorsal peduncular cortex. A faint but specific signal is observed at this stage in the hypothalamic ventral medial nucleus, a region that will become strongly labeled in the adult brain, while binding in the lateral septum and bed nucleus of the stria terminalis will undergo an intra-regional reshaping during post-natal development. Of relevance, between PN10 and PN25, is the disappearance of binding in the dorsal subiculum, accompanied by the concomitant appearance of increasingly strong binding in the ventral subiculum. During the same period, binding drops in the thalamus, cingulate cortex and CA1 but increases sharply in the accumbens, where it peaks at PN20 to subsequently decline during the second phase of transition to the adult brain. Changes in selected brain regions between week 5 and week 8 have been reported, such as an increase in OTR binding in the ventromedial hypothalamus and a decrease in the lateral septum (Lukas et al., 2010). However, a detailed, comprehensive study of OTR expression trajectories around weaning in males and females is, at present, missing.

Unfortunately, the studies available in literature for mice, voles and humans do not allow for similar comprehensive compilation of OTR expression trajectories during development. Nevertheless, a recent autoradiography study in mice revealed that region-specific trajectories of OTR expression are present in this species as well (Hammock and Levitt, 2013). A qualitative inspection of OTR binding from P0 to PN60 outlined a progressive strong increase of OTR from P0 to PN14, followed by region-specific up and down regulation of receptor expression. Different temporal expression profiles were reported in the three areas of the brain in which the OTR binding profile was quantified (hippocampus, lateral septum, and neocortex) with no significant differences between sexes. A very high degree of individual variability in OTR expression during ontogenesis was also reported in prairie voles, hampering the detailed delineation of developmental trajectories in this species; however as observed in mice and rats, a higher density of OTR was observed in some forebrain regions (the septo-hippocampal nucleus and the hippocampus) between PN6 and PN21 as compared to PN1 and PN60 (Prounis and Ophir, 2013). Similarly, in the lateral septum, OTR density increased during the post-natal age, reaching the adult level at weaning; in particular, the binding increased more rapidly in mountain than in prairie voles, resulting in species differences at weaning and adulthood (Wang and Young, 1997). Finally, it is worth noting that in the different species, the overall pattern of the OTR expression during development does not match completely. The

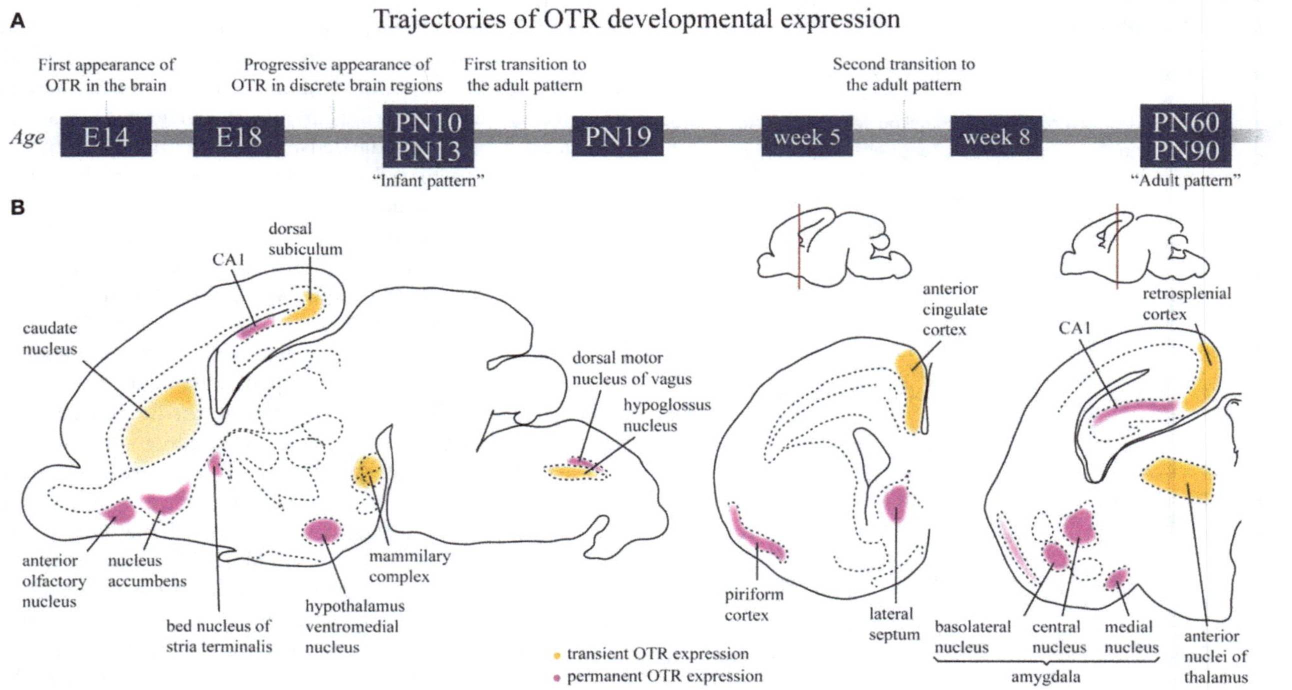

FIGURE 4 | Developmental trajectories of OTR in the rat brain. **(A)** Schematic time course of OTR expression in the developing brain. **(B)** OTR expression in the infant brain around P10–P13. Regions in which a transient OTR expression is observed are colored in yellow; regions in which OTR expression is maintained to adult life are colored in magenta.

strong transient expression of OTR in the neocortex reported in mice was suggested to account for a species-specific role played by OTR during brain development (Hammock and Levitt, 2013). However, it should be mentioned that a transient OTR expression in the parietal cortex has also been reported in the rat brain (Snijdewint et al., 1989).

As in humans, the transcriptomic analysis of OTR reported a progressive increase in OTR mRNA during embryonic life in five out of six brain areas analyzed (Kang et al., 2011 and http://hbatlas.org/). Remarkably, the receptor level appeared to reach a maximum already before birth and to remain quite stable thereafter, at least in the first 5 years of life, although with some wide individual variations.

An important consideration when comparing developmental trajectories in translational medicine approaches is that the neurodevelopmental stage of the human brain at birth corresponds to rat and mouse brain at PN10 (Workman et al., 2013 and related web tool at http://www.translatingtime.net/home). Consistently, the human infant pattern of OTR expression is achieved before parturition while, in the rat, the infant pattern of OTR expression is achieved around PN10, and, in mice, between PN7 and PN14. To extrapolate the effects of pharmacological and environmental manipulation of the OT/OTR system in the human newborn brain from experiments performed in mice and rats, treatments should thus be performed in rodents around PN10, when a comparable maturation of the brain and of the OTR system has been reached in these species.

Several environmental factors have been reported to affect OTR expression in embryogenesis and early postnatal life, among which a predominant role is played by social and sensorial experiences, as more extensively discussed in the next paragraph. Furthermore, exposure to drugs and toxic agents can also modulate the OT/OTR system, as outlined by the interesting finding that nicotine and ethanol administration to pregnant rats increases OTR binding in the nucleus accumbens and in the CA3 region of the hippocampus of male offspring (Williams et al., 2009). Recently, an up-regulation of OTR in the nucleus accumbens, medial anterior olfactory nucleus and central and medial nuclei of amygdala has been reported in μ-opioid receptor knock out mice (Gigliucii et al., 2014), which suggests a close link between OTR expression and the opioid reward system.

OT AND SOCIAL EXPERIENCE IN DEVELOPMENT

Effects of OT during embryogenesis and early postnatal ontogenesis on social life are extensively summarized in recent reviews (Carter, 2014; Hammock, 2014), but the reverse—i.e., the effects of social stimuli on maturation of OT system—are less explored. It has been reported that early social experience tremendously affects physiology of the OT system (Bales and Perkeybile, 2012; Hammock, 2014). Recently it has been demonstrated that early sensory experience (in the newborn) regulates development of sensory cortices via OT-signaling (Zheng et al., 2014).

This oxytocin early regulation may have long-term consequences in adults. It has been known for many years that exogenous OT in neonates can revert the long-term behavioral effects of prenatal stress (Lee et al., 2007b) and has consequences on other endocrine systems (i.e., the estrogen receptor, Pournajafi-Nazarloo et al., 2007) as well as on blood pressure (Holst et al., 2002) in adults. The effects of OT, or of the environmental and familial circumstances resulting in increased production of mature neonatal OT, on adult social behavior mainly remain to be investigated. With respect to OTR expression, increased levels have been observed in offspring after communal rearing (Curley et al., 2012), increased maternal licking/grooming (Champagne et al., 2001) and social enrichment (Champagne and Meaney, 2007). On the contrary, late weaning has been reported to reduce OTR density in selected, socially relevant, brain regions (Curley et al., 2009). Furthermore, maternal separation has been found to induce a complex modulation of OTR expression with region-specific up and down regulation of OTR (Lukas et al., 2010). It is important to note, at the end of this section, that exploration of early life experience on OT/OTR system in animals provides a scientific basis for child care and new therapeutical approaches to ameliorating social alterations occurring in adult patients afflicted with Autism Spectrum Disorders or the PWS (see below).

OT AND DEVELOPMENTAL NEUROLOGICAL DISORDERS

Many reviews are exhaustive on the involvement of OT in shaping and regulating the social brain (Meyer-Lindenberg et al., 2011; Striepens et al., 2011; McCall and Singer, 2012) or in learning and memory (Chini et al., 2014). The strongest line of demonstration of the OT system in social behavior, feeding behavior and maternal care is via the study of knockout mice in which either the *OT* or the *OTR* genes are inactivated (**Table 4**). Mice constitutively lacking OT ($Oxt^{-/-}$) are unable to release milk and have impaired social memory (Ferguson et al., 2000). Mice with constitutive ablation of the OTR gene ($Oxtr^{-/-}$) display a behavior very similar to the $Oxt^{-/-}$ mouse, mainly marked by social deficits (Takayanagi et al., 2005). In addition, although learning is normal in *Oxtr-/-* mice, reversal learning is strongly decreased, indicating impaired cognitive flexibility reminiscent of the ASD syndrome (Sala et al., 2011). Importantly, even a 50% loss of the OTRs also leads to an impairment of social behavior, suggesting that a fine tuning of the OT system is necessary to control behavior (Sala et al., 2013). Other mouse models, in which the knock-out of a specific gene induced a disruption in the OT system that has been linked to a pathological phenotype, reinforce the role of OT in neurodevelopmental disorders (**Table 4**). Recently, it has been shown that disruption of the neonatal surge of OT coming from the mother during delivery results in autistic-like features in the adults (Tyzio et al., 2014). All these data suggest that an early postnatal injury or dysfunction of the OT system has consequences in infant and adult behaviors. Unfortunately, the contribution of early life experience to OT signaling, in a pathological context or following a trauma, has not been extensively studied in the brain of highly social mammalian species such as voles or monkeys. A limited number of reports (Bales et al., 2007, 2011; Ahern and Young, 2009) demonstrated that social deprivation and enrichment paradigms induce changes in OT synthesis and OTR binding in voles (Bales et al., 2007, 2011; Ahern and Young, 2009). While it is not yet clear how these changes occur, the most likely scenario is the environmental influence on the gene expression through epigenetic mechanisms.

In humans, autistic spectrum disorder (ASD) is a broadly-defined disorder that mainly affects behavior and cognition. Social interaction impairments are the most characteristic deficits in ASD. Interestingly, several lines of evidence suggest a role of OT in the etiology of ASD (Harony and Wagner, 2010; LoParo and

Table 4 | OT and neurodevelopmental disorders.

Alteration	Mouse models	Human (early neurodevelopmental disorders)
Feeding problems: Early impairment of feeding (suckling activity) Obesity	*Magel2* KO (Schaller et al., 2010) *Oxt*-KO (Camerino, 2009) *Oxt*-KO (Takayanagi et al., 2008) *Sim1*-KO (heterozygotes) (Kublaoui et al., 2008)	Prader-Willi syndrome (McAllister et al., 2011; Miller et al., 2011) Autistic patients with *MAGEL2* mutations (Schaaf et al., 2013)
Social and emotional defects ASD	*Oxtr*-KO (Takayanagi et al., 2005; Sala et al., 2011, 2013) *Oxt*-KO (Ferguson et al., 2000) *CD38*-KO (Jin et al., 2007) BTBR T+ tf/J (Silverman et al., 2010) *Magel2* KO (FM, submitted) *FraX* KO (Mineur et al., 2006; Pietropaolo et al., 2011; Francis et al., 2014) *MageD1*-KO (Dombret et al., 2012) Haploinsufficient *reeler* (Liu et al., 2005)	ASD (Li et al., 2012; Aoki et al., 2014; LoParo and Waldman, 2014) Prader-Willi syndrome (Swaab et al., 1995; Dykens et al., 2011; Tauber et al., 2011) Williams syndrome (Dai et al., 2012; Jarvinen and Bellugi, 2013) Autistic patients with *MAGEL2* mutations (Schaaf et al., 2013)
Maternal care and/or social development of the progeny	*Oxt*-KO (Winslow et al., 2000) *CD38*-KO (Liu et al., 2008) *Oxtr*-KO (Higashida et al., 2010; Rilling and Young, 2014) *Peg3*-KO (Champagne et al., 2009)	*OTR* risk allele *CD38* risk allele (Feldman et al., 2012; Rilling and Young, 2014)
Neurodegenerative diseases	*CD157(BST1)* KO Lopatina et al., 2014	No clear data

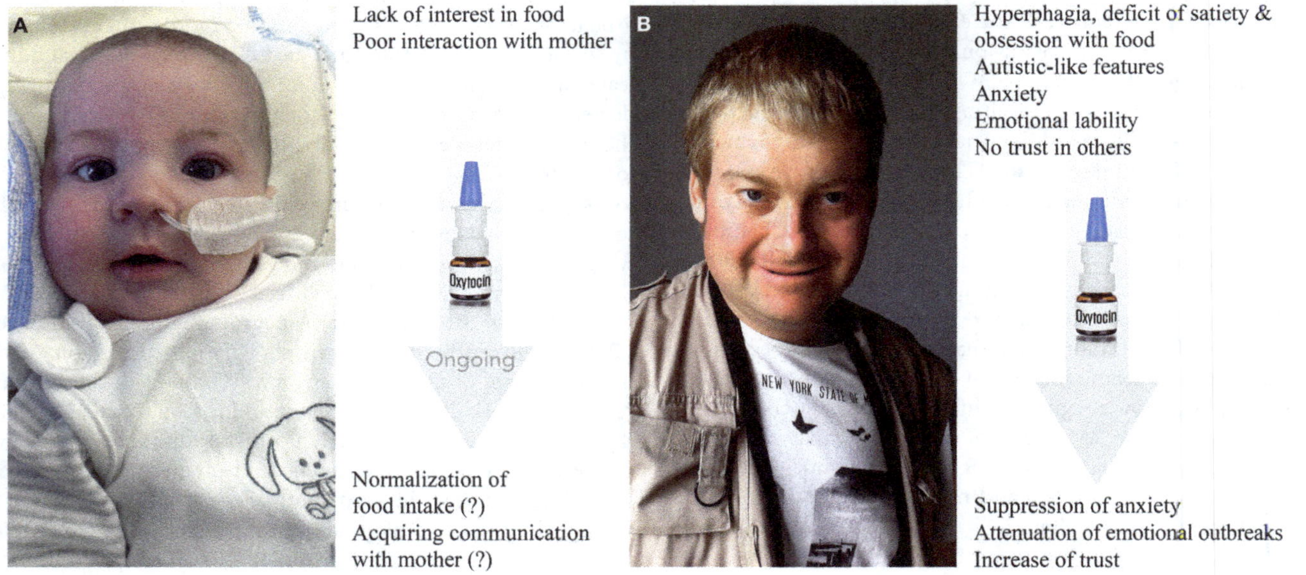

FIGURE 5 | Prader-Willi syndrome: clinical features and effects of OT. **(A)** Three-month-old baby born at term has symptoms of hypotonia, deficit of suckling and poor interest in food. Nasogastric tube, which is shown in the photo, is used in almost all PWS neonates to prevent failure to thrive for a mean of 1 month. Baby also exhibits facial dysmorphism, such as almond-shaped eyes, thin upper lip, down-turned corner of the mouth, narrow bi-frontal diameter and slight facial assymetria. Behaviorally, the baby shows low interest in mother and poor social skills in general. Ongoing treatment with OT shows positive trends in both stimulation of food intake and social bonding with the mother (further confirmation is needed). **(B)** Twenty-three-year-old male patient has a record of hyperphagia, deficit of satiety, obsession with food, dysmorphic features (scoliosis, kyphosis), autistic-like features (stereotype and repetitive movements, deficit of social skills and poor trust in others), anxiety, emotional liability (including emotional outbreaks), creation of stories filled with fantasies (termed as "fabulation") and compulsive skin picking. The patient is under psychotropic treatments. First applications of OT seem to result in increase of trust, decrease in anxiety and attenuation of emotional outbreaks (further confirmation is needed). Photos are reproduced here with permission of Prof. Maithé Tauber.

Waldman, 2014) and OT's therapeutic effects have been observed in social communication (Aoki et al., 2014), however, they are still debated (Guastella et al., 2014). Furthermore, it is also acknowledged that an alteration in the OT-system might be involved in neurodevelopmental disorders marked by social cue deficits such as Fragile X Syndrome, Williams Syndrome and PWS (see **Table 3** and Francis et al., 2014).

PWS is one of the best reported examples of a neurodevelopmental disease characterized mainly as an eating disorder with behavioral and social disturbances (**Figure 5**; Butler et al., 2011; Dykens et al., 2011; McAllister et al., 2011; Cassidy et al., 2012; Jauregi et al., 2013). PWS is a rare genetic disease with an estimated prevalence worldwide of 1 in 10,000–30,000 individuals (Cassidy et al., 2012). Patients with PWS exhibit a complex and progressive phenotype. Their eating behavior is mainly characterized by two opposite stages (Butler et al., 2010; Miller et al., 2011). During phase I of the syndrome, apparent at birth, the suckling activity is weak or absent and babies show little interest in feeding during the first few months of their lives. After 2 years, it is characterized by a true hyperphagia with obesity. In fact, PWS children initially display anorexia as neonates and then switch to hyperphagia with obesity (Tauber et al., 2014).

In parallel with the eating problem, PWS patients have mild to moderate intellectual disability and behavioral alterations (Ho and Dimitropoulos, 2010; Chevalere et al., 2013), including emotional outbreaks (temper tantrums) and compulsive traits (Dimitropoulos et al., 2006). Repetitive and ritualistic behaviors and difficulty with routine changes (Holland et al., 2003; Greaves et al., 2006; Dykens et al., 2011), similar to those found in autistic spectrum conditions, have also been described. Indeed all PW patients share some features of ASD (Koenig et al., 2004). Some patients, who are diagnosed as autists, share some features observed in PWS and are defined as PWS-like patients (Schaaf et al., 2013).

Nevertheless, only a few patients with PWS are diagnosed as autists. Patients with PWS present greater overall behavior disturbance than age-matched mentally retarded patients, but score comparably to patients with psychiatric disorders. Indeed, they frequently display anxiety traits and anxious mood comparable to those of patients presenting anxiety disorder or schizophrenia. They also show pronounced emotional liability and a striking inability to control their emotions, which results in frequent emotional outbreaks (temper tantrums), which can occur due to an impaired capacity to understand the motivations of others in the social environment, possibly indicating deficits in "theory of mind" (the ability to attribute mental states to others) and empathy (the ability to infer emotional experiences) (Lo et al., 2013). Importantly, Tauber et al. (2011) reported the first clinical trial on OT that showed that a single intranasal administration of OT rescue some behavioral features, such as increased trust and decreased signs of depression as well as emotional outbreaks, in patients with PWS (**Figure 5**). However, a double-blind randomized cross-over trial of OT nasal spray performed in 22 PWS patients (12–29 years old) did not find statistically significant effects using 18–40 IU of intranasal OT twice daily for 8 weeks (Einfeld et al., 2014). The authors reported an increased number of temper tantrums in the patients receiving the high dose of OT and no effect was observed in patients treated with low doses. The discrepancies between these two studies may be explained by the dose used, the short wash-out period (15 days), the duration of treatment and the sex ratio (most patients were male in the report of Einfeld and colleagues compared to the report of Tauber's team).

Much of the phenotype of PWS is consistent with a hypothalamic defect (Swaab et al., 1995; Swaab, 1997a,b) characterized by a reduction of OT expressing neurons in the PVN, mostly represented by parvocellular OT neurons (Swaab et al., 1995; Swaab, 1997a,b). These cells project to the brainstem nuclei, including the nucleus of the solitary tract, where OT acts as a powerful anorexic peptide (Atasoy et al., 2012). Normal OT plasma levels have been detected in 17 PWS adult patients (Höybye et al., 2003), but elevated cerebrospinal fluid (CSF) OT levels have been reported in five PWS patients (Martin et al., 1998). This high level of OT in the CSF most likely relies on OT released from magnocellular neurons, contacting both the vasculature of the posterior pituitary and the lumen of the third ventricle (Knobloch and Grinevich, 2014). However, such discrepancy between OT released into the blood and CSF needs further clarification, especially with respect to methodological limitations for measuring OT in biological samples (McCullough et al., 2013).

Genetically, PWS results from the lack of expression of several contiguous imprinted genes located in the 15q11–q13 region. These genes are regulated by genomic imprinting: a mechanism leading to the transcriptional expression of the paternal alleles of these genes only, the maternal alleles being silent (i.e., not expressed). Recently, pathogenic mutations of *MAGEL2* alone have been reported in four patients (Schaaf et al., 2013), causing a classical PWS in one patient and PWS-like phenotypes in the other three. All of the cases described were also diagnosed with early feeding problems and ASD, without severe obesity. These results underline *MAGEL2's* contributing role in cognitive and behavioral alterations in PWS and early feeding in general.

Francoise Muscatelli's group created a mouse model deficient for *Magel2*. These mice showed an altered onset of suckling activity and subsequent impaired feeding leading to 50% of neonatal lethality, affecting both males and females (Schaller et al., 2010). Impressively, there is an obvious alteration of production of mature OT in the PVN of *Magel2*-deficient pups, while a single administration of OT, in a restricted time window after birth, allows resetting of the feeding behavior and consequently rescues the life of all pups (Schaller et al., 2010, p. 24). Furthermore, inactivation of *Magel2* induces in adult males (but not in females) a deficit in social recognition and social interaction as well as a reduced learning ability with an alteration of social and spatial memory. A daily administration of oxytocin (OT) in the first week of life is sufficient to restore suckling activity at birth and to restore a normal social behavior and learning abilities in adult mutant males (Meziane et al., in press).

Altogether, these results suggest that an alteration of the OT system around birth has early and long term consequences on feeding and social behaviors and on cognition. Importantly, an OT treatment of Magel2-deficient pups in the first post-natal week partially restores a normal anatomy of the OT system and prevents deficits in social behavior and learning in adults. This concept opens the door to a powerful pharmacological therapy in early infancy for the PWS and might be considered for other pathologies such as autism spectrum disorders. Importantly, a clinical trial on OT treatment of PWS infants has been initiated by Maithé Tauber and her team.

OT PATHWAYS IN PERINATAL ONTOGENESIS: PHYSIOLOGY, PATHOLOGY, AND TREATMENT

While the picture of OT pathways development is far from complete, at least three conclusions can be made (see **Figure 6**):

1) OT neurons start to produce a mature form of OT in rodents much later than other neurons express AVP and hypophyseotrophic neuropeptides (Markakis and Swanson, 1997; Markakis, 2002). In fact, in mice, the mature form of OT appears on the day of delivery, suggesting that maternal OT can promote synthesis of mature OT in newborns.
2) OT neurons (magnocellular) at birth have immature morphological ("spindle-like morphology") and physiological properties (including intrinsic electrophysiological properties and synaptic inputs). Furthermore, many OT neurons project axons to the posterior pituitary only after birth (Makarenko et al., 2002) and no collaterals of OT axons have been reported in extrahypothalamic brain regions of neonates in contrast to those in adult rodents (Knobloch and Grinevich, 2014).
3) OT receptors are widely expressed in the brain well before the synthesis of mature OT, suggesting their receptivity either for immature forms of OT, maternal OT, maternal/neonatal AVP or uncharacterized peptides. During maturation of the system (i.e., postweaning period > P60), the expression of OTR is restricted to several brain regions, most of which are innervated by OT axons at this age (Knobloch et al., 2012; Dölen et al., 2013).

The delayed maturation of the central OT system in rodents (and humans) may be caused or may correlate with the feature of these species, which are born relatively immature (termed "altricial" species). From a comparative point of view, it would be interesting to compare the dynamics of OT system maturation with the animals which are relatively mature and mobile from the moment of birth (termed "precocial" species, such as guinea pigs).

Since the distant/extrahypothalamic OT axons during neonatal period in studied (altricial) species are absent (at least not reported), but OT neurons were responsive to externally applied OT, it is most likely that neonate rodents operate by endogenous OT released from somato-dendritic compartments of OT cells. While PVN OT cells are closely located to the ependymal layer of the third ventricle, OT may diffuse also to the cerebrospinal fluid, resembling the evolutionarily old "transventricular" pathway of OT action (Knobloch and Grinevich, 2014). Moreover, OT can

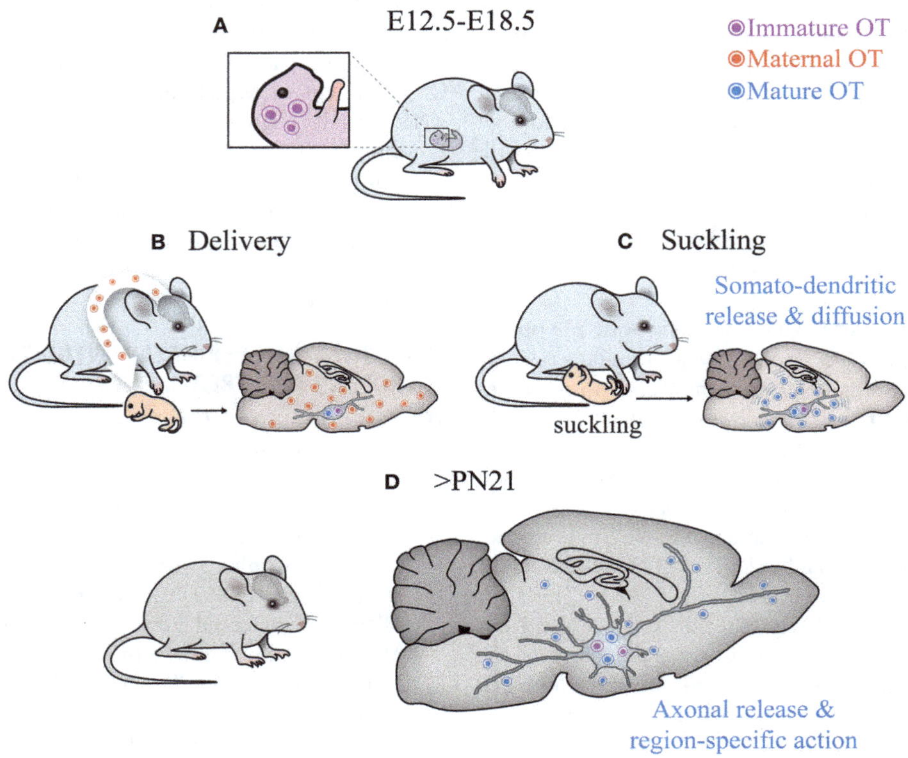

FIGURE 6 | Central OT pathways in development. (A) The hypothalamus of embryos produces immature OT. **(B)** After birth, the cells start to generate mature (amidated) OT. Although it is unclear why this switch occurs, the fact that it happens after parturition suggests that perinatal maternal OT (of extremely high concentrations!), passing via the placental barrier (Malek et al., 1996) to the hypothalamus of newborns, may initiate the activation respective enzyme (see **Figure 2**) and, hence, appearance of the mature form of OT. **(C)** After birth, the suckling activity of pups transmitted to the activation of sensory pathways converging on OT neurons, may stimulate somatodendritic OT release. Such mode of release leads to "ubiquitous filling" of the brain with OT. **(D)** Later on, starting from the fourth week, OT neurons establish axonal projections to various brain areas to release OT into selective targets to modulate specific behaviors, especially social behaviors (Knobloch and Grinevich, 2014).

reach the brain directly via brain capillaries, as the blood brain barrier is not formed at that age (Ugrumov, 2010 and references therein), allowing peripherally administered OT to efficiently reach the brain (Meziane et al., in press).

In line with the "diffusion-like" mode of OT action, the report on newborn and young mice (P0–P14; Zheng et al., 2014) showed no axonal projections in the somatosensory cortex, while the effects of OT on electrical activity of cortical neurons as well as on sensory processing were very prominent (Zheng et al., 2014). Keeping this contradiction in mind, the authors speculated about "diffusible" OT reaching the cortex from the hypothalamus. Despite the lack of literature, it is tempting to speculate that magnocellular OT axons will grow to forebrain regions and parvocellular OT neuronal axons to brain stem/spinal cord only after weaning, to execute addressed OT release aimed to orchestrate autonomic and behavioral responses respectively (see above).

Animal models of social deficiency (such as OT and OTR knockout mice) and human cases of OTR gene duplication (Bittel et al., 2006) support the critical role of neonatal OT signaling in the development of an adequate social skill. The model of PWS—Magel2 knockout mice has pronounced OT deficiency with delayed expression of mature OT on the day of birth.

The discovery that peripheral OT administration to neonate Magel2 knockout mice rescues both the feeding problem in neonates and social impairments in adults, gives the reason to dissect alteration in sequences of OT signaling (i.e., in steps of OT expression in OT cells, OT transport via axons and their releasing capacity, expression of OTR etc.), which can be considered as target(s) for exogenous OT. Keeping in mind the potential OT sensitivity of OT neurons, and many other brain cells, as well as long-lasting OT effects, someone may hypothesize that exogenous OT stimulates transcriptional, electric and secretory activity of OT neurons, which start to release larger amounts of OT to fill in the brain. Additionally, upregulation of central OTR expression can facilitate OT signaling. However, the testing of these scenarios requires further comprehensive research.

ACKNOWLEDGMENTS

The preparation of this review was supported by the Chica and Heinz Schaller Research Foundation, German Research Foundation (DFG) grant GR 3619/4-1, SFB 1134, Royal Society Edinburgh Award, and German Academic Exchange service (DAAD) program for partnership between German and Japanese Universities, PHC PROCOP program (DAAD and Campus France) (to Valery Grinevich), Telethon Foundation grant GGP12207 (to Bice Chini), ANR and MESR (to Michel G. Desarménien), INSERM, the European community (grant #512136 PWS), Prader-Willi France (to Maithé Tauber and Françoise Muscatelli) and Fondation Jerôme LeJeune (to Françoise Muscatelli). The authors thank Thomas Splettstoesser (SciStyle; www.scistyle.com), Vivien Chevaleyre, and Muriel Asary for their help with the preparation of Figures and Anne Seller for proof reading the manuscript.

REFERENCES

Adan, R. A., Van Leeuwen, F. W., Sonnemans, M. A., Brouns, M., Hoffman, G., Verbalis, J. G., et al. (1995). Rat oxytocin receptor in brain, pituitary, mammary gland, and uterus: partial sequence and immunocytochemical localization. *Endocrinology* 136, 4022–4028.

Ahern, T. H., and Young, L. J. (2009). The impact of early life family structure on adult social attachment, alloparental behavior, and the neuropeptide systems regulating affiliative behaviors in the monogamous prairie vole (*Microtus ochrogaster*). *Front. Behav. Neurosci.* 3:17. doi: 10.3389/neuro.08.017.2009

Altman, J., and Bayer, S. A. (1978a). Development of the diencephalon in the rat. I. Autoradiographic study of the time of origin and settling patterns of neurons of the hypothalamus. *J. Comp. Neurol.* 182, 945– 971.

Altman, J., and Bayer, S. A. (1978b). Development of the diencephalon in the rat. II. Correlation of the embryonic development of the hypothalamus with the time of origin of its neurons. *J. Comp. Neurol.* 182, 973–993.

Altman, J., and Bayer, S. A. (1978c). Development of the diencephalon in the rat. III. Ontogeny of the specialized ventricular linings of the hypothalamic third ventricle. *J. Comp. Neurol.* 182, 995–1015.

Altstein, M., and Gainer, H. (1988). Differential biosynthesis and posttranslational processing of vasopressin and oxytocin in rat brain during embryonic and postnatal development. *J. Neurosci.* 8, 3967–3977.

Aoki, Y., Yahata, N., Watanabe, T., Takano, Y., Kawakubo, Y., Kuwabara, H., et al. (2014). Oxytocin improves behavioural and neural deficits in inferring others' social emotions in autism. *Brain* 137, 3073–3086. doi: 10.1093/brain/awu231

Atasoy, D., Betley, J. N., Su, H. H., and Sternson, S. M. (2012). Deconstruction of a neural circuit for hunger. *Nature* 488, 172–177. doi: 10.1038/nature11270

Bales, K. L., Boone, E., Epperson, P., Hoffman, G., and Carter, C. S. (2011). Are behavioral effects of early experience mediated by oxytocin? *Front. Psychiatry* 2:24. doi: 10.3389/fpsyt.2011.00024

Bales, K. L., Lewis-Reese, A. D., Pfeifer, L. A., Kramer, K. M., and Carter, C. S. (2007). Early experience affects the traits of monogamy in a sexually dimorphic manner. *Dev. Psychobiol.* 49, 335–342. doi: 10.1002/dev.20216

Bales, K. L., and Perkeybile, A. M. (2012). Developmental experiences and the oxytocin receptor system. *Horm. Behav.* 61, 313–319. doi: 10.1016/j.yhbeh.2011.12.013

Bartz, J., Simeon, D., Hamilton, H., Kim, S., Crystal, S., Braun, A., et al. (2011). Oxytocin can hinder trust and cooperation in borderline personality disorder. *Soc. Cogn. Affect. Neurosci.* 6, 556–563. doi: 10.1093/scan/nsq085

Belenky, M., Castel, M., Young, W. S. 3rd, Gainer, H., and Cohen, S. (1992). Ultrastructural immunolocalization of rat oxytocin-neurophysin in transgenic mice expressing the rat oxytocin gene. *Brain Res.* 583, 279–286. doi: 10.1016/S0006-8993(10)80034-4

Bittel, D. C., Kibiryeva, N., Dasouki, M., Knoll, J. H. M., and Butler, M. (2006). A 9-year old male with duplication of chromosome 3p25.3p26.2: clinical report and gene expression analysis. *Am. J. Med. Gen.* 140A, 573–579. doi: 10.1002/ajmg.a.31132

Blaess, S., Szabo, N., Haddad-Tóvolli, R., Zhou, X., and Alvarez-Bolado, G. (2014). Sonic hedgehog signaling in the development of the mouse hypothalamus. *Front. Neuroanat.* 8:156. doi: 10.3389/fnana.2014.00156

Boer, K., Dogterom, J., and Pronker, H. F. (1980). Pituitary content of oxytocin, vasopressin and alpha-melanocyte-stimulating hormone in the fetus of the rat during labour. *J. Endocrinol.* 86, 221–229. doi: 10.1677/joe.0.0860221

Brooks, L. R., Chung, W. C., and Tsai, P. S. (2010). Abnormal hypothalamic oxytocin system in fibroblast growth factor 8-deficient mice. *Endocrine* 38, 174–180. doi: 10.1007/s12020-010-9366-9

Buijs, R. M., Velis, D. N., and Swaab, D. F. (1980). Ontogeny of vasopressin and oxytocin in the fetal rat: early vasopressinergic innervation of the fetal brain. *Peptides* 1, 315–324. doi: 10.1016/0196-9781(80)90009-1

Butler, M. G., Sturich, J., Lee, J., Myers, S. E., Whitman, B. Y., Gold, J. A., et al. (2011). Growth standards of infants with Prader-Willi syndrome. *Pediatrics* 127, 687–695. doi: 10.1542/peds.2010-2736

Butler, J. V., Whittington, J. E., Holland, A. J., McAllister, C. J., and Goldstone, A. P. (2010). The transition between the phenotypes of Prader-Willi syndrome during infancy and early childhood. *Dev. Med. Child Neurol.* 52, e88–93. doi: 10.1111/j.1469-8749.2009.03530.x

Camerino, C. (2009). Low sympathetic tone and obese phenotype in oxytocin-deficient mice. *Obesity* 17, 980–984. doi: 10.1038/oby.2009.12

Caqueret, A., Boucher, F., and Michaud, J. L. (2006). Laminar organization of the early developing anterior hypothalamus. *Dev. Biol.* 298, 95–106. doi: 10.1016/j.ydbio.2006.06.019

Carrel, A. L., and Allen, D. B. (2000). Effects of growth hormone on adipose tissue. *J. Pediatr. Endocrinol. Metab.* 13, 1003–1009.

Carter, C. S. (2014). Oxytocin pathways and the evolution of human behavior. *Annu. Rev. Psychol.* 65, 17–39. doi: 10.1146/annurev-psych-010213-115110

Cassidy, S. B., Schwartz, S, Miller, J. L., and Driscoll, D. J. (2012). Prader-Willi syndrome. *Gen. Med.* 14, 10–26. doi: 10.1038/gim.0b013e31822bead0

Champagne, F. A., Curley, J. P., Swaney, W. T., Hasen, N. S., and Keverne, E. B. (2009). Paternal influence on female behavior: the role of Peg3 in exploration, olfaction, and neuroendocrine regulation of maternal behavior of female mice. *Behav. Neurosci.* 123, 469–480. doi: 10.1037/a0015060

Champagne, F., Diorio, J., Sharma, S., and Meaney, M. J. (2001). Naturally occurring variations in maternal behavior in the rat are associated with differences in estrogen-inducible central oxytocin receptors. *Proc. Natl. Acad. Sci. U.S.A.* 98, 12736–12741. doi: 10.1073/pnas.221224598

Champagne, F. A., and Meaney, M. J. (2007). Transgenerational effects of social environment on variations in maternal care and behavioral response to novelty. *Behav. Neurosci.* 121, 1353–1363. doi: 10.1037/0735-7044.121.6.1353

Chevalere, J., Postal, V., Jauregui, J., Copet, P., Laurier, V., and Thuilleaux, D. (2013). Assessment of executive functions in Prader-Willi syndrome and relationship with intellectual level. *J. Appl. Res. Intellect. Disabil.* 26, 309–318. doi: 10.1111/jar.12044

Chevaleyre, V., Dayanithi, G., Moos, F. C., and Desarmenien, M. G. (2000). Developmental regulation of a local positive autocontrol of supraoptic neurons. *J. Neurosci.* 20, 5813–5819.

Chevaleyre, V., Moos, F. C., and Desarmenien, M. G. (2001). Correlation between electrophysiological and morphological characteristics during maturation of rat supraoptic neurons. *Eur. J. Neurosci.* 13, 1136–1146. doi: 10.1046/j.0953-816x.2001.01489.x

Chevaleyre, V., Moos, F. C., and Desarmenien, M. G. (2002). Interplay between presynaptic and postsynaptic activities is required for dendritic plasticity and synaptogenesis in the supraoptic nucleus. *J. Neurosci.* 22, 265–273.

Chini, B., Leonzino, M., Braida, D., and Sala, M. (2014). Learning about oxytocin: pharmacologic and behavioral issues. *Biol. Psychiatry* 76, 360–366. doi: 10.1016/j.biopsych.2013.08.029

Crespo, D., Viadero, C. F., Villegas, J., and Lafarga, M. (1988). Nucleoli numbers abd neuronal growth in supraoptic nucleus neurons during postnatal development in the rat. *Dev. Brain Res.* 44, 151–155. doi: 10.1016/0165-3806(88)90126-5

Curley, J. P., Jensen, C. L., Franks, B., and Champagne, F. A. (2012). Variation in maternal and anxiety-like behavior associated with discrete patterns of oxytocin and vasopressin 1a receptor density in the lateral septum. *Horm. Behav.* 61, 454–461. doi: 10.1016/j.yhbeh.2012.01.013

Curley, J. P., Jordan, E. R., Swaney, W. T., Izraelit, A., Kammel, S., and Champagne, F. A. (2009). The meaning of weaning: influence of the weaning period on behavioral development in mice. *Dev. Neurosci.* 31, 318–331. doi: 10.1159/000216543

Dai, L., Carter, C. S., Ying, J., Bellugi, U., Pournajafi-Nazarloo, H., and Korenberg, J. R. (2012). Oxytocin and vasopressin are dysregulated in Williams Syndrome, a genetic disorder affecting social behavior. *PloS ONE* 7:e38513. doi: 10.1371/journal.pone.0038513

De Dreu, C. K., Greer, L. L., Van Kleef, G. A., Shalvi, S., and Handgraaf, M. J. (2011). Oxytocin promotes human ethnocentrism. *Proc. Natl. Acad. Sci. U.S.A.* 108, 1262–1266. doi: 10.1073/pnas.1015316108

Dimitropoulos, A., Blackford, J., Walden, T., and Thompson, T. (2006). Compulsive behavior in Prader-Willi syndrome: examining severity in early childhood. *Res. Dev. Disabil.* 27, 190–202. doi: 10.1016/j.ridd.2005.01.002

Dombret, C., Nguyen, T., Schakman, O., Michaud, J. L., Hardin-Pouzet, H., Bertrand, M. J., et al. (2012). Loss of Maged1 results in obesity, deficits of social interactions, impaired sexual behavior and severe alteration of mature oxytocin production in the hypothalamus. *Hum. Mol. Gen.* 21, 4703–4717. doi: 10.1093/hmg/dds310

Dongen, V. P. A. M., and Nieuwenhuys, R. (1989). "Diencephalon," in *The Central Nervous System of Vertebrates*, Vol. 3, eds J. L. Dubbeldam, P. A. M. Van Dongen, and J. Voogd (Berlin; Heidelberg; New York; Tokyo: Springer-Verlag), 1844–1871.

Dölen, G., Darvishzadeh, A., Huang, K. W., and Malenka, R. C. (2013). Social reward requires coordinated activity of nucleus acumbens oxytocin and serotonin. *Nature* 501, 179–184. doi: 10.1038/nature12518

Dörner, G., and Staudt, J. (1972). Vergleichende morphologische Untersuchugen der Hypothalamusdifferenzierung bei Ratte und Mensch. *Endocrinologie* 59, S152–155.

Dykens, E. M., Lee, E., and Roof, E. (2011). Prader-Willi syndrome and autism spectrum disorders: an evolving story. *J. Neurodev. Disord.* 3, 225–237. doi: 10.1007/s11689-011-9092-5

Einfeld, S. L., Smith, E., McGregor, I. S., Steinbeck, K., Taffe, J., Rice, L. J., et al. (2014). A double-blind randomized controlled trial of oxytocin nasal spray in Prader Willi syndrome. *Am. J. Med. Genet.* 164A. 2232–2239. doi: 10.1002/ajmg.a.36653

Feldman, R., Zagoory-Sharon, O., Weisman, O., Schneiderman, I., Gordon, I., Maoz, R., et al. (2012). Sensitive parenting is associated with plasma oxytocin and polymorphisms in the OXTR and CD38 genes. *Biol. Psychiatry* 72, 175–181. doi: 10.1016/j.biopsych.2011.12.025

Ferguson, J. N., Young, L. J., Hearn, E. F., Matzuk, M. M., Insel, T. R., and Winslow, J. T. (2000). Social amnesia in mice lacking the oxytocin gene. *Nat. Gen.* 25, 284–288. doi: 10.1038/77040

Fertuzinhos, S., Li, M., Kawasawa, Y. I., Ivic, V., Franjic, D., Singh, D., et al. (2014). Laminar and temporal expression dynamics of coding and noncoding RNAs in the mouse neocortex. *Cell Rep.* 13, 938–950. doi: 10.1016/j.celrep.2014.01.036

Fields, R. L., Ponzio, T. A., Kaeasaki, M., and Gainer, H. (2012). Cell-type specific oxytocin gene expression from adeno-associated virus delivered promoter deletion constructs into the rat supraoptic nucleus *in vivo*. *PLoS ONE* 7:e32085. doi: 10.1371/annotation/2d183615-8b34-4ea4-ae9b-9833d6079d11

Francis, S. M., Sagar, A., Levin-Decanini, T., Liu, W., Carter, C. S., and Jacob, S. (2014). Oxytocin and vasopressin systems in genetic syndromes and neurodevelopmental disorders. *Brain Res.* 1580, 199–218. doi: 10.1016/j.brainres.2014.01.021

Freund-Mercier, M. J., Stoeckel, M. E., Palacios, J. M., Pazos, A., Reichhart, J. M., Porte, A., et al. (1987). Pharmacological characteristics and anatomical distribution of [3H]oxytocin-binding sites in the Wistar rat brain studied by autoradiography. *Neuroscience* 20, 599–614. doi: 10.1016/0306-4522(87)90113-8

Gainer, H. (2012). Cell-type specific expression of oxytocin and vasopressin genes: an experimental Odyssey. *J. Neuroendocrinol.* 24, 528–538. doi: 10.1111/j.1365-2826.2011.02236.x

Gigliucii, V., Leonzino, M., Busnelli, M., Luchetti, A., Palladino, V. S., Amato, F. R., et al. (2014). Region specific up-regulation of oxytocin receptors in the Oprm1-/- mouse model of autism. *Front. Pediatrics* 2:91. doi: 10.3389/fped.2014.00091

Goudsmit, E., Neijmeijer-Leloux, A., and Swaab, D. F. (1992). The human hypothalamo-neurohypophyseal system in relation to development, aging and Alzheimer's disease. *Prog. Brain Res.* 93, 237–247. doi: 10.1016/S0079-6123(08)64575-6

Greaves, N., Prince, E., Evans, D. W., and Charman, T. (2006). Repetitive and ritualistic behaviour in children with Prader-Willi syndrome and children with autism. *J. Intellect. Dosabil. Res.* 50, 92–100. doi: 10.1111/j.1365-2788.2005.00726.x

Guastella, A. J., Gray, K. M., Rinehart, N. J., Alvares, G. A., Tonge, B. J., Hickie, I. B., et al. (2014). The effects of a course of intranasal oxytocin on social behaviors in youth diagnosed with autism spectrum disorders: a randomized controlled trial. *J. Child Psychol. Psychiatry.* doi: 10.1111/jcpp.12305. [Epub ahead of print].

Gutnick, A., Blechman, J., Kaslin, J., Herwig, L., Belting, H. G., Affolter, M., et al. (2011). The hypothalamic neuropeptide oxytocin is required for formation of the neurovascular interface of the pituitary. *Dev. Cell.* 21, 642–654. doi: 10.1016/j.devcel.2011.09.004

Hammock, E. A. (2014). Developmental perspectives on oxytocin and vasopressin. *Neuropsychopharmacology* 40, 24–42. doi: 10.1038/npp.2014.120

Hammock, E. A., and Levitt, P. (2013). Oxytocin receptor ligand binding in embryonic tissue and postnatal brain development of the C57BL/6J mouse. *Front. Behav. Neurosci.* 7:195. doi: 10.3389/fnbeh.2013.00195

Harony, H., and Wagner, S. (2010). The contribution of oxytocin and vasopressin to mammalian social behavior: potential role in autism spectrum disorder. *Neurosignals* 18, 82–97. doi: 10.1159/000321035

Higashida, H., Lopatina, O., Yoshihara, T., Pichugina, Y. A., Soumarokov, A. A., Munesue, T., et al. (2010). Oxytocin signal and social behaviour: comparison among adult and infant oxytocin, oxytocin receptor and CD38 gene knockout mice. *J. Neuroendocrinol.* 22, 373–379. doi: 10.1111/j.1365-2826.2010.01976.x

Ho, A. Y., and Dimitropoulos, A. (2010). Clinical management of behavioral characteristics of Prader-Willi syndrome. *Neuropsychiatr. Dis. Treat.* 6, 107–118. doi: 10.2147/NDT.S5560

Holland, A. J., Whittington, J. E., Butler, J., Webb, T., Boer, H., and Clarke, D. (2003). Behavioural phenotypes associated with specific genetic disorders: evidence from a population-based study of people with Prader-Willi syndrome. *Psychol. Med.* 33, 141–153. doi: 10.1017/S0033291702006736

Holst, S., Uvnas-Moberg, K., and Petersson, M. (2002). Postnatal oxytocin treatment and postnatal stroking of rats reduce blood pressure in adulthood. *Auton. Neurosci.* 99, 85–90. doi: 10.1016/S1566-0702(02)00134-0

Hosoya, T., Oda, Y., Takahashi, S., Morita, M., Kawauchi, S., Ema, M., et al. (2001). Defective development of secretory neurones in the hypothalamus of Arnt2-knockout mice. *Genes Cells* 6, 361–374. doi: 10.1046/j.1365-2443.2001.00421.x

Höybye, C., Barkeling, B., Espelund, U., Petersson, M., and Thoren, M. (2003). Peptides associated with hyperphagia in adults with Prader-Willi syndrome before and during GH treatment. *Growth Horm. IGF Res.* 13, 322–327. doi: 10.1016/S1096-6374(03)00077-7

Hussy, N., Boissin-Agasse, L., Richard, P., and Desarmenien, M. G. (1997). NMDA receptor properties in rat supraoptic magnocellular neurons: characterization and postnatal development. *Eur. J. Neurosci.* 9, 1439–1449. doi: 10.1111/j.1460-9568.1997.tb01498.x

Jarvinen, A. M., and Bellugi, U. (2013). What does Williams syndrome reveal about the determinants of social behavior? *Front. Hum. Neurosci.* 7:321. doi: 10.3389/fnhum.2013.00321

Jauregi, J., Laurier, V., Copet, P., Tauber, M., and Thuilleaux, D. (2013). Behavioral profile of adults with Prader-Willi syndrome: correlations with individual and environmental variables. *J. Neurodev. Disord.* 5:18. doi: 10.1186/1866-1955-5-18

Jin, D., Liu, H. X., Hirai, H., Torashima, T., Nagai, T., Lopatina, O., et al. (2007). CD38 is critical for social behaviour by regulating oxytocin secretion. *Nature* 446, 41–45. doi: 10.1038/nature05526

Jing, X., Ratty, A. K., and Murphy, D. (1998). Ontogeny of the vasopressin and oxytocin RNAs in the mouse hypothalamus. *Neurosci. Res.* 30, 343–349. doi: 10.1016/S0168-0102(98)00017-0

Kang, H. J., Kawasawa, Y. I., Cheng, F., Zhu, Y., Xu, X., Li, M., et al. (2011). Spatio-temporal transcriptome of the human brain. *Nature* 478, 483–489. doi: 10.1038/nature10523

Knobloch, H. S., Charlet, A., Hoffmann, L. C., Eliava, M., Khrulev, S., Cetin, A. H., et al. (2012). Evoked axonal oxytocin release in the central amygdala attenuates fear response. *Neuron* 73, 553–566. doi: 10.1016/j.neuron.2011.11.030

Knobloch, S., and Grinevich, V. (2014). Evolution of central oxytocin pathways in vertebrates. *Front. Behav. Neurosci.* 8:31. doi: 10.3389/fnbeh.2014.00031

Koenig, K., Klin, A., and Schultz, R. (2004). Deficits in social attribution ability in Prader-Willi syndrome. *J. Autism Dev. Disord.* 34, 573–582. doi: 10.1007/s10803-004-2551-z

Kosfeld, M., Heinrichs, M., Zak, P. J., Fischbacher, U., and Fehr, E. (2005). Oxytocin increases trust in humans. *Nature* 435, 673–676. doi: 10.1038/nature 03701

Kublaoui, B. M., Gemelli, T., Tolson, K. P., Wang, Y., and Zinn, A. R. (2008). Oxytocin deficiency mediates hyperphagic obesity of Sim1 haploinsufficient mice. *Mol. Endocrinol.* 22, 1723–1734. doi: 10.1210/me.2008-0067

Landgraf, R., and Neumann, I. (2004). Vasopressin and oxytocin release within the brain: a dynamic concept of multiple and variable models of neuropeptide communication. *Front. Neuroendocrinol.* 25, 150–176. doi: 10.1016/j.yfrne.2004.05.001

Laurent, F. M., Hindelang, C., Klein, M. J., Stoeckel, M. E., and Felix, J. M. (1989). Expression of the oxytocin and vasopressin genes in the rat hypothalamus during development: an *in situ* hybridization study. *Brain Res. Dev. Brain Res.* 46, 145–154. doi: 10.1016/0165-3806(89)90152-1

Lee, P. R., Brady, D. L., Shapiro, R. A., Dorsa, D. M., and Koenig, J. I. (2007a). Prenatal stress generates deficits in rat social behavior: Reversal by oxytocin. *Brain Res.* 1156, 152–167. doi: 10.1016/j.brainres.2007.04.042

Lee, H.-J., Macbeth, A. H., Pagani, J. H., and Young, W. S. 3rd (2009). Oxytocin: the great facilitator of life. *Prog. Neurobiol.* 88, 127–151. doi: 10.1016/j.pneurobio.2009.04.001

Lee, S. H., Park, K. H., and Ho, W. K. (2007b). Postnatal developmental changes in Ca2+ homeostasis in supraoptic magnocellular neurons. *Cell Calcium* 41, 441–450. doi: 10.1016/j.ceca.2006.08.003

Li, X., Zou, H., and Brown, W. T. (2012). Genes associated with autism spectrum disorder. *Brain Res. Bull.* 88, 543–552. doi: 10.1016/j.brainresbull.2012.05.017

Liu, H. X., Lopatina, O., Higashida, C., Tsuji, T., Kato, I., Takasawa, S., et al. (2008). Locomotor activity, ultrasonic vocalization and oxytocin levels in infant CD38 knockout mice. *Neurosci. Lett.* 448, 67–70. doi: 10.1016/j.neulet.2008.09.084

Liu, W., Pappas, G. D., and Carter, C. S. (2005). Oxytocin receptors in brain cortical regions are reduced in haploinsufficient (+/-) reeler mice. *Neurol. Res.* 27, 339–345. doi: 10.1179/016164105X35602

Lo, S. T., Siemensma, E., Collin, P., and Hokken-Koelega, A. (2013). Impaired theory of mind and symptoms of Autism Spectrum Disorder in children with Prader-Willi syndrome. *Res. Dev. Disabil.* 34, 2764–2773. doi: 10.1016/j.ridd.2013.05.024

LoParo, D., and Waldman, I. D. (2014). The oxytocin receptor gene (OXTR) is associated with autism spectrum disorder: a meta-analysis. *Mol. Psychiatry.* doi: 10.1038/mp.2014.77. [Epub ahead of print].

Lopatina, O., Yoshihara, T., Nishimura, T., Zhong, J., Akther, S., Fakhrul, A. A., et al. (2014). Anxiety- and depression-like behavior in mice lacking the CD157/BST1 gene, a risk factor for Parkinson's disease. *Front. Behav. Neurosci.* 8:133. doi: 10.3389/fnbeh.2014.00133

Lukas, M., Bredewold, R., Neumann, I. D., and Veenema, A. H. (2010). Maternal separation interferes with developmental changes in brain vasopressin and oxytocin receptor binding in male rats. *Neuropharmacology* 58, 78–87. doi: 10.1016/j.neuropharm.2009.06.020

Malek, A., Blann, E., and Mattison, D. R. (1996). Human plancental transport of oxytocin. *J. Matern. Fetal Med.* 5, 245–255.

Makarenko, I. G., Ugrumov, M. V., and Calas, A. (2002). Involvement of accessory neurosecretory nuclei of hypothalamus in the formation of hypothalamohypophysial system during prenatal and postnatal development in rats. *Rus. J. Dev. Biol.* 33, 37–42. doi: 10.1023/A:1013873012416

Makarenko, I. G., Ugrumov, M. V., Derer, P., and Calas, A. (2000). Projections from the hypothalamus to the posterior loob in rats during ontogenesis: 1,1'-Dioctadecyl-3,3,3',3'-Tetramethylindocarbocyanine perchlorate tracing study. *J. Comp. Neurol.* 422, 327–337. doi: 10.1016/j.devbrainres.2004.12.007

Markakis, E. A. (2002). Development of the neuroendocrine hypothalamus. *Front. Neuroendocrinol.* 23, 257–291. doi: 10.1016/S0091-3022(02)00003-1

Markakis, E. A., and Swanson, L. W. (1997). Spatiotemporal patterns of secretomotor neuron generation in the parvicellular neuroendocrine system. *Brain Res. Brain Res. Rev.* 24, 255–291. doi: 10.1016/S0165-0173(97)00006-4

Martin, A., State, M., Koenig, K., Schultz, R., Dykens, E. M., Cassidy, S. B., et al. (1998). Prader-Willi syndrome [clinical conference]. *Am. J. Psychiatry* 155, 1265–1273. doi: 10.1176/ajp.155.9.1265

Mathieu, J., Barth, A., Rosa, F. M., Wilson, S. W., and Peyrieras, N. (2002). Distinct and cooperative roles for Nodal and Hedgehog signals during hypothalamic development. *Development* 129, 3055–3065.

McAllister, C. J., Whittington, J. E., and Holland, A. J. (2011). Development of the eating behaviour in Prader-Willi Syndrome: advances in our understanding. *Intern. J. Obesity* 35, 188–197. doi: 10.1038/ijo.2010.139

McCall, C., and Singer, T. (2012). The animal and human neuroendocrinology of social cognition, motivation and behavior. *Nat. Neurosci.* 15, 681–688. doi: 10.1038/nn.3084

McCullough, M. E., Churchland, P. S., and Mendez, A. J. (2013). Problems with measuring peripheral oxytocin: can the data on oxytocin and human behavior be trusted? *J. Neurosci. Biobehav. Rev.* 37, 1485–1492. doi: 10.1016/j.neubiorev.2013.04.018

Meyer-Lindenberg, A., Domes, G., Kirsch, P., and Heinrichs, M. (2011). Oxytocin and vasopressin in the human brain: social neuropeptides for translational medicine. *Nat. Rev. Neurosci.* 12, 524–538. doi: 10.1038/nrn3044

Meziane, H., Schaller, F., Bauer, S., Villard, C., Matarazzo, V., Riet, F., et al. (in press). An early postnatal oxytocin treatment prevents social and learning deficits in adult mice deficient for Magel 2, a gene involved in Prader-Willi syndrome and autism. *Biol. Psychiatry.* doi: 10.1016/j.biopsych.2014.11.010

Michaud, J. L., DeRossi, C., May, N. R., Holdener, B. C., and Fan, C. M. (2000). ARNT2 acts as the dimerization partner of SIM1 for the development of the hypothalamus. *Mech. Dev.* 90, 253–261. doi: 10.1016/S0925-4773(99)00328-7

Miller, J. L., Lynn, C. H., Driscoll, D. C., Goldstone, A. P., Gold, J. A., Kimonis, V., et al. (2011). Nutritional phases in Prader-Willi syndrome. *Am. J. Med. Gen.* 155A, 1040–1049. doi: 10.1002/ajmg.a.33951

Mineur, Y. S., Huynh, L. X., and Crusio, W. E. (2006). Social behavior deficits in the Fmr1 mutant mouse. *Behav. Brain Res.* 168, 172–175. doi: 10.1016/j.bbr.2005.11.004

Nakai, S., Kawano, H., Yudate, T., Nishi, M., Kuno, J., Nagata, A., et al. (1995). The POU domain transcription factor Brn-2 is required for the determination of specific neuronal lineages in the hypothalamus of the mouse. *Genes Dev.* 9, 3109–3121. doi: 10.1101/gad.9.24.3109

Ohyama, K., Das, R., and Placzek, M. (2008). Temporal progression of hypothalamic patterning by a dual action of BMP. *Development* 135, 3325–3331. doi: 10.1242/dev.027078

Pietropaolo, S., Guilleminot, A., Martin, B., D'Amato, F. R., and Crusio, W. E. (2011). Genetic-background modulation of core and variable autistic-like symptoms in Fmr1 knock-out mice. *PloS ONE* 6:e17073. doi: 10.1371/journal.pone.0017073

Pournajafi-Nazarloo, H., Carr, M. S., Papademeteriou, E., Schmidt, J. V., and Cushing, B. S. (2007). Oxytocin selectively increases ERalpha mRNA in the neonatal hypothalamus and hippocampus of female prairie voles. *Neuropeptides* 41, 39–44. doi: 10.1016/j.npep.2006.10.002

Prounis, G., and Ophir, A. (2013). *The Influence of Socio-Spatial Experience on Dynamics of Oxytocin Receptor Development in the Prairie Voles.* Abstract 37806/III46. San Diego, CA: Society for Neuroscience. Available online at: http://www.abstractsonline.com/plan/ViewAbstract.aspx?cKey=920330d5-a2d2-46a3-b4a2-70cb0d5dd279&mID=3236&mKey=8d2a5bec-4825-4cd6-9439-b42bb151d1cf&sKey=4e6bd5c0-f881-4c4c-b017-727347369718

Randle, J. C., Bourque, C. W., and Renaud, L. P. (1986). Serial reconstruction of Lucifer yellow-labeled supraoptic nucleus neurons in perfused rat hypothalamic explants. *Neuroscience* 17, 453–467. doi: 10.1016/0306-4522(86)90259-9

Richard, P., Moos, F., Dayanithi, G., Gouzenes, L., and Sabatier, N. (1997). Rhythmic activities of hypothalamic magnocellular neurons: autocontrol mechanisms. *Biol. Cell* 89, 555–560. doi: 10.1111/j.1768-322X.1997.tb01032.x

Rinaman, L. (2007). Visceral sensory inputs to the endocrine hypothalamus. *Front. Neuroendocrinol.* 28, 50–60. doi: 10.1016/j.yfrne.2007.02.002

Rilling, J. K., and Young, L. J. (2014). The biology of mammalian parenting and its effect on offspring social development. *Science* 345, 771–776. doi: 10.1126/science.1252723

Rinne, U. K., Kivalo, E., and Talanti, S. (1962). Maturation of human hypothalamic neurosecretion. *Biol. Neonat.* 4, 351–364. doi: 10.1159/000239845

Ross, H. E., Cole, C. D., Smith, Y., Neumann, I. D., Landgraf, R., Murphy, A. Z., et al. (2009). Characterization of the oxytocin system regulating affiliative behavior in female prairie voles. *Neuroscience* 162, 892–903. doi: 10.1016/j.neuroscience.2009.05.055

Ross, H. E., and Young, L. J. (2009). Oxytocin and the neural mechanisms regulating social condition and affiliative behavior. *Front. Neuroendocrinol.* 30, 534–547. doi: 10.1016/j.yfrne.2009.05.004

Sala, M., Braida, D., Donzelli, A., Martucci, R., Busnelli, M., Bulgheroni, E., et al. (2013). Mice heterozygous for the oxytocin receptor gene (Oxtr(+/-)) show impaired social behaviour but not increased aggression or cognitive inflexibility: evidence of a selective haploinsufficiency gene effect. *J. Neuroendocrinol.* 25, 107–118. doi: 10.1111/j.1365-2826.2012.02385.x

Sala, M., Braida, D., Lentini, D., Busnelli, M., Bulgheroni, E., Capurro, V., et al. (2011). Pharmacologic rescue of impaired cognitive flexibility, social deficits, increased aggression, and seizure susceptibility in oxytocin receptor null mice: a neurobehavioral model of autism. *Biol. Psychiatry* 69, 875–882. doi: 10.1016/j.biopsych.2010.12.022

Sawchenko, P. E., and Swanson, L. W. (1982). Immunohistochemical identification of neurons in the paraventricular nucleus of the hypothalamus that project to the medulla or to the spinal cord in the rat. *J. Comp. Neurol.* 205, 260–272. doi: 10.1002/cne.902050306

Schaaf, C. P., Gonzalez-Garay, M. L., Xia, F., Potocki, L., Gripp, K. W., Zhang, B., et al. (2013). Truncating mutations of MAGEL2 cause Prader-Willi phenotypes and autism. *Nat. Genet.* 45, 1405–1408. doi: 10.1038/ng.2776

Schaller, F., Watrin, F., Sturny, R., Massacrier, A., Szepetowski, P., and Muscatelli, F., A (2010). Single postnatal injection of oxytocin rescues the lethal feeding behaviour in mouse newborns deficient for the imprinted Magel2 gene. *Hum. Mol. Gen.* 19, 4895–4905. doi: 10.1093/hmg/ddq424

Schoneman, M. D., Ryan, A. K., McEvilli, R. J., O'Conell, S. M., Arias, C. A., Kalla, K. A., et al. (1995). Development and survival of the endocrine hypothalamus and posterior pituitary gland requires the neuronal POU domain factor Brn-2. *Genes Dev.* 9, 3122–3135.

Schubert, F., George, J. M., and Rao, M. B. (1981). Vasopressin and oxytocin content of human fetal brain at different stages of gestation. *Brain Res.* 213, 111–117. doi: 10.1016/0006-8993(81)91251-8

Shamay-Tsoory, S. G., Fischer, M., Dvash, J., Harari, H., Perach-Bloom, N., and Levkovitz, Y. (2009). Intranasal administration of oxytocin increases envy and schadenfreude (gloating). *Biol. Psychiatry* 66, 864–870. doi: 10.1016/j.biopsych.2009.06.009

Shapiro, L. E., and Insel, T. R. (1989). Ontogeny of oxytocin receptors in rat forebrain: a quantitative study. *Synapse* 4, 259–266. doi: 10.1002/syn.890040312

Silverman, A.-J., Glodstein, R., and Gadde, C. A. (1980). The ontogenesis of neurophysin-containing neurons in the mouse hypothalamus. *Peptides* 1, 27–44. doi: 10.1016/0196-9781(80)90101-1

Silverman, J. L., Yang, M., Turner, S. M., Katz, A. M., Bell, D. B., Koenig, J. I., et al. (2010). Low stress reactivity and neuroendocrine factors in the BTBR T+tf/J mouse model of autism. *Neuroscience* 171, 1197–1208. doi: 10.1016/j.neuroscience.2010.09.059

Sinding, C., Robinson, A. G., Seif, S. M., and Schmid, P. G. (1980). Neurohypophyseal peptides in the developing rat fetus. *Brain Res.* 195, 177–186. doi: 10.1016/0006-8993(80)90875-6

Snijdewint, F. G., Van Leeuwen, F. W., and Boer, G. J. (1989). Ontogeny of vasopressin and oxytocin binding sites in the brain of Wistar and Brattleboro rats as demonstrated by lightmicroscopical autoradiography. *J. Chem. Neuroanat.* 2, 3–17.

Striepens, N., Kendrick, K. M., Maier, W., and Hurlemann, R. (2011). Prosocial effects of oxytocin and clinical evidence for its therapeutic potential. *Front. Neuroendocrinol.* 32, 426–450. doi: 10.1016/j.yfrne.2011.07.001

Swaab, D. F. (1995). Development of the human hypothalamus. *Neurochem. Res.* 20, 509–519. doi: 10.1007/BF01694533

Swaab, D. F. (1997a). Prader-Willi syndrome and the hypothalamus. *Acta Paediatr. Suppl.* 423, 50–54.

Swaab, D. F. (1997b). Neurobiology and neuropathology of human hypothalamus. *Handbook Chem. Neuroanat.* 13, 39–137.

Swaab, D. F., Purba, J. S., and Hofman, M. A. (1995). Alterations in the hypothalamic paraventricular nucleus and its oxytocin neurons (putative satiety cells) in Prader-Willi syndrome: a study of five cases. *J. Clin. Endocrinol. Metab.* 80, 573–579.

Szarek, E., Cheah, P. S., Schwartz, J., and Thomas, P. (2010). Molecular genetics of the developing neuroendocrine hypothalamus. *Mol. Cell. Endocrinol.* 323, 115–123. doi: 10.1016/j.mce.2010.04.002

Takayanagi, Y., Kasahara, Y., Onaka, T., Takahashi, N., Kawada, T., and Nishimori, K. (2008). Oxytocin receptor-deficient mice developed late-onset obesity. *Neuroreport* 19, 951–955. doi: 10.1097/WNR.0b013e3283021ca9

Takayanagi, Y., Yoshida, M., Bielsky, I. F., Ross, H. E., Kawamata, M., Onaka, T., et al. (2005). Pervasive social deficits, but normal parturition, in oxytocin receptor-deficient mice. *Proc. Natl. Acad. Sci. U.S.A.* 102, 16096–16101. doi: 10.1073/pnas.0505312102

Tauber, M., Diene, G., Mimoun, E., Cabal-Berthoumieu, S., Mantoulan, C., Molinas, C., et al. (2014). Prader-Willi syndrome as a model of human hyperphagia. *Front. Horm Res.* 42, 93–106. doi: 10.1159/000358317

Tauber, M., Mantoulan, C., Copet, P., Jauregui, J., Demeer, G., Diene, G., et al. (2011). Oxytocin may be useful to increase trust in others and decrease disruptive behaviours in patients with Prader-Willi syndrome: a randomised placebo-controlled trial in 24 patients. *Orphanet. J. Rare Dis.* 6:47. doi: 10.1186/1750-1172-6-47

Tobin, V. A., Arechaga, G., Brunton, P. J., Russell, J. A., Leng, G., Ludwig, M., et al. (2014). Oxytocinase in the female rat hypothalamus: a novel mechanism controlling oxytocin neurones during lactation. *J. Neuroendocrinol.* 26, 205–216. doi: 10.1111/jne.12141

Trembleau, A., Ugrumov, M., Roche, D., and Calas, A. (1995). Vasopressin and oxytocin gene expression in intact rats and under catecholamine deficiency during ontogenesis. *Brain Res. Bull.* 37, 437–448. doi: 10.1016/0361-9230(95)00020-F

Tribollet, E., Barberis, C., Jard, S., Dubois-Dauphin, M., and Dreifuss, J. J. (1988). Localization and pharmacological characterization of high affinity binding sites for vasopressin and oxytocin in the rat brain by light microscopic autoradiography. *Brain Res.* 442, 105–118. doi: 10.1016/0006-8993(88)91437-0

Tribollet, E., Charpak, S., Schmidt, A., Dubois-Dauphin, M., and Dreifuss, J. J. (1989). Appearance and transient expression of oxytocin receptors in fetal, infant, and peripubertal rat brain studied by autoradiography and electrophysiology. *J. Neurosci.* 9, 1764–1773.

Tyzio, R., Nardou, R., Ferrari, D. C., Tsintsadze, T., Shahrokhi, A., Eftekhari, S., et al. (2014). Oxytocin-mediated GABA inhibition during delivery attenuates autism pathogenesis in rodent offspring. *Science* 343, 675–679. doi: 10.1126/science.1247190

Ugrumov, M. V. (2010). Developing brain as endocrine organ: a paradoxical reality. *Neurochem. Res.* 35, 837–850. doi: 10.1007/s11064-010-0127-1

Van der Woude, P. F., Goudsmit, E., Wierda, M., Purba, J. S., Hofman, M. A., Bogte, H., et al. (1995). No vasopressin cell loss in the human paraventricular and supraoptic nucleus during aging and in Alzheimer's disease. *Neurobiol. Aging* 16, 11–18. doi: 10.1016/0197-4580(95)80003-A

van Eerdenburg, F. J., and Rakic, P. (1994). Early neurogenesis in the anterior hypothalamus of the rhesus monkey. *Brain Res. Dev. Brain Res.* 79, 290–296. doi: 10.1016/0165-3806(94)90134-1

van Leeuwen, F. W., van Heerikhuize, J., van der Meulen, G., and Wolters, P. (1985). Light microscopic autoradiographic localization of [3H]oxytocin binding sites in the rat brain, pituitary and mammary gland. *Brain Res.* 359, 320–325. doi: 10.1016/0006-8993(85)91443-X

Wang, Z., and Young, L. J. (1997). Ontogeny of oxytocin and vasopressin receptor binding in the lateral septum in prairie and montane voles. *Brain Res. Dev. Brain Res.* 104, 191–195. doi: 10.1016/S0165-3806(97)00138-7

Whitnall, M. H., Key, S., Ben-Barak, Y., Ozato, K., and Gainer, H. (1985). Neurophysin in the hypothalamo-neurohypophysial system. II. Immunocytochemical studies of the ontogeny of oxytocinergic and vasopressinergic neurons. *J. Neurosci.* 5, 98–109.

Widmer, H., Amerdeil, H., Fontanaud, P., and Desarmenien, M. G. (1997). Postnatal maturation of rat hypothalamoneurohypophysial neurons: evidence for a developmental decrease in calcium entry during action potentials. *J. Neurophysiol.* 77, 260–271.

Wierda, M., Goudsmit, E., Van der Woude, P. F., Purba, J. S., Hofman, M. A., Bogte, H., et al. (1991). Oxytocin cell number in the human paraventricular nucleus remains constant with aging and Alzheimer's disease. *Neurobiol. Aging* 12, 511–516. doi: 10.1016/0197-4580(91)90081-T

Williams, S. K., Cox, E. T., McMurray, M. S., Fay, E. E., Jarrett, T. M., et al. (2009). Simultaneous prenatal ethanol and nicotine exposure affect ethanol consumption, ethanol preference and oxytocin receptor binding in adolescent and adult rats. *Neurotoxicol. Teratol.* 31, 291–302. doi: 10.1016/j.ntt.2009.06.001

Winslow, J. T., Hearn, E. F., Ferguson, J., Young, L. J., Matzuk, M. M., and Insel, T. R. (2000). Infant vocalization, adult aggression, and fear behavior of an oxytocin null mutant mouse. *Horm. Behav.* 37, 145–155. doi: 10.1006/hbeh.1999.1566

Workman, A. D., Charvet, C. J., Clancy, B., Darlington, R. B., and Finlay, B. L. (2013). Modeling transformations of neurodevelopmental sequences across mammalian species. *J. Neurosci.* 24, 7368–7383. doi: 10.1523/JNEUROSCI.5746-12.2013

Yoshimura, R., Kimura, T., Watanabe, D., and Kiyama, H. (1996). Differential expression of oxytocin receptor mRNA in the developing rat brain. *Neurosci. Res.* 24, 291–304. doi: 10.1016/0168-0102(95)01003-3

Yoshimura, R., Kiyama, H., Kimura, T., Araki, T., Maeno, H., Tanizawa, O., et al. (1993). Localization of oxytocin receptor messenger ribonucleic acid in the rat brain. *Endocrinology* 133, 1239–1246.

Young, W. S. 3rd, Reynolds, K., Shepard, E. A., Gainer, H., and Castel, M. (1990). Cell-specific expression of the rat oxytocin gene in transgenic mice. *J. Neuroendocrinol.* 2, 917–925. doi: 10.1111/j.1365-2826.1990.tb00660.x

Zheng, J.-J., Li, S.-J., Zhang, X.-D., Miao, W.-Y., Zhang, D., Yao, H., et al. (2014). Oxytocin mediates early experience-dependent cross-modal plasticity in the sensory cortices. *Nat. Neurosci.* 17, 391–399. doi: 10.1038/nn.3634

6

A unifying computational framework for stability and flexibility of arousal

***Christin Kosse*[1] *and Denis Burdakov*[1,2]*

[1] *Neurophysiology, MRC National Institute for Medical Research, London, UK*
[2] *MRC Centre for Developmental Neurobiology, King's College London, London, UK*

***Correspondence:**
Denis Burdakov, Neurophysiology, MRC National Institute for Medical Research, The Ridgeway, Mill Hill, London NW7 1AA, UK
e-mail: denis.burdakov@kcl.ac.uk

Arousal and consciousness flexibly adjust to salient cues, but remain stable despite noise and disturbance. Diverse, highly interconnected neural networks govern the underlying transitions of behavioral state; these networks are robust but very complex. Frameworks from systems engineering provide powerful tools for understanding functional logic behind component complexity. From a general systems viewpoint, a minimum of three communicating control modules may enable flexibility and stability to coexist. Comparators would subtract current arousal from desired arousal, producing an error signal. Regulators would compute control signals from this error. Generators would convert control signals into arousal, which is fed back to comparators, to make the system noise-proof through self-correction. Can specific neurons correspond to these control elements? To explore this, here we consider the brain-wide orexin/hypocretin network, which is experimentally established to be vital for flexible and stable arousal. We discuss whether orexin neurons may act as comparators, and their target neurons as regulators and generators. Experiments are proposed for testing such predictions, based on computational simulations showing that comparators, regulators, and generators have distinct temporal signatures of activity. If some regulators integrate orexin-communicated errors, robust arousal control may be achieved via integral feedback (a basic engineering strategy for tracking a set-point despite noise). An integral feedback view also suggests functional roles for specific molecular aspects, such as differing life-spans of orexin peptides. The proposed framework offers a unifying logic for molecular, cellular, and network details of arousal systems, and provides insight into behavioral state transitions, complex behavior, and bases for disease.

Keywords: arousal, hypothalamus, narcolepsy, orexin, hypocretin, histamine, computation, control

INTRODUCTION

In many everyday situations, it is vital for arousal and consciousness to remain stable despite changes in mental state. Failure of such arousal "cruise-control" can produce deleteriously unstable arousal, as seen in narcoleptic patients who lose consciousness during emotional disturbances such as laughter. On the other hand, it is also important for the arousal drive to be flexible and modifiable by salient features of the environment, such as metabolic needs or the time of day. This presumably evolved because the energy cost of arousal (Dworak et al., 2010) makes it more economical to tune arousal to demand, rather than switch it on and off in a binary, flip-flop manner. Failure of arousal to be flexible can lead to debilitating disorders such as insomnia. The subject of this article is to explore the currently unclear mechanisms through which brain arousal systems may combine stability/robustness with flexibility.

We shall present a systems perspective on this subject. To define our terms, consciousness and arousal will be used to simply refer to brain states distinct from sleep/unconsciousness. By systems perspective, we mean a level of description lying between generalized mathematics and specialized jargons of neuroscience subfields. Systems views help understanding, because translating a specific problem (e.g., a molecularly defined disease) into a more general "systems" language makes it understandable to other fields and thus addressable by more tools than typically available in one specialized field (Wiener, 1965; Csete and Doyle, 2002, 2004; Doyle and Csete, 2011; von Bertalanffy, 2013). Many specific health problems today are linked to the hypothalamus (obesity, sleep disorders, e.g., Mignot et al., 2002; Yeo and Heisler, 2012; Horvath et al., 2014). Despite huge advances in specialized knowledge (Sohn et al., 2013), these problems remain unsolved and might benefit from additional tools.

From classic clinical studies to modern genetic work, increasingly detailed evidence emerged that the lateral hypothalamus provides a critical part of the brain hardware required for stable consciousness. Almost a century ago, based on post-mortem studies of brains of patients with "sleeping sickness", von Economo suggested that the lateral hypothalamus is critical for the control of wakefulness and arousal (Saper et al., 2001). Around 70 years later, the lateral hypothalamus was discovered to be the unique location of neurons containing neuropeptide transmitters orexins/hypocretins (de Lecea et al., 1998; Sakurai et al., 1998). Loss of orexin neurons, orexin type-2 (OXR2) receptors, or orexin peptides leads to the narcoleptic inability to maintain stable wakefulness (Sakurai, 2007). Most cases of human narcolepsy, a relatively frequent neurological disorder (1:2000 people, Nishino and Kanbayashi, 2005), are thought to be due to loss of orexin neurons (Nishino et al., 2000; Thannickal et al., 2000; Dauvilliers et al., 2007). Without orexin neurons, arousal can still be generated in normal amounts, but it is neither flexible nor robust (see Section "Are Orexin Neurons Comparators?" below). Orexin neurons are now seen as vital orchestrators of other arousal systems distributed throughout the brain, such as the aminergic systems (see Section "A Modular Model for Neural Control of Arousal in An Uncertain World" below).

From their cell bodies in the lateral hypothalamus, orexin neurons project to almost the entire brain, and their projections largely mirror the distribution of OXR1 and OXR2, the two G-protein coupled receptors for orexin (Peyron et al., 1998; Sakurai, 2007). The firing of orexin neurons stimulates awakening (Adamantidis et al., 2007), and the classic arousal neurons of the brain are innervated by orexin fibers and excited by orexin peptides (histamine, serotonin, noradrenaline neurons, Sakurai, 2007).

These and other experimental studies of orexin networks (reviewed in de Lecea et al., 2006; Sakurai, 2007) define brain hardware required for robust-yet-flexible arousal. However, how these components are arranged to implement wakefulness-stabilizing mechanisms is still unclear. In this review, we consider how experimentally-discovered components can be generalized to operations, and how this may improve understanding of arousal control, including diagnosis and arousal malfunction in sleep disorders. We argue that in the real world, arousal control would be inaccurate if brain arousal generators varied their activity in simple proportion to the environment-controlled activity of orexin neurons. We discuss how different neurons and their connections may implement better mechanisms (e.g., integration, feedback) that are needed for robust-yet-flexible arousal. We produce experimental predictions for testing which neurons implement which aspects of control, and conclude with limitations of the presented models. In broader terms, this article considers a conceptual unification of specific biology of stable wakefulness and general mechanisms for stability as studied in non-biological sciences (e.g., in fields variously known as cybernetics, general systems theory, and control theory, Wiener, 1965; Csete and Doyle, 2002; von Bertalanffy, 2013).

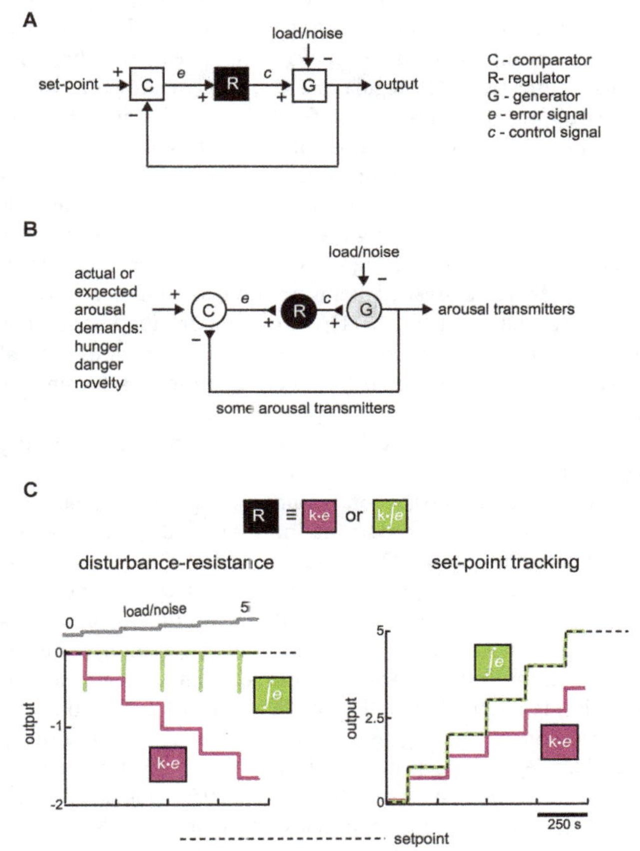

FIGURE 1 | Functional connectivity for making a stable-yet-flexible signal. (A) A general mechanism (feedback loop) for tracking a set-point despite disturbance (after Csete and Doyle, 2002). For simplicity, load/noise is modeled as entering at a final summing point, but it can enter the system at any point. **(B)** An equivalent representation of a neural circuit for producing appropriate levels of arousal-enhancing neurotransmitters. **(C)** System performance with and without integral control. Computational simulations of temporal dynamics of the system shown in **(A)**, in the face of changes in load/noise or changes in desired set-point. Left, effect of escalating disturbance on system output with (green) and without (magenta) integration in the module R (k = 1 in both cases). Right, response of system output to changes in desired set-point for the two types of control. Integration here had a time window longer than the simulation time; effects of varying the integration window are described in the text and **Figure 2A**. See Supplementary Figure for more information on computational simulations.

CIRCUIT MOTIFS FOR STABLE-YET-FLEXIBLE CONTROL

From a general systems point of view, it can be argued that pressure to develop good policies for stable-yet-flexible function is not unique to biological evolution (Csete and Doyle, 2002, 2004). For example, under consumer pressure, in recent decades diverse robotic devices (thermostats, car cruise-controllers) also evolved remarkably effective strategies to make their controlled variables (temperature, speed, etc.) follow set-points despite disturbance. For example, a car cruise-controller can defend set-point speed despite unpredictable variations in slope, wind, or component function, by employing a feedback mechanism (**Figure 1A**). It has been proposed that, faced with similar general problems (i.e., tracking a set-point despite unpredictable noise), biological and engineering systems undergo a convergent evolution and arrive at similar solutions, such as self-correction via feedback (Csete and Doyle, 2002, 2004). Reverse engineering of biology may therefore benefit from broader frameworks in engineering (Csete and Doyle, 2002; Franklin and Wolpert, 2011).

From considerations of convergent evolution, appropriate arousal in an uncertain world may also require a feedback mechanism. In its simplest form, this may be implemented by three elements: comparator (C), regulator (R), and generator (G), which achieve appropriate output via a feedback loop (**Figure 1B**). The comparator computes an error signal, which tells the regulator how much generator output is deviating from desired performance. The regulator is useful, because it can compensate for disturbance without affecting the final (generator) output of the system (see simulation in **Figure 3B**). There has been debate in some hypothalamus-related literature about set-points vs. settling points (Speakman et al., 2011); in our model the set-point is variable and can be viewed as a settling-point of various arousal demands listed in **Figure 1B** (but we use the term set-point for brevity).

Theoretical and practical studies suggest that, for tracking despite noise, a particularly effective signal that regulators can send to generators is based on temporal integration of the error signal (integral feedback, Aström and Hagglund, 1995; Yi et al., 2000; Csete and Doyle, 2002; DiStefano et al., 2012). In qualitative terms, error integration enables perfect control based on an accumulated history ("past"), rather than the instantaneous value ("present"), of errors. The quantitative advantage of error integration for precision-tracking of a set-point is demonstrated by a simple simulation in **Figure 1C**. Control speed (but not the precision of keeping to a set-point) can also be improved by adding regulator actions based on "future", i.e., time derivative, of error (Aström and Hagglund, 1995; DiStefano et al., 2012). For example, glutamate released by orexin cells can create derivative-like control signals (**Figure 2B**; see Schöne et al., 2014), but unlike orexin release considered below, glutamate release is insufficient for consciousness stability (Chemelli et al., 1999).

If convergent evolution exists, considerations of general models for control (**Figure 1A**) may illuminate the function of different types of neurons underlying stable-yet-flexible arousal. In Section "A Modular Model for Neural Control of Arousal in An Uncertain World", we discuss literature suggesting that some elements of brain orexin circuits are similar to control schemes in **Figures 1A,B**. In Section "Model Predictions", we use computational simulations to generate experimentally-testable predictions to evaluate whether specific neurons may indeed behave as specific control modules.

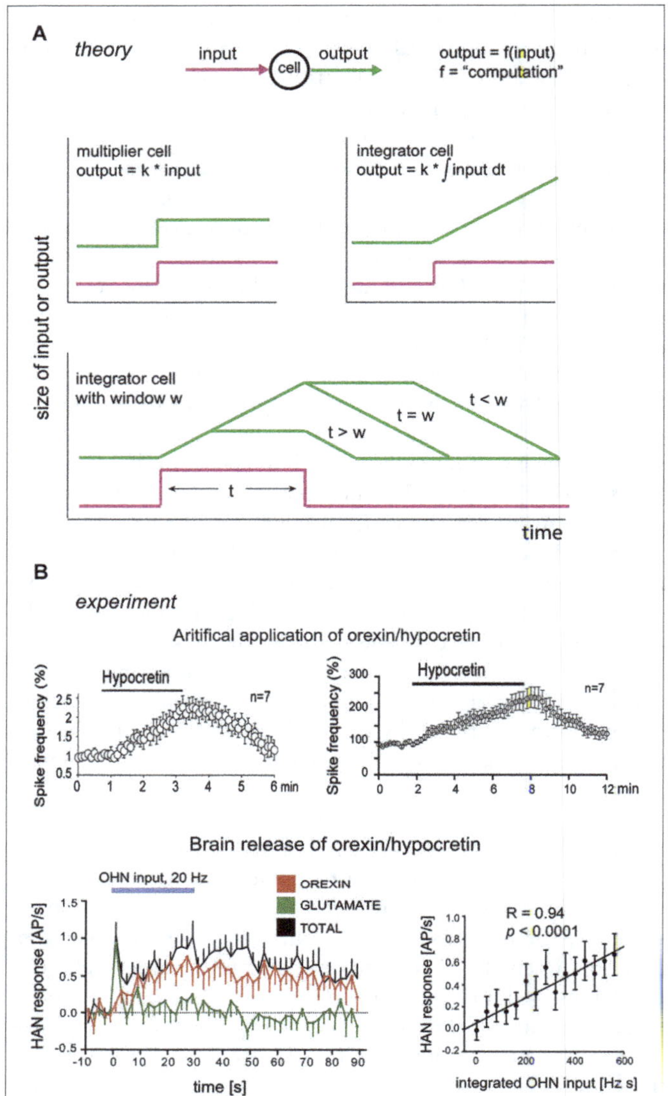

FIGURE 2 | Integrators and their hypothetical neural correlates. **(A)** Theoretical input-output dynamics of neurons that act as multipliers (top left graph), or integrators (top right graph) with different integration windows (bottom graph). W here is defined as the duration of integration window, i.e., given $\int_b^a input\ dt$, $w = a - b$. Input is shown in magenta, and output in green. **(B)** Experimental input-output relations of neurons in brain orexin circuits. Top row, firing outputs of orexin/hypocretin neurons (OHNs) in response to bath application of 1 μM (left) and 200 nM (right) orexin/hypocretin peptides (from Li and van den Pol, 2006, reproduced with permission from The Society for Neuroscience). Bottom row, firing outputs of histamine neurons (HAN) in response to optogenetic stimulation of OHNs at 20 Hz (blue bar). Responses due to orexin transmission are in red (data from Schöne et al., 2014).

A MODULAR MODEL FOR NEURAL CONTROL OF AROUSAL IN AN UNCERTAIN WORLD

We note that brain arousal-control systems resemble the schemes in **Figures 1A,B** in some general respects:

1. Distinct modules are involved, including classic arousal-controling clusters (noradrenaline, histamine, serotonin neurons) and more recently discovered clusters (orexin neurons).
2. These modules are non-redundant (if the few thousands of orexin cells are missing, remaining billions of neurons cannot compensate (Hara et al., 2001). This argues for serial, non-redundant control loops, rather than grossly redundant parallel networks.
3. There is evidence for feedback signals to orexin cells from "arousal generator" chemicals such as some aminergic transmitters (see Section Are Orexin Neurons Comparators?).

The canonical feedback loop (**Figure 1A**) may therefore be implemented in the brain by specific neurons that are wired together and controlled by physiologically relevant inputs (**Figures 1B, 3B**). In this context, load/noise (**Figures 1A,B, 3B**) would correspond to anything that opposes the function of the arousal neurons (e.g., a spontaneous inhibitory input from sleep neurons). A definite mapping of cell types to control modules (C-R-G, **Figure 3B**) needs more experimental tests, as suggested in section "Model Predictions". However, existing data raise the following questions:

ARE OREXIN NEURONS COMPARATORS?

Studies of narcolepsy (in dogs, mice, humans) caused by loss of orexin neurons, type-2 receptors, or orexin peptides, illustrate that orexin cells are vital for arousal cruise-control (Chemelli et al., 1999; Lin et al., 1999; Peyron et al., 2000; Willie et al., 2003). First, orexin neurons and receptors are essential for protecting consciousness from instability during emotional excitement (Dauvilliers et al., 2007). In orexin-deficient brains, emotional load, e.g., excitement from a funny joke, winning a game, playing, or exposure to a favorite food, can inappropriately reduce normal wakefulness and produce sleep attacks (Dauvilliers et al., 2007). Second, the orexin system ensures that arousal levels track environmentally-relevant set-points. Knockout of orexin peptides greatly reduces normal arousal responses (such as elevated locomotion, heart rate, breathing) to food shortage, high CO_2, or stress (Yamanaka et al., 2003a; Sakurai, 2007; Kuwaki, 2011). However, orexin neurons are not essential for wakefulness *per se*: their loss fragments wakefulness but does not change its total amount per day (Hara et al., 2001). This suggests that orexin neurons are not themselves generators of wakefulness (if this were the case, animals lacking orexin would sleep more). Indeed, during wakefulness *in vivo*, orexin cells are not constantly firing, but become stimulated by signals that demand increased wakefulness, such as sudden sounds, stress, hypoglycaemia or CO_2 (**Figure 3A**; Yamanaka et al., 2003a; Mileykovskiy et al., 2005; Sakurai, 2007; Williams et al., 2007).

We believe that several experiments are consistent with a comparator (error-generator) role for orexin neurons in wake-control circuitry (module C in **Figure 1**). *In vitro*, orexin neurons appear to be excited by signals indicative of wakefulness demand (higher set-point), and inhibited by some of the signals indicative of current wakefulness drive. The excitatory signals include CO_2, unexpected noises, low glucose, stress; and the inhibitory signals include serotonin and, under some circumstances, noradrenaline (Sakurai et al., 1998; Liu et al., 2002; Winsky-Sommerer et al., 2004; Grivel et al., 2005; Mileykovskiy et al., 2005; Sakurai, 2007; Williams et al., 2007, 2008). Noradrenaline effects on orexin cells are currently a subject of discussion: some groups report excitation and propose noradrenaline-induced inhibition to occur only after sleep deprivation (Bayer et al., 2005; Grivel et al., 2005; Uschakov et al., 2011), whereas other groups report only inhibition (Li et al., 2002; Yamanaka et al., 2003b; Williams et al., 2011). In any case, it is still unclear how these *in vitro* studies reflect the effects of noradrenaline cell firing *in vivo*, since orexin-projecting noradrenaline neurons may co-release fast transmitter such as glutamate or GABA (as recently reported for different subpopulations of dopamine neurons, Tecuapetla et al., 2010; Tritsch et al., 2012).

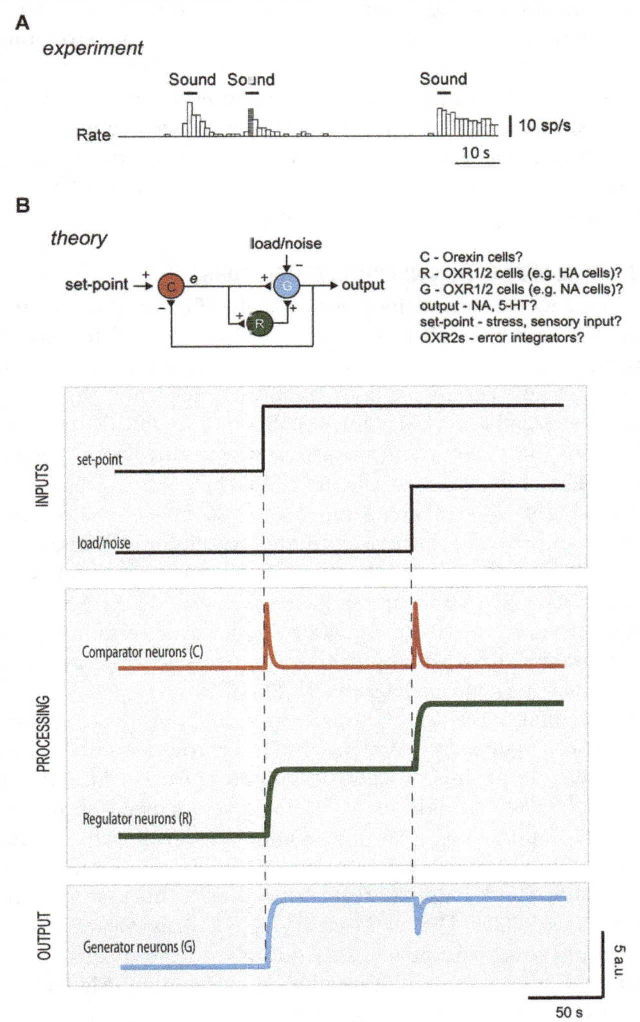

FIGURE 3 | Diagnosing control roles of neurons from temporal activity pattern. (A) Firing of an orexin neuron in the hypothalamus of an awake rat experiencing sensory inputs (reproduced with permission from Cell Press from Mileykovskiy et al., 2005). **(B)** Top drawing, hypothetical mapping of control elements to neuronal types in brain orexin circuits. To protect the output (arousal drive) from instability, R could correspond to OXR2-expressing cells (e.g., histamine neurons), and e could come from orexin neurons driven by positive inputs (e.g., sounds, Mileykovskiy et al., 2005) and negative feedback inputs (e.g., serotonin and/or noradrenaline, Li et al., 2002; Yamanaka et al., 2003b). G could correspond to noradrenaline cells, that express OXR1 and are expected to be excited by HANs (Haas et al., 2008). The intermittent firing of orexin cells during wakefulness *in vivo* (Mileykovskiy et al., 2005) is broadly consistent with this placement in the feedback loop. Bottom plots, computational predictions of temporal variations in activity of the different neurons to changes in set-point or in load/noise (R is modeled as an integrator with a time window that exceeded simulation duration; C and G are modeled as algebraic summing points of the inputs they receive, DiStefano et al., 2012). See Supplementary Figure for more information on computational simulations.

Thus at least some aspect of orexin cell activity may reflect what would be considered an (arousal) error signal in control engineering, since they sum/compare some positive inputs requiring arousal (e.g., sounds) and at least some negative feedback signals of current arousal networks activity (e.g., serotonin). This suggests that orexin neurons might be comparators, but we also note that orexin neurons themselves express functional OXR2s, and are excited by orexin (**Figure 2B**; see Li and van den Pol, 2006; Yamanaka et al., 2010). Although we do not consider it here, this may mean that some orexin cells (or a subpopulation of them) act as regulators as well as comparators.

ARE OXR2-EXPRESSION NEURONS REGULATORS?

In the generic control loop for stability (**Figure 1**), comparators send error signals to regulators. May such regulators correspond to some of the neurons expressing orexin type-2 receptors (OXR2)? Like orexin peptides (or orexin neurons), the OXR2 cells are essential for wakefulness stability, since OXR2 knockout (but not OXR1 knockout) causes a severe narcoleptic phenotype (Lin et al., 1999; Willie et al., 2003; Mieda et al., 2011). However, like orexin knockout, the OXR2 knockout does not significantly change the total amount of wakefulness (Willie et al., 2003). This seems to imply that, like orexin neurons, OXR2s are not themselves wakefulness generators. Could OXR2 neurons (e.g., histamine cells) be regulators, which receive inputs from comparators and send outputs to wakefulness generators such as noradrenaline neurons (Haas et al., 2008)?

Intriguingly, relations between inputs and outputs (i.e., computations, **Figure 2A**) of some OXR2 neurons resemble those of regulators in integral control loops (**Figure 2B**; Li and van den Pol, 2006; Schöne et al., 2014). As discussed above, an integral control loop may be necessary and sufficient for the type of robust flexibility that orexins give to arousal. In an integral feedback loop, the regulator acts as an integrator (Csete and Doyle, 2002; DiStefano et al., 2012). This means that it has a linear relation between its output and the integral of its input, i.e., its response increases during steady input (**Figure 2A**). Experimentally, when a constant firing input from orexin neurons is optogenetically replayed to histamine neurons (HANs; which express OXR2 and are a key anti-narcoleptic target of orexin cells, Yamanaka et al., 2002; Mochizuki et al., 2011), they increase their firing rate linearly for at least 30 s (**Figure 2B**; Schöne et al., 2014). In turn, when constant concentrations of orexin are applied by bath to orexin neurons (which express OXR2, Yamanaka et al., 2010), they also keep increasing their firing rate linearly, for at least 6 min (**Figure 2B**; Li and van den Pol, 2006). Although these data are consistent with OXR2s acting as integrators, they do not yet rule out that OXR2s instead act as low-pass filters, whose input-output relations can be similar to those of integrators. While placing a low-pass filter in the regulator position may achieve reasonable feedback control, such a regulator may require considerably more gain (i.e., be more expensive to implement) than integral feedback.

Some OXR2-expressing neurons may therefore integrate orexin cell input at time scales relevant for processing the durations of orexin cell firing bursts seen *in vivo* (reported to last from seconds to minutes, Mileykovskiy et al., 2005). The computational outcome of this integration will be passed on to downstream arousal generators. We note that, *in vivo* in the brain, orexin peptides will be subject to diffusion/degradation and so postsynaptic effects of neurotransmission may saturate during constant firing of orexin axons. This is likely to constrain integration to a finite time window (i.e., the firing rate of an OXR2 cell may no longer be affected by orexin release from a day ago). Experimentally measurable consequences of this are illustrated in **Figure 2A** (bottom). A neuron integrating an orexin signal will give different temporal patterns of spiking, depending on how long the input is relative to how fast orexin is removed from receptors (by degradation/diffusion) (**Figure 2A**). It should therefore be possible to estimate the integration window by experimentally varying input duration (e.g., time for which orexin is applied) and analyzing output dynamics (e.g., temporal variation in OXR2 cell firing). In Section "Model Predictions" below, we speculate that by varying half-lives of orexins (e.g., by adjusting the relative proportions of orexin-A and orexin-B) it may theoretically be possible to tune the integration window for optimal control responses.

GENERATORS OF AROUSAL DRIVE

Generator neurons for arousal would have the following operational features: (1) their activity should promote arousal; (2) their activity would be essential for the signal from comparators (or regulators) to be converted into wakefulness/arousal; (3) their direct modulation by comparators would be insufficient for appropriate arousal; and (4) some aspects of their activity would be sent to comparators as negative feedback. At present, at least some of these properties seem to be exhibited by noradrelanine neurons in the brain's locus coeruleus. Their activity promotes arousal (Carter et al., 2010). Their activity is essential for the signals from orexin neurons to produce awakening (Carter et al., 2012). Their direct modulation by orexin cell inputs, via OXR1 expressed by noradrenaline neurons (Hagan et al., 1999; Sakurai, 2007), cannot rescue unstable arousal caused by loss of OXR2 from other neural modules (Lin et al., 1999; Willie et al., 2003). Finally, noradrenaline has been shown to inhibit orexin neurons (Li et al., 2002; Yamanaka et al., 2003b), although this effect could change as a function of prior sleep history (Grivel et al., 2005). However, negative feedback to orexin neurons can be mediated by other chemicals indicative of arousal drive, in particular serotonin which robustly inhibits orexin neurons via 5-HT_{1A} receptors (Muraki et al., 2004).

In summary, although specific details remain to be elucidated, we suggest that the above experimental data could be interpreted as consistent with control of arousal by non-redundant modules similar to those in **Figure 1A**. However, based on current evidence, it cannot be excluded that real control circuits also contain redundant wiring (e.g., parallel connections from several comparator and regulator neurons to several generators).

MODEL PREDICTIONS

A major advantage of expressing theories as formal control diagrams (**Figure 1A**) is that they can be analyzed computationally, to make quantitative experimental predictions to test the theories. **Figure 3B** shows computational predictions for temporal activity patterns of different neurons (comparator, regulator, generator). The circuit diagram in **Figure 3B** has been altered slightly from the basic control scheme in **Figure 1A**: comparator C now communicates directly with both regulator R and generator G, **Figure 3B**. This alteration is not critical for conclusions presented here, and was introduced to make the circuit more similar to orexin circuit, in which orexin cells synapse with both putative regulators (e.g., histamine cells) and putative generators (e.g., noradrenaline cells) (Sakurai, 2007).

In response to a step change in set-point, the activities of the interconnected neurons C-G-R rearrange to make the output of G exactly match the new set-point (**Figure 3B**). Note that temporal response of neuron C (i.e., error signal) is transient, in contrast to sustained responses of neurons R and G, since the system is wired to eliminate the error.

While responses of regulator and generator to a change in set-point are broadly similar (**Figure 3B**), they can be operationally differentiated by looking at their responses to load/noise (i.e., the type of input that the system is designed to resist). Introduction of a sustained load/noise causes the regulator neurons to produce a sustained change in activity which opposes the load, while the generator neuron activity is unsettled only transiently and then goes back to set-point (**Figure 3A**). This illustrates why both regulator and generator are important for robust performance. The regulator deals with unwanted signals, so that the generator is not distracted from delivering a set-point.

Experimental activity signatures of different neurons may thus point to their specific control roles and mutual interconnections in a network. Neurophysiological correlates of brain's set-points remain elusive, but selective manipulations of specific hypothalamic neurons have effects that can be interpreted as changes of vital set-points (Gropp et al., 2005; Luquet et al., 2005; Aponte et al., 2011; Krashes et al., 2011). A load/noise can also be introduced into arousal circuits, e.g., by activating opposing sleep circuits. It should thus be experimentally possible to impose changes in set-points or loads on the brain, to measure consequent responses of different cells, and to compare them with predictions associated with different control architectures and computations, such as those shown in **Figure 3B**. At present, such investigations are complicated by the lack of universal agreement of how to measure the final output of the system, the level of arousal. For example, the level of arousal can be measured as cortical gamma activity (EEG), and/or as muscle tone and movement (EMG), and/or as sympathetic parameters such as heart rate, blood pressure, and respiration. Choice of most appropriate measure of the level of arousal may ultimately improve our understanding of activity in different arousal-related neurons in relation to EEG, EMG, and sympathetic measures.

Do existing *in vivo* recordings from orexin, histamine, and noradrenaline networks correspond to the predictions in **Figure 3B**? From the limited number of such recordings that exist in the literature, it is difficult to infer this definitively, without precisely controlled and quantified inputs the system, e.g., introducing a constant level of disturbance such as that shown in **Figure 3B** (Aston-Jones and Bloom, 1981; Lee et al., 2005; Takahashi et al., 2006). The interpretation of existing data in the context of our model is thus unclear, but there is some evidence that orexin neurons fire transiently in response to disturbances (Mileykovskiy et al., 2005), while histamine and noradrenaline neurons discharge in a tonic fashion (Aston-Jones and Bloom, 1981; Takahashi et al., 2006). This issue needs to be revisited with more quantified experimental stimuli, and with recordings from a greater number of neurons to assess the net output of the networks.

A special note is warranted about the time window integrated by the regulator neurons. As mentioned above, this may correspond to physiological variables such as the active life-span of neurotransmitter molecules (i.e., diffusion/degradation/half-life). A short life-span would mean a brief integration window, and vice versa. A full computational treatment is beyond the scope of this article, but because the integration time window determines the regulator response (**Figure 2A**), it also determines how quickly the integral feedback circuit deals with changes in set-point or noise. If the life-span of a transmitter is overly short, the circuit will behave like a proportional controller, giving rise to problems illustrated in **Figure 1C**. If the life-span is overly long, a control signal will persist much longer than the error signal, causing the generator to deviate from set-point for unacceptable amounts of time. Ideally the life-span would thus be tuned to typical durations of inputs (set-point or noise) experienced by the system in real life. Physiologically, for arousal systems these input durations would correspond to durations of salient signals (e.g., 10 s of crossing a busy street) and random disturbances (e.g., 5 min of laughter). Typical durations of these features would obviously vary vastly depending on the environment. It is tempting to speculate that the environment might tune the half-life of the mix of orexin-A and -B released by orexin neurons, in order to optimize the integration window and control. Orexin-A and -B are equally potent activators of the anti-narcoleptic OXR2s, but two disulfide bonds in orexin-A would presumably make it much less easily degradable than orexin-B (Sakurai et al., 1998). If the brain could vary the proportions of orexin-A and -B released onto OXR2 neurons, we predict that an environment filled with rapidly changing inputs should increase orexin-B/orexin-A ratio (e.g., by environment-dependent processing of the pre-proorexin precursor peptide). This would result in a shorter integration window and better tracking of error signals by the control system (**Figure 2A**).

CONCLUSIONS AND LIMITATIONS

We have presented a systems framework that unifies biologically-plausible neurophysiology and appropriate cruise-control of arousal. This framework highlights the need for at least three types of neurons with specific connections and response properties. Several types of arousal-promoting neurons have been discovered in the brain (Saper et al., 2001; Jones, 2003). We suggest that these distinct neurons may implement distinct, non-redundant algorithms (**Figure 1A**). The proposed framework also highlights weak-points in the system. If an irrelevant input/noise enters the system at the level of regulator or generator, it may be reasonably counteracted by the feedback loop so that the generator output remains appropriate (as in **Figure 2B**). However, if disruption enters at the level of the comparator, the consequences could be disastrous, since the system would process it as a salient set-point (i.e., generator output will be disrupted). These considerations are useful for at least two reasons. First, for interpreting experiments aimed at identifying roles of neurons (comparator, regulator, generator) in behavior, e.g., during targeted optogenetic interventions combined with behavioral readouts (Adamantidis et al., 2010; Atasoy et al., 2012). Second, for understanding why disrupting a tiny fraction of certain brain cells (e.g., few thousand orexin neurons out of billions of neurons in the brain) can have such dramatic impact on brain state control.

The proposed model is intended as a useful guide for rationalizing the vast complexity of arousal control components in the brain, and for designing new experiments. We acknowledge that it does not explicitly consider many fundamental aspects of brain state control, and has other limitations. For example, aspects such as plasticity (learning and memory) in the cruise-control circuit remain relatively unexplored. We also neglected the potentially intricate dynamics of sleep-promoting signals (Achermann and Borbély, 2003; Fulcher et al., 2014) by viewing such signals as noise during wakefulness. Our model focuses on wakefulness only and does not deal with sleep; other engineering analogies, such as flip-flop control circuits, have been proposed for sleep state control (Lu et al., 2006).

Despite these limitations, the proposed framework highlights the importance of specific computations for arousal control in the real world. Current (drug) therapies for arousal disorders (insomnia, narcolepsy) are essentially aimed at increasing brain concentrations of chemicals that suppress or promote arousal (Saper and Scammell, 2013). Such drug strategies may not replay brain computations required for proper arousal control (**Figures 1C, 2B**). Indeed, current drug therapies for narcolepsy and insomnia have mild therapeutic success with many unwanted side-effects (Bhat et al., 2008; Saper and Scammell, 2013). An alternative therapy would be to compute and re-introduce appropriate brain activity through electroceuticals and closed-loop control of brain function (Armstrong et al., 2013; Famm et al., 2013). Computational frameworks such as those presented here would be critical for success of such therapies, when tools for targeted closed-loop control of the human brain become sufficiently developed.

ACKNOWLEDGMENTS

This work was supported by UK Medical Research Council (Denis Burdakov, ref. MC_UP_1202/2), and Human Frontiers Science Foundation (Denis Burdakov, ref. RGY0076/2012). We thank the reviewers for their constructive comments on the manuscript.

REFERENCES

Achermann, P., and Borbély, A. A. (2003). Mathematical models of sleep regulation. *Front. Biosci.* 8, s683–s693. doi: 10.2741/1064

Adamantidis, A., Carter, M. C., and de Lecea, L. (2010). Optogenetic deconstruction of sleep-wake circuitry in the brain. *Front. Mol. Neurosci.* 2:31. doi: 10.3389/neuro.02.031.2009

Adamantidis, A. R., Zhang, F., Aravanis, A. M., Deisseroth, K., and de Lecea, L. (2007). Neural substrates of awakening probed with optogenetic control of hypocretin neurons. *Nature* 450, 420–424. doi: 10.1038/nature06310

Aponte, Y., Atasoy, D., and Sternson, S. M. (2011). AGRP neurons are sufficient to orchestrate feeding behavior rapidly and without training. *Nat. Neurosci.* 14, 351–355. doi: 10.1038/nn.2739

Armstrong, C., Krook-Magnuson, E., Oijala, M., and Soltesz, I. (2013). Closed-loop optogenetic intervention in mice. *Nat. Protoc.* 8, 1475–1493. doi: 10.1038/nprot.2013.080

Aston-Jones, G., and Bloom, F. E. (1981). Norepinephrine-containing locus coeruleus neurons in behaving rats exhibit pronounced responses to non-noxious environmental stimuli. *J. Neurosci.* 1, 887–900.

Aström, K., and Hagglund, T. (1995). *PID Controllers Theory, Design and Tuning.* Intrument Society of America.

Atasoy, D., Betley, J. N., Su, H. H., and Sternson, S. M. (2012). Deconstruction of a neural circuit for hunger. *Nature* 488, 172–177. doi: 10.1038/nature11270

Bayer, L., Eggermann, E., Serafin, M., Grivel, J., Machard, D., Muhlethaler, M., et al. (2005). Opposite effects of noradrenaline and acetylcholine upon hypocretin/orexin versus melanin concentrating hormone neurons in rat hypothalamic slices. *Neuroscience* 130, 807–811. doi: 10.1016/j.neuroscience.2004.10.032

Bhat, A., Shafi, F., and El Solh, A. A. (2008). Pharmacotherapy of insomnia. *Expert Opin. Pharmacother.* 9, 351–362. doi: 10.1517/14656566.9.3.351

Carter, M. E., Brill, J., Bonnavion, P., Huguenard, J. R., Huerta, R., and de Lecea, L. (2012). Mechanism for hypocretin-mediated sleep-to-wake transitions. *Proc. Natl. Acad. Sci. U S A* 109, E2635–E2644. doi: 10.1073/pnas.1202526109

Carter, M. E., Yizhar, O., Chikahisa, S., Nguyen, H., Adamantidis, A., Nishino, S., et al. (2010). Tuning arousal with optogenetic modulation of locus coeruleus neurons. *Nat. Neurosci.* 13, 1526–1533. doi: 10.1038/nn.2682

Chemelli, R. M., Willie, J. T., Sinton, C. M., Elmquist, J. K., Scammell, T., Lee, C., et al. (1999). Narcolepsy in orexin knockout mice: molecular genetics of sleep regulation. *Cell* 98, 437–451. doi: 10.1016/s0092-8674(00)81973-x

Csete, M. E., and Doyle, J. C. (2002). Reverse engineering of biological complexity. *Science* 295, 1664–1669. doi: 10.1126/science.1069981

Csete, M., and Doyle, J. (2004). Bow ties, metabolism and disease. *Trends Biotechnol.* 22, 446–450. doi: 10.1016/j.tibtech.2004.07.007

Dauvilliers, Y., Arnulf, I., and Mignot, E. (2007). Narcolepsy with cataplexy. *Lancet* 369, 499–511. doi: 10.1016/S0140-6736(07)60237-2

de Lecea, L., Jones, B. E., Boutrel, B., Borgland, S. L., Nishino, S., Bubser, M., et al. (2006). Addiction and arousal: alternative roles of hypothalamic peptides. *J. Neurosci.* 26, 10372–10375. doi: 10.1523/jneurosci.3118-06.2006

de Lecea, L., Kilduff, T. S., Peyron, C., Gao, X., Foye, P. E., Danielson, P. E., et al. (1998). The hypocretins: hypothalamus-specific peptides with neuroexcitatory activity. *Proc. Natl. Acad. Sci. U S A* 95, 322–327. doi: 10.1073/pnas.95.1.322

DiStefano, J., Stubberud, A., and Williams, I. (2012). *Feedback and Control Systems.* New York: McGrawHill.

Doyle, J. C., and Csete, M. (2011). Architecture, constraints and behavior. *Proc. Natl. Acad. Sci. U S A* 108(Suppl. 3), 15624–15630. doi: 10.1073/pnas.1103557108

Dworak, M., McCarley, R. W., Kim, T., Kalinchuk, A. V., and Basheer, R. (2010). Sleep and brain energy levels: ATP changes during sleep. *J. Neurosci.* 30, 9007–9016. doi: 10.1523/JNEUROSCI.1423-10.2010

Famm, K., Litt, B., Tracey, K. J., Boyden, E. S., and Slaoui, M. (2013). Drug discovery: a jump-start for electroceuticals. *Nature* 496, 159–161. doi: 10.1038/496159a

Franklin, D. W., and Wolpert, D. M. (2011). Computational mechanisms of sensorimotor control. *Neuron* 72, 425–442. doi: 10.1016/j.neuron.2011.10.006

Fulcher, B. D., Phillips, A. J., Postnova, S., and Robinson, P. A. (2014). A physiologically based model of orexinergic stabilization of sleep and wake. *PLoS One* 9:e91982. doi: 10.1371/journal.pone.0091982

Grivel, J., Cvetkovic, V., Bayer, L., Machard, D., Tobler, I., Mühlethaler, M., et al. (2005). The wake-promoting hypocretin/orexin neurons change their response to noradrenaline after sleep deprivation. *J. Neurosci.* 25, 4127–4130. doi: 10.1523/jneurosci.0666-05.2005

Gropp, E., Shanabrough, M., Borok, E., Xu, A. W., Janoschek, R., Buch, T., et al. (2005). Agouti-related peptide-expressing neurons are mandatory for feeding. *Nat. Neurosci.* 8, 1289–1291. doi: 10.1038/nn1548

Haas, H. L., Sergeeva, O. A., and Selbach, O. (2008). Histamine in the nervous system. *Physiol. Rev.* 88, 1183–1241. doi: 10.1152/physrev.00043.2007

Hagan, J. J., Leslie, R. A., Patel, S., Evans, M. L., Wattam, T. A., Holmes, S., et al. (1999). Orexin a activates locus coeruleus cell firing and increases arousal in the rat. *Proc. Natl. Acad. Sci. U S A* 96, 10911–10916. doi: 10.1073/pnas.96.19.10911

Hara, J., Beuckmann, C. T., Nambu, T., Willie, J. T., Chemelli, R. M., Sinton, C. M., et al. (2001). Genetic ablation of orexin neurons in mice results in narcolepsy, hypophagia and obesity. *Neuron* 30, 345–354. doi: 10.1016/s0896-6273(01)00293-8

Horvath, T. L., Stachenfeld, N. S., and Diano, S. (2014). A temperature hypothesis of hypothalamus-driven obesity. *Yale J. Biol. Med.* 87, 149–158.

Jones, B. E. (2003). Arousal systems. *Front. Biosci.* 8, s438–s451. doi: 10.2741/1074

Krashes, M. J., Koda, S., Ye, C., Rogan, S. C., Adams, A. C., Cusher, D. S., et al. (2011). Rapid, reversible activation of AgRP neurons drives feeding behavior in mice. *J. Clin. Invest.* 121, 1424–1428. doi: 10.1172/JCI46229

Kuwaki, T. (2011). Orexin links emotional stress to autonomic functions. *Auton. Neurosci.* 161, 20–27. doi: 10.1016/j.autneu.2010.08.004

Lee, M. G., Hassani, O. K., and Jones, B. E. (2005). Discharge of identified orexin/hypocretin neurons across the sleep-waking cycle. *J. Neurosci.* 25, 6716–6720. doi: 10.1523/jneurosci.1887-05.2005

Li, Y., Gao, X. B., Sakurai, T., and van den Pol, A. N. (2002). Hypocretin/Orexin excites hypocretin neurons via a local glutamate neuron-A potential mechanism for orchestrating the hypothalamic arousal system. *Neuron* 36, 1169–1181. doi: 10.1016/s0896-6273(02)01132-7

Li, Y., and van den Pol, A. N. (2006). Differential target-dependent actions of coexpressed inhibitory dynorphin and excitatory hypocretin/orexin neuropeptides. *J. Neurosci.* 26, 13037–13047. doi: 10.1523/jneurosci.3380-06.2006

Lin, L., Faraco, J., Li, R., Kadotani, H., Rogers, W., Lin, X., et al. (1999). The sleep disorder canine narcolepsy is caused by a mutation in the hypocretin (orexin) receptor 2 gene. *Cell* 98, 365–376. doi: 10.1016/s0092-8674(00)81965-0

Liu, R. J., van den Pol, A. N., and Aghajanian, G. K. (2002). Hypocretins (orexins) regulate serotonin neurons in the dorsal raphe nucleus by excitatory direct and inhibitory indirect actions. *J. Neurosci.* 22, 9453–9464.

Lu, J., Sherman, D., Devor, M., and Saper, C. B. (2006). A putative flip-flop switch for control of REM sleep. *Nature* 441, 589–594. doi: 10.1038/nature04767

Luquet, S., Perez, F. A., Hnasko, T. S., and Palmiter, R. D. (2005). NPY/AgRP neurons are essential for feeding in adult mice but can be ablated in neonates. *Science* 310, 683–685. doi: 10.1126/science.1115524

Mieda, M., Hasegawa, E., Kisanuki, Y. Y., Sinton, C. M., Yanagisawa, M., and Sakurai, T. (2011). Differential roles of orexin receptor-1 and -2 in the regulation of non-REM and REM sleep. *J. Neurosci.* 31, 6518–6526. doi: 10.1523/JNEUROSCI.6506-10.2011

Mignot, E., Taheri, S., and Nishino, S. (2002). Sleeping with the hypothalamus: emerging therapeutic targets for sleep disorders. *Nat. Neurosci.* 5(Suppl.), 1071–1075. doi: 10.1038/nn944

Mileykovskiy, B. Y., Kiyashchenko, L. I., and Siegel, J. M. (2005). Behavioral correlates of activity in identified hypocretin/orexin neurons. *Neuron* 46, 787–798. doi: 10.1016/j.neuron.2005.04.035

Mochizuki, T., Arrigoni, E., Marcus, J. N., Clark, E. L., Yamamoto, M., Honer, M., et al. (2011). Orexin receptor 2 expression in the posterior hypothalamus rescues sleepiness in narcoleptic mice. *Proc. Natl. Acad. Sci. U S A* 108, 4471–4476. doi: 10.1073/pnas.1012456108

Muraki, Y., Yamanaka, A., Tsujino, N., Kilduff, T. S., Goto, K., and Sakurai, T. (2004). Serotonergic regulation of the orexin/hypocretin neurons through the 5-HT1A receptor. *J. Neurosci.* 24, 7159–7166. doi: 10.1523/jneurosci.1027-04.2004

Nishino, S., and Kanbayashi, T. (2005). Symptomatic narcolepsy, cataplexy and hypersomnia and their implications in the hypothalamic hypocretin/orexin system. *Sleep Med. Rev.* 9, 269–310. doi: 10.1016/j.smrv.2005.03.004

Nishino, S., Ripley, B., Overeem, S., Lammers, G. J., and Mignot, E. (2000). Hypocretin (orexin) deficiency in human narcolepsy. *Lancet* 355, 39–40. doi: 10.1016/s0140-6736(99)05582-8

Peyron, C., Faraco, J., Rogers, W., Ripley, B., Overeem, S., Charnay, Y., et al. (2000). A mutation in a case of early onset narcolepsy and a generalized absence of hypocretin peptides in human narcoleptic brains. *Nat. Med.* 6, 991–997. doi: 10.1038/79690

Peyron, C., Tighe, D. K., van den Pol, A. N., de lecea, L., Heller, H. C., Sutcliffe, J. G., et al. (1998). Neurons containing hypocretin (orexin) project to multiple neuronal systems. *J. Neurosci.* 18, 9996–10015.

Sakurai, T. (2007). The neural circuit of orexin (hypocretin): maintaining sleep and wakefulness. *Nat. Rev. Neurosci.* 8, 171–181. doi: 10.1038/nrn2092

Sakurai, T., Amemiya, A., Ishii, M., Matsuzaki, I., Chemelli, R. M., Tanaka, H., et al. (1998). Orexins and orexin receptors: a family of hypothalamic neuropeptides and G protein-coupled receptors that regulate feeding behavior. *Cell* 92, 573–585. doi: 10.1016/s0092-8674(00)80949-6

Saper, C. B., Chou, T. C., and Scammell, T. E. (2001). The sleep switch: hypothalamic control of sleep and wakefulness. *Trends Neurosci.* 24, 726–731. doi: 10.1016/s0166-2236(00)02002-6

Saper, C. B., and Scammell, T. E. (2013). Emerging therapeutics in sleep. *Ann. Neurol.* 74, 435–440. doi: 10.1002/ana.24000

Schöne, C., Apergis-Schoute, J., Sakurai, T., Adamantidis, A., and Burdakov, D. (2014). Coreleased orexin and glutamate evoke nonredundant spike outputs and computations in histamine neurons. *Cell Rep.* 7, 697–704. doi: 10.1016/j.celrep.2014.03.055

Sohn, J. W., Elmquist, J. K., and Williams, K. W. (2013). Neuronal circuits that regulate feeding behavior and metabolism. *Trends Neurosci.* 36, 504–512. doi: 10.1016/j.tins.2013.05.003

Speakman, J. R., Levitsky, D. A., Allison, D. B., Bray, M. S., De Castro, J. M., Clegg, D. J., et al. (2011). Set points, settling points and some alternative models: theoretical options to understand how genes and environments combine to regulate body adiposity. *Dis. Model. Mech.* 4, 733–745. doi: 10.1242/dmm.008698

Takahashi, K., Lin, J. S., and Sakai, K. (2006). Neuronal activity of histaminergic tuberomammillary neurons during wake-sleep states in the mouse. *J. Neurosci.* 26, 10292–10298. doi: 10.1523/jneurosci.2341-06.2006

Tecuapetla, F., Patel, J. C., Xenias, H., English, D., Tadros, I., Shah, F., et al. (2010). Glutamatergic signaling by mesolimbic dopamine neurons in the nucleus accumbens. *J. Neurosci.* 30, 7105–7110. doi: 10.1523/JNEUROSCI.0265-10.2010

Thannickal, T. C., Moore, R. Y., Nienhuis, R., Ramanathan, L., Gulyani, S., Aldrich, M., et al. (2000). Reduced number of hypocretin neurons in human narcolepsy. *Neuron* 27, 469–474. doi: 10.1016/s0896-6273(00)00058-1

Tritsch, N. X., Ding, J. B., and Sabatini, B. L. (2012). Dopaminergic neurons inhibit striatal output through non-canonical release of GABA. *Nature* 490, 262–266. doi: 10.1038/nature11466

Uschakov, A., Grivel, J., Cvetkovic-Lopes, V., Bayer, L., Bernheim, L., Jones, B. E., et al. (2011). Sleep-deprivation regulates alpha-2 adrenergic responses of rat hypocretin/orexin neurons. *PLoS One* 6:e16672. doi: 10.1371/journal.pone.0016672

von Bertalanffy, L. (2013). *General Systems Theory.* New York: George Braziller.

Wiener, N. (1965). *Cybernetics: Or Control and Communication in the Animal and the Machine.* Cambridge, Massachusetts: The MIT Press.

Williams, R. H., Alexopoulos, H., Jensen, L. T., Fugger, L., and Burdakov, D. (2008). Adaptive sugar sensors in hypothalamic feeding circuits. *Proc. Natl. Acad. Sci. U S A* 105, 11975–11980. doi: 10.1073/pnas.0802687105

Williams, R. H., Jensen, L. T., Verkhratsky, A., Fugger, L., and Burdakov, D. (2007). Control of hypothalamic orexin neurons by acid and CO2. *Proc. Natl. Acad. Sci. U S A* 104, 10685–10690. doi: 10.1073/pnas.0702676104

Williams, R. H., Morton, A. J., and Burdakov, D. (2011). Paradoxical function of orexin/hypocretin circuits in a mouse model of Huntington's disease. *Neurobiol. Dis.* 42, 438–455. doi: 10.1016/j.nbd.2011.02.006

Willie, J. T., Chemelli, R. M., Sinton, C. M., Tokita, S., Williams, S. C., Kisanuki, Y. Y., et al. (2003). Distinct narcolepsy syndromes in orexin receptor-2 and orexin null mice: molecular genetic dissection of Non-REM and REM sleep regulatory processes. *Neuron* 38, 715–730. doi: 10.1016/s0896-6273(03)00330-1

Winsky-Sommerer, R., Yamanaka, A., Diano, S., Borok, E., Roberts, A. J., Sakurai, T., et al. (2004). Interaction between the corticotropin-releasing factor system and hypocretins (orexins): a novel circuit mediating stress response. *J. Neurosci.* 24, 11439–11448. doi: 10.1523/jneurosci.3459-04.2004

Yamanaka, A., Beuckmann, C. T., Willie, J. T., Hara, J., Tsujino, N., Mieda, M., et al. (2003a). Hypothalamic orexin neurons regulate arousal according to energy balance in mice. *Neuron* 38, 701–713. doi: 10.1016/s0896-6273(03)00331-3

Yamanaka, A., Muraki, Y., Tsujino, N., Goto, K., and Sakurai, T. (2003b). Regulation of orexin neurons by the monoaminergic and cholinergic systems. *Biochem. Biophys. Res. Commun.* 303, 120–129. doi: 10.1016/s0006-291x(03)00299-7

Yamanaka, A., Tabuchi, S., Tsunematsu, T., Fukazawa, Y., and Tominaga, M. (2010). Orexin directly excites orexin neurons through orexin 2 receptor. *J. Neurosci.* 30, 12642–12652. doi: 10.1523/JNEUROSCI.2120-10.2010

Yamanaka, A., Tsujino, N., Funahashi, H., Honda, K., Guan, J. L., Wang, Q. P., et al. (2002). Orexins activate histaminergic neurons via the orexin 2 receptor. *Biochem. Biophys. Res. Commun.* 290, 1237–1245. doi: 10.1006/bbrc.2001.6318

Yeo, G. S., and Heisler, L. K. (2012). Unraveling the brain regulation of appetite: lessons from genetics. *Nat. Neurosci.* 15, 1343–1349. doi: 10.1038/nn.3211

Yi, T. M., Huang, Y., Simon, M. I., and Doyle, J. (2000). Robust perfect adaptation in bacterial chemotaxis through integral feedback control. *Proc. Natl. Acad. Sci. U S A* 97, 4649–4653. doi: 10.1073/pnas.97.9.4649

7

The contribution of hypothalamic macroglia to the regulation of energy homeostasis

Laura B. Buckman*[1,2] *and Kate L. J. Ellacott*[3]

[1] Department of Molecular Physiology and Biophysics, Vanderbilt University Medical Center, Nashville, TN, USA
[2] Division of Infectious Disease, School of Medicine, University of North Carolina at Chapel Hill, Chapel Hill, NC, USA
[3] Biomedical Neuroscience Research Group, University of Exeter Medical School, Hatherly Laboratories, Exeter, UK

***Correspondence:**
Kate L. J. Ellacott, Biomedical Neuroscience Research Group, University of Exeter Medical School, Hatherly Laboratories, Prince of Wales Rd, Exeter, EX4 4PS, UK
e-mail: k.ellacott@exeter.ac.uk

The hypothalamus is critical for the regulation of energy homeostasis. Genetic and pharmacologic studies have identified a number of key hypothalamic neuronal circuits that integrate signals controlling food intake and energy expenditure. Recently, studies have begun to emerge demonstrating a role for non-neuronal cell types in the regulation of energy homeostasis. In particular the potential importance of different glial cell types is increasingly being recognized. A number of studies have described changes in the activity of hypothalamic macroglia (principally astrocytes and tanycytes) in response to states of positive and negative energy balance, such as obesity and fasting. This article will review these studies and discuss how these findings are changing our understanding of the cellular mechanisms by which energy homeostasis is regulated.

Keywords: astrocyte, tanycyte, fasting, obesity, high-fat diet, inflammation, hypothalamus

ENERGY HOMEOSTASIS

Energy homeostasis, the balance between food intake and energy expenditure, is an exquisitely sensitive process regulated by the central nervous system (CNS). Mediated by nutritional, humoral and nervous inputs into the brain from the periphery, information on energy status is integrated by hypothalamic and brainstem nuclei, and relayed to other neural circuits such as those of the mesolimbic dopaminergic pathway. To date the vast majority of research on the hypothalamic regulation of energy homeostasis has focused on the involvement of neuronal signaling with the contribution of other cell types only beginning to be addressed (Yi et al., 2011; Chowen et al., 2013). This mini-review will summarize and discuss the emerging evidence for a role of one of these cellular classes, hypothalamic macroglia, in the regulation of energy homeostasis focusing on states of both positive (e.g., obesity and neonatal overnutrition) and negative energy balance (e.g., fasting).

MACROGLIA

In the adult CNS glia are broadly categorized into two main classes: (1) macroglia—including astrocytes, oligodendrocytes, NG-2 glia, tanycytes and other ependymal cells; and (2) microglia. Originally thought to be largely structural cells acting as "glue" in the CNS it is now widely accepted that glia are critical regulators of parenchymal homeostasis and directly influence neuronal communication (Tasker et al., 2012). As will be discussed in more detail below, changes in hypothalamic glial cell activity have been reported in states of positive and negative energy balance in rodents (Hsuchou et al., 2009a; Horvath et al., 2010; García-Cáceres et al., 2011; Thaler et al., 2012; Buckman et al., 2013; Langlet et al., 2013) and non-human primates (Grayson et al., 2010), suggestive of an active role in the regulation of energy homeostasis. Furthermore, consistent with data from animal models, evidence of gliosis, a condition associated with increased numbers of activated glia, has been discovered in humans with elevated body mass index using neuroimaging techniques (Drake et al., 2011; Thaler et al., 2012). Due to space constraints this mini-review is focused on the contribution of macroglia, primarily astrocytes and tanycytes, to the regulation of energy homeostasis; however, it is not our intention to underplay the importance of microglia to this area which is likely to be highly significant (Bilbo and Schwarz, 2012).

ASTROCYTES

Astrocytes are macroglial cells of ectodermal origin. In the human brain, astrocytes constitute nearly half of the cells in the CNS, in some brain regions outnumbering neurons by a factor of ten to one. The functions of astrocytes in the CNS are diverse (extensively reviewed by Abbott et al., 2006; Sofroniew and Vinters, 2010; Tasker et al., 2012) and include: (1) modulating neuronal activity; (2) energy storage and supply to neurons; and (3) regulation of blood-brain barrier (BBB) permeability and cerebral blood flow. Astrocytes play a critical role in regulating other neuroendocrine processes in the hypothalamus including activity of gonadotrophin-releasing hormone (Prevot et al., 2007) and magnocellular (Panatier, 2009; Tasker et al., 2012) neurons. Intriguingly, hypothalamic astrocytes also show diurnal variation in their morphology and gene expression (reviewed in Jackson,

2011) and play a critical role in the control of circadian rhythms (Ng et al., 2011).

OLIGODENDROCYTES AND NG-2 GLIA

In common with astrocytes, oligodendrocytes are derived from the ectoderm; however, their principal function is believed to be the formation of myelin which insulates neuronal axons, facilitating salutatory conduction. A third type of macroglia, NG-2 glia, are more recently described, and as such are less well characterized. NG-2 glia act as oligodendrocyte precursors but also have functional similarities to astrocytes (Nishiyama et al., 2005). To date there is minimal published evidence for a role for oligodendrocytes or NG-2 glia in the regulation of energy homeostasis. However, given the recent focus on the functional role of astrocytes in the modulation of energy homeostasis and the potential functional overlap between NG-2 glia and astrocytes, it is likely that time will reveal that these cells also contribute to the regulation of neuroendocrine circuitry. Indeed, recent evidence suggests that NG-2 glia are capable of differentiating into neurons within the hypothalamus (Robins et al., 2013b). Furthermore, specific deletion of the NG-2 proteoglycan from oligodendrocytes results in a lean phenotype in mice (Chang et al., 2012), but whether this occurs due to specific alterations in oligodendrocyte action or as a result of a global deficit in neuronal function as a consequence of hypomyelination is not known.

EPENDYMAL CELLS/TANYCYTES

Ependymal cells are dedicated glia lining the cerebral ventricles. Tight-junctions between cells of the ependymal layer regulate the exchange of substances between the cerebral-spinal fluid and CNS parenchyma. Within the third and fourth ventricles there is a specialist population of ependymal cells called tanycytes which are divided into four subclasses ($\alpha 1$, $\alpha 2$, $\beta 1$ and $\beta 2$) distinguished by their morphology and localization (for review see Rodríguez et al., 2005). In the hypothalamus a subpopulation of α-tanycytes is believed to have the capacity to act as neural stem cells in the adult brain (Robins et al., 2013a). The reader is referred to a comprehensive review by Bolborea and Dale published in 2013 on the potential role of hypothalamic tanycytes in the regulation of food intake and energy homeostasis (Bolborea and Dale, 2013). In light of this we have tried to focus our discussion of tanycytes to pertinent work that has been published subsequent to their review article.

MACROGLIAL CHANGES IN STATES OF POSITIVE ENERGY BALANCE

ASTROCYTES ARE RESPONSIVE TO HIGH-FAT FEEDING, OBESITY AND NEONATAL OVERNUTRITION

Diet-induced obesity causes activation of hypothalamic inflammatory signaling pathways (De Souza et al., 2005). In part due to their intimate relationship with neurons and the BBB, astrocytes have fundamental roles in the innate immune response of the CNS and undergo key morphological changes in CNS pathologies. In the context of inflammation, astrocytes respond by a process referred to as reactive astrogliosis, characterized by cellular hypertrophy, proliferation, and increased expression of the intermediate filaments: glial-fibrillary acidic protein (GFAP), vimentin, and nestin (Sofroniew, 2009). Reactive astrogliosis is a graded phenomenon, ranging from mild alterations in gene expression and cellular morphology to severe (sometimes permanent) tissue reorganization leading to glial scars (Sofroniew, 2009). Changes in astrocyte morphology indicative of reactive astrogliosis have been reported in rodent models of chronic-diet induced obesity (Hsuchou et al., 2009a; Horvath et al., 2010; Thaler et al., 2012; Buckman et al., 2013), genetic obesity (Hsuchou et al., 2009a; Buckman et al., 2013) and neonatal overnutrition (García-Cáceres et al., 2011; Fuente-Martín et al., 2012). In adult animals obesity-associated reactive astrogliosis has been implicated in altering the firing of neurons of the central melanocortin system (Horvath et al., 2010); thus, potentially contributing to the perpetuation of obesity by modulating the tone of this neuronal circuit critical for the regulation of energy homeostasis (Cone, 2005). However, further work is required to determine the precise molecular mechanism(s) by which astrocytes influence neuronal activity in the context of obesity. The extensive structural changes in hypothalamic astrocytes seen during obesity and neonatal overnutrition suggests that these cells may directly contribute to synaptic rewiring physically by changing glial ensheathment of neurons and also by altering the ability of neurons to receive direct humoral inputs from the periphery (Horvath et al., 2010). Additionally, astrocytes might directly modulate neuronal activity during obesity *via* the action of glial-derived factors, commonly referred to as gliotransmitters, or the modulation of glutamate availability in the synaptic cleft. The presence of astrogliosis in a rodent model of neonatal overnutrition (García-Cáceres et al., 2011; Fuente-Martín et al., 2012) likely has significant implications for the developmental wiring of hypothalamic feeding circuitry, which influences the propensity of these animals to go on to develop obesity in adulthood.

Recent immunohistochemical data suggests that obesity-associated morphologic changes in glial cells of adult rodents are reversible following weight-loss (Berkseth et al., 2014); however, it remains to be fully determined how obesity functionally alters glial-cell activity and whether these changes are restored following weight-loss.

In addition to modulation by chronic high-fat feeding and neonatal overnutrition, changes in markers of astrocyte activation have been reported as early as twenty-four hours after introduction of a high-fat diet to rodents (Thaler et al., 2012). This suggests that astrocytes may also be involved in modulating the acute homeostatic response to high-fat feeding. Indeed, recent work by Le Foll et al. suggests that ketone bodies produced by astrocytes of the ventromedial hypothalamus contribute to the regulation of acute high-fat chow intake in a restricted feeding paradigm (Le Foll et al., 2013). This indicates that astrocytes directly contribute to the regulation of food intake in response to acute high-fat feeding in part by modulating energy availability to key hypothalamic neurons.

The molecular trigger(s) for astrocyte activation/astrogliosis in response to high-fat feeding and obesity are still unclear. It is intriguing that obesity associated-astrogliosis does not occur uniformly across the hypothalamus (Buckman et al., 2013) suggesting that regional factors such as proximity to the third ventricle, BBB permeability, neuronal activity and neurochemical identity may factor in the response. The inflammatory constituents in obesogenic diets are unlikely to be the sole stimuli for obesity-associated astrogliosis. The finding that in addition to diet-induced obesity, hypothalamic astrogliosis is present in rodent models of genetic obesity (Hsuchou et al., 2009a; Buckman et al., 2013) when the animals are maintained on standard laboratory chow, suggests that other humoral and molecular changes associated with obesity contribute to this response. The potential importance of humoral signaling in glial cell activation is further supported by studies in microglia (Gao et al., 2014). Data from *in vitro* studies indicate that saturated fatty acids activate inflammatory signaling in primary astrocyte cultures (Gupta et al., 2012); however, other potential triggers for obesity-associated astrogliosis include: metabolic endotoxemia as a result of changes in the gut microbiome (Cani et al., 2007); endoplasmic reticulum stress (Zhang et al., 2008); neuronal injury (Thaler et al. 2012) and potentially neurogenic neuroinflammation arising from increased neuronal activity (Xanthos and Sandkühler, 2014). Further work is required elucidate the molecular triggers for obesity-associated astrogliosis; however, it is likely to be a highly complex process involving the integration of multiple signals and cues.

MACROGLIA ARE DIRECTLY RESPONSIVE TO KEY METABOLIC HORMONES

Astrocytes can directly respond to humoral stimuli further supporting the hypothesis that these cells contribute to the regulation of energy homeostasis under normal physiologic conditions as well as during pathologic states such as obesity. For example, astrocytes express receptors for the key adipostatic hormone leptin (Hsuchou et al., 2009a,b; Kim et al., 2014) suggesting that astrocytes may be capable of directly responding to changes in adipose tissue energy stores by modulating the activity of hypothalamic neuronal circuitry. Indeed, experimental evidence indicates that chronic intracerebroventricular leptin treatment regulates the expression of both structural astrocyte proteins, vimentin and GFAP (García-Cáceres et al., 2011), and key glutamate and glucose transporters on hypothalamic astrocytes (Fuente-Martín et al., 2012). Furthermore, mice with germ-line deletion of leptin-receptors from astrocytes show a modest protection from diet-induced obesity (Jayaram et al., 2013); however, in this study it was not determined whether this was the result of a failure of the astrocytes to become reactive in response to high-fat feeding or due to other alterations in the astrocyte activity.

A more recent study utilizing a mouse model with tamoxifen-inducible deletion of leptin receptors from astrocytes of adult mice indicates that intact leptin signaling in astrocytes important for the actions of this hormone in the regulation of energy homeostasis (Kim et al., 2014). For example, it was demonstrated in this study that the ability of leptin to reduce food intake is partially inhibited following was loss of astrocytic leptin-receptor signaling in adult mice. Furthermore, mice with loss of astrocytic leptin signaling show reduced astrocytic coverage of ARC melanocortin neurons leading to altered synaptic inputs to these neuronal populations that are critical for the regulation of feeding behavior.

In addition to leptin receptors, astrocytes have also been reported to express insulin (Albrecht et al., 1982) and melanocortin-4 receptors (Selkirk et al., 2007) *in vitro* in primary culture. Furthermore, in astrocytes insulin has been shown to directly regulate cell surface expression of the glutamate transporter, excitatory amino acid transporter 2 (EAAT2/GLT1; Ji et al., 2011) providing a potential humoral mechanism for the astrocytic-regulation of synaptic activity during obesity.

Emerging evidence suggests that in common with neurons, macroglia develop hormone resistance during chronic obesity. A recent study by Balland and colleagues demonstrates that median eminence tanycytes of diet-induced obese mice show reduced STAT3 phosphorylation in response to leptin treatment (Balland et al., 2014). The investigators also go on to show that intact leptin signaling in tanycytes is required for leptin transport into the medial basal hypothalamus, which may represent a new regulatory node for central hormone sensitivity. Moreover, it is likely that astrocytes are also capable of developing leptin and/or insulin resistance; however direct *in vivo* evidence of astrocytic hormone resistance during obesity is lacking.

THE NEUROGENIC CAPACITY OF TANYCYTES IS REGULATED BY HIGH-FAT FEEDING

In 2005 Kokoeva et al. first reported neurogenesis of hypothalamic neurons in adult mice, suggestive of a role for these cells in the regulation of energy homeostasis (Kokoeva et al., 2005). In a subsequent study the same group demonstrated that turn-over of hypothalamic neurons was suppressed in diet-induced obese mice, linked to a reduction in neurogenesis and an increase in apoptosis of the newly divided cells (McNay et al., 2012). Activation of the inflammatory IκKβ/NFκB pathway in neural stem cells *in vitro* and *in vivo* reduces their neurogenic capacity and subsequent survival (Li et al., 2012) providing a novel mechanistic link between CNS inflammation and the regulation of energy homeostasis. Recent work shows that tanycytes are key components of this neurogenic niche (Lee et al., 2012; Robins et al., 2013a) suggestive of a unique role for these macroglia in the regulation of energy homeostasis.

MACROGLIAL CHANGES IN STATES OF NEGATIVE ENERGY BALANCE

ASTROCYTES ARE CRITICAL MEDIATORS OF THE RESPONSE TO HYPOGLYCEMIA

The energy needs of the brain are prioritized at all costs during states of low energy availability. Indeed, astrocytic glycogen stores are critical to sustain neurons under these conditions (Suh et al., 2007). Thus, due to their roles in glucose uptake into the CNS and in providing energy to neurons it is logical that macroglia must be superbly sensitive to glycemic state, and this is supported by published data. For example, pharmacologic inhibition of metabolic activity in hypothalamic glia reduces neuronal activation in response 2-deoxyglucose induced glucoprivation (Young et al., 2000) establishing that glia are critical for the neuronal response to low glucose. Subsequently, expression of the glucose transporter GLUT-2 in astrocytes was discovered to be vital for CNS sensing of hypoglycemia when it was shown that overexpression of GLUT-2 in astrocytes was sufficient to restore hypoglycemia-induced peripheral glucagon release in animals with GLUT-2 deficiency (*Ripglut1;glut2-/-* mice; Marty et al.,

2005). Further studies also implicate the type 1 glucose transporter (GLUT-1) in hypothalamic astrocytes in sensing changes in peripheral glucose homeostasis (Chari et al., 2011).

Recent data suggests that in addition to astrocyte-neuronal interactions, intact astrocyte-astrocyte networks in the medial-basal hypothalamus are also important for glucose sensing. Allard and colleagues demonstrated that reducing cell-cell transfer of small molecules *via* gap-junctions in hypothalamic astroglial networks *via* inhibition of connexin-43, results in reduced hypothalamic glucose sensitivity (Allard et al., 2014). Further studies in this area are necessary to fully elucidate the molecular mechanisms by which astrocytes communicate information on glycemic status to neurons. Is it due to astrocyte mediated changes in substrate availability as suggested by the work of Arrieta-Cruz et al. (2013)? Alternatively, are there also direct regulatory roles for astrocytes in modulating the activity of glucose sensing neurons in the hypothalamus *via* the release of gliotransmitters, the modulation of neurotransmitter reuptake, and/or alterations in synaptic plasticity?

TANYCYTES ARE DIRECTLY RESPONSIVE TO FASTING

The localization of tanycytes at the base of the third ventricle, proximal to the median eminence, makes them ideally positioned to act as gatekeepers between the periphery and the brain *via* the cerebroventricular system. Tanycytes are glucose sensitive (for review see Bolborea and Dale, 2013) and respond to reduced circulating glucose levels associated with fasting by altering the permeability of their tight-junctions which subsequently increases access of circulating factors to the CNS (Langlet et al., 2013).

In addition to a role in altering permeability of the blood-hypothalamus barrier in response to fasting, there is also evidence that tanycytes modulate energy homeostasis *via* their neurogenic capacity. Median eminence Fgf10-expressing tanycytes (thought to be largely of the β-subtype) have been demonstrated to repopulate the arcuate nucleus of the hypothalamus in the fasted state where they become NPY expressing neurons (Haan et al., 2013); thus, promoting a rise in food intake by increasing orexigenic drive.

EVIDENCE FOR A ROLE OF GLIOTRANSMITTERS IN REGULATION OF FOOD INTAKE

Endozepines are endogenous proteins with "benzodiazepine-like" binding capacity and include the diazepam-binding inhibitor (DBI) and its cleavage products including the octadecaneuropeptide (ODN; DBI_{33-50}). Expressed at high levels in hypothalamic macroglia (astrocytes and tanycytes; Tonon et al., 1990), endozepine expression is down-regulated by fasting in mice and rats (Compère et al., 2010; Lanfray et al., 2013), providing evidence of metabolic control of this system. The finding that CNS administration of ODN significantly reduces food intake in rodents further supports a potential role in the regulation of energy homeostasis (de Mateos-Verchere et al., 2001; Compère et al., 2003; Lanfray et al., 2013). While the mechanisms remain to be fully elucidated, there is some data to suggest that the anorexigenic actions of endozepines are not mediated *via* a classical benzodiazepine receptor but *via* a metabotropic receptor (do Rego et al., 2007) and also require intact central melanocortin-3/4 receptor signaling (Lanfray et al., 2013). Moreover, as astrocytic DBI is known to potentiate inhibitory GABAergic transmission (Christian and Huguenard, 2013) it is likely that modulation of this important neurotransmitter pathway may contribute to the anorexigenic actions of this peptide. In addition to binding the $GABA_A$ receptor, endozepines also show high binding affinity for the mitochondrial translocator protein (TSPO). Intriguing, in the CNS TSPO is largely localized within glia and is highly upregulated by glial cell activation leading to the widespread use of TSPO ligands as *in vivo* neuroimaging agents for CNS pathologies (Venneti et al., 2013). This indicates that another potential mechanism for the anorexigenic activity of endozepines may be *via* direct modulation of glial cell activity. Further studies, including examining the phenotype of animal models with alterations in endozepine signaling are necessary to clarify the physiologic role for this pathway in the regulation of energy homeostasis.

SUMMARY

It is apparent from the wealth of emerging evidence that, in addition to their role in other neuroendocrine processes, hypothalamic macroglia have a critical role in the regulation of energy homeostasis. While much of the current research is focused on macroglial-neuronal interactions in the regulation of energy homeostasis, it is highly likely that the interaction between glial cell types, such as microglia and astrocytes, also represents a key regulatory node. Important work remains to be done to determine the roles of hypothalamic macroglia in the physiologic maintenance of energy balance as well as their contribution to disease pathology when an organism is out of homeostasis in disease states such as obesity and cachexia.

REFERENCES

Abbott, N. J., Rönnbäck, L., and Hansson, E. (2006). Astrocyte-endothelial interactions at the blood-brain barrier. *Nat. Rev. Neurosci.* 7, 41–53. doi: 10.1038/nrn1824

Albrecht, J., Wróblewska, B., and Mossakowski, M. J. (1982). The binding of insulin to cerebral capillaries and astrocytes of the rat. *Neurochem. Res.* 7, 489–494. doi: 10.1007/bf00965500

Allard, C., Carneiro, L., Grall, S., Cline, B. H., Fioramonti, X., Chrétien, C., et al. (2014). Hypothalamic astroglial connexins are required for brain glucose sensing-induced insulin secretion. *J. Cereb. Blood Flow Metab.* 34, 339–346. doi: 10.1038/jcbfm.2013.206

Arrieta-Cruz, I., Su, Y., Knight, C. M., Lam, T. K., and Gutiérrez-Juárez, R. (2013). Evidence for a role of proline and hypothalamic astrocytes in the regulation of glucose metabolism in rats. *Diabetes* 62, 1152–1158. doi: 10.2337/db12-0228

Balland, E., Dam, J., Langlet, F., Caron, E., Steculorum, S., Messina, A., et al. (2014). Hypothalamic tanycytes are an ERK-gated conduit for leptin into the brain. *Cell Metab.* 19, 293–301. doi: 10.1016/j.cmet.2013.12.015

Berkseth, K. E., Guyenet, S. J., Melhorn, S. J., Lee, D., Thaler, J. P., Schur, E. A., et al. (2014). Hypothalamic gliosis associated with high-fat diet feeding is reversible in mice: a combined immunohistochemical and magnetic resonance imaging study. *Endocrinology* 155, 2858–2867. doi: 10.1210/en.2014-1121

Bilbo, S. D., and Schwarz, J. M. (2012). The immune system and developmental programming of brain and behavior. *Front. Neuroendocrinol.* 33, 267–286. doi: 10.1016/j.yfrne.2012.08.006

Bolborea, M., and Dale, N. (2013). Hypothalamic tanycytes: potential roles in the control of feeding and energy balance. *Trends Neurosci.* 36, 91–100. doi: 10.1016/j.tins.2012.12.008

Buckman, L. B., Thompson, M. M., Moreno, H. N., and Ellacott, K. L. (2013). Regional astrogliosis in the mouse hypothalamus in response to obesity. *J. Comp. Neurol.* 521, 1322–1333. doi: 10.1002/cne.23233

Cani, P. D., Amar, J., Iglesias, M. A., Poggi, M., Knauf, C., Bastelica, D., et al. (2007). Metabolic endotoxemia initiates obesity and insulin resistance. *Diabetes* 56, 1761–1772. doi: 10.2337/db06-1491

Chang, Y., She, Z. G., Sakimura, K., Roberts, A., Kucharova, K., Rowitch, D. H., et al. (2012). Ablation of NG2 proteoglycan leads to deficits in brown fat function and to adult onset obesity. *PLoS One* 7:e30637. doi: 10.1371/journal.pone.0030637

Chari, M., Yang, C. S., Lam, C. K., Lee, K., Mighiu, P., Kokorovic, A., et al. (2011). Glucose transporter-1 in the hypothalamic glial cells mediates glucose sensing to regulate glucose production in vivo. *Diabetes* 60, 1901–1906. doi: 10.2337/db11-0120

Chowen, J. A., Argente, J., and Horvath, T. L. (2013). Uncovering novel roles of nonneuronal cells in body weight homeostasis and obesity. *Endocrinology* 154, 3001–3007. doi: 10.1210/en.2013-1303

Christian, C. A., and Huguenard, J. R. (2013). Astrocytes potentiate GABAergic transmission in the thalamic reticular nucleus via endozepine signaling. *Proc. Natl. Acad. Sci. U S A* 110, 20278–20283. doi: 10.1073/pnas.1318031110

Compère, V., Lanfray, D., Castel, H., Morin, F., Leprince, J., Dureuil, B., et al. (2010). Acute food deprivation reduces expression of diazepam-binding inhibitor, the precursor of the anorexigenic octadecaneuropeptide ODN, in mouse glial cells. *J. Mol. Endocrinol.* 44, 295–299. doi: 10.1677/jme-09-0176

Compere, V., Li, S., Leprince, J., Tonon, M. C., Vaudry, H., and Pelletier, G. (2003). Effect of intracerebroventricular administration of the octadecaneuropeptide on the expression of pro-opiomelanocortin, neuropeptide Y and corticotropin-releasing hormone mRNAs in rat hypothalamus. *J. Neuroendocrinol.* 15, 197–203. doi: 10.1046/j.1365-2826.2003.00970.x

Cone, R. D. (2005). Anatomy and regulation of the central melanocortin system. *Nat. Neurosci.* 8, 571–578. doi: 10.1038/nn1455

de Mateos-Verchere, J. G., Leprince, J., Tonon, M. C., Vaudry, H., and Costentin, J. (2001). The octadecaneuropeptide [diazepam-binding inhibitor (33-50)] exerts potent anorexigenic effects in rodents. *Eur. J. Pharmacol.* 414, 225–231. doi: 10.1016/s0014-2999(01)00771-3

De Souza, C. T., Araujo, E. P., Bordin, S., Ashimine, R., Zollner, R. L., Boschero, A. C., et al. (2005). Consumption of a fat-rich diet activates a proinflammatory response and induces insulin resistance in the hypothalamus. *Endocrinology* 146, 4192–4199. doi: 10.1210/en.2004-1520

do Rego, J. C., Orta, M. H., Leprince, J., Tonon, M. C., Vaudry, H., and Costentin, J. (2007). Pharmacological characterization of the receptor mediating the anorexigenic action of the octadecaneuropeptide: evidence for an endozepinergic tone regulating food intake. *Neuropsychopharmacology* 32, 1641–1648. doi: 10.1038/sj.npp.1301280

Drake, C., Boutin, H., Jones, M. S., Denes, A., Mccoll, B. W., Selvarajah, J. R., et al. (2011). Brain inflammation is induced by co-morbidities and risk factors for stroke. *Brain Behav. Immun.* 25, 1113–1122. doi: 10.1016/j.bbi.2011.02.008

Fuente-Martín, E., García-Cáceres, C., Granado, M., De Ceballos, M. L., Sánchez-Garrido, M. A., Sarman, B., et al. (2012). Leptin regulates glutamate and glucose transporters in hypothalamic astrocytes. *J. Clin. Invest.* 122, 3900–3913. doi: 10.1172/jci64102

Gao, Y., Ottaway, N., Schriever, S. C., Legutko, B., García-Cáceres, C., De La Fuente, E., et al. (2014). Hormones and diet, but not body weight, control hypothalamic microglial activity. *Glia* 62, 17–25. doi: 10.1002/glia.22580

García-Cáceres, C., Fuente-Martín, E., Burgos-Ramos, E., Granado, M., Frago, L. M., Barrios, V., et al. (2011). Differential acute and chronic effects of leptin on hypothalamic astrocyte morphology and synaptic protein levels. *Endocrinology* 152, 1809–1818. doi: 10.1210/en.2010-1252

Grayson, B. E., Levasseur, P. R., Williams, S. M., Smith, M. S., Marks, D. L., and Grove, K. L. (2010). Changes in melanocortin expression and inflammatory pathways in fetal offspring of nonhuman primates fed a high-fat diet. *Endocrinology* 151, 1622–1632. doi: 10.1210/en.2009-1019

Gupta, S., Knight, A. G., Keller, J. N., and Bruce-Keller, A. J. (2012). Saturated long-chain fatty acids activate inflammatory signaling in astrocytes. *J. Neurochem.* 120, 1060–1071. doi: 10.1111/j.1471-4159.2012.07660.x

Haan, N., Goodman, T., Najdi-Samiei, A., Stratford, C. M., Rice, R., El Agha, E., et al. (2013). Fgf10-expressing tanycytes add new neurons to the appetite/energy-balance regulating centers of the postnatal and adult hypothalamus. *J. Neurosci.* 33, 6170–6180. doi: 10.1523/jneurosci.2437-12.2013

Horvath, T. L., Sarman, B., García-Cáceres, C., Enriori, P. J., Sotonyi, P., Shanabrough, M., et al. (2010). Synaptic input organization of the melanocortin system predicts diet-induced hypothalamic reactive gliosis and obesity. *Proc. Natl. Acad. Sci. U S A* 107, 14875–14880. doi: 10.1073/pnas.1004282107

Hsuchou, H., He, Y., Kastin, A. J., Tu, H., Markadakis, E. N., Rogers, R. C., et al. (2009a). Obesity induces functional astrocytic leptin receptors in hypothalamus. *Brain* 132, 889–902. doi: 10.1093/brain/awp029

Hsuchou, H., Pan, W., Barnes, M. J., and Kastin, A. J. (2009b). Leptin receptor mRNA in rat brain astrocytes. *Peptides* 30, 2275–2280. doi: 10.1016/j.peptides.2009.08.023

Jackson, F. R. (2011). Glial cell modulation of circadian rhythms. *Glia* 59, 1341–1350. doi: 10.1002/glia.21097

Jayaram, B., Pan, W., Wang, Y., Hsuchou, H., Mace, A., Cornelissen-Guillaume, G. G., et al. (2013). Astrocytic leptin-receptor knockout mice show partial rescue of leptin resistance in diet-induced obesity. *J. Appl. Physiol. (1985)* 114, 734–741. doi: 10.1152/japplphysiol.01499.2012

Ji, Y. F., Xu, S. M., Zhu, J., Wang, X. X., and Shen, Y. (2011). Insulin increases glutamate transporter GLT1 in cultured astrocytes. *Biochem. Biophys. Res. Commun.* 405, 691–696. doi: 10.1016/j.bbrc.2011.01.105

Kim, J. G., Suyama, S., Koch, M., Jin, S., Argente-Arizon, P., Argente, J., et al. (2014). Leptin signaling in astrocytes regulates hypothalamic neuronal circuits and feeding. *Nat. Neurosci.* 17, 908–910. doi: 10.1038/nn.3725

Kokoeva, M. V., Yin, H., and Flier, J. S. (2005). Neurogenesis in the hypothalamus of adult mice: potential role in energy balance. *Science* 310, 679–683. doi: 10.1126/science.1115360

Lanfray, D., Arthaud, S., Ouellet, J., Compère, V., Do Rego, J. L., Leprince, J., et al. (2013). Gliotransmission and brain glucose sensing: critical role of endozepines. *Diabetes* 62, 801–810. doi: 10.2337/db11-0785

Langlet, F., Levin, B. E., Luquet, S., Mazzone, M., Messina, A., Dunn-Meynell, A. A., et al. (2013). Tanycytic VEGF-A boosts blood-hypothalamus barrier plasticity and access of metabolic signals to the arcuate nucleus in response to fasting. *Cell Metab.* 17, 607–617. doi: 10.1016/j.cmet.2013.03.004

Lee, D. A., Bedont, J. L., Pak, T., Wang, H., Song, J., Miranda-Angulo, A., et al. (2012). Tanycytes of the hypothalamic median eminence form a diet-responsive neurogenic niche. *Nat. Neurosci.* 15, 700–702. doi: 10.1038/nn.3079

Le Foll, C., Dunn-Meynell, A. A., Miziorko, H. M., and Levin, B. E. (2013). Regulation of hypothalamic neuronal sensing and food intake by ketone bodies and fatty acids. *Diabetes* 63, 1259–1269. doi: 10.2337/db13-1090

Li, J., Tang, Y., and Cai, D. (2012). IKKβ/NF-kappaB disrupts adult hypothalamic neural stem cells to mediate a neurodegenerative mechanism of dietary obesity and pre-diabetes. *Nat. Cell Biol.* 14, 999–1012. doi: 10.1038/ncb2562

Marty, N., Dallaporta, M., Foretz, M., Emery, M., Tarussio, D., Bady, I., et al. (2005). Regulation of glucagon secretion by glucose transporter type 2 (glut2) and astrocyte-dependent glucose sensors. *J. Clin. Invest.* 115, 3545–3553. doi: 10.1172/jci26309

McNay, D. E., Briançon, N., Kokoeva, M. V., Maratos-Flier, E., and Flier, J. S. (2012). Remodeling of the arcuate nucleus energy-balance circuit is inhibited in obese mice. *J. Clin. Invest.* 122, 142–152. doi: 10.1172/jci43134

Ng, F. S., Tangredi, M. M., and Jackson, F. R. (2011). Glial cells physiologically modulate clock neurons and circadian behavior in a calcium-dependent manner. *Curr. Biol.* 21, 625–634. doi: 10.1016/j.cub.2011.03.027

Nishiyama, A., Yang, Z., and Butt, A. (2005). Astrocytes and NG2-glia: what's in a name? *J. Anat.* 207, 687–693 doi: 10.1111/j.1469-7580.2005.00489.x

Panatier, A. (2009). Glial cells: indispensable partners of hypothalamic magnocellular neurones. *J. Neuroendocrinol.* 21, 665–672. doi: 10.1111/j.1365-2826.2009.01884.x

Prevot, V., Dehouck, B., Poulain, P., Beauvillain, J. C., Buée-Scherrer, V., and Bouret, S. (2007). Neuronal-glial-endothelial interactions and cell plasticity in the postnatal hypothalamus: implications for the neuroendocrine control of reproduction. *Psychoneuroendocrinology* 32(Suppl. 1), S46–S51. doi: 10.1016/j.psyneuen.2007.03.018

Robins, S. C., Stewart, I., Mcnay, D. E., Taylor, V., Giachino, C., Goetz, M., et al. (2013a). α-Tanycytes of the adult hypothalamic third ventricle include distinct populations of FGF-responsive neural progenitors. *Nat. Commun.* 4:2049. doi: 10.1038/ncomms3049

Robins, S. C., Trudel, E., Rotondi, O., Liu, X., Djogo, T., Kryzskaya, D., et al. (2013b). Evidence for NG2-glia derived, adult-born functional neurons in the hypothalamus. *PLoS One* 8:e78236. doi: 10.1371/journal.pone.0078236

Rodríguez, E. M., Blázquez, J. L., Pastor, F. E., Peláez, B., Peña, P., Peruzzo, B., et al. (2005). Hypothalamic tanycytes: a key component of brain-endocrine interaction. *Int. Rev. Cytol.* 247, 89–164. doi: 10.1016/s0074-7696(05)47003-5

Selkirk, J. V., Nottebaum, L. M., Lee, J., Yang, W., Foster, A. C., and Lechner, S. M. (2007). Identification of differential melanocortin 4 receptor agonist profiles at natively expressed receptors in rat cortical astrocytes and recombinantly expressed receptors in human embryonic kidney cells. *Neuropharmacology* 52, 459–466. doi: 10.1016/j.neuropharm.2006.08.015

Sofroniew, M. V. (2009). Molecular dissection of reactive astrogliosis and glial scar formation. *Trends Neurosci.* 32, 638–647. doi: 10.1016/j.tins.2009.08.002

Sofroniew, M. V., and Vinters, H. V. (2010). Astrocytes: biology and pathology. *Acta Neuropathol.* 119, 7–35. doi: 10.1007/s00401-009-0619-8

Suh, S. W., Bergher, J. P., Anderson, C. M., Treadway, J. L., Fosgerau, K., and Swanson, R. A. (2007). Astrocyte glycogen sustains neuronal activity during hypoglycemia: studies with the glycogen phosphorylase inhibitor CP-316,819 ([R-R*,S*]-5-chloro-N-[2-hydroxy-3-(methoxymethylamino)-3-oxo-1-(phenylmethyl)pro pyl]-1H-indole-2-carboxamide). *J. Pharmacol. Exp. Ther.* 321, 45–50. doi: 10.1124/jpet.106.115550

Tasker, J. G., Oliet, S. H., Bains, J. S., Brown, C. H., and Stern, J. E. (2012). Glial regulation of neuronal function: from synapse to systems physiology. *J. Neuroendocrinol.* 24, 566–576. doi: 10.1111/j.1365-2826.2011.02259.x

Thaler, J. P., Yi, C. X., Schur, E. A., Guyenet, S. J., Hwang, B. H., Dietrich, M. O., et al. (2012). Obesity is associated with hypothalamic injury in rodents and humans. *J. Clin. Invest.* 122, 153–162. doi: 10.1172/JCI59660

Tonon, M. C., Désy, L., Nicolas, P., Vaudry, H., and Pelletier, G. (1990). Immunocytochemical localization of the endogenous benzodiazepine ligand octadecaneuropeptide (ODN) in the rat brain. *Neuropeptides* 15, 17–24. doi: 10.1016/0143-4179(90)90155-r

Venneti, S., Lopresti, B. J., and Wiley, C. A. (2013). Molecular imaging of microglia/macrophages in the brain. *Glia* 61, 10–23. doi: 10.1002/glia.22357

Xanthos, D. N., and Sandkühler, J. (2014). Neurogenic neuroinflammation: inflammatory CNS reactions in response to neuronal activity. *Nat. Rev. Neurosci.* 15, 43–53. doi: 10.1038/nrn3617

Yi, C. X., Habegger, K. M., Chowen, J. A., Stern, J., and Tschöp, M. H. (2011). A role for astrocytes in the central control of metabolism. *Neuroendocrinology* 93, 143–149. doi: 10.1159/000324888

Young, J. K., Baker, J. H., and Montes, M. I. (2000). The brain response to 2-deoxy glucose is blocked by a glial drug. *Pharmacol. Biochem. Behav.* 67, 233–239. doi: 10.1016/s0091-3057(00)00315-4

Zhang, X., Zhang, G., Zhang, H., Karin, M., Bai, H., and Cai, D. (2008). Hypothalamic IKKbeta/NF-kappaB and ER stress link overnutrition to energy imbalance and obesity. *Cell* 135, 61–73. doi: 10.1016/j.cell.2008.07.043

8

Notch signaling and proneural genes work together to control the neural building blocks for the initial scaffold in the hypothalamus

Michelle Ware, Houda Hamdi-Rozé and Valérie Dupé *

Institut de Génétique et Développement de Rennes, Faculté de Médecine, CNRS UMR6290, Université de Rennes 1, Rennes, France

***Correspondence:**
Valérie Dupé, Institut de Génétique et Développement de Rennes, Faculté de Médecine, CNRS UMR6290, Université de Rennes 1, IFR140 GFAS, 2 Avenue du Pr. Léon Bernard, 35043 Rennes Cedex, France
e-mail: valerie.dupe@univ-rennes1.fr

The vertebrate embryonic prosencephalon gives rise to the hypothalamus, which plays essential roles in sensory information processing as well as control of physiological homeostasis and behavior. While patterning of the hypothalamus has received much attention, initial neurogenesis in the developing hypothalamus has mostly been neglected. The first differentiating progenitor cells of the hypothalamus will give rise to neurons that form the nucleus of the tract of the postoptic commissure (nTPOC) and the nucleus of the mammillotegmental tract (nMTT). The formation of these neuronal populations has to be highly controlled both spatially and temporally as these tracts will form part of the ventral longitudinal tract (VLT) and act as a scaffold for later, follower axons. This review will cumulate and summarize the existing data available describing initial neurogenesis in the vertebrate hypothalamus. It is well-known that the Notch signaling pathway through the inhibition of proneural genes is a key regulator of neurogenesis in the vertebrate central nervous system. It has only recently been proposed that loss of Notch signaling in the developing chick embryo causes an increase in the number of neurons in the hypothalamus, highlighting an early function of the Notch pathway during hypothalamus formation. Further analysis in the chick and mouse hypothalamus confirms the expression of Notch components and *Ascl1* before the appearance of the first differentiated neurons. Many newly identified proneural target genes were also found to be expressed during neuronal differentiation in the hypothalamus. Given the critical role that hypothalamic neural circuitry plays in maintaining homeostasis, it is particularly important to establish the targets downstream of this Notch/proneural network.

Keywords: early axon scaffold, forebrain, differentiation, tract of the postoptic commissure, mammillotegmental tract, hypothalamus patterning, ASCL1

INTRODUCTION

The hypothalamus is an evolutionary ancient structure in the rostral brain that plays a central role in the regulation of physiological processes such as hunger, thermoregulation, reproduction and behavior in adult vertebrates. The adult hypothalamus is subdivided into regions, each containing well documented clusters of neurons with defined functions (Simerly, 2004). Countless work involving physiological and genetic studies has focused on signaling molecules and transcription factors that control hypothalamus morphogenesis and the emergence of different neuronal subtypes (Shimogori et al., 2010). However, relatively little attention has been paid to the process through which the initial neurons are induced and specified in the primordium of the vertebrate hypothalamus, despite their key roles in pioneering the major axon pathways in the forebrain (Wilson et al., 1990; Mastick and Easter, 1996; Ware and Schubert, 2011). The first differentiating cells of the hypothalamus will give rise to neurons that form the nucleus of the tract of the postoptic commissure (nTPOC) and the nucleus of the mammillotegmental tract (nMTT). Recent advances in the chick model has established that a Notch/proneural regulatory loop is implicated very early during the differentiation of these neurons (Ratié et al., 2013). The aim of this review is to highlight a role for Notch signaling during nTPOC and nMTT differentiation; including key findings from zebrafish, chick and mouse models, which has contributed to our understanding of this field. A potential cascade involving *Ascl1* and target genes will be discussed to determine the possible regulation of these initial hypothalamic neurons.

Abbreviations: AH, anterior hypothalamus; bHLH, basic helix-loop-helix; MH, mammillary hypothalamus; MTT, mammillotegmental tract; TH, tuberal hypothalamus; NPC, neural progenitor cell; nTPOC, nucleus of the tract of the postoptic commissure; nMTT, nucleus of mamillo-tegmental tract; TPOC, tract of the postoptic commissure.

PATTERNING OF THE VERTEBRATE HYPOTHALAMIC PRIMORDIUM

During early embryogenesis the hypothalamus develops within the secondary prosencephalon (Puelles and Rubenstein, 2003;

Martinez-Ferre and Martinez, 2012; Puelles et al., 2012). Developmental studies performed in zebrafish, chick and mouse indicate Sonic Hedgehog (SHH), secreted by the underlying prechordal plate mesendoderm, induces the formation of the hypothalamus (Dale et al., 1997; Mathieu et al., 2002; Aoto et al., 2009). Loss of *Shh* leads to missing ventral structures including the hypothalamus in zebrafish (Varga et al., 2001) and mouse (Chiang et al., 1996). In humans, mutations in the *Shh* gene results in holoprosencephaly, the most frequent human brain malformation that includes hypothalamic defects (Mercier et al., 2011). However, SHH alone is not sufficient to induce specific hypothalamus identity. The prechordal plate expresses numerous other secreted proteins that are involved in the development of the overlying hypothalamus primordium including Wnt antagonists, NODAL and Bone Morophogenic Proteins (BMP; Pera and Kessel, 1997; Kiecker and Niehrs, 2001; Mathieu et al., 2002; Manning et al., 2006; Cavodeassi and Houart, 2012).

Specific patterning of the hypothalamus begins when the hypothalamic primordium expresses the transcription factor *Nkx2.1* from Hamburger and Hamilton stage (HH)8 in chick and embryonic day (E)8 in mouse (Shimamura et al., 1995; Pera and Kessel, 1998; Sussel et al., 1999; Crossley et al., 2001). This expression of *Nkx2.1*, along with *Nkx2.2* is dependent on the presence of *Shh* in the prechordal plate (Barth and Wilson, 1995; Pera and Kessel, 1997; Rohr et al., 2001; Mathieu et al., 2002). SHH is then required to coordinate tissue growth and acquisition of anteroposterior (AP), dorsoventral (DV) and mediolateral patterning of the hypothalamus (Manning et al., 2006; Szabó et al., 2009).

At HH10, *Shh*, *Nkx2.1* and *Nkx2.2* expression expands in the basal plate of the chick prosencephalon, with the same rostral expression at the level of the presumptive anterior hypothalamus (AH) that corresponds to the prospective chiasmatic area (also called suboptical domain) (Crossley et al., 2001). A new *Nkx2.1* expression domain develops at HH12, just rostral to the hypothalamus in the basal telencephalon called the postoptic area (POA). In zebrafish and mouse, the same dynamic expression patterns of *Shh*, *Nkx2.1* and *Nkx2.2* is present within the hypothalamus (**Figure 1**). By HH13 in chick and E9.5 in the mouse, *Shh* and *Nkx2.1* expression has expanded further and the hypothalamic primordium is morphologically evident. Studies in chick show that once the hypothalamic primordium is established, SHH down-regulation mediated by local production of BMPs is necessary for establishing region-specific transcriptional profiles (Patten and Placzek, 2002; Manning et al., 2006; Ohyama et al., 2008). This leads to the subdivisions of the primordial hypothalamus into three regions, the AH, the tuberal hypothalamus (TH) and the mammillary hypothalamus (MH), with each region expressing specific markers (**Figure 1**; Alvarez-Bolado et al., 2012; Wolf and Ryu, 2013).

INITIAL NEUROGENESIS IN THE VERTEBRATE HYPOTHALAMUS

The first neurons that differentiate in the vertebrate brain give rise to the highly conserved early axon scaffold (Chitnis and Kuwada, 1990; Wilson et al., 1990; Easter et al., 1993; Mastick and Easter, 1996; Barreiro-Iglesias et al., 2008; Ware and Schubert, 2011; Ware et al., 2014). This is an important structure for the guidance of later, follower axons allowing more complex connections to form. Predating the mature hypothalamic neuronal clusters, two small GABAergic positive populations differentiate within the hypothalamus (**Figure 1**; Patel et al., 1994). The first neurons in the hypothalamic primordium differentiate to give rise to the nTPOC (also termed the ventro-rostral cluster (vrc) in anamniotes) at 16 hpf in zebrafish (**Figure 1A**; Chitnis and Kuwada, 1990; Ross et al., 1992) and HH13 in chick (**Figure 1B**; Ware and Schubert, 2011). An early birth-dating study has shown that hypothalamic neurogenesis in the mouse begins at E10 (Shimada and Nakamura, 1973). However, it is well-known that the initial nTPOC neurons arise at E9.5, suggesting neurogenesis begins earlier than previously thought (**Figure 1C**; Easter et al., 1993; Mastick and Easter, 1996; Ricaño-Cornejo et al., 2011). From the nTPOC neurons, axons extend and project caudally within the basal plate. The tract of the postoptic commissure (TPOC) axons project into the mesencephalon where these axons form part of the ventral longitudinal tract (VLT) along with the medial longitudinal fascicle (MLF) and later the mammillotegmental tract (MTT; Ware and Schubert, 2011). The MTT forms from a second set of neurons (nMTT) that differentiate later in the caudal hypothalamus of amniotes from HH14 in chick and E10 in mouse (**Figures 1E,F**; Puelles et al., 1987; Easter et al., 1993; Mastick and Easter, 1996). While the presence and location of the nTPOC is conserved in all vertebrates studied, the nMTT is not present in zebrafish, at least during early development (Barreiro-Iglesias et al., 2008). Neurons do however form later in the zebrafish MH, but it is not possible to comment on the homology with the nMTT (Wolf and Ryu, 2013). The postoptic commissure (POC) forms by 24 hpf, projecting axons from the nTPOC rostrally to form a commissure across the rostral midline connecting the left and right sides of the neural tube (**Figure 1D**; Ross et al., 1992; Bak and Fraser, 2003). The POC is likely to form in chick and mouse at later stages but has not been studied exhaustively (Croizier et al., 2011; Ware and Schubert, 2011).

The prosomeric model and hypothalamic markers such as *Shh*, *Nkx2.1* and *Nkx2.2* confirms the nTPOC and nMTT neurons form within the hypothalamus (**Figure 1**; Hjorth and Key, 2001; Puelles and Rubenstein, 2003). The nTPOC arises just below the optic stalk at the midline of the AH area and the nMTT in the lateral edge of the caudal hypothalamus in the MH (**Figure 1**; Easter et al., 1993). The nTPOC neurons differentiate along the boundaries of many gene expression areas in zebrafish (Macdonald et al., 1994), however the mechanism by which these neurons differentiate has been overlooked.

Some zebrafish and mouse mutants are available where the formation of these hypothalamic axon tracts is affected. Some genes are implicated in the differentiation of the neurons such as *Six3* (Ando et al., 2005), but many studies focus on the effect of gene inactivation on axon guidance, including *Fgf8* (Shanmugalingam et al., 2000), *Pax6* (Mastick et al., 1997; Nural and Mastick, 2004), Slits and Robos (Ricaño-Cornejo et al., 2011)

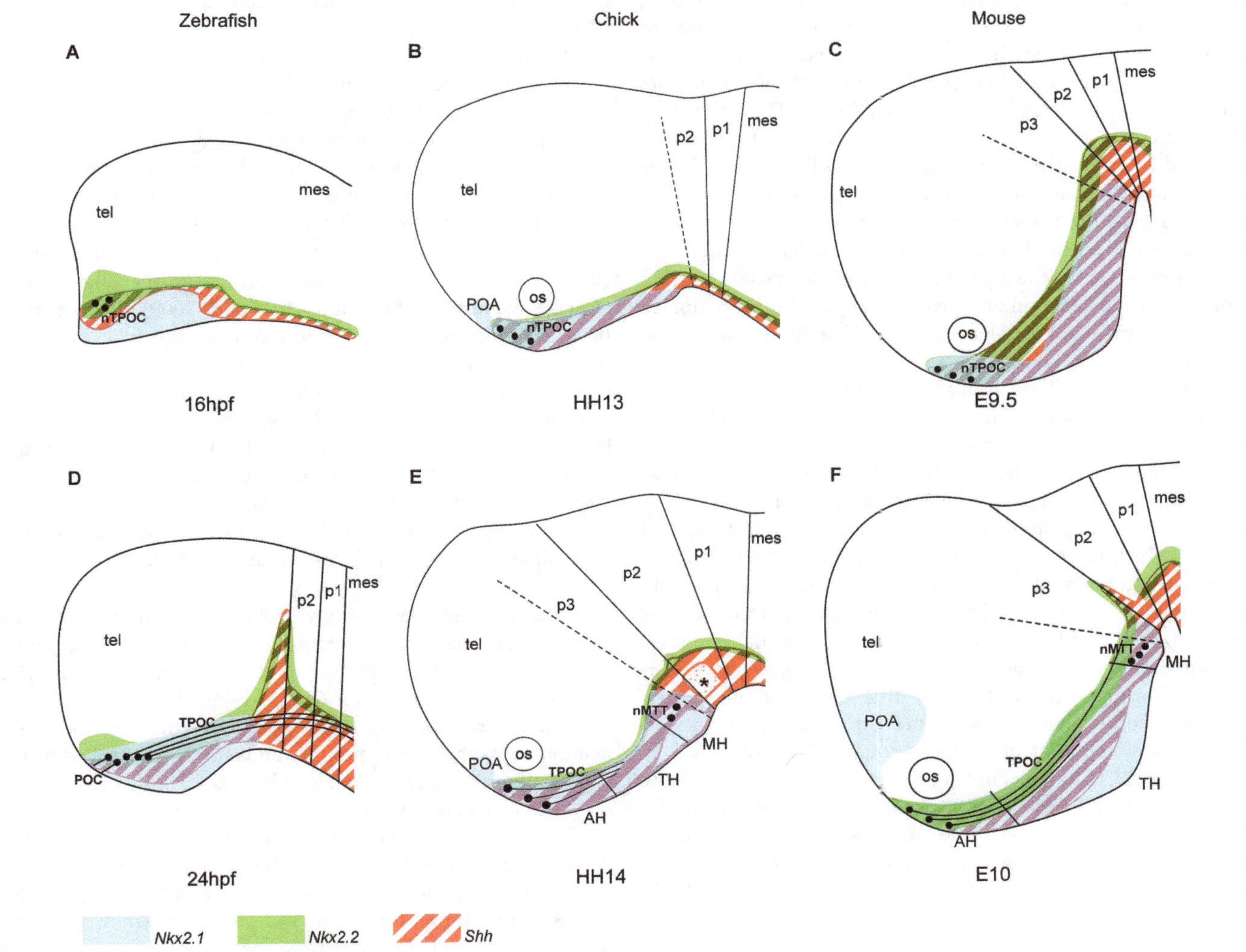

FIGURE 1 | Organization of the hypothalamic primordium in the rostral vertebrate brain. (A–C) The first nTPOC neurons arise in the hypothalamus in zebrafish **(A)** at 16 hpf, chick **(B)** at HH13 and mouse **(C)** at E9.5. **(D)** Axons project caudally from the nTPOC forming the TPOC and rostrally from the nTPOC to form the POC in zebrafish at 24 hpf. **(E, F)** The nTPOC neurons begin projecting axons and the first nMTT neurons arise in chick at HH14 **(E)** and in mouse **(F)** at E10. The hypothalamus is specifically marked by three genes, *Nkx2.1* (light blue), *Nkx2.2* (green) and *Shh* (red stripes). **(A, D)** Gene expression in zebrafish is based on the following studies: *Shh, Nkx2.2* (Barth and Wilson, 1995; Hjorth and Key, 2001) and *Nkx2.1a* (Rohr and Concha, 2000; Rohr et al., 2001). **(B, E)** Gene expression in chick is based on the following studies: *Shh* (Bardet et al., 2010), *Nkx2.1* (Ratié et al., 2013) and *Nkx2.2* (Gimeno and Martinez, 2007). **(C, F)** Gene expression in mouse is based on the following studies: *Shh* (Shimamura et al., 1995; Alvarez-Bolado et al., 2012), *Nkx2.1* and *Nkx2.2* (Shimamura et al., 1995). **(E, F)** The three subdivisions of the hypothalamus (AH, TH and MH) in chick and mouse is based on *Shh* expression (Alvarez-Bolado et al., 2012; Ratié et al., 2013). **(E)** Asterisk, *Shh* negative region, overlapping where the ventral MLF neurons differentiate. For all schematics, subdivisions of the brain is based on the prosomeric model (Mastick and Easter, 1996; Hauptmann et al., 2002; Puelles and Rubenstein 2003; Ware and Schubert, 2011). **(D–F)** Zona limitans intrathalamica (ZLI) marks the p2/p3 boundary. Although other neuronal populations are present in the brain at these stages, they are not added to focus on the hypothalamic neurons. AH, anterior hypothalamus; mes, mesencephalon; MH, mammillary hypothalamus; nMTT, nucleus of the tract of the mammillotegmental tract; nTPOC, nucleus of the tract of the postoptic commissure; os, optic stalk; POA, postoptic area; POC, postoptic commissure; p1–p3, prosomeres 1–3; TPOC, tract of the postoptic commissure; TH, tuberal hypothalamus; tel, telencephalon.

and *Sim1/Sim2* (Marion et al., 2005). Functionally, the TPOC is important for the guidance of other axon tracts. Ablation of the TPOC axons in the zebrafish embryo affects the patterning of the early axon scaffold (Chitnis and Kuwada, 1991). In zebrafish *Cyclops* mutants, the TPOC does not form, leading to the misguidance of the tract of the posterior commissure (TPC) axons (Patel et al., 1994). More recently, a study in the embryonic mouse has shown later hypothalamic axons from the melanin-concentrating hormone (MCH) neurons use the TPOC for guidance (Croizier et al., 2011). While the potential function of the TPOC neurons is not known, lypophilic tracing shows that the TPOC axons project into the hindbrain, although the target of these axons remains a mystery (Ware and Schubert, 2011). It is also unclear whether these neurons are still present postnatally, it could be that their sole purpose is to provide axons for guidance and then simply die after connections are made in the adult brain (Easter et al., 1993). The MTT may also function in the guidance of other tracts but this has not been studied exhaustively. In mouse, the MTT is likely to guide the mammillothalamic tract (MTH) that forms later in mouse contributing to the principle mammillary tract (Marion et al., 2005). The MTH is not known to form in zebrafish or chick. The MTT axons project to the tegmentum and are described as having a role in visceral function and processing special information in the adult human brain (Alpeeva and Makarenko, 2007; Kwon et al., 2011).

No attention has been brought to the mechanism by which the nTPOC and nMTT neurons differentiate, until 2013, when Notch components were first described as being present very early in the hypothalamus of the developing chick embryo (Ratié et al., 2013). A basic PubMed search of the key words Notch and hypothalamus generated very few publications and many of which are based in adult models or describe differentiation of late forming embryonic neurons (Chapouton et al., 2011; Aujla et al., 2013). This indicates a surprising lack of investigations surrounding neurogenesis of the initial hypothalamus neurons, when considering these early neurons have been described through-out the 1990s in different vertebrate species. As these neurons contribute to the early axon scaffold and are essential for the set-up of more complex connections, it is surely essential to understand how they differentiate and how they are specified. Finally, considering Notch along with the proneural network is a well-known signaling pathway, little is known about the implication of Notch signaling or neurogenic factors involved in the formation of the nTPOC and nMTT neurons.

NEUROGENESIS AND THE NOTCH/PRONEURAL NETWORK

Notch signaling is an evolutionary conserved signaling pathway involved in cell-cell communication regulating multiple processes throughout development. The Notch signaling pathway has previously been reviewed in detail, here a brief outline is described (Pierfelice et al., 2011). First identified in *Drosophila*, the Notch pathway has been confirmed to have similar roles in vertebrates (Coffman et al., 1990; Artavanis-Tsakonas and Simpson, 1991; Artavanis-Tsakonas et al., 1999). The core pathway consists of the interaction between a transmembrane Notch receptor anchored in one cell, with a transmembrane Notch ligand (Delta or Serrate/Jagged) in a neighboring cell. Upon receptor-ligand binding a series of proteolytic cleavages are triggered that releases the intracellular domain of Notch (NICD), which forms a nuclear complex with recombination signal binding protein for immunoglobulin kappa J region (RBPJ). This complex activates the transcription of target genes (Tamura et al., 1995; Fortini, 2009). The best characterized direct targets of the NICD/RBPJ complex are the Hes (Hairy-Enhancer of Split) and Hey (Hes related type) genes (Jarriault et al., 1995; Maier and Gessler, 2000). They are class-C basic helix-loop-helix (bHLH) proteins that function as transcriptional repressors and can function together as homodimers or heterodimers (Iso et al., 2003).

One function of Notch relies on lateral induction, which is defined as the process by which a ligand-expressing cell stimulates those cells nearby to upregulate ligand expression, promoting ligand propagation and coordinated cell behavior (Eddison et al., 2000). The other function of Notch is lateral inhibition, whereby a ligand-expressing cell inhibits the expression of the ligand in the neighboring cells, therefore preventing those cells from adopting the same fate and generating a patched cellular pattern (Bray, 2006). It is associated with salt-and-pepper like patterns of gene expression (Fior and Henrique, 2009). For example, these two modes of Notch pathway operation coexist during inner ear development. Each mode relies on an associated gene regulatory network (Kiernan, 2013; Neves et al., 2013). Expression and functional studies suggest that lateral induction and lateral inhibition are associated with different Notch ligands that initiate signaling (Brooker et al., 2006; Saravanamuthu et al., 2009; Petrovic et al., 2014). The association of DLL1 with lateral inhibition is a general theme during neural development (Henrique et al., 1995; Adam et al., 1998; Kageyama et al., 2010).

Notch signaling has a very well-known role in neurogenesis, controlling the balance between proliferation of neural progenitor cells (NPCs) and differentiation of NPCs into neuronal and glial cells (Campos-Ortega, 1993; Chitnis et al., 1995; de La Pompa et al., 1997; reviewed by Paridaen and Huttner, 2014). In the neuroepithelium, neuron production is mostly controlled by lateral inhibition, where a regulatory loop is formed, with proneural genes controlling the expression of Notch ligands (Bertrand et al., 2002). The ligand, DLL1, can bind and active NOTCH in neighboring cells. When the Notch signaling pathway is activated, transcriptional repressors (such as Hes or Hey genes) are expressed that prevent expression of proneural genes, inhibiting differentiation and therefore cells remain as progenitors. Cells expressing the ligand and therefore lacking Notch signaling can no longer express transcriptional repressors, leading to the upregulation of bHLH proneural transcription factors such as *Ascl1* or *Neurog1/2*. Under this Notch/proneural network the cell can exit the cell cycle and undergoes neural differentiation (Bertrand et al., 2002). This differentiation step is controlled by several classes of transcription factors that determine the identity of the neuron produced. Among them, a number of bHLH differentiation genes are switched on, such as *Nhlh1* or *NeuroD4*, followed by specific neuronal genes.

NOTCH SIGNALING IN THE VERTEBRATE HYPOTHALAMUS PRIMORDIUM

There are numerous studies investigating the expression and function of Notch components, proneural genes and downstream targets. However, as mentioned previously there is very little data describing the role of Notch signaling during the differentiation of the nTPOC and nMTT neurons. When Notch signaling is inhibited in the developing chick embryo, the number of nTPOC neurons increases, along with ectopic expression of many genes within the hypothalamus, confirming Notch has a role during hypothalamic neurogenesis at this early stage (Ratié et al., 2013).

This study describes a typical neurogenic phenotype expected for the loss of Notch function, working by lateral inhibition.

For the first time, the Notch components *Dll1*, *Hes5* and *Hey1* are shown to be expressed just before HH11 in the presumptive AH of the chick embryonic brain where the first nTPOC neurons will differentiate at HH13 (Ware and Schubert, 2011; Ratié et al., 2013). Expression of Notch components during initial neurogenesis in the zebrafish and mouse has been extensively studied, however for much of the data, it is difficult to interpret the expression in the hypothalamic primordium as no special attention was given to this area at early stages. The expression of Notch receptors in zebrafish are first described at 16 hpf in the prosencephalon and appear to overlap in the area where the nTPOC forms (Bierkamp and Campos-Ortega, 1993; Dyer et al., 2014). In mouse, while *Notch3* is ubiquitously expressed in the neuroectoderm from E8.0, *Notch2* and *Hes1* are expressed in the ventral prosencephalon from E8.5 and *Notch1* is expressed from E9.5 (Reaume et al., 1992; Williams et al., 1995; Koop et al., 1996). Remarkably, little information is present in the literature about when these genes are first expressed in the developing hypothalamus (Bettenhausen et al., 1995; de La Pompa et al., 1997; Leimeister et al., 1999; Barsi et al., 2005). Therefore, in this review, expression of Notch components are analyzed using *in situ* hybridization data to deal with this deficiency (**Figure 2**). *Dll1, Hes5* and *Hey1* mRNA probes are used to show the presence of Notch activity, focusing more specifically in the hypothalamus. At E8.0, *Dll1*, *Hes5* and *Hey1* are not expressed in the mouse presumptive hypothalamus (**Figures 2A–C**), it is only from E8.5, before the initial neurons differentiate that *Dll1* and *Hes5* expression is first observed (**Figures 2E,E',F,F'**, arrowheads). Flat-mounted preparations of the ventral midline reveal a salt-and-pepper like pattern for these genes in the rostral hypothalamus (**Figures 2E',F'**). Expression continues in the AH at E9 for *Dll1* and *Hes5* (**Figures 2I,J**, arrowhead), while *Hey1* expression first starts to be expressed in the same region (**Figure 2K**, arrowhead). At E9.5, *Dll1*, *Hes5* and *Hey1* are first expressed in the MH where the nMTT neurons will differentiate at E10 (**Figures 2M–O**, unfilled arrowhead). It is important to note that the genes analyzed here are not specific for either the nTPOC or nMTT, but are also expressed by other early developing neurons such as those in the nucleus of the mesencephalic tract of the trigeminal nerve (nmesV; **Figure 2**). This is not surprising as Notch is a very general pathway involved in neuron progenitor expansion (Kageyama et al., 2009). Flat-mounted preparations performed at E9.5 confirm the localized expression of *Hes5* (**Figure 2N**) and *Hey1* (**Figure 2O**) in the AH.

Bringing together the data from the literature and *in situ* hybridization of mouse embryos presented here, this highlights that Notch signaling is active very early in the AH and MH where the nTPOC and nMTT neurons will develop respectively (Mastick and Easter, 1996; Ratié et al., 2013). The data also suggests that redundancy could be strong between the direct Notch target genes as multiple transcriptional repressors such as *Hes1*, *Hes5* and *Hey1* are expressed in the developing hypothalamus.

Like with the expression studies described in this section, no functional data about neurogenesis in the early hypothalamus is available in zebrafish and mouse. There are several models lacking Notch signaling, which exhibit an increase in neurons throughout the embryo (de La Pompa et al., 1997; Itoh et al., 2003). For example, in the zebrafish and mouse mindbomb/Mib1 mutants, *Dll1* ubiquitination is affected and aberrant neurogenesis due to lower expression of *Hes1* and *Hes5* is observed throughout the embryo (Itoh et al., 2003; Barsi et al., 2005; Koo et al., 2005). A similar phenotype is also present in RBPj mutant mice, where Notch activity is absent (Oka et al., 1995; de La Pompa et al., 1997). As all these mutant mice display early lethality, no description is available to indicate whether neurogenesis is disturbed in the hypothalamus. Conditional loss-of-function mice lacking RBPJ, using *Nkx2.1*-Cre to specifically knock-out Notch signaling in the hypothalamus, shows that Notch signaling is essential for the differentiation of late arcuate hypothalamic neurons in the mouse from E13.5 (Aujla et al., 2013). This study did not identify a role in the initial neurons, but we would assume there would be an increase in the number of nTPOC and nMTT neurons in these mutant mice.

Many other knock-out or ectopic expression studies of Notch components describe an effect on neurogenesis throughout the embryo. The *Dll1* mutant mouse has not been well studied for a neurogenesis phenotype (Hrabe de Angelis et al., 1997; Przemeck et al., 2003). However, *Dll1* does regulate primary neurogenesis in the *Xenopus* embryo (Chitnis et al., 1995).

There appears to be much redundancy between genes of the Notch pathway, which could explain why a function for Notch during nTPOC neuronal differentiation has not been described before in the mouse. For example, *Hes5* does not show any phenotype in single mutants (Cau et al., 2000). Double or triple knock-out mice produce more obvious phenotypes and prove redundancy occurs between these genes (Hatakeyama et al., 2004; Kageyama et al., 2008a). The absence of both *Hes1* and *Hes5* leads to aberrant neuronal localization. Interestingly, expression of *Dll1* and *Ascl1* is highly upregulated in the ventral diencephalon of E9.5 *Hes1/Hes5* double mutants as are the number of βIII-tubulin (Tuj1) positive cells (Hatakeyama et al., 2004). The capacity of these bHLH proteins to do the same job, may also explain why there is discrepancy between their expressions in chick compared with mouse. For example, flat-mounted preparations of chick embryos at HH15 (**Figure 3A**, arrowhead) and HH14 (Ratié et al., 2013) confirm specific expression of *Hey1* in the AH, whereas expression is throughout the developing hypothalamus in the mouse (**Figures 2O,O'**).

PRONEURAL GENE EXPRESSION IN THE VERTEBRATE HYPOTHALAMUS PRIMORDIUM

Induction of the Notch/proneural loop is essential in the developing hypothalamus as this will eventually lead to the correct number of cells differentiating into nTPOC and nMTT neurons as well as maintaining the progenitor population.

Ascl1 is a well-studied proneural bHLH transcription factor, its expression and function during early embryogenesis has been well described in many vertebrates (Johnson et al., 1990; Ferreiro et al., 1993; Guillemot and Joyner, 1993; Jasoni et al., 1994; Mcnay et al., 2006). In zebrafish, *Ascl1* expression appears early

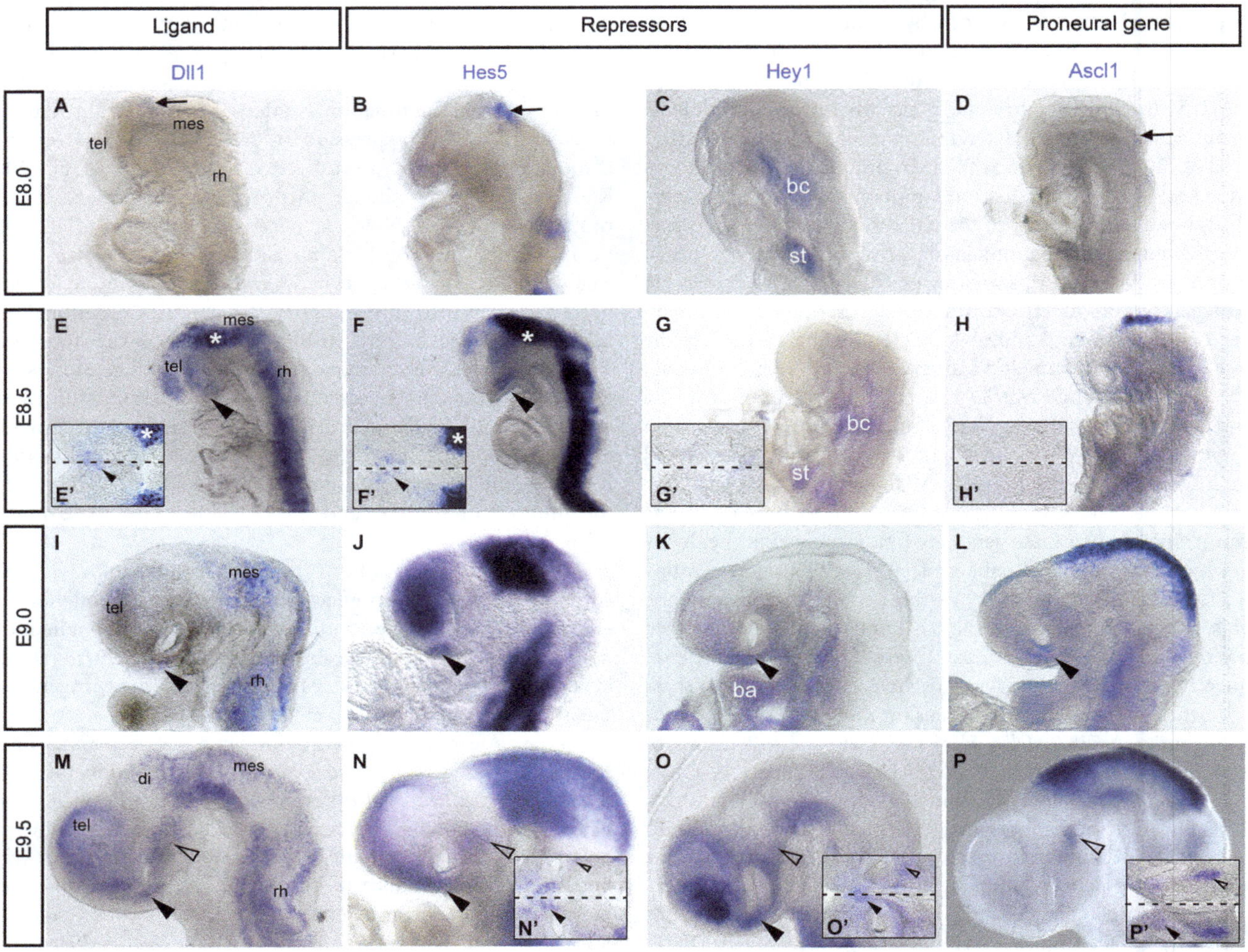

FIGURE 2 | Notch components *Dll1*, *Hes5*, *Hey1* and the proneural gene, *Ascl1* are expressed in the developing mouse hypothalamus. Whole mount *in situ* hybridization was performed on mouse embryos as previously described (Chapman et al., 2002). Digoxigenin labeled mRNA probes were made from the following plasmids *Dll1*, *Hes5*, *Hey1* and *Ascl1* (Guillemot and Joyner, 1993). **(A–D)** E8.0, no expression of *Dll1* **(A)**, *Hes5* **(B)**, *Hey1* **(C)** and *Ascl1* **(D)** in the ventral prosencephalon. Arrows indicate dorsal expression that corresponds to NPCs and early differentiating descending tract of the mesencephalic nucleus of the trigeminal nerve (DTmesV) neurons. **(E–H)** E8.5, expression of *Dll1* **(E)** and *Hes5* **(F)** throughout the neural tube and in the AH (arrowhead). Asterisks in **(E)** and **(F)** correspond to dorsal staining in flat-mounted preparations in **(E')** and **(F')**. Expression of *Hey1* **(G)** and *Ascl1* **(H)** is not yet present in the AH. **(E'–H')** Flat-mounted preparation of the hypothalamus in the same embryo at E8.5. Expression of *Dll1* **(E')** and *Hes5* **(F')** in the AH (arrowhead). Dashed line represents ventral midline. **(I–L)** E9.0, expression of *Dll1* **(I)**, *Hes5* **(J)** in the AH (arrowhead). Expression of *Hey1* **(K)** and *Ascl1* **(L)** begin in the AH (arrowhead). **(C, G, K)** Expression of *Hey1* in the branchial cleft (bc), septum transversum (st) and branchial arch (ba) (Leimeister et al., 1999). (M-P) E9.5, expression of *Dll1* **(M)**, *Hes5* **(N)**, *Hey1* **(O)** and *Ascl1* **(P)** in the AH (arrowhead) and in the MH (unfilled arrowhead). **(M'–P')** Flat-mounted preparations of the hypothalamus at E9.5, arrowheads indicate expression in the AH and unfilled arrowheads indicate expression in the MH. Dashed lines represent ventral midline. mes, mesencephalon; tel, telencephalon; rh, rhombencephalon.

at 12 hpf in cells prior to the appearance of markers indicative of overt differentiation, by 16 hpf, *Ascl1* expression overlaps with the nTPOC (Allende and Weinberg, 1994; Ando et al., 2005). In the Notch inhibited chick model, embryos display an upregulation of *Ascl1* expression in the AH, overlapping the nTPOC (Ratié et al., 2013). Flat-mounted preparations of HH15 chick hypothalamus show that *Ascl1* expression overlaps with *Shh* expression in the AH (**Figure 3B**, arrowhead). The expression of *Ascl1* in the hypothalamus is examined further by *in situ* hybridization between E8 and E9.5 in the mouse embryo, like with the Notch components, expression of *Ascl1* has been badly interpreted in this region (**Figures 2D,H,L,P**). *Ascl1* starts to be expressed in the developing hypothalamus at E9.0 (**Figure 2L**, arrowhead). At E9.5, flat-mounted preparations indicate that *Ascl1* is specifically expressed in a salt-and-pepper like pattern in the AH (**Figures 2P,P'**, arrowhead) and in the MH (**Figures 2P,P'**, unfilled arrowhead). *Ascl1* is important for the differentiation of late hypothalamic neurons because in *Ascl1* knock-out mice differentiation of neuroendocrine neurons is disturbed (Mcnay et al., 2006). Although the authors did not specifically look at the

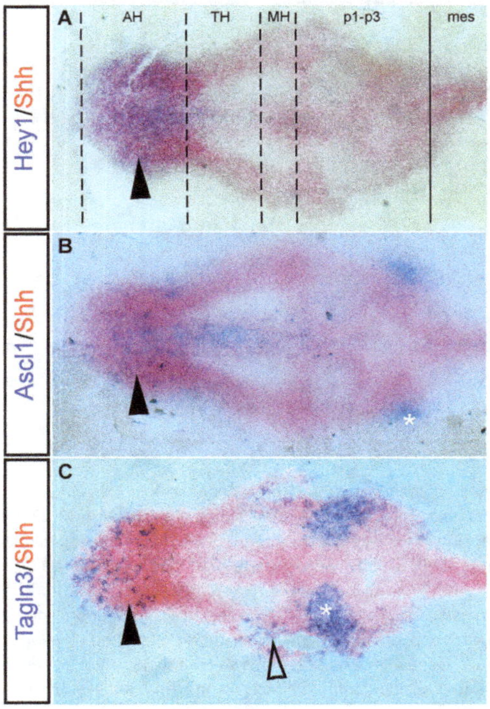

FIGURE 3 | *Hey1*, *Ascl1* and *Tagln3* expression overlaps with *Shh* in the chick hypothalamus primordium. Double labeling of *Hey1*, *Ascl1* and *Tagln3* (Purple, Digoxigenin labeled probes) at HH15 with the dynamic hypothalamic marker, *Shh* (Red, Fluorescein labeled mRNA probe) in chick confirms expression of these genes in the hypothalamic domains. **(A)** *Hey1* expression is specifically expressed in the anterior hypothalamus (AH) (arrowhead), overlapping the area where the nTPOC neurons will differentiate. Dashed lines indicate the boundaries of the hypothalamic domains, while the solid line marks the diencephalic-mesencephalic boundary (DMB). **(B)** *Ascl1* expression is located in the AH (arrowhead). Asterisk labels the nTPOC located in p1 (Ware and Schubert, 2011). **(C)** *Tagln3* expression is located in the AH (arrowhead) and in the mammillary hypothalamus (MH), overlapping where the nMTT neurons differentiate (unfilled arrowhead). Asterisk labels the ventral medial longitudinal fascicle (nMLF) located in p2 (Ware and Schubert, 2011). mes, mesencephalon; p1-p3, prosomeres 1–3; TH; tuberal hypothalamus.

nTPOC or nMTT neurons it can be assumed these neurons will be affected.

During initiation of neuronal differentiation various proneural genes are recruited, but the specific proneural genes involved could be different between species and neuronal populations. Here, the expression of other proneural genes has been researched in the developing hypothalamus. Remarkably, as *Neurog1/2* are not expressed in the hypothalamus (Ratié et al., 2013), *Ascl1* appears to be the only proneural gene expressed in the ventral chick AH, at least during early development. Lateral inhibition is the process controlling differentiation of these neurons but the precise mechanisms is different between chick and mouse. There are several lines of evidence to suggest this including restriction of *Ascl1* expression to the AH in chick (**Figure 2B**), where in mouse *Ascl1* is expressed in both the AH and MH (**Figure 2P**). To date, no other proneural gene has been described in the developing chick MH. *Neurog1* and *Neurog2* are not found in the ventral hypothalamus of zebrafish and mouse (Ando et al., 2005; Mcnay et al., 2006; Osório et al., 2010), but a third member of the neurogenin family, *Neurog3* has been identified, specifically expressed in the AH (Wang et al., 2001; Villasenor et al., 2008; Pelling et al., 2011). *Neurog3* expression is regulated by *Ascl1* (Mcnay et al., 2006), but in *Neurog3* mutant mice there is no effect on early neurogenesis in the hypothalamus (Pelling et al., 2011; Anthwal et al., 2013). This lack of phenotype could be due to redundancy between the two proneural genes. It would be interesting to analyses *Ascl1/Neurog3* mutant mice to determine whether there is an additional defect in the formation of the nTPOC.

Additionally, in zebrafish and mouse, *Ascl1* and *Neurog3* may act together to control the processes of lateral inhibition leading to the differentiation of the nTPOC, whereas in chick differentiation is specifically regulated by *Ascl1*.

As the capacity to regulate differentiation steps during neurogenesis is shared by all the proneural genes (Guillemot, 2007), it may explain why neuronal differentiation in the vertebrate hypothalamus is not conserved.

DESCRIPTION OF PRONEURAL TARGET GENES WITHIN THE HYPOTHALAMIC PRIMORDIUM

In the absence of Notch activity during nTPOC differentiation in the chick hypothalamus, *Ascl1* is upregulated and induces expression of a wide spectrum of neuron specific genes (Castro et al., 2011; Ratié et al., 2013). While upregulation of some neuronal genes like *Nhlh1* or *Stmn2* is expected in tissue lacking Notch signaling, other genes identified are not associated with a role in hypothalamic development, such as Transgelin 3 (*Tagln3*) and Chromogranin A (*Chga*). *Nhlh1* and *Chga* mutant mice are available, but there is no phenotype or effect on neurogenesis, suggesting redundancy with other genes (Krüger and Braun, 2002; Hendy et al., 2006; Schmid et al., 2007). *Tagln3* appears to be a good marker because it is strongly expressed in the areas where both the nTPOC and nMTT form. In a flat-mounted preparation of HH15 chick hypothalamus, double labeling with *Shh* and *Tagln3* reveals expression of *Tagln3* in the AH and MH where the nTPOC and nMTT neurons are respectively located (**Figure 3C**, arrowhead and unfilled arrowhead). *Tagln3* is also expressed in the ventral MLF population, which are the first neurons to develop in the brain (**Figure 3C**, asterisk). While these target genes are all expressed in post-mitotic neurons (Theodorakis et al., 2002; Pape et al., 2008; Xie et al., 2008; Burzynski et al., 2009; Ratié et al., under review) no specific function can be attributed to these genes during nTPOC and nMTT development.

Another set of genes are specifically upregulated in the chick AH when Notch signaling is inhibited, *Slit1* and *Robo2*, which are well-known components involved in axon guidance (Chisholm and Tessier-Lavigne, 1999). They guide the TPOC axons through the hypothalamus (Devine and Key, 2008; Ricaño-Cornejo et al., 2011) and the regulation of these genes is Notch dependent (Ratié et al., 2013).

Analysis of the promoter regions in *Slit1*, *Robo2*, *Tagln3* and *Chga* reveal binding sites of *Hes5*, *Hey1*, *Ascl1* and *Nhlh1*

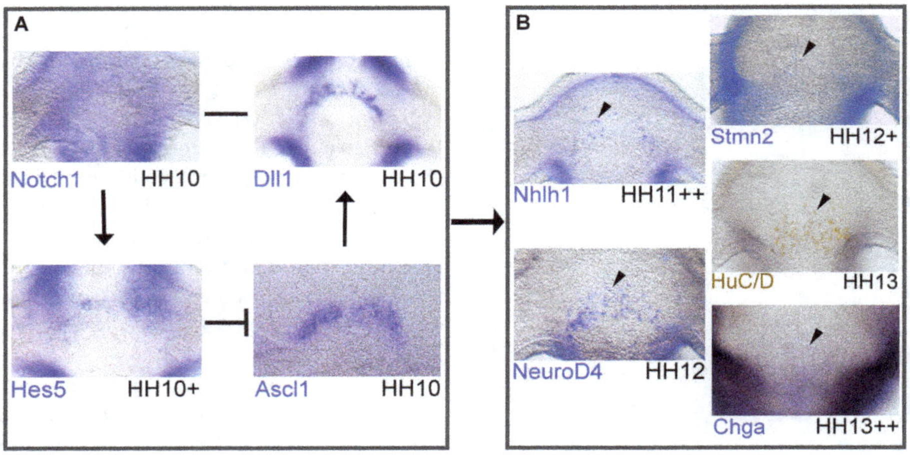

FIGURE 4 | Network of Notch/proneural genes and initial expression of downstream targets in the developing chick hypothalamus. Whole-mount *in situ* hybridization or immunohistochemistry of markers in chick. Immunohistochemistry protocol has been described elsewhere (Lumsden and Keynes, 1989). Anti-HuC/D mouse (1:500; molecular probes; A21271) primary antibody was detected with a peroxidase-conjugated rabbit-anti-mouse secondary antibody (1:2000; Jackson ImmunoResearch; 315-035-045). Probes were obtained from cDNA and subcloned into pCRII-TOPO (Invitrogen) to make RNA probes or plasmids were obtained from other sources: *Dll1* and *Notch1* (kind gifts from Dr Frank Schubert). **(A, B)** Frontal view of the AH in the developing hypothalamus where the nTPOC neurons will differentiate. This network of genes is based on *in silico* results and data from Ratié et al., 2013. Expression of all markers, except *Notch1* have a horseshoe shape. **(A)** Notch network loop in NPCs. *Notch1* expression is ubiquitous throughout the hypothalamus at HH10. *Dll1* and *Ascl1* expression in the hypothalamus at HH10. *Hes5* expression in the hypothalamus at HH10^{+}. **(B)** Genes are upregulated in post-mitotic differentiating neurons. Expression of *Nhlh1* at HH11^{+} and *NeuroD4* at HH12. *Stmn2* expression at HH12^{+}, HuC/D expression at HH13 and *Chga* expression, first appears at HH13^{++} in very few cells in the developing hypothalamus. Genes are expressed in a salt-and-pepper like pattern (arrowhead). Expression confirms Notch components and *Ascl1* are expressed first, followed by the expression of downstream targets. Arrows represent activation of downstream targets. Barred lines represent repression of downstream targets. A single line represents direct binding between ligand and receptor.

providing further evidence these target genes are part of the Notch/proneural regulatory network involved in neuronal differentiation in the hypothalamus (Ratié et al., 2013).

MOLECULAR CASCADE OF NEUROGENESIS ONSET IN THE CHICK HYPOTHALAMUS PRIMORDIUM

In order to corroborate this network of genes, the expression of Notch components and target genes is analyzed by *in situ* hybridization in the chick hypothalamus to provide further evidence for the existence of a molecular cascade that is Notch/proneural dependent.

The molecular cascade begins with the expression of Notch components and proneural genes followed by other bHLH transcription factors, target genes and well-known neuronal markers (**Figure 4**). *Notch1*, *Hes5*, *Dll1*, *Ascl1*, *Nhlh1*, *NeuroD4*, *Stmn2*, HuC/D and *Chga* are examples chosen to evaluate the stage of their first expression in the AH (**Figure 4**). At HH10, the first components to be expressed in the developing hypothalamus are *Notch1*, *Dll1* and *Ascl1*, followed by *Hes5* that form a regulatory loop (**Figure 4A**; Ratié et al., 2013). This mechanism has been well described in the literature for the induction of neurogenesis by lateral inhibition (Bertrand et al., 2002; Kageyama et al., 2008b).

Notch1 is present in the AH, ubiquitously expressed (**Figure 4A**) compared with *Dll1*, *Ascl1* and *Hes5* that are expressed in a salt-and-pepper like pattern with a horseshoe shape (**Figure 4**). This is in agreement with a lateral inhibition model taking place in the AH. In this model, when *Ascl1* is active in a NPC, this can upregulate other bHLH genes such as *Nhlh1* (Ratié et al., 2013). *Nhlh1* and *NeuroD4* are analyzed as they are known markers of differentiation and expressed in the hypothalamus (Murdoch et al., 1999; Abu-Elmagd et al., 2001; Ratié et al., 2013). These genes are expressed from HH12, with *Nhlh1* expression appearing slightly earlier at HH11++ (**Figure 4B**). Other genes are upregulated from around HH13 such as, the well-known neuronal markers *Stmn2* and HuC/D but also new markers such as *Chga* (**Figure 4B**; Ratié et al., 2013).

BrdU labeling suggests *Dll1* expressing cells have exited the cell cycle (Henrique et al., 1995; Myat et al., 1996) therefore NPCs destined to become nTPOC neurons exit the cell cycle around HH10 as seen with *Dll1* expression (**Figure 4A**). It suggests that as early as HH10, the *Dll1* positive cells of the hypothalamus are destined to become neurons several stages before they become mature neurons expressing markers such as *Stmn2* or HuC/D at HH13. These results provide further evidence that the Notch/proneural loop is active in the hypothalamus from a very early stage before the first neurons appear.

CONCLUDING REMARKS

In this review, data has been discussed implicating the Notch/proneural network with a role during the differentiation of the first two groups of neurons that develop in the hypothalamus, the nTPOC and nMTT. There is still specific functional data lacking in the hypothalamus to conclude the specific mechanisms in which these neurons differentiate, but a general picture using expression data and interpretation of other functional models has been achieved. The same Notch/proneural network is likely to regulate differentiation of nTPOC neurons in zebrafish, chick and mouse. Considering the conservation of the TPOC axon tract and the Notch signaling pathway, this is not surprising. Data regarding proneural gene expression in the chick MH is still too scarce to conclude, but some of the components of the Notch/proneural network are expressed in the mouse MH before the nMTT neurons differentiate. This expression suggests the same mechanisms occur between the nTPOC and nMTT, only the players for nMTT differentiation are yet to be found in chick.

It is still not known what triggers this Notch/proneural loop in these hypothalamic NPCs. Neuronal specification during spinal cord development is initially generated by activities of two competing signaling pathways: SHH and BMP/Wnt (Ericson et al., 1997; Jessell, 2000; Liem et al., 2000). Evidence is emerging to suggest that SHH and BMP may play a similar role in the differentiation of the early hypothalamic neurons (Manning et al., 2006; Ahsan et al., 2007; Szabó et al., 2009; Alvarez-Bolado et al., 2012). However, how these signaling pathways integrate the Notch/proneural network has to be investigated in the developing hypothalamus. Future work will require a study to identify transcription factors that are necessary for the patterning of the AH and MH very early during vertebrate development.

One thing is clear, this review highlights lots of open questions regarding initial neuronal differentiation in the hypothalamus as well as general patterning of the hypothalamic regions. We hope that this review will encourage the scientific communities to investigate the phenotype of their mutants during earlier stages when the nTPOC and nMTT neurons develop.

A final thought, distinct late hypothalamic cell types dysfunction can lead to metabolic or homeostatic disorders and there is evidence that this is the case in congenital obesity (Gibson et al., 2004; Bingham et al., 2008). Therefore, could a defect in the induction and specification of the initial neurons lead to such disorders as these neurons are essential to the axon tract formation of the late hypothalamic neurons (such as the MCH neurons) (Croizier et al., 2011).

AUTHOR CONTRIBUTIONS

Michelle Ware and Valérie Dupé set up and designed the experiments. Michelle Ware and Houda Hamdi-Rozé performed the experiments. Michelle Ware and Valérie Dupé wrote the manuscript. All authors read, discussed and edited the manuscript.

ACKNOWLEDGMENTS

We would like to thank the members of the David laboratory for suggestions and comments. This work was supported by the Agence Nationale de la Recherche (grant no. ANR-12-BSV1-0007-01, Valérie Dupé). We also thank the animal house platform ARCHE (SFR Biosit, Rennes, France). We are grateful to receive the following plasmids: mouse *Ascl1* (Dr Francois Guillemot, London, UK), chick *Dll1* and *Notch1* (Dr Frank Schubert, Portsmouth, UK).

REFERENCES

Abu-Elmagd, M., Ishii, Y., Cheung, M., Rex, M., Le Rouëdec, D., and Scotting, P. J. (2001). cSox3 expression and neurogenesis in the epibranchial placodes. *Dev. Biol.* 237, 258–269. doi: 10.1006/dbio.2001.0378

Adam, J., Myat, A., Le Roux, I., Eddison, M., Henrique, D., Ish-Horowicz, D., et al. (1998). Cell fate choices and the expression of Notch, Delta and Serrate homologues in the chick inner ear: parallels with Drosophila sense-organ development. *Development* 125, 4645–4654.

Ahsan, M., Riley, K. L., and Schubert, F. R. (2007). Molecular mechanisms in the formation of the medial longitudinal fascicle. *J. Anat.* 211, 177–187. doi: 10.1111/j.1469-7580.2007.00774.x

Allende, M. L., and Weinberg, E. S. (1994). The expression pattern of two zebrafish achaete-scute homolog (ash) genes is altered in the embryonic brain of the cyclops mutant. *Dev. Biol.* 166, 509–530. doi: 10.1006/dbio.1994.1334

Alpeeva, E. V., and Makarenko, I. G. (2007). [Perinatal development of mammillotegmental connections in rats]. *Ontogenez* 38, 86–93.

Alvarez-Bolado, G., Paul, F. A., and Blaess, S. (2012). Sonic hedgehog lineage in the mouse hypothalamus: from progenitor domains to hypothalamic regions. *Neural Dev.* 7:4. doi: 10.1186/1749-8104-7-4

Ando, H., Kobayashi, M., Tsubokawa, T., Uyemura, K., Furuta, T., and Okamoto, H. (2005). Lhx2 mediates the activity of Six3 in zebrafish forebrain growth. *Dev. Biol.* 287, 456–468. doi: 10.1016/j.ydbio.2005.09.023

Anthwal, N., Pelling, M., Claxton, S., Mellitzer, G., Collin, C., Kessaris, N., et al. (2013). Conditional deletion of neurogenin-3 using Nkx2.1iCre results in a mouse model for the central control of feeding, activity and obesity. *Dis. Model. Mech.* 6, 1133–1145. doi: 10.1242/dmm.011916

Aoto, K., Shikata, Y., Imai, H., Matsumaru, D., Tokunaga, T., Shioda, S., et al. (2009). Mouse Shh is required for prechordal plate maintenance during brain and craniofacial morphogenesis. *Dev. Biol.* 327, 106–120. doi: 10.1016/j.ydbio.2008.11.022

Artavanis-Tsakonas, S., Rand, M. D., and Lake, R. J. (1999). Notch signaling: cell fate control and signal integration in development. *Science* 284, 770–776. doi: 10.1126/science.284.5415.770

Artavanis-Tsakonas, S., and Simpson, P. (1991). Choosing a cell fate: a view from the Notch locus. *Trends Genet.* 7, 403–408. doi: 10.1016/0168-9525(91)90264-Q

Aujla, P. K., Naratadam, G. T., Xu, L., and Raetzman, L. T. (2013). Notch/Rbpjkappa signaling regulates progenitor maintenance and differentiation of hypothalamic arcuate neurons. *Development* 140, 3511–3521. doi: 10.1242/dev.098681

Bak, M., and Fraser, S. E. (2003). Axon fasciculation and differences in midline kinetics between pioneer and follower axons within commissural fascicles. *Development* 130, 4999–5008. doi: 10.1242/dev.00713

Bardet, S. M., Ferran, J. L., Sanchez-Arrones, L., and Puelles, L. (2010). Ontogenetic expression of sonic hedgehog in the chicken subpallium. *Front. Neuroanat.* 4:28. doi: 10.3389/fnana.2010.00028

Barreiro-Iglesias, A., Villar-Cheda, B., Abalo, X. M., Anadón, R., and Rodicio, M. C. (2008). The early scaffold of axon tracts in the brain of a primitive vertebrate, the sea lamprey. *Brain Res. Bull.* 75, 42–52. doi: 10.1016/j.brainresbull.2007.07.020

Barsi, J. C., Rajendra, R., Wu, J. I., and Artzt, K. (2005). Mind bomb1 is a ubiquitin ligase essential for mouse embryonic development and Notch signaling. *Mech. Dev.* 122, 1106–1117. doi: 10.1016/j.mod.2005.06.005

Barth, K. A., and Wilson, S. W. (1995). Expression of zebrafish nk2.2 is influenced by sonic hedgehog/vertebrate hedgehog-1 and demarcates a zone of neuronal differentiation in the embryonic forebrain. *Development* 121, 1755–1768.

Bertrand, N., Castro, D. S., and Guillemot, F. (2002). Proneural genes and the specification of neural cell types. *Nat. Rev. Neurosci.* 3, 517–530. doi: 10.1038/nrn874

Bettenhausen, B., Hrabe De Angelis, M., Simon, D., Guénet, J. L., and Gossler, A. (1995). Transient and restricted expression during mouse embryogenesis of Dll1, a murine gene closely related to Drosophila Delta. *Development* 121, 2407–2418.

Bierkamp, C., and Campos-Ortega, J. (1993). A zebrafish homologue of the Drosophila neurogenic gene Notch and its pattern of transcription during early embryogenesis. *Mech. Dev.* 43, 87–100. doi: 10.1016/0925-4773(93)90027-U

Bingham, N. C., Anderson, K. K., Reuter, A. L., Stallings, N. R., and Parker, K. L. (2008). Selective loss of leptin receptors in the ventromedial hypothalamic nucleus results in increased adiposity and a metabolic syndrome. *Endocrinology* 149, 2138–2148. doi: 10.1210/en.2007-1200

Bray, S. J. (2006). Notch signalling: a simple pathway becomes complex. *Nat. Rev. Mol. Cell Biol.* 7, 678–689. doi: 10.1038/nrm2009

Brooker, R., Hozumi, K., and Lewis, J. (2006). Notch ligands with contrasting functions: Jagged1 and Delta1 in the mouse inner ear. *Development* 133, 1277–1286. doi: 10.1242/dev.02284

Burzynski, G. M., Delalande, J. M., and Shepherd, I. (2009). Characterization of spatial and temporal expression pattern of SCG10 during zebrafish development. *Gene Expr. Patterns* 9, 231–237. doi: 10.1016/j.gep.2008.12.010

Campos-Ortega, J. A. (1993). Mechanisms of early neurogenesis in Drosophila melanogaster. *J. Neurobiol.* 24, 1305–1327. doi: 10.1002/neu.480241005

Castro, D. S., Martynoga, B., Parras, C., Ramesh, V., Pacary, E., Johnston, C., et al. (2011). A novel function of the proneural factor Ascl1 in progenitor proliferation identified by genome-wide characterization of its targets. *Genes Dev.* 25, 930–945. doi: 10.1101/gad.627811

Cau, E., Gradwohl, G., Casarosa, S., Kageyama, R., and Guillemot, F. (2000). Hes genes regulate sequential stages of neurogenesis in the olfactory epithelium. *Development* 127, 2323–2332.

Cavodeassi, F., and Houart, C. (2012). Brain regionalization: of signaling centers and boundaries. *Dev. Neurobiol.* 72, 218–233. doi: 10.1002/dneu.20938

Chapman, S. C., Schubert, F. R., Schoenwolf, G. C., and Lumsden, A. (2002). Analysis of spatial and temporal gene expression patterns in blastula and gastrula stage chick embryos. *Dev. Biol.* 245, 187–199. doi: 10.1006/dbio.2002.0641

Chapouton, P., Webb, K. J., Stigloher, C., Alunni, A., Adolf, B., Hesl, B., et al. (2011). Expression of hairy/enhancer of split genes in neural progenitors and neurogenesis domains of the adult zebrafish brain. *J. Comp. Neurol.* 519, 1748–1769. doi: 10.1002/cne.22599

Chiang, C., Litingtung, Y., Lee, E., Young, K. E., Corden, J. L., Westphal, H., et al. (1996). Cyclopia and defective axial patterning in mice lacking sonic hedgehog gene function. *Nature* 383, 407–413. doi: 10.1038/383407a0

Chisholm, A., and Tessier-Lavigne, M. (1999). Conservation and divergence of axon guidance mechanisms. *Curr. Opin. Neurobiol.* 9, 603–615. doi: 10.1016/S0959-4388(99)00021-5

Chitnis, A., Henrique, D., Lewis, J., Ish-Horowicz, D., and Kintner, C. (1995). Primary neurogenesis in Xenopus embryos regulated by a homologue of the Drosophila neurogenic gene Delta. *Nature* 375, 761–766. doi: 10.1038/375761a0

Chitnis, A. B., and Kuwada, J. Y. (1990). Axonogenesis in the brain of zebrafish embryos. *J. Neurosci.* 10, 1892–1905.

Chitnis, A. B., and Kuwada, J. Y. (1991). Elimination of a brain tract increases errors in pathfinding by follower growth cones in the zebrafish embryo. *Neuron* 7, 277–285. doi: 10.1016/0896-6273(91)90266-3

Coffman, C., Harris, W., and Kintner, C. (1990). Xotch, the xenopus homolog of Drosophila notch. *Science* 249, 1438–1441. doi: 10.1126/science.2402639

Croizier, S., Amiot, C., Chen, X., Presse, F., Nahon, J.-L., Wu, J. Y., et al. (2011). Development of posterior hypothalamic neurons enlightens a switch in the prosencephalic basic plan. *PLoS One* 6:e28574. doi: 10.1371/journal.pone.0028574

Crossley, P. H., Martinez, S., Ohkubo, Y., and Rubenstein, J. L. (2001). Coordinate expression of Fgf8, Otx2, Bmp4 and Shh in the rostral prosencephalon during development of the telencephalic and optic vesicles. *Neuroscience* 108, 183–206. doi: 10.1016/S0306-4522(01)00411-0

Dale, J. K., Vesque, C., Lints, T. J., Sampath, T. K., Furley, A., Dodd, J., et al. (1997). Cooperation of BMP7 and SHH in the induction of forebrain ventral midline cells by prechordal mesoderm. *Cell* 90, 257–269. doi: 10.1016/S0092-8674(00)80334-7

de La Pompa, J. L., Wakeham, A., Correia, K. M., Samper, E., Brown, S., Aguilera, R. J., et al. (1997). Conservation of the Notch signalling pathway in mammalian neurogenesis. *Development* 124, 1139–1148.

Devine, C. A., and Key, B. (2008). Robo-slit interactions regulate longitudinal axon pathfinding in the embryonic vertebrate brain. *Dev. Biol.* 313, 371–383. doi: 10.1016/j.ydbio.2007.10.040

Dyer, C., Linker, C., Graham, A., and Knight, R. (2014). Specification of sensory neurons occurs through diverse developmental programs functioning in the brain and spinal cord. *Dev. Dyn.* 243, 1429–1439. doi: 10.1002/dvdy.24184

Easter, S. S. Jr., Ross, L. S., and Frankfurter, A. (1993). Initial tract formation in the mouse brain. *J. Neurosci.* 13, 285–299.

Eddison, M., Le Roux, I., and Lewis, J. (2000). Notch signaling in the development of the inner ear: lessons from Drosophila. *Proc. Natl. Acad. Sci. U S A* 97, 11692–11699. doi: 10.1073/pnas.97.22.11692

Ericson, J., Briscoe, J., Rashbass, P., Van Heyningen, V., and Jessell, T. M. (1997). Graded sonic hedgehog signaling and the specification of cell fate in the ventral neural tube. *Cold Spring Harb. Symp. Quant. Biol.* 62, 451–466. doi: 10.1101/SQ7.1997.062.01.053

Ferreiro, B., Skoglund, P., Bailey, A., Dorsky, R., and Harris, W. A. (1993). XASH1, a xenopus homolog of achaete-scute: a proneural gene in anterior regions of the vertebrate CNS. *Mech. Dev.* 40, 25–36. doi: 10.1016/0925-4773(93)90085-C

Fior, R., and Henrique, D. (2009). "Notch-Off": a perspective on the termination of Notch signalling. *Int. J. Dev. Biol.* 53, 1379–1384. doi: 10.1387/ijdb.072309rf

Fortini, M. E. (2009). Notch signaling: the core pathway and its posttranslational regulation. *Dev. Cell* 16, 633–647. doi: 10.1016/j.devcel.2009.03.010

Gibson, W. T., Pissios, P., Trombly, D. J., Luan, J., Keogh, J., Wareham, N. J., et al. (2004). Melanin-concentrating hormone receptor mutations and human obesity: functional analysis. *Obes. Res.* 12, 743–749. doi: 10.1038/oby.2004.89

Gimeno, L., and Martinez, S. (2007). Expression of chick Fgf19 and mouse Fgf15 orthologs is regulated in the developing brain by Fgf8 and Shh. *Dev. Dyn.* 236, 2285–2297. doi: 10.1002/dvdy.21237

Guillemot, F. (2007). Spatial and temporal specification of neural fates by transcription factor codes. *Development* 134, 3771–3780. doi: 10.1242/dev.006379

Guillemot, F., and Joyner, A. L. (1993). Dynamic expression of the murine Achaete-Scute homologue Mash-1 in the developing nervous system. *Mech. Dev.* 42, 171–185. doi: 10.1016/0925-4773(93)90006-J

Hatakeyama, J., Bessho, Y., Katoh, K., Ookawara, S., Fujioka, M., Guillemot, F., et al. (2004). Hes genes regulate size, shape and histogenesis of the nervous system by control of the timing of neural stem cell differentiation. *Development* 131, 5539–5550. doi: 10.1242/dev.01436

Hauptmann, G., Söll, I., and Gerster, T. (2002). The early embryonic zebrafish forebrain is subdivided into molecularly distinct transverse and longitudinal domains. *Brain Res. Bull.* 57, 371–375. doi: 10.1016/S0361-9230(01)00691-8

Hendy, G. N., Li, T., Girard, M., Feldstein, R. C., Mulay, S., Desjardins, R., et al. (2006). Targeted ablation of the chromogranin a (Chga) gene: normal neuroendocrine dense-core secretory granules and increased expression of other granins. *Mol. Endocrinol.* 20, 1935–1947. doi: 10.1210/me.2005-0398

Henrique, D., Adam, J., Myat, A., Chitnis, A., Lewis, J., and Ish-Horowicz, D. (1995). Expression of a Delta homologue in prospective neurons in the chick. *Nature* 375, 787–790. doi: 10.1038/375787a0

Hjorth, J. T., and Key, B. (2001). Are pioneer axons guided by regulatory gene expression domains in the zebrafish forebrain? High-resolution analysis of the patterning of the zebrafish brain during axon tract formation. *Dev. Biol.* 229, 271–286. doi: 10.1006/dbio.2000.9980

Hrabe de Angelis, M., Mcintyre, J. 2nd, and Gossler, A. (1997). Maintenance of somite borders in mice requires the Delta homologue DII1. *Nature* 386, 717–721. doi: 10.1038/386717a0

Iso, T., Kedes, L., and Hamamori, Y. (2003). HES and HERP families: multiple effectors of the notch signaling pathway. *J. Cell. Physiol.* 194, 237–255. doi: 10.1002/jcp.10208

Itoh, M., Kim, C. H., Palardy, G., Oda, T., Jiang, Y. J., Maust, D., et al. (2003). Mind bomb is a ubiquitin ligase that is essential for efficient activation of Notch signaling by Delta. *Dev. Cell* 4, 67–82. doi: 10.1016/S1534-5807(02)00409-4

Jarriault, S., Brou, C., Logeat, F., Schroeter, E. H., Kopan, R., and Israel, A. (1995) Signalling downstream of activated mammalian Notch. *Nature* 377, 355–358. doi: 10.1038/377355a0

Jasoni, C. L., Walker, M. B., Morris, M. D., and Reh, T. A. (1994). A chicken achaete-scute homolog (CASH-1) is expressed in a temporally and spatially discrete manner in the developing nervous system. *Development* 120, 769–783.

Jessell, T. M. (2000). Neuronal specification in the spinal cord: inductive signals and transcriptional codes. *Nat. Rev. Genet.* 1, 20–29. doi: 10.1038/35049541

Johnson, J. E., Birren, S. J., and Anderson, D. J. (1990). Two rat homologues of Drosophila achaete-scute specifically expressed in neuronal precursors. *Nature* 346, 858–861. doi: 10.1038/346858a0

Kageyama, R., Niwa, Y., Shimojo, H., Kobayashi, T., and Ohtsuka, T. (2010). "Chapter Ten - Ultradian oscillations in Notch signaling regulate dynamic biological events," in *Current Topics in Developmental Biology*, ed K. Raphael (San Diego: Academic Press), 311–331.

Kageyama, R., Ohtsuka, T., and Kobayashi, T. (2008a). Roles of Hes genes in neural development. *Dev. Growth Differ.* 50(Suppl. 1), S97–S103. doi: 10.1111/j.1440-169X.2008.00993.x

Kageyama, R., Ohtsuka, T., Shimojo, H., and Imayoshi, I. (2008b). Dynamic Notch signaling in neural progenitor cells and a revised view of lateral inhibition. *Nat. Neurosci.* 11, 1247–1251. doi: 10.1038/nn.2208

Kageyama, R., Ohtsuka, T., Shimojo, H., and Imayoshi, I. (2009). Dynamic regulation of Notch signaling in neural progenitor cells. *Curr. Opin. Cell Biol.* 21, 733–740. doi: 10.1016/j.ceb.2009.08.009

Kiecker, C., and Niehrs, C. (2001). The role of prechordal mesendoderm in neural patterning. *Curr. Opin. Neurobiol.* 11, 27–33. doi: 10.1016/S0959-4388(00)00170-7

Kiernan, A. E. (2013). Notch signaling during cell fate determination in the inner ear. *Semin. Cell Dev. Biol.* 24, 470–479. doi: 10.1016/j.semcdb.2013.04.002

Koo, B. K., Lim, H. S., Song, R., Yoon, M. J., Yoon, K. J., Moon, J. S., et al. (2005). Mind bomb 1 is essential for generating functional Notch ligands to activate Notch. *Development* 132, 3459–3470. doi: 10.1242/dev.01922

Koop, K. E., Macdonald, L. M., and Lobe, C. G. (1996). Transcripts of Grg4, a murine groucho-related gene, are detected in adjacent tissues to other murine neurogenic gene homologues during embryonic development. *Mech. Dev.* 59, 73–87. doi: 10.1016/0925-4773(96)00582-5

Krüger, M., and Braun, T. (2002). The neuronal basic helix-loop-helix transcription factor NSCL-1 is dispensable for normal neuronal development. *Mol. Cell. Biol.* 22, 792–800. doi: 10.1128/MCB.22.3.792-800.2002

Kwon, H. G., Hong, J. H., and Jang, S. H. (2011). Mammillotegmental tract in the human brain: diffusion tensor tractography study. *Neuroradiology* 53, 623–626. doi: 10.1007/s00234-011-0858-y

Leimeister, C., Externbrink, A., Klamt, B., and Gessler, M. (1999). Hey genes: a novel subfamily of hairy- and Enhancer of split related genes specifically expressed during mouse embryogenesis. *Mech. Dev.* 85, 173–177. doi: 10.1016/S0925-4773(99)00080-5

Liem, K. F. Jr., Jessell, T. M., and Briscoe, J. (2000). Regulation of the neural patterning activity of sonic hedgehog by secreted BMP inhibitors expressed by notochord and somites. *Development* 127, 4855–4866.

Lumsden, A., and Keynes, R. (1989). Segmental patterns of neuronal development in the chick hindbrain. *Nature* 337, 424–428. doi: 10.1038/337424a0

Macdonald, R., Xu, Q., Barth, K. A., Mikkola, I., Holder, N., Fjose, A., et al. (1994). Regulatory gene expression boundaries demarcate sites of neuronal differentiation in the embryonic zebrafish forebrain. *Neuron* 13, 1039–1053. doi: 10.1016/0896-6273(94)90044-2

Maier, M. M., and Gessler, M. (2000). Comparative analysis of the human and mouse Hey1 promoter: hey genes are new Notch target genes. *Biochem. Biophys. Res. Commun.* 275, 652–660. doi: 10.1006/bbrc.2000.3354

Manning, L., Ohyama, K., Saeger, B., Hatano, O., Wilson, S. A., Logan, M., et al. (2006). Regional morphogenesis in the hypothalamus: a BMP-Tbx2 pathway coordinates fate and proliferation through Shh downregulation. *Dev. Cell* 11, 873–885. doi: 10.1016/j.devcel.2006.09.021

Marion, J. F., Yang, C., Caqueret, A., Boucher, F., and Michaud, J. L. (2005). Sim1 and Sim2 are required for the correct targeting of mammillary body axons. *Development* 132, 5527–5537. doi: 10.1242/dev.02142

Martinez-Ferre, A., and Martinez, S. (2012). Molecular regionalization of the diencephalon. *Front. Neurosci.* 6:73. doi: 10.3389/fnins.2012.00073

Mastick, G. S., Davis, N. M., Andrew, G. L., and Easter, S. S. Jr. (1997). Pax-6 functions in boundary formation and axon guidance in the embryonic mouse forebrain. *Development* 124, 1985–1997.

Mastick, G. S., and Easter, S. S. Jr. (1996). Initial organization of neurons and tracts in the embryonic mouse fore- and midbrain. *Dev. Biol.* 173, 79–94. doi: 10.1006/dbio.1996.0008

Mathieu, J., Barth, A., Rosa, F. M., Wilson, S. W., and Peyriéras, N. (2002). Distinct and cooperative roles for Nodal and Hedgehog signals during hypothalamic development. *Development* 129, 3055–3065.

Mcnay, D. E., Pelling, M., Claxton, S., Guillemot, F., and Ang, S. L. (2006). Mash1 is required for generic and subtype differentiation of hypothalamic neuroendocrine cells. *Mol. Endocrinol.* 20, 1623–1632. doi: 10.1210/me.2005-0518

Mercier, S., Dubourg, C., Garcelon, N., Campillo-Gimenez, B., Gicquel, I., Belleguic, M., et al. (2011). New findings for phenotype-genotype correlations in a large European series of holoprosencephaly cases. *J. Med. Genet.* 48, 752–760. doi: 10.1136/jmedgenet-2011-100339

Murdoch, J. N., Eddleston, J., Leblond-Bourget, N., Stanier, P., and Copp, A. J. (1999). Sequence and expression analysis of Nhlh1: a basic helix-loop-helix gene implicated in neurogenesis. *Dev. Genet.* 24, 165–177. doi: 10.1002/(SICI)1520-6408(1999)24:1/2<165::AID-DVG15>3.0.CO;2-V

Myat, A., Henrique, D., Ish-Horowicz, D., and Lewis, J. (1996). A chick homologue of serrate and its relationship with Notch and Delta homologues during central neurogenesis. *Dev. Biol.* 174, 233–247. doi: 10.1006/dbio.1996.0069

Neves, J., Abelló, G., Petrovic, J., and Giraldez, F. (2013). Patterning and cell fate in the inner ear: a case for Notch in the chicken embryo. *Dev. Growth Differ.* 55, 96–112. doi: 10.1111/dgd.12016

Nural, H. F., and Mastick, G. S. (2004). Pax6 guides a relay of pioneer longitudinal axons in the embryonic mouse forebrain. *J. Comp. Neurol.* 479, 399–409. doi: 10.1002/cne.20317

Ohyama, K., Das, R., and Placzek, M. (2008). Temporal progression of hypothalamic patterning by a dual action of BMP. *Development* 135, 3325–3331. doi: 10.1242/dev.027078

Oka, C., Nakano, T., Wakeham, A., de la Pompa, J. L., Mori, C., Sakai, T., et al. (1995). Disruption of the mouse RBP-J kappa gene results in early embryonic death. *Development* 121, 3291–3301.

Osório, J., Mueller, T., Rétaux, S., Vernier, P., and Wullimann, M. F. (2010). Phylotypic expression of the bHLH genes neurogenin2, neurod and Mash1 in the mouse embryonic forebrain. *J. Comp. Neurol.* 518, 851–871. doi: 10.1002/cne.22247

Pape, M., Doxakis, E., Reiff, T., Duong, C. V., Davies, A., Geissen, M., et al. (2008). A function for the calponin family member NP25 in neurite outgrowth. *Dev. Biol.* 321, 434–443. doi: 10.1016/j.ydbio.2008.07.001

Paridaen, J. T., and Huttner, W. B. (2014). Neurogenesis during development of the vertebrate central nervous system. *EMBO Rep.* 15, 351–364. doi: 10.1002/embr.201438447

Patel, C. K., Rodriguez, L. C., and Kuwada, J. Y. (1994). Axonal outgrowth within the abnormal scaffold of brain tracts in a zebrafish mutant. *J. Neurobiol.* 25, 345–360. doi: 10.1002/neu.480250402

Patten, I., and Placzek, M. (2002). Opponent activities of Shh and BMP signaling during floor plate induction in vivo. *Curr. Biol.* 12, 47–52. doi: 10.1016/S0960-9822(01)00631-5

Pelling, M., Anthwal, N., Mcnay, D., Gradwohl, G., Leiter, A. B., Guillemot, F., et al. (2011). Differential requirements for neurogenin 3 in the development of POMC and NPY neurons in the hypothalamus. *Dev. Biol.* 349, 406–416. doi: 10.1016/j.ydbio.2010.11.007

Pera, E. M., and Kessel, M. (1997). Patterning of the chick forebrain anlage by the prechordal plate. *Development* 124, 4153–4162.

Pera, E. M., and Kessel, M. (1998). Demarcation of ventral territories by the homeobox gene NKX2.1 during early chick development. *Dev. Genes Evol.* 208, 168–171. doi: 10.1007/s004270050170

Petrovic, J., Formosa-Jordan, P., Luna-Escalante, J. C., Abelló, G., Ibañes, M., Neves, J., et al. (2014). Ligand-dependent Notch signaling strength orchestrates lateral induction and lateral inhibition in the developing inner ear. *Development* 141, 2313–2324. doi: 10.1242/dev.108100

Pierfelice, T., Alberi, L., and Gaiano, N. (2011). Notch in the vertebrate nervous system: an old dog with new tricks. *Neuron* 69, 840–855. doi: 10.1016/j.neuron.2011.02.031

Przemeck, G. K., Heinzmann, U., Beckers, J., and Hrabe De Angelis, M. (2003). Node and midline defects are associated with left-right development in Delta1 mutant embryos. *Development* 130, 3–13. doi: 10.1242/dev.00176

Puelles, L., Amat, J. A., and Martinez-de-la-Torre, M. (1987). Segment-related, mosaic neurogenetic pattern in the forebrain and mesencephalon of early chick embryos: I. Topography of AChE-positive neuroblasts up to stage HH18. *J. Comp. Neurol.* 266, 247–268. doi: 10.1002/cne.902660210

Puelles, L., Martinez-De-La-Torre, M., Bardet, S., and Rubenstein, J. L. R. (2012). "Chapter 8 - Hypothalamus," in *The Mouse Nervous System*, ed C. W. P. Puelles (San Diego: Academic Press), 221–312.

Puelles, L., and Rubenstein, J. L. (2003). Forebrain gene expression domains and the evolving prosomeric model. *Trends Neurosci.* 26, 469–476. doi: 10.1016/S0166-2236(03)00234-0

Ratié, L., Ware, M., Barloy-Hubler, F., Romé, H., Gicquel, I., Dubourg, C., et al. (2013). Novel genes upregulated when NOTCH signalling is disrupted during hypothalamic development. *Neural Dev.* 8:25. doi: 10.1186/1749-8104-8-25

Reaume, A. G., Conlon, R. A., Zirngibl, R., Yamaguchi, T. P., and Rossant, J. (1992). Expression analysis of a Notch homologue in the mouse embryo. *Dev. Biol.* 154, 377–387. doi: 10.1016/0012-1606(92)90076-S

Ricaño-Cornejo, I., Altick, A. L., García-Peña, C. M., Nural, H. F., Echevarría, D., Miquelajáuregui, A., et al. (2011). Slit-Robo signals regulate pioneer axon pathfinding of the tract of the postoptic commissure in the mammalian forebrain. *J. Neurosci. Res.* 89, 1531–1541. doi: 10.1002/jnr.22684

Rohr, K. B., Barth, K. A., Varga, Z. M., and Wilson, S. W. (2001). The nodal pathway acts upstream of hedgehog signaling to specify ventral telencephalic identity. *Neuron* 29, 341–351. doi: 10.1016/S0896-6273(01)00210-0

Rohr, K. B., and Concha, M. L. (2000). Expression of nk2.1a during early development of the thyroid gland in zebrafish. *Mech. Dev.* 95, 267–270. doi: 10.1016/S0925-4773(00)00345-2

Ross, L. S., Parrett, T., and Easter, S. S. Jr. (1992). Axonogenesis and morphogenesis in the embryonic zebrafish brain. *J. Neurosci.* 12, 467–482.

Saravanamuthu, S. S., Gao, C. Y., and Zelenka, P. S. (2009). Notch signaling is required for lateral induction of Jagged1 during FGF-induced lens fiber differentiation. *Dev. Biol.* 332, 166–176. doi: 10.1016/j.ydbio.2009.05.566

Schmid, T., Krüger, M., and Braun, T. (2007). NSCL-1 and -2 control the formation of precerebellar nuclei by orchestrating the migration of neuronal precursor cells. *J. Neurochem.* 102, 2061–2072. doi: 10.1111/j.1471-4159.2007.04694.x

Shanmugalingam, S., Houart, C., Picker, A., Reifers, F., Macdonald, R., Barth, A., et al. (2000). Ace/Fgf8 is required for forebrain commissure formation and patterning of the telencephalon. *Development* 127, 2549–2561.

Shimada, M., and Nakamura, T. (1973). Time of neuron origin in mouse hypothalamic nuclei. *Exp. Neurol.* 41, 163–173. doi: 10.1016/0014-4886(73)90187-8

Shimamura, K., Hartigan, D. J., Martinez, S., Puelles, L., and Rubenstein, J. L. (1995). Longitudinal organization of the anterior neural plate and neural tube. *Development* 121, 3923–3933.

Shimogori, T., Lee, D. A., Miranda-Angulo, A., Yang, Y., Wang, H., Jiang, L., et al. (2010). A genomic atlas of mouse hypothalamic development. *Nat. Neurosci.* 13, 767–775. doi: 10.1038/nn.2545

Simerly, R. B. (2004). "Anatomical substrates of hypothalamic integration," in *The Rat Nervous System*, ed G. Paxinos (Amsterdam: Elsevier Science), 335–368.

Sussel, L., Marin, O., Kimura, S., and Rubenstein, J. L. (1999). Loss of Nkx2.1 homeobox gene function results in a ventral to dorsal molecular respecification within the basal telencephalon: evidence for a transformation of the pallidum into the striatum. *Development* 126, 3359–3370.

Szabó, N. E., Zhao, T., Cankaya, M., Theil, T., Zhou, X., and Alvarez-Bolado, G. (2009). Role of neuroepithelial sonic hedgehog in hypothalamic patterning. *J. Neurosci.* 29, 6989–7002. doi: 10.1523/JNEUROSCI.1089-09.2009

Tamura, K., Taniguchi, Y., Minoguchi, S., Sakai, T., Tun, T., Furukawa, T., et al. (1995). Physical interaction between a novel domain of the receptor Notch and the transcription factor RBP-Jκ/Su(H). *Curr. Biol.* 5, 1416–1423. doi: 10.1016/S0960-9822(95)00279-X

Theodorakis, K., Kyriakopoulou, K., Wassef, M., and Karagogeos, D. (2002). Novel sites of expression of the bHLH gene NSCL1 in the developing nervous system. *Mech. Dev.* 119(Suppl. 1), S103–S106. doi: 10.1016/S0925-4773(03)00100-X

Varga, Z. M., Amores, A., Lewis, K. E., Yan, Y. L., Postlethwait, J. H., Eisen, J. S., et al. (2001). Zebrafish smoothened functions in ventral neural tube specification and axon tract formation. *Development* 128, 3497–3509.

Villasenor, A., Chong, D. C., and Cleaver, O. (2008). Biphasic Ngn3 expression in the developing pancreas. *Dev. Dyn.* 237, 3270–3279. doi: 10.1002/dvdy.21740

Wang, X., Chu, L. T., He, J., Emelyanov, A., Korzh, V., and Gong, Z. (2001). A novel zebrafish bHLH gene, neurogenin3, is expressed in the hypothalamus. *Gene* 275, 47–55. doi: 10.1016/S0378-1119(01)00648-5

Ware, M., and Schubert, F. R. (2011). Development of the early axon scaffold in the rostral brain of the chick embryo. *J. Anat.* 219, 203–216. doi: 10.1111/j.1469-7580.2011.01389.x

Ware, M., Waring, C. P., and Schubert, F. R. (2014). Development of the early axon scaffold in the rostral brain of the small spotted cat shark (Scyliorhinus canicula) embryo. *Int. Sch. Res. Not.* 2014:8. doi: 10.1155/2014/196594

Williams, R., Lendahl, U., and Lardelli, M. (1995). Complementary and combinatorial patterns of Notch gene family expression during early mouse development. *Mech. Dev.* 53, 357–368. doi: 10.1016/0925-4773(95)00451-3

Wilson, S. W., Ross, L. S., Parrett, T., and Easter, S. S. Jr. (1990). The development of a simple scaffold of axon tracts in the brain of the embryonic zebrafish, Brachydanio rerio. *Development* 108, 121–145.

Wolf, A., and Ryu, S. (2013). Specification of posterior hypothalamic neurons requires coordinated activities of Fezf2, Otp, Sim1a and Foxb1.2. *Development* 140, 1762–1773. doi: 10.1242/dev.085357

Xie, J., Wang, W. Q., Liu, T. X., Deng, M., and Ning, G. (2008). Spatio-temporal expression of chromogranin a during zebrafish embryogenesis. *J. Endocrinol.* 198, 451–458. doi: 10.1677/JOE-08-0221

9

Neurons containing orexin or melanin concentrating hormone reciprocally regulate wake and sleep

Roda Rani Konadhode[1], Dheeraj Pelluru[1] and Priyattam J. Shiromani[1,2]*

[1] Departments of Psychiatry and Behavioral Sciences, Medical University of South Carolina, Charleston, SC, USA
[2] Ralph H. Johnson VA Medical Center, Medical University of South Carolina, Charleston, SC, USA

Correspondence:
Priyattam J. Shiromani, Ralph H. Johnson VA Medical Center and Departments of Psychiatry and Behavioral Sciences, Medical University of South Carolina, 114 Doughty Street, Room 404, Charleston, SC 29425, USA
e-mail: shiroman@musc.edu

Neurons containing orexin (hypocretin), or melanin concentrating hormone (MCH) are intermingled with each other in the perifornical and lateral hypothalamus. Each is a separate and distinct neuronal population, but they project to similar target areas in the brain. Orexin has been implicated in regulating arousal since loss of orexin neurons is associated with the sleep disorder narcolepsy. Microinjections of orexin into the brain or optogenetic stimulation of orexin neurons increase waking. Orexin neurons are active in waking and quiescent in sleep, which is consistent with their role in promoting waking. On the other hand, the MCH neurons are quiet in waking but active in sleep, suggesting that they could initiate sleep. Recently, for the first time the MCH neurons were stimulated optogenetically and it increased sleep. Indeed, optogenetic activation of MCH neurons induced sleep in both mice and rats at a circadian time when they should be awake, indicating the powerful effect that MCH neurons have in suppressing the wake-promoting effect of not only orexin but also of all of the other arousal neurotransmitters. Gamma-Aminobutyric acid (GABA) is coexpressed with MCH in the MCH neurons, although MCH is also inhibitory. The inhibitory tone of the MCH neurons is opposite to the excitatory tone of the orexin neurons. We hypothesize that strength in activity of each determines wake vs. sleep.

Keywords: sleep, melanin concentrating hormone, optogenetics, hypothalamus

EARLY HISTORY OF SLEEP RESEARCH

In the last 100 years significant progress has been made in identifying the neurons that wake us up and make us fall asleep. The history behind the research effort is quite fascinating and involves the influenza epidemic of 1918. It was during that epidemic that a young Viennese physician named Baron von Economo concluded that sleep and waking were generated from specific areas of the brain (Economo, 1930). von Economo's conclusions were revolutionary since at that time it was believed that sleep occurred because people simply closed their eyes. Von Economo performed autopsies on some of the patients who had succumbed to the disease and from his observations he concluded that there was a region in the rostral part of the hypothalamus that was responsible for sleep and a region in the posterior hypothalamus that was responsible for wake.

At that time many distinguished scientists were intrigued by sleep and wake centers in the brain and were actively involved in trying to unravel the mysteries of the sleeping brain. One such investigator was Walle Nauta who was conducting his studies during the height of the Second World War in Holland. He wanted to determine whether rats with lesions in the brain, similar to those found in humans by von Economo, could have changes in sleep and wake. He did not have an electroencephalogram to record brain activity, but solely from behavioral observations he came to the same conclusion as von Economo (Nauta, 1946). Moruzzi and Magoun then showed that a sedated animal without any lesions could be aroused by electrically stimulating the brainstem reticular core (Moruzzi and Magoun, 1949).

DISCOVERY OF REM SLEEP

Everything changed in 1953 when REM sleep was discovered (Aserinsky and Kleitman, 1953). The discovery was made by Eugene Aserinsky, a graduate student in the laboratory of Nathaniel Kleitman at the University of Chicago. Aserinsky's doctoral thesis was to describe the pattern of eye movements in infants. He connected his 8 year-old son Armond to an EEG machine and noticed that at various points in the night, the pattern of the EEG activity and the eye movements began to resemble what one would notice during waking (Brown, 2003). He rushed in to the room to see if the boy was awake and much to his surprise he was fast asleep, but yet the EEG looked as if he was awake. He could not readily explain why there would be a sudden shift in the EEG to a waking EEG even though the boy was behaviorally asleep. His mentor was equally skeptical and both felt that they were recording some sort of artifact. Aserinsky methodically eliminated all doubts and once Kleitman was convinced, they published their paper in the journal Science. It was a simple paper that described regularly occurring periods of eye movements every 90 min or so, and that these periods occurred with a waking EEG.

Their discovery was a landmark in neuroscience research because it clearly showed for the first time that every 90 min the brain awakened itself during sleep. This new sleep state was called rapid eye movement sleep or REM sleep because of the occurrence of eye movements. The other phase of sleep was called non-REM sleep. REM sleep represents a paradox in that behaviorally one can see that the person is asleep, yet the pattern of the EEG activity resembles what is seen during waking. Another name for REM sleep is "paradoxical sleep". Indeed, it is now very clear that the activity of the brain during a REM sleep episode is similar to waking.

Very quickly other researchers began to investigate this new phase of sleep and it was discovered that it was present in lower animal species as well. By the late 1950's a French neuroscientist, Michel Jouvet, determined that REM sleep was generated from the brainstem (Jouvet, 1962, 1972). We now know that there are neurons in the pontine brainstem that are responsible for generating REM sleep (Kaur et al., 2009). However the signal that initiates REM sleep emanates from the hypothalamus. In other words, we have now come full circle to von Economo.

OREXIN, WAKING AND NARCOLEPSY

In 1998 two independent groups using different approaches discovered orexin (also known as hypocretin) (de Lecea et al., 1998; Sakurai et al., 1998). The distribution of orexin-containing neurons has been plotted in the mouse, rat (de Lecea et al., 1998; Peyron et al., 1998; Sakurai et al., 1998; Nambu et al., 1999) and humans (Elias et al., 1998; Thannickal et al., 2000), and we have plotted its distribution in the cat (Wagner et al., 2000). Orexin neurons project to virtually the entire brain and spinal cord, providing especially heavy innervation to regions implicated in the regulation of wakefulness such as the tuberomammillary nucleus (TMN) and the locus coeruleus (LC; Peyron et al., 1998). There are two orexin receptors (orexin-1 and orexin-2 receptors; or hypocretin 1 and hypocretin-2 receptors) and their distribution in the brain has been determined (Greco and Shiromani, 2001; Marcus et al., 2001). These receptors are especially heavy in areas implicated in wakefulness such as the LC (mainly orexin-1 receptors), TMN (mainly orexin-2 receptors), the dorsal raphe, and the basal forebrain.

In 1999 these peptides were linked to narcolepsy, a sleep disorder characterized by excessive daytime sleepiness and sudden muscle paralysis (called cataplectic attacks). Canines with narcolepsy were found to have a mutation in the orexin-2 (hypocretin-2) receptor (Lin et al., 1999) while mice lacking the orexin peptide (Chemelli et al., 1999) or the neurons containing orexin (hypocretin) (Hara et al., 2001) displayed behavioral and EEG signs of narcolepsy. Human narcoleptics have low to negligible levels of orexin-A in the cerebrospinal fluid (CSF) (Nishino et al., 2000), indicating a defect in release of the peptide, or actual loss of the orexin neurons. That same year, examination of post-mortem tissue revealed massive loss of the orexin neurons in the brains of subjects with narcolepsy (Peyron et al., 2000; Thannickal et al., 2000). In narcolepsy the orexin neurons are likely destroyed since other markers that colocalize with orexin, such as dynorphin and NARP, are also absent in humans with narcolepsy (Blouin et al., 2005; Crocker et al., 2005).

WHAT KILLS OREXIN NEURONS IN NARCOLEPSY?

It is not clear what kills the orexin neurons. Human narcolepsy is considered to be an autoimmune disease because of its linkage with the human leukocyte antigen-DQB1*0602 (Mignot et al., 1995, 1997). There appears to be a link with influenza based on the evidence that the influenza epidemic of 1918 caused people to be excessively sleepy and those that died were found to have lesions in the posterior hypothalamus (Economo, 1930). Indeed, in 2009 an H1N1 influenza strain appeared and a vaccine was created to prevent a global epidemic. The vaccine contained three genes derived from H1N1 and batches were made with and without adjuvants. By 2010 there emerged a cluster of cases in Europe, especially children, who displayed sudden-onset narcolepsy. An initial report (De la Herrán-Arita et al., 2013) suggesting a possible mimicry between epitopes on endogenous orexin (hypocretin) and the influenza protein has not been borne out.

OREXIN, AROUSAL AND CATAPLEXY

Orexin neurons discharge only during waking, especially with movement (Lee et al., 2005; Mileykovskiy et al., 2005). Thus, it is not surprising that when these neurons are lost, as in narcolepsy, patients have excessive daytime sleepiness and frequent sleep attacks. Narcoleptic patients also suddenly lose motor tone and collapse, especially in response to emotional stimuli, such as laughter or anger (Aldrich, 1991). These bouts are referred to as cataplexy. Canines with narcolepsy have a mutation in the orexin-2 (hypocretin-2) receptor and display cataplexy (Lin et al., 1999). The orexin control of muscle tone is through a specific pathway in the pons and medulla (Peever et al., 2014). Mice that lack orexin (Chemelli et al., 1999) or the orexin neurons (Hara et al., 2001) display all of the symptoms of narcolepsy. Mice that lack the orexin-1 (hypocretin-1) receptor have excessive sleepiness, albeit cataplexy is not as severe as the ligand knockouts (Willie et al., 2003). Mice with deletions of the orexin-2 receptor have a severe cataplexy as the ligand knockouts (Kalogiannis et al., 2011). We have linked orexin-B to the neurotoxin saporin to kill the orexin neurons and find that the rats display narcoleptic symptoms (Gerashchenko et al., 2001).

Because the orexin neurons are nestled with neurons that control other behaviors new genetically engineered tools are necessary to selectively manipulate only the orexin neurons. These new tools include optogenetics and DREDD (Designer Receptors Excitated by Designer Drugs). Optogenetic activation of the orexin neurons produces arousal (Adamantidis et al., 2007; Carter et al., 2010; Tsunematsu et al., 2011) and inhibition with DREDD produces sleep (Sasaki et al., 2011).

Based on the converging evidence from human narcolepsy, neuroanatomy, electrophysiology, pharmacology, knockout (ligand and receptor), and the new optogenetic/DREDD data a network model has emerged that hypothesizes that the orexin neurons regulate arousal and muscle tone by activating downstream arousal neurons in the basal forebrain, TMN, dorsal raphe, and the LC.

OREXIN GENE TRANSFER TO RESCUE NARCOLEPSY SYMPTOMS

We pioneered the use of gene therapy to rescue narcolepsy symptoms in mouse models of the disease. In three studies we reinserted the gene for orexin into surrogate neurons and convincingly demonstrated that it decreased cataplexy (Liu et al., 2008, 2011; Blanco-Centurion et al., 2013). We demonstrated that there is site-specificity in that the orexin gene must be inserted into surrogate neurons that are part of the circuit regulating cataplexy. Moreover, the surrogate neurons must be active during the cataplexy bout because that would release the orexin onto target neurons and stabilize the circuit (Bourgin et al., 2000; Huang et al., 2001). Another group transferred the gene for the orexin receptors into mice that lacked both the orexin receptors (Hasegawa et al., 2014). Reinsertion of the orexin-2 receptor specifically into the serotonergic dorsal raphe neurons decreased cataplexy while insertion of the orexin-1 receptor only in noradrenergic LC neurons increased waking. Such, mapping studies using genetically engineered tools are elucidating specific circuits regulating sleep and wake.

SLEEP-ACTIVE NEURONS

Much of the research in sleep neurobiology has focused on the arousal neurons. However, what shuts-off the arousal neurons so that sleep can ensue? One possibility is that during waking endogenous factors such as adenosine, cytokines and prostaglandins accumulate and inhibit the waking neurons (Krueger et al., 2011). Glia may also release adenosine to increase sleep pressure (Halassa et al., 2009). The decrease in activity of arousal neurons allows sleep-active neurons to become active and generate sleep. These sleep-active neurons begin to fire in drowsiness and then increase their firing during non-REM sleep and REM sleep (Jones, 2011). The increase in activity of the sleep-active neurons potently shuts off the wake-active neurons to induce sleep. Sleep-active neurons have been identified in the preoptic area (Sherin et al., 1996), the cortex (Gerashchenko et al., 2008), and in the lateral hypothalamus (Hassani et al., 2009).

THE GALANIN-POSITIVE SLEEP-ACTIVE NEURONS IN THE PREOPTIC AREA

The preoptic area was initially identified by von Economo and Nauta as being important for sleep since discrete lesions of this region produced insomnia. It is now known that stimulation of this region by small electrical currents, warming or by pharmacological means will produce sleep (McGinty and Szymusiak, 2000). c-Fos, an immediate early gene and a marker of neuronal activity, has helped to identify the phenotype of the sleep-active neurons and define the region and the connection to arousal neurons (Sherin et al., 1996). c-Fos expressing sleep-active neurons are present in the ventral lateral preoptic area (VLPO; Sherin et al., 1996) and the median preoptic area (MnPN; Alam et al., 1995; Szymusiak et al., 1998; Gong et al., 2000; Suntsova et al., 2002). These sleep-active neurons contain Gamma-Aminobutyric acid (GABA) and galanin and are inhibitory to major arousal populations (Chou et al., 2002). The VLPO neurons are inhibited by acetylcholine, serotonin and norepinephrine (NE), but are unaffected by histamine (Gallopin et al., 2000).

Electrophysiology studies have confirmed that neurons in the VLPO and MnPN begin to fire during drowsiness and peak activity is seen during non-REM sleep. The sleep-active cells comprise about 25% of the recorded cells in the basal forebrain-preoptic area and are intermixed with wake-active cells which predominate. Thus, the activity of the sleep-active neurons would release inhibitory agents at target wake-active neurons, shutting them off and triggering sleep (McGinty and Szymusiak, 2000). Lesions of the VLPO decrease sleep and increase wake (Lu et al., 2000), thereby replicating Nauta's and von Economo's observations. When the lesions extend dorsally then REM sleep is decreased, suggesting that this region influences pontine REM sleep generator neurons. The VLPO and MnPN neurons may become active in response to sleep pressure (Gvilia et al., 2006a,b). The preoptic area sleep-active neurons in the VLPO and MnPN may convey light-dark information since they receive input from the retina (Lu et al., 1999). Since the sleep-active neurons are in a minority and are nestled with neurons regulating waking it is important to selectively stimulate phenotypically identified GABA/galanin sleep-active neurons. This will provide direct evidence linking them to sleep generation. The new methods, such as optogenetics and DREDD, enable selective manipulation of neurons, which is an advantage over non-selective neuronal activation with electrical studies.

NEURONS CONTAINING MELANIN CONCENTRATING HORMONE (MCH)

The sleep-active neurons in the preoptic area (VLPO and MnPN) are still considered to be the only neurons responsible for sleep in current models of sleep-wake regulation (Saper et al., 2010).

However, sleep-active neurons outside the preoptic area have been found (Jones, 2011). Some of these neurons contain melanin concentrating hormone (MCH; Hassani et al., 2009). In head restrained rats MCH neurons are quiet during waking, begin firing during non-REM and are most active during REM sleep (Hassani et al., 2009).

Mammalian MCH is a 19 amino acid hormone synthesized as a prepro-hormone encoding two additional peptides neuropeptide EI and neuropeptide GE (NGE) which are cleaved by post-translational modification (Nahon, 1994). MCH neurons co-express GABA (Elias et al., 2008), CART (cocaine- and amphetamine-regulated transcript; Broberger, 1999), and nesfatin (Fort et al., 2008).

However, GABA, nesfatin and CART are also found in non-MCH neurons. MCH expressing neurons are present in the zona incerta, dorsomedial hypothamus and lateral hypothalamus (Elias et al., 1998; See **Figure 1**). Overall, MCH neurons project to the same targets as orexin neurons (Bittencourt and Elias, 1993, 1998; Elias and Bittencourt, 1997; Elias et al., 2008). MCH neurons have been shown by *in situ* hybridization, to co-localize with nociceptin/orphanin FQ opioid receptor (NOP), MCHR1, both orexin receptors (ORX), somatostatin receptors 1 and 2

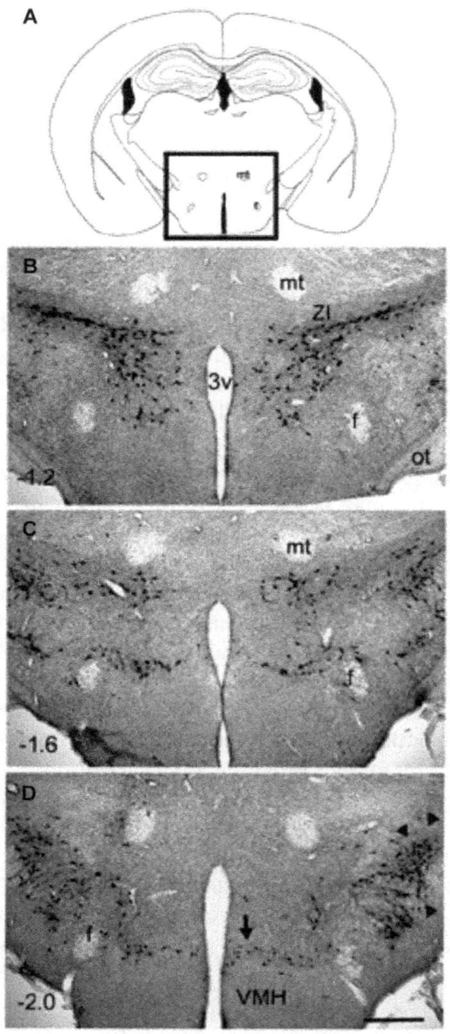

FIGURE 1 | Distribution of MCH-immunoreactive neurons in wildtype C57Bl6/j mice (3 months old). Coronal sections (40 μm thick) were processed for immunohistochemical detection of MCH-immunoreactivity (rabbit anti-MCH; 1:5000 dilution; overnight incubation) and visualized using the avidin-biotin -diaminobenzidene method. The MCH-ir neurons were present only in the hypothalamus (boxed area in photo **A**). A major cluster is located in the zona incerta (photo **B**) and extends medially to the ventricle. Another major cluster is located laterally (arrowheads in **D**). Minor clusters are located around the fornix (photo **C**) and ventrally along the dorsal border of the VMH (arrow in photo **D**). The numbers in **(B–D)** represent distance (millimeters) caudal to bregma. The calibration bar in **(D)** = 250 μm. Abbreviations: 3v= third ventricle; f = fornix; mt = mammillothalamic tract; ot = optic tract; ZI = zona incerta.

(SSTR1, SSTR2), kisspeptin receptor (KissR1), neurotensin receptor 1 (NTSR1), neuropeptide S receptor (NPSR), cholecystokinin receptor A (CCKAR), and the κ-opioid receptor (Parks et al., 2014b).

There are two MCH receptors, but only MCH receptor-1 is present in rodents (Chambers et al., 1999; Tan et al., 2002). MCHR1 is expressed in hippocampus, subiculum, basolateral amygdala, shell of the nucleus accumbens, hypothalamus (ventromedial nucleus, arcuate nucleus, and zona incerta), TMN, dorsolateral pons, including the dorsal raphe, and LC (Saito et al., 2001). MCH couples to the Gi alpha subunit and inhibits production of cAMP (Saito et al., 2001).

MCH knockout mice are awake and more active, have less non-REM, and are lean (Zhou et al., 2005; Willie et al., 2008). MCHR1 knockout mice have overall normal sleep levels and a normal sleep rebound after sleep deprivation (Adamantidis et al., 2008). Transgenic mice overexpressing prepro-MCH are hyperphagic and develop mild obesity with insulin-resistance (Ludwig et al., 2001). Ablation of the MCH neurons (MCH-ataxin; 60–70% loss) results in mice that are lean, hypophagic, having increased temperature and energy expenditure (Alon and Friedman, 2006), but sleep has not been recorded in these mice.

Effects of MCH on sleep

Intracerebroventricular (ICV) injection of MCH during the dark period dose dependently increases REM sleep by 200% and non-REM by 70% (Verret et al., 2003). MCH injection into sleep promoting areas such as VLPO significantly increase non-REM (Benedetto et al., 2013) while injection into REM sleep areas such as nucleus pontis oralis or dorsal raphe increase REM sleep (Torterolo et al., 2009; Lagos et al., 2011). Luppi's group has suggested that MCH neurons regulate REM sleep based on c-Fos expression in MCH neurons after REM sleep deprivation (Verret et al., 2003; Hanriot et al., 2007).

We have measured CSF levels of MCH in rats and find that it is highest during the day when the rats have the most sleep (Pelluru et al., 2013). In the same rats, orexin levels were highest at night, which is when the rats are awake. In humans, MCH is also associated with sleep and orexin with waking (Blouin et al., 2013). Thus, orexin and MCH levels are reciprocal to each other just like their firing pattern. They also have opposite effect on sleep-wake.

Pharmacology of MCH neurons (partial list; Figure 3)

MCH neurons are excited by orexin directly, and indirectly by enhancing glutamate release from excitatory neurons synapsing on MCH neurons (van den Pol et al., 2004; Huang and van den Pol, 2007). MCH neurons are excited by AMPA agonists and NMDA (van den Pol et al., 2004; Huang and van den Pol, 2007). MCH neurons are also excited by cannabinoid type-1 receptor (CB1R) agonist (Huang et al., 2007). This might explain the sleep-inducing effects of marijuana (Huang et al., 2007).

The peptide MCH inhibits orexin neurons, an effect not seen in MCHR1KO (Rao et al., 2008). MCH also inhibits neighboring GABA neurons (Gao and van den Pol, 2001). MCH neurons are inhibited by MCH, GABA, NE (effect mediated by alpha-2 receptor), serotonin, acetylcholine (muscarinic), Neuropeptide Y (NPY; Gao et al., 2003; van den Pol et al., 2004) and Histamine (Parks et al., 2014a). Dopamine (DA) inhibits MCH neurons through alpha-2 receptor (Alberto et al., 2011) and also D1 and D2 like receptors (Conductier et al., 2011).

Optogenetic activation of MCH neurons

The MCH neurons are virtually silent during waking, increase their discharge rates during sleep and reach their peak activity during REM sleep (Hassani et al., 2009). Based on their activity patterns we hypothesized that activating the neurons during waking should hasten sleep onset. To test this hypothesis we inserted the gene for the light-sensitive cation channel, channelrhodopsin-2, into MCH neurons in wildtype C57Bl6/j mice (**Figure 2**). We chose not to use the MCH-Cre mice, which have limited testing the hypothesis only in mice. Instead, we created our own MCH-promoter driven vector (supplied by Anthony van den Pol) to insert the ChR2+EYFP into MCH neurons in all vertebrate species. Three weeks after gene insertion, we recorded sleep for 48 h and then stimulated the MCH neurons with 473 nm blue light pulses (10 ms; 1 min on every 5 min; Konadhode et al., 2013). The stimulation began at lights-off, which is the start of the active phase of nocturnal rodents. We found that such stimulation reduced the length of waking bouts and increased both non-REM and REM sleep. The increase in sleep was most robust when the lights pulses were given at 10 Hz compared to 0 Hz or 5 Hz. The 10 Hz stimulation also increased delta power, a marker of sleep intensity. We did not find that optogenetic activation of MCH neurons during the light phase, which is the rest phase of nocturnal rodents, had any effect on sleep. We concluded that because the mice are normally asleep during the day it is not possible to generate more sleep. In other words, during the light phase there is a ceiling effect.

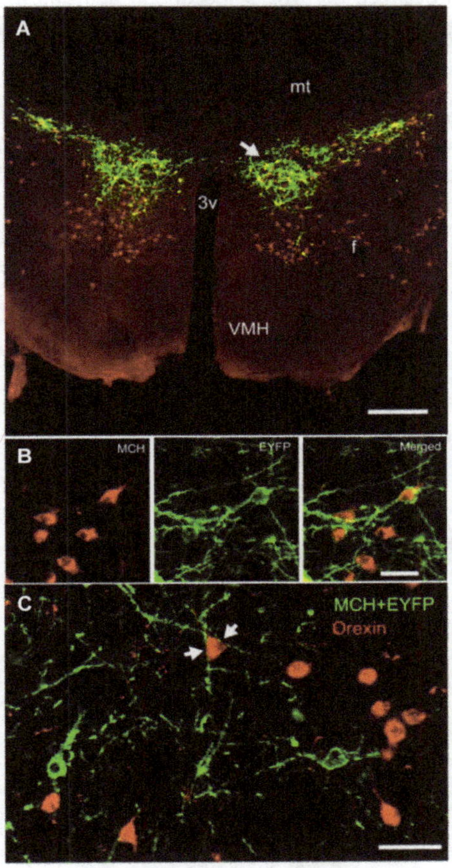

FIGURE 2 | Expression of ChR2-eYFP in MCH-immunoreactive neurons in the lateral hypothalamus of a representative wildtype C57BL/6J mouse. Compare with **Figure 1**. Panel **(A)** depicts the expression of ChR2-eYFP (green) in MCH neurons (red). Notice that the MCH neurons are diffusely distributed around the fornix and many MCH neurons located medial and ventral to the fornix did not contain the light-sensitive opsin. Panel **(B)** is a higher magnification view of a cluster of MCH neurons (arrow in panel **A**) that also contain ChR2-EYFP. Panel **(C)** depicts the close relationship between the orexin neurons (red) and MCH neurons (green ChR2-eYFP). The arrows in panel **(C)** show the encirclement of an orexin soma by MCH-ChR2-EYFP processes. Scale bar in **(A)** is 250 μm, **(B)** is 50 μm and **(C)** is 60 μm. Abbreviations: 3V = third ventricle; mt = mammillothalamic tract; mfb = medial forebrain bundle; f = fornix; VMH = ventromedial hypothalamus.

Another group (Jego et al., 2013) used MCH-Cre mice, and used a different stimulation paradigm compared to ours. They stimulated only during the second half of the light phase and only once the mice entered into REM sleep. They found that such stimulation during REM sleep prolonged the REM sleep bout. They also used light-sensitive halorhodopsin, eNpHR3.0, to inhibit the MCH neurons but it did not abort REM sleep bouts. They did not stimulate during waking or at night.

A third group expressed the gene for diphtheria toxin in the MCH neurons to selectively kill the MCH neurons (Tsunematsu et al., 2014). When the MCH neurons were ablated the mice were awake more during the day and night and had a selective decrease in non-REM sleep, but no change in amount of REM sleep. That study also found that optogenetic stimulation of the MCH neurons at night decreased the length of waking bouts at night and increased the number of non-REM sleep bouts (Figures 2A,B in Tsunematsu et al., 2014). In their study inhibition of the MCH neurons during the day had no effect on sleep, which confirms what was found by Jego et al. (2013).

The difference between levels of non-REM and REM sleep between the three studies might be related to activation of specific population of MCH neurons. As seen in **Figure 1** the MCH neurons extend about 1 mm along the anterior posterior plane, and are diffusely distributed about 1.5 mm laterally from the midline, and about 1 mm along the dorsal-ventral plane. MCH neurons are located densely in the zona incerta, in the lateral portions of the lateral hypothalamus, along the perifornical area, and ventrally along dorsal ridge of the ventromedial hypothalamus. In our study ChR2 was robustly expressed in the MCH neurons in the zona incerta, and less so in the lateral divisions (see **Figures 1, 2**). Moreover, in our study, we stimulated about half of the total population of MCH neurons, and found robust increases in both non-REM and REM sleep. In particular, the increase in sleep occurred against a strong waking drive indicating that MCH neurons can suppress the combined activity of all of the arousal neurons. The other two studies infected about 88% of the MCH neurons but given the diffuse distribution of the MCH neurons, and the fact that mammalian brain tissue heavily scatters light so that only about 10% of light reaches to about 500 μm (Adamantidis et al., 2007; Aravanis et al., 2007), it is very difficult to reliably stimulate all MCH+ChR2-positive neurons with optogenetics. Nevertheless, these three studies underscore the importance of MCH neurons in both non-REM and REM sleep. It is likely that a pharmacogenetic approach with DREDD may reach all the MCH neurons. However, the drawback of

DREDD is that it is short-lived (because of half-life of the drug), and does not provide millisecond control of targeted neurons.

The MCH peptide is inhibitory and inhibits orexin neurons (Rao et al., 2008). It also inhibits neighboring GABA neurons (Gao and van den Pol, 2001). MCH neurons also co-express GABA. Thus, both MCH and GABA are likely to inhibit target neurons. Thus, it is not surprising that activation of MCH neurons is able to shut-off the arousal neurons and induce sleep. When they are lost, as in the Tsunematsu et al. (2014) study, then the orexin neurons are likely to be more active resulting in increasing waking.

MCH has been implicated in feeding but optogenetic activation of MCH neurons induced sleep, not feeding (Jego et al., 2013; Konadhode et al., 2013). In our study, we found that mice slept rather than eat at a circadian time point when they normally should be eating (Konadhode et al., 2013). In our study, the mice had satiated their sleep need and undoubtedly were hungry. Nevertheless, they slept in response to MCH neuron stimulation. However, normal sucrose preference was reversed to sucralose in response to 20 Hz optogenetic stimulation of MCH neurons (Domingos et al., 2013).

Theoretical framework for the regulation of wake, non-REM and REM sleep

Based on data from optogenetics, c-Fos, electrophysiology, and lesion studies we hypothesize that sleep begins with activity of the sleep-active neurons (preoptic and MCH). The MCH neurons prevent the activation of the local orexin neurons which likely decreases orexin's drive of downstream arousal neurons. The preoptic sleep-active neurons are also inhibiting the arousal neurons. REM sleep occurs when the sleep-active neurons inhibit GABA neurons in the pons (see our model for REM sleep in Kaur et al., 2009) which then allows REM sleep-active neurons to fire and REM sleep ensues. We hypothesize that sleep ends because the MCH neurons are self-inhibiting and the wake state ends when the orexin neurons activate the MCH neurons (see **Figure 3**). There is support for this possibility because we find that with MCH stimulation length of wake bouts is cut in half but the length of non-REM or REM sleep bouts is unchanged. We suggest that this is because with progressive activity MCH neurons shut-off (self-inhibiting) and non-REM sleep ends. The interaction between the MCH and orexin neurons still needs to be investigated, but it provides a heuristic model of sleep-wake regulation.

Our position based on existing data is that the MCH neurons are a separate sleep promoting group that *partners* with the preoptic sleep-active neurons in generating sleep. Can sleep occur without the MCH neurons? Yes, since the preoptic area sleep-active neurons are intact. Which dominates: preoptic or MCH neurons? We think that each influences sleep based on their input. For instance, preoptic sleep-active neurons receive direct input from retina (Lu et al., 1999), are entrained to the light-dark cycle and could control timing of sleep. MCH neurons are within an area serving energy metabolism and respond to glucose

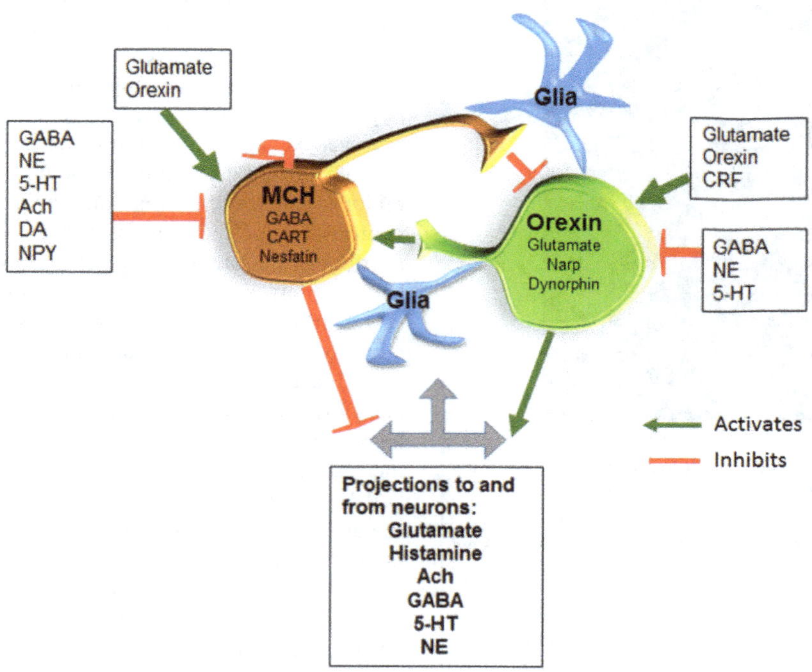

FIGURE 3 | MCH/GABA neurons are antagonistic to the orexin neurons. We hypothesize that local interaction between these two opposing neurons regulate sleep and wake. Glia are also likely to interact with neurons along the lines hypothesized by Haydon's studies. Abbreviations: Gamma-Aminobutyric acid (GABA); Norepinephrine (NE); Serotonin (5-HT); Acetylcholine (Ach); Dopamine (DA); Neuropeptide Y (NPY); Corticotropin releasing factor (CRF); Cocaine-Amphetamine-Regulated Transcript (CART); Neuronal activity regulated pentraxin (Narp).

(Burdakov et al., 2005). Both the MCH and the hypocretin/orexin neurons are located in a region sensing energy metabolism. A rise in glucose activates MCH neurons (Burdakov et al., 2005; Kong et al., 2010), which may explain post-prandial sleep.

CONCLUSIONS

More work needs to be done to fully identify the interaction between the sleep-active and arousal neurons in regulating sleep and wake. Important questions remain. For instance: How does the suprachiasmatic nucleus regulate these neurons? What is the relationship of energy metabolism and sleep-wake neurons? It is also important to mechanistically demonstrate that turning on sleep-active neurons shuts-off the wake-active neurons. This can now be done with optogenetics, a powerful tool that allows the neuroscientist to selectively manipulate specific neurons.

ACKNOWLEDGMENTS

We thank Dr. Carlos Blanco-Centurion and Dr. Meng Liu for helpful comments during the writing of the manuscript. Supported by NIH grants MH055772, NS052287, NS079940, NS084477 and Medical Research Service of the Department of Veterans Affairs.

REFERENCES

Adamantidis, A., Salvert, D., Goutagny, R., Lakaye, B., Gervasoni, D., Grisar, T., et al. (2008). Sleep architecture of the melanin-concentrating hormone receptor 1-knockout mice. *Eur. J. Neurosci.* 27, 1793–1800. doi: 10.1111/j.1460-9568.2008.06129.x

Adamantidis, A. R., Zhang, F., Aravanis, A. M., Deisseroth, K., and De Lecea, L. (2007). Neural substrates of awakening probed with optogenetic control of hypocretin neurons. *Nature* 450, 420–424. doi: 10.1038/nature06310

Alam, M. N., McGinty, D., and Szymusiak, R. (1995). Neuronal discharge of preoptic/anterior hypothalamic thermosensitive neurons: relation to NREM sleep. *Am. J. Physiol.* 269, R1240–1249.

Alberto, C. O., Trask, R. B., and Hirasawa, M. (2011). Dopamine acts as a partial agonist for alpha2A adrenoceptor in melanin-concentrating hormone neurons. *J. Neurosci.* 31, 10671–10676. doi: 10.1523/jneurosci.6245-10.2011

Aldrich, M. S. (1991). The neurobiology of narcolepsy. *Trends Neurosci.* 14, 235–239.

Alon, T., and Friedman, J. M. (2006). Late-onset leanness in mice with targeted ablation of melanin concentrating hormone neurons. *J. Neurosci.* 26, 389–397. doi: 10.1523/jneurosci.1203-05.2006

Aravanis, A. M., Wang, L. P., Zhang, F., Meltzer, L. A., Mogri, M. Z., Schneider, M. B., et al. (2007). An optical neural interface: in vivo control of rodent motor cortex with integrated fiberoptic and optogenetic technology. *J. Neural Eng.* 4, S143–S156. doi: 10.1088/1741-2560/4/3/s02

Aserinsky, E., and Kleitman, N. (1953). Regularly occurring periods of eye motility and concomitant phenomena, during sleep. *Science* 118, 273–274. doi: 10.1126/science.118.3062.273

Benedetto, L., Rodriguez-Servetti, Z., Lagos, P., D'almeida, V., Monti, J. M., and Torterolo, P. (2013). Microinjection of melanin concentrating hormone into the lateral preoptic area promotes non-REM sleep in the rat. *Peptides* 39, 11–15. doi: 10.1016/j.peptides.2012.10.005

Bittencourt, J. C., and Elias, C. F. (1993). Diencephalic origins of melanin-concentrating hormone immunoreactive projections to medial septum/diagonal band complex and spinal cord using two retrograde fluorescent tracers. *Ann. N Y Acad. Sci.* 680, 462–465. doi: 10.1111/j.1749-6632.1993.tb19708.x

Bittencourt, J. C., and Elias, C. F. (1998). Melanin-concentrating hormone and neuropeptide EI projections from the lateral hypothalamic area and zona incerta to the medial septal nucleus and spinal cord: a study using multiple neuronal tracers. *Brain Res.* 805, 1–19. doi: 10.1016/s0006-8993(98)00598-8

Blanco-Centurion, C., Liu, M., Konadhode, R., Pelluru, D., and Shiromani, P. J. (2013). Effects of orexin gene transfer in the dorsolateral pons in orexin knockout mice. *Sleep* 36, 31–40. doi: 10.5665/sleep.2296

Blouin, A. M., Fried, I., Wilson, C. L., Staba, R. J., Behnke, E. J., Lam, H. A., et al. (2013). Human hypocretin and melanin-concentrating hormone levels are linked to emotion and social interaction. *Nat. Commun.* 4:1547. doi: 10.1038/ncomms2461

Blouin, A. M., Thannickal, T. C., Worley, P. F., Baraban, J. M., Reti, I. M., and Siegel, J. M. (2005). Narp immunostaining of human hypocretin (orexin) neurons: loss in narcolepsy. *Neurology* 65, 1189–1192. doi: 10.1212/01.wnl.0000175219.01544.c8

Bourgin, P., Huitrón-Résendiz, S., Spier, A. D., Fabre, V., Morte, B., Criado, J. R., et al. (2000). Hypocretin-1 modulates rapid eye movement sleep through activation of locus coeruleus neurons. *J. Neurosci.* 20, 7760–7765.

Broberger, C. (1999). Hypothalamic cocaine- and amphetamine-regulated transcript (CART) neurons: histochemical relationship to thyrotropin-releasing hormone, melanin-concentrating hormone, orexin/hypocretin and neuropeptide Y. *Brain Res.* 848, 101–113. doi: 10.1016/s0006-8993(99)01977-0

Brown, C. (2003). The stubborn scientist who unraveled a mystery of night. *Smithsonian Magazine.* http://www.smithsonianmag.com/science-nature/the-stubborn-scientist-who-unraveled-a-mystery-of-the-night-91514538/?no-ist

Burdakov, D., Gerasimenko, O., and Verkhratsky, A. (2005). Physiological changes in glucose differentially modulate the excitability of hypothalamic melanin-concentrating hormone and orexin neurons in situ. *J. Neurosci.* 25, 2429–2433. doi: 10.1523/jneurosci.4925-04.2005

Carter, M. E., Yizhar, O., Chikahisa, S., Nguyen, H., Adamantidis, A., Nishino, S., et al. (2010). Tuning arousal with optogenetic modulation of locus coeruleus neurons. *Nat. Neurosci.* 13, 1526–1533. doi: 10.1038/nn.2682

Chambers, J., Ames, R. S., Bergsma, D., Muir, A., Fitzgerald, L. R., Hervieu, G., et al. (1999). Melanin-concentrating hormone is the cognate ligand for the orphan G-protein-coupled receptor SLC-1. *Nature* 400, 261–265.

Chemelli, R. M., Willie, J. T., Sinton, C. M., Elmquist, J. K., Scammell, T., Lee, C., et al. (1999). Narcolepsy in orexin knockout mice: molecular genetics of sleep regulation. *Cell* 98, 437–451. doi: 10.1016/s0092-8674(00)81973-x

Chou, T. C., Bjorkum, A. A., Gaus, S. E., Lu, J., Scammell, T. E., and Saper, C. B. (2002). Afferents to the ventrolateral preoptic nucleus. *J. Neurosci.* 22, 977–990.

Conductier, G., Nahon, J. L., and Guyon, A. (2011). Dopamine depresses melanin concentrating hormone neuronal activity through multiple effects on alpha2-noradrenergic, D1 and D2-like dopaminergic receptors. *Neuroscience* 178, 89–100. doi: 10.1016/j.neuroscience.2011.01.030

Crocker, A., España, R. A., Papadopoulou, M., Saper, C. B., Faraco, J., Sakurai, T., et al. (2005). Concomitant loss of dynorphin, NARP and orexin in narcolepsy. *Neurology* 65, 1184–1188. doi: 10.1212/01.wnl.0000168173.71940.ab

De la Herrán-Arita, A. K., Kornum, B. R., Mahlios, J., Jiang, W., Lin, L., Hou, T., et al. (2013). CD4+ T cell autoimmunity to hypocretin/orexin and cross-reactivity to a 2009 H1N1 influenza A epitope in narcolepsy. *Sci. Transl. Med.* 5:216ra176. doi: 10.1126/scitranslmed.3007762

de Lecea, L., Kilduff, T. S., Peyron, C., Gao, X., Foye, P. E., Danielson, P. E., et al. (1998). The hypocretins: hypothalamus-specific peptides with neuroexcitatory activity. *Proc. Natl. Acad. Sci. U S A* 95, 322–327. doi: 10.1073/pnas.95.1.322

Domingos, A. I., Sordillo, A., Dietrich, M. O., Liu, Z. W., Tellez, L. A., Vaynshteyn, J., et al. (2013). Hypothalamic melanin concentrating hormone neurons communicate the nutrient value of sugar. *Elife* 2:e01462. doi: 10.7554/elife.01462

Economo, C. V. (1930). Sleep as a problem of localization. *J. Nerv. Mental Dis.* 71, 249–259. doi: 10.1097/00005053-193003000-00001

Elias, C. F., and Bittencourt, J. C. (1997). Study of the origins of melanin-concentrating hormone and neuropeptide EI immunoreactive projections to the periaqueductal gray matter. *Brain Res.* 755, 255–271. doi: 10.1016/s0006-8993(97)00104-2

Elias, C. F., Saper, C. B., Maratos-Flier, E., Tritos, N. A., Lee, C., Kelly, J., et al. (1998). Chemically defined projections linking the mediobasal hypothalamus and the lateral hypothalamic area. *J. Comp. Neurol.* 402, 442–459. doi: 10.1002/(sici)1096-9861(19981228)402:4<442::aid-cne2>3.3.co;2-i

Elias, C. F., Sita, L. V., Zambon, B. K., Oliveira, E. R., Vasconcelos, L. A., and Bittencourt, J. C. (2008). Melanin-concentrating hormone projections to areas involved in somatomotor responses. *J. Chem. Neuroanat.* 35, 188–201. doi: 10.1016/j.jchemneu.2007.10.002

Fort, P., Salvert, D., Hanriot, L., Jego, S., Shimizu, H., Hashimoto, K., et al. (2008). The satiety molecule nesfatin-1 is co-expressed with melanin concentrating hormone in tuberal hypothalamic neurons of the rat. *Neuroscience* 155, 174–181. doi: 10.1016/j.neuroscience.2008.05.035

Gallopin, T., Fort, P., Eggermann, E., Cauli, B., Luppi, P. H., Rossier, J., et al. (2000). Identification of sleep-promoting neurons in vitro. *Nature* 404, 992–995. doi: 10.1038/35010109

Gao, X. B., Ghosh, P. K., and van den Pol, A. N. (2003). Neurons synthesizing melanin-concentrating hormone identified by selective reporter gene expression after transfection in vitro: transmitter responses. *J. Neurophysiol.* 90, 3978–3985. doi: 10.1152/jn.00593.2003

Gao, X. B., and van den Pol, A. N. (2001). Melanin concentrating hormone depresses synaptic activity of glutamate and GABA neurons from rat lateral hypothalamus. *J. Physiol.* 533, 237–252. doi: 10.1111/j.1469-7793.2001.0237b.x

Gerashchenko, D., Kohls, M. D., Greco, M., Waleh, N. S., Salin-Pascual, R., Kilduff, T. S., et al. (2001). Hypocretin-2-saporin lesions of the lateral hypothalamus produce narcoleptic-like sleep behavior in the rat. *J. Neurosci.* 21, 7273–7283.

Gerashchenko, D., Wisor, J. P., Burns, D., Reh, R. K., Shiromani, P. J., Sakurai, T., et al. (2008). Identification of a population of sleep-active cerebral cortex neurons. *Proc. Natl. Acad. Sci. U S A* 105, 10227–10232. doi: 10.1073/pnas.0803125105

Gong, H., Szymusiak, R., King, J., Steininger, T., and Mcginty, D. (2000). Sleep-related c-Fos protein expression in the preoptic hypothalamus: effects of ambient warming. *Am. J. Physiol. Regul. Integr. Comp. Physiol.* 279, R2079–2088.

Greco, M. A., and Shiromani, P. J. (2001). Hypocretin receptor protein and mRNA expression in the dorsolateral pons of rats. *Brain Res. Mol. Brain Res.* 88, 176–182. doi: 10.1016/s0169-328x(01)00039-0

Gvilia, I., Turner, A., Mcginty, D., and Szymusiak, R. (2006a). Preoptic area neurons and the homeostatic regulation of rapid eye movement sleep. *J. Neurosci.* 26, 3037–3044. doi: 10.1523/jneurosci.4827-05.2006

Gvilia, I., Xu, F., Mcginty, D., and Szymusiak, R. (2006b). Homeostatic regulation of sleep: a role for preoptic area neurons. *J. Neurosci.* 26, 9426–9433. doi: 10.1523/jneurosci.2012-06.2006

Halassa, M. M., Florian, C., Fellin, T., Munoz, J. R., Lee, S. Y., Abel, T., et al. (2009). Astrocytic modulation of sleep homeostasis and cognitive consequences of sleep loss. *Neuron* 61, 213–219. doi: 10.1016/j.neuron.2008.11.024

Hanriot, L., Camargo, N., Courau, A. C., Leger, L., Luppi, P. H., and Peyron, C. (2007). Characterization of the melanin-concentrating hormone neurons activated during paradoxical sleep hypersomnia in rats. *J. Comp. Neurol.* 505, 147–157. doi: 10.1002/cne.21482

Hara, J., Beuckmann, C. T., Nambu, T., Willie, J. T., Chemelli, R. M., Sinton, C. M., et al. (2001). Genetic ablation of orexin neurons in mice results in narcolepsy, hypophagia and obesity. *Neuron* 30, 345–354. doi: 10.1016/s0896-6273(01)00293-8

Hasegawa, E., Yanagisawa, M., Sakurai, T., and Mieda, M. (2014). Orexin neurons suppress narcolepsy via 2 distinct efferent pathways. *J. Clin. Invest.* 124, 604–616. doi: 10.1172/jci71017

Hassani, O. K., Lee, M. G., and Jones, B. E. (2009). Melanin-concentrating hormone neurons discharge in a reciprocal manner to orexin neurons across the sleep-wake cycle. *Proc. Natl. Acad. Sci. U S A* 106, 2418–2422. doi: 10.1073/pnas.0811400106

Huang, H., Acuna-Goycolea, C., Li, Y., Cheng, H. M., Obrietan, K., and van den Pol, A. N. (2007). Cannabinoids excite hypothalamic melanin-concentrating hormone but inhibit hypocretin/orexin neurons: implications for cannabinoid actions on food intake and cognitive arousal. *J. Neurosci.* 27, 4870–4881. doi: 10.1523/jneurosci.0732-07.2007

Huang, Z. L., Qu, W. M., Li, W. D., Mochizuki, T., Eguchi, N., Watanabe, T., et al. (2001). Arousal effect of orexin A depends on activation of the histaminergic system. *Proc. Natl. Acad. Sci. U S A* 98, 9965–9970. doi: 10.1073/pnas.181330998

Huang, H., and van den Pol, A. N. (2007). Rapid direct excitation and long-lasting enhancement of NMDA response by group I metabotropic glutamate receptor activation of hypothalamic melanin-concentrating hormone neurons. *J. Neurosci.* 27, 11560–11572. doi: 10.1523/jneurosci.2147-07.2007

Jego, S., Glasgow, S. D., Herrera, C. G., Ekstrand, M., Reed, S. J., Boyce, R., et al. (2013). Optogenetic identification of a rapid eye movement sleep modulatory circuit in the hypothalamus. *Nat. Neurosci.* 16, 1637–1643. doi: 10.1038/nn.3522

Jones, B. E. (2011). Neurobiology of waking and sleeping. *Handb. Clin. Neurol.* 98, 131–149. doi: 10.1016/b978-0-444-52006-7.00009-5

Jouvet, M. (1962). Research on the neural structures and responsible mechanisms in different phases of physiological sleep. *Arch. Ital. Biol.* 100, 125–206.

Jouvet, M. (1972). The role of monoamines and acetylcholine-containing neurons in the regulation of the sleep-waking cycle. *Ergeb. Physiol.* 64, 166–307.

Kalogiannis, M., Hsu, E., Willie, J. T., Chemelli, R. M., Kisanuki, Y. Y., Yanagisawa, M., et al. (2011). Cholinergic modulation of narcoleptic attacks in double orexin receptor knockout mice. *PLoS One* 6:e18697. doi: 10.1371/journal.pone.0018697

Kaur, S., Thankachan, S., Begum, S., Liu, M., Blanco-Centurion, C., and Shiromani, P. J. (2009). Hypocretin-2 saporin lesions of the ventrolateral periaquaductal gray (vlPAG) increase REM sleep in hypocretin knockout mice. *PLoS One* 4:e6346. doi: 10.1371/journal.pone.0006346

Konadhode, R. R., Pelluru, D., Blanco-Centurion, C., Zayachkivsky, A., Liu, M., Uhde, T., et al. (2013). Optogenetic stimulation of MCH neurons increases sleep. *J. Neurosci.* 33, 10257–10263. doi: 10.1523/jneurosci.1225-13.2013

Kong, D., Vong, L., Parton, L. E., Ye, C., Tong, Q., Hu, X., et al. (2010). Glucose stimulation of hypothalamic MCH neurons involves K(ATP) channels, is modulated by UCP2 and regulates peripheral glucose homeostasis. *Cell Metab.* 12, 545–552. doi: 10.1016/j.cmet.2010.09.013

Krueger, J. M., Clinton, J. M., Winters, B. D., Zielinski, M. R., Taishi, P., Jewett, K. A., et al. (2011). Involvement of cytokines in slow wave sleep. *Prog. Brain Res.* 193, 39–47. doi: 10.1016/b978-0-444-53839-0.00003-x

Lagos, P., Torterolo, P., Jantos, H., and Monti, J. M. (2011). Immunoneutralization of melanin-concentrating hormone (MCH) in the dorsal raphe nucleus: effects on sleep and wakefulness. *Brain Res.* 1369, 112–118. doi: 10.1016/j.brainres.2010.11.027

Lee, M. G., Hassani, O. K., and Jones, B. E. (2005). Discharge of identified orexin/hypocretin neurons across the sleep-waking cycle. *J. Neurosci.* 25, 6716–6720. doi: 10.1523/jneurosci.1887-05.2005

Lin, L., Faraco, J., Li, R., Kadotani, H., Rogers, W., Lin, X., et al. (1999). The sleep disorder canine narcolepsy is caused by a mutation in the hypocretin (orexin) receptor 2 gene. *Cell* 98, 365–376. doi: 10.1016/s0092-8674(00)81965-0

Liu, M., Blanco-Centurion, C., Konadhode, R., Begum, S., Pelluru, D., Gerashchenko, D., et al. (2011). Orexin gene transfer into zona incerta neurons suppresses muscle paralysis in narcoleptic mice. *J. Neurosci.* 31, 6028–6040. doi: 10.1523/jneurosci.6069-10.2011

Liu, M., Thankachan, S., Kaur, S., Begum, S., Blanco-Centurion, C., Sakurai, T., et al. (2008). Orexin (hypocretin) gene transfer diminishes narcoleptic sleep behavior in mice. *Eur. J. Neurosci.* 28, 1382–1393. doi: 10.1111/j.1460-9568.2008.06446.x

Lu, J., Greco, M. A., Shiromani, P., and Saper, C. B. (2000). Effect of lesions of the ventrolateral preoptic nucleus on NREM and REM sleep. *J. Neurosci.* 20, 3830–3842.

Lu, J., Shiromani, P., and Saper, C. B. (1999). Retinal input to the sleep-active ventrolateral preoptic nucleus in the rat. *Neuroscience* 93, 209–214. doi: 10.1016/s0306-4522(99)00094-9

Ludwig, D. S., Tritos, N. A., Mastaitis, J. W., Kulkarni, R., Kokkotou, E., Elmquist, J., et al. (2001). Melanin-concentrating hormone overexpression in transgenic mice leads to obesity and insulin resistance. *J. Clin. Invest.* 107, 379–386. doi: 10.1172/jci10660

Marcus, J. N., Aschkenasi, C. J., Lee, C. E., Chemelli, R. M., Saper, C. B., Yanagisawa, M., et al. (2001). Differential expression of orexin receptors 1 and 2 in the rat brain. *J. Comp. Neurol.* 435, 6–25. doi: 10.1002/cne.1190

McGinty, D., and Szymusiak, R. (2000). The sleep-wake switch: a neuronal alarm clock. *Nat. Med.* 6, 510–511. doi: 10.1038/74988

Mignot, E., Hayduk, R., Black, J., Grumet, F. C., and Guilleminault, C. (1997). HLA DQB1*0602 is associated with cataplexy in 509 narcoleptic patients. *Sleep* 20, 1012–1020. doi: 10.1212/wnl.48.6.1550

Mignot, E., Tafti, M., and Dement, W. C. (1995). Narcolepsy and immunity. *Adv. Neuroimmunol.* 5, 23–37. doi: 10.1016/0960-5428(94)00043-n

Mileykovskiy, B. Y., Kiyashchenko, L. I., and Siegel, J. M. (2005). Behavioral correlates of activity in identified hypocretin/orexin neurons. *Neuron* 46, 787–798. doi: 10.1016/j.neuron.2005.04.035

Moruzzi, G., and Magoun, H. W. (1949). Brain stem reticular formation and activation of the EEG. *Electroencephalogr. Clin. Neurophysiol.* 1, 455–473. doi: 10.1016/0013-4694(49)90219-9

Nahon, J. L. (1994). The melanin-concentrating hormone: from the peptide to the gene. *Crit. Rev. Neurobiol.* 8, 221–262.

Nambu, T., Sakurai, T., Mizukami, K., Hosoya, Y., Yanagisawa, M., and Goto, K. (1999). Distribution of orexin neurons in the adult rat brain. *Brain Res.* 827, 243–260. doi: 10.1016/s0006-8993(99)01336-0

Nauta, W. J. (1946). Hypothalamic regulation of sleep in rats; an experimental study. *J. Neurophysiol.* 9, 285–316.

Nishino, S., Ripley, B., Overeem, S., Lammers, G. J., and Mignot, E. (2000). Hypocretin (orexin) deficiency in human narcolepsy. *Lancet* 355, 39–40. doi: 10.1016/s0140-6736(99)05582-8

Parks, G. S., Olivas, N. D., Ikrar, T., Sanathara, N. M., Wang, L., Wang, Z., et al. (2014a). Histamine inhibits the melanin-concentrating hormone system: implications for sleep and arousal. *J. Physiol.* 592, 2183–2196. doi: 10.1113/jphysiol.2013.268771

Parks, G. S., Wang, L., Wang, Z., and Civelli, O. (2014b). Identification of neuropeptide receptors expressed by melanin-concentrating hormone neurons. *J. Comp. Neurol.* 522, 3817–3833. doi: 10.1002/cne.23642

Peever, J., Luppi, P. H., and Montplaisir, J. (2014). Breakdown in REM sleep circuitry underlies REM sleep behavior disorder. *Trends Neurosci.* 37, 279–288. doi: 10.1016/j.tins.2014.02.009

Pelluru, D., Konadhode, R., and Shiromani, P. J. (2013). MCH neurons are the primary sleep-promoting group. *Sleep* 36, 1779–1781. doi: 10.5665/sleep.3196

Peyron, C., Faraco, J., Rogers, W., Ripley, B., Overeem, S., Charnay, Y., et al. (2000). A mutation in a case of early onset narcolepsy and a generalized absence of hypocretin peptides in human narcoleptic brains. *Nat. Med.* 6, 991–997. doi: 10.1038/79690

Peyron, C., Tighe, D. K., van den Pol, A. N., De Lecea, L., Heller, H. C., Sutcliffe, J. G., et al. (1998). Neurons containing hypocretin (orexin) project to multiple neuronal systems. *J. Neurosci.* 18, 9996–10015.

Rao, Y., Lu, M., Ge, F., Marsh, D. J., Qian, S., Wang, A. H., et al. (2008). Regulation of synaptic efficacy in hypocretin/orexin-containing neurons by melanin concentrating hormone in the lateral hypothalamus. *J. Neurosci.* 28, 9101–9110. doi: 10.1523/jneurosci.1766-08.2008

Saito, Y., Cheng, M., Leslie, F. M., and Civelli, O. (2001). Expression of the melanin-concentrating hormone (MCH) receptor mRNA in the rat brain. *J. Comp. Neurol.* 435, 26–40. doi: 10.1002/cne.1191

Sakurai, T., Amemiya, A., Ishii, M., Matsuzaki, I., Chemelli, R. M., Tanaka, H., et al. (1998). Orexins and orexin receptors: a family of hypothalamic neuropeptides and G protein-coupled receptors that regulate feeding behavior. *Cell* 92, 573–585. doi: 10.1016/s0092-8674(00)80949-6

Saper, C. B., Fuller, P. M., Pedersen, N. P., Lu, J., and Scammell, T. E. (2010). Sleep state switching. *Neuron* 68, 1023–1042. doi: 10.1016/j.neuron.2010.11.032

Sasaki, K., Suzuki, M., Mieda, M., Tsujino, N., Roth, B., and Sakurai, T. (2011). Pharmacogenetic modulation of orexin neurons alters sleep/wakefulness states in mice. *PLoS One* 6:e20360. doi: 10.1371/journal.pone.0020360

Sherin, J. E., Shiromani, P. J., Mccarley, R. W., and Saper, C. B. (1996). Activation of ventrolateral preoptic neurons during sleep. *Science* 271, 216–219. doi: 10.1126/science.271.5246.216

Suntsova, N., Szymusiak, R., Alam, M. N., Guzman-Marin, R., and Mcginty, D. (2002). Sleep-waking discharge patterns of median preoptic nucleus neurons in rats. *J. Physiol.* 543, 665–677. doi: 10.1113/jphysiol.2002.023085

Szymusiak, R., Alam, N., Steininger, T. L., and Mcginty, D. (1998). Sleep-waking discharge patterns of ventrolateral preoptic/anterior hypothalamic neurons in rats. *Brain Res.* 803, 178–188. doi: 10.1016/s0006-8993(98)00631-3

Tan, C. P., Sano, H., Iwaasa, H., Pan, J., Sailer, A. W., Hreniuk, D. L., et al. (2002). Melanin-concentrating hormone receptor subtypes 1 and 2: species-specific gene expression. *Genomics* 79, 785–792. doi: 10.1006/geno.2002.6771

Thannickal, T. C., Moore, R. Y., Nienhuis, R., Ramanathan, L., Gulyani, S., Aldrich, M., et al. (2000). Reduced number of hypocretin neurons in human narcolepsy. *Neuron* 27, 469–474. doi: 10.1016/s0896-6273(00)00058-1

Torterolo, P., Sampogna, S., and Chase, M. H. (2009). MCHergic projections to the nucleus pontis oralis participate in the control of active (REM) sleep. *Brain Res.* 1268, 76–87. doi: 10.1016/j.brainres.2009.02.055

Tsunematsu, T., Kilduff, T. S., Boyden, E. S., Takahashi, S., Tominaga, M., and Yamanaka, A. (2011). Acute optogenetic silencing of orexin/hypocretin neurons induces slow-wave sleep in mice. *J. Neurosci.* 31, 10529–10539. doi: 10.1523/jneurosci.0784-11.2011

Tsunematsu, T., Ueno, T., Tabuchi, S., Inutsuka, A., Tanaka, K. F., Hasuwa, H., et al. (2014). Optogenetic manipulation of activity and temporally controlled cell-specific ablation reveal a role for MCH neurons in sleep/wake regulation. *J. Neurosci.* 34, 6896–6909. doi: 10.1523/JNEUROSCI.5344-13.2014

van den Pol, A. N., Acuna-Goycolea, C., Clark, K. R., and Ghosh, P. K. (2004). Physiological properties of hypothalamic MCH neurons identified with selective expression of reporter gene after recombinant virus infection. *Neuron* 42, 635–652. doi: 10.1016/s0896-6273(04)00251-x

Verret, L., Goutagny, R., Fort, P., Cagnon, L., Salvert, D., Leger, L., et al. (2003). A role of melanin-concentrating hormone producing neurons in the central regulation of paradoxical sleep. *BMC Neurosci.* 4:9. doi: 10.1186/1471-2202-4-19.

Wagner, D., Salin-Pascual, R., Greco, M. A., and Shiromani, P. J. (2000). Distribution of hypocretin-containing neurons in the lateral hypothalamus and C-fos-immunoreactive neurons in the VLPO. *Sleep Res. Online* 3, 35–42.

Willie, J. T., Chemelli, R. M., Sinton, C. M., Tokita, S., Williams, S. C., Kisanuki, Y. Y., et al. (2003). Distinct narcolepsy syndromes in Orexin receptor-2 and Orexin null mice: molecular genetic dissection of Non-REM and REM sleep regulatory processes. *Neuron* 38, 715–730. doi: 10.1016/s0896-6273(03)00330-1

Willie, J. T., Sinton, C. M., Maratos-Flier, E., and Yanagisawa, M. (2008). Abnormal response of melanin-concentrating hormone deficient mice to fasting: hyperactivity and rapid eye movement sleep suppression. *Neuroscience* 156, 819–829. doi: 10.1016/j.neuroscience.2008.08.048

Zhou, D., Shen, Z., Strack, A. M., Marsh, D. J., and Shearman, L. P. (2005). Enhanced running wheel activity of both Mch1r- and Pmch-deficient mice. *Regul. Pept.* 124, 53–63. doi: 10.1016/j.regpep.2004.06.026

10

Thyroid hormone and the developing hypothalamus

Anneke Alkemade *

Amsterdam Brain and Cognition Center, University of Amsterdam, Amsterdam, Netherlands

Correspondence:
Anneke Alkemade, Amsterdam Brain and Cognition Center, University of Amsterdam, Nieuwe Achtergracht 129, 1018WS Amsterdam, Netherlands
e-mail: jmalkemade@gmail.com

Thyroid hormone (TH) plays an essential role in normal brain development and function. Both TH excess and insufficiency during development lead to structural brain abnormalities. Proper TH signaling is dependent on active transport of the prohormone thyroxine (T4) across the blood-brain-barrier and into brain cells. In the brain T4 undergoes local deiodination into the more active 3,3′,5-triiodothyronine (T3), which binds to nuclear TH receptors (TRs). TRs are already expressed during the first trimester of pregnancy, even before the fetal thyroid becomes functional. Throughout pregnancy, the fetus is largely dependent on the maternal TH supply. Recent studies in mice have shown that normal hypothalamic development requires intact TH signaling. In addition, the development of the human lateral hypothalamic zone coincides with a strong increase in T3 and TR mRNA concentrations in the brain. During this time the fetal hypothalamus already shows evidence for TH signaling. Expression of components crucial for central TH signaling show a specific developmental timing in the human hypothalamus. A coordinated expression of deiodinases in combination with TH transporters suggests that TH concentrations are regulated to prevent untimely maturation of brain cells. Even though the fetus depends on the maternal TH supply, there is evidence suggesting a role for the fetal hypothalamus in the regulation of TH serum concentrations. A decrease in expression of proteins involved in TH signaling towards the end of pregnancy may indicate a lower fetal TH demand. This may be relevant for the thyrotropin (TSH) surge that is usually observed after birth, and supports a role for the hypothalamus in the regulation of TH concentrations during the fetal period anticipating birth.

Keywords: hypothalamus, brain development, thyroid hormone, paraventricular nucleus, deiodinase

INTRODUCTION

Thyroid hormone (TH) is crucial for normal fetal growth and maturation including the brain (Eayrs and Taylor, 1951; Morreale de Escobar et al., 1983; Legrand, 1984). Developmental TH deficiency impairs growth, and compromises adaptation to life outside the womb (Forhead et al., 1998; Hillman et al., 2012; Sferruzzi-Perri et al., 2013; Forhead and Fowden, 2014). The importance of TH during development is widely recognized and reflected in government interventions, such as iodine supplementation programs, as recommended by the World Health Organization (e.g., universal salt iodisation), and population wide screening for TH deficiency via the heel prick (Ford and LaFranchi, 2014). TH deficiency during development causes irreversible damage, which can largely be prevented by TH replacement therapy (Dubuis et al., 1996; Grüters and Krude, 2011).

During uterine development the fetus is largely dependent on the maternal TH supply, and TH receptors (TRs) are already present before the thyroid gland becomes functional (Morreale de Escobar et al., 2004, 2007). TH is implicated in many developmental processes in the brain including cell cycling, synaptogenesis, migration, plasticity, and myelination (Bernal, 2007). In both humans and rodents, brain development is not completed at, and continues after birth. From the moment of birth, the offspring no longer benefits from maternal TH supply. Insufficient TH availability, also during the postnatal developmental period, leads to severe neurological damage and mental retardation. TH insufficiency can be the result of iodine deficiency, or of defective formation of the thyroid gland (Deladoëy et al., 2007; Nilsson and Fagman, 2013; Szinnai, 2014). Interestingly, many studies have focused on the importance of TH in brain development, but much less is known about the development of the hypothalamic feedback loop of TH. When studying intrauterine development, it is not only the fetal hypothalamus that is in play, it is also that of the mother. In view of the cross-talk between systems it is often not possible to distinguish between the different (neuro-)endocrine systems in play. Rodent studies have been crucial for understanding TH signaling, but the research is complicated by interspecies differences that are observed between rodents, humans and other mammals. In the present review I will focus mainly on TH signaling in the developing human hypothalamus.

TH SIGNALING IN THE HYPOTHALAMUS

Under normal conditions, TH signaling is controlled via a classic negative feedback pathway at the level of the anterior

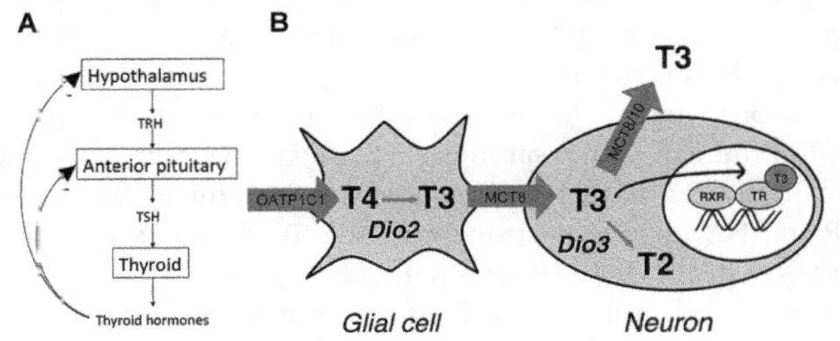

FIGURE 1 | (A) Classic thyroid hormone (TH) feedback loop. TH exerts a negative feedback at the level of the hypothalamus and anterior pituitary. **(B)** Model for thyroid hormone (TH) transport and metabolism in the human hypothalamus. The model indicates distinct roles for the different TH transporters in hypothalamic TH action by affecting intracellular TH concentrations through import and efflux. T2 = 3,3′-T2 (Adapted from Alkemade et al., 2011).

pituitary and hypothalamus (**Figure 1A**). Hypothalamic TH signaling is also involved in circadian rhythmicity, feeding and adaptation to environmental challenges (Costa-e-Sousa and Hollenberg, 2012). Interestingly, studies in anencephalic humans have shown that when the hypothalamus is not formed at all, pituitary-thyroid function still develops (Beck-Peccoz et al., 1992). Following normal brain development, hypophysiotropic neurons of the paraventricular nucleus (PVN) of the hypothalamus expressing thyrotropin releasing hormone (TRH) project to the portal system, via which it reaches the thyrotropin (TSH) producing cells of the anterior pituitary. TSH, which is subsequently released, binds to its receptor in the thyroid where TH is produced and released. TH is released predominantly as thyroxine (T4), a prohormone, and to a lesser extent as the active 3,3′,5-triiodothyronine (T3). T4 is converted locally into T3 providing a negative feedback at the level of the pituitary as well as the hypothalamus (**Figure 1A**). T3 mainly acts by regulation of gene expression via binding of nuclear TRs, although nongenomic effects of T3 have been described as well (Cheng et al., 2010; Davis et al., 2013).

A number of specific proteins are required for normal TH signaling in the brain including the hypothalamus. These proteins have been studied mainly in humans and rodents. TH cannot enter or exit the cell via passive diffusion and requires facilitated transport across the cell membrane, as well as the membrane of the cell nucleus (Visser et al., 2008; Heuer and Visser, 2009; Wirth et al., 2014). Proteins capable of transporting TH belong to a number of families including the sodium dependent organic anion tranporters (NTCP), organic anion transporting polypeptides (OATP), heterodimeric amino acid transporters (HAT) including light chains LAT1 and 2, and the monocarboxylate transporters MCT8 and 10 (Friesema et al., 1999, 2001; Hennemann et al., 2001; Roberts et al., 2008). The distribution patterns of these transporters throughout the body show significant overlap, and most of them are able to transport other molecules than iodothyronines as well. MCT8 appears to be specific for transporting iodothyronines (Friesema et al., 2003). OATP1C1 is expressed in endothelial cells of the blood brain barrier, as well as the choroid plexus (Roberts et al., 2008). MCT8 is also expressed in the human as well as the rodent choroid plexus (Heuer et al., 2005; Friesema et al., 2012). LAT1 and 2 do not appear to play any major role in the human brain (Wirth et al., 2014).

T4 is converted to T3 via intracellular outer ring deiodination. In the central nervous system conversion of T4 into T3 is mainly dependent on type 2 deiodinase (D2), and inactivation of T4 and T3 is dependent on inner ring deiodination by type 3 deiodinase (D3). Type 1 deiodinase (D1) does not appear to play a major role in rodent or human brain (Bianco et al., 2002). Interestingly, D2 is mainly expressed in glial cells of the hypothalamus. These include astrocytes and specialized glial cells called tanycytes, which are located at the ependymal layer of the third ventricle (Tu et al. 1997; Alkemade et al., 2005a). *Dio2 mRNA* expression in tanycytes shows a clear increase in response to hypothyroidism and iodine deficiency (Tu et al., 1997; Peeters et al., 2001).

In the cell nucleus, T3 binds the nuclear receptors encoded by the THRA and THRB genes, which give rise to TRα1, α2, β1 and β2 (Sap et al., 1986; Weinberger et al., 1986; Benbrook and Pfahl, 1987; König and Moura Neto, 2002). TRα2 does not bind T3, but exerts dominant negative effects on TRH transcription (Guissouma et al., 2014). Studies in knockout mice indicate that TRβ2 is crucial for the negative feedback loop controlling TH concentrations in the body (Abel et al., 2001). In addition, TRβ1 is also involved in regulating serum TSH (Guissouma et al., 2006). It is not entirely clear what the role for TRα in the negative feedback loop is. In the human and rat hypothalamus TRs are expressed in a number of nuclei, including the PVN where the hypophysiotropic TRH neurons are located (Lechan et al., 1994; Alkemade et al., 2005b). We, and others have proposed models for TH signaling in the hypothalamus, which involves both glial cells and neurons (Guadaño-Ferraz et al., 1997; Tu et al., 1997; Diano et al., 2003; Lechan and Fekete, 2004; Alkemade et al., 2005a; **Figure 1B**).

Hypothalamic TH signaling extends beyond the classical feedback loop affecting the TRH neurons of the PVN. In addition, functioning of other nuclear receptors such as the liver X receptor is dependent on thyroid status (Ghaddab-Zroud et al., 2014). We found in our previous studies on the human hypothalamus that the individual TR isoforms are expressed in a number of hypothalamic nuclei and studies in rats have shown comparable results. In addition, the supraoptic (SON), infundibular (IFN), tuberomamillary (TMN), and the lateral tuberal nucleus (NTL) express TRs. In rodents, TR isoforms have been described in the arcuate nucleus (ARC), the rodent equivalent of the IFN, as well as SON and PVN (Bradley et al., 1989; Cook et al., 1992; Lechan et al., 1994). The SON showed higher TRα than TRβ expression (Bradley et al., 1989). Studies in a transgenic mouse line with a GFP-labeled TRα1 (Wallis et al., 2010) have shown that the distribution of the TRα1 is even more widespread than we concluded from our studies on the human hypothalamus. In mice TRα1 was expressed in the majority of cerebral neurons, including many hypothalamic nuclei, as well as in tanycytes. Several explanations are possible for the discrepancy between our findings and findings in this transgenic mouse strain. It is possible that the antibodies we used for studying TR expression in the human hypothalamus lacked sensitivity to detect all TRs in the human hypothalamus, or, alternatively, interspecies differences may exist. Wallis et al. (2010) further showed TRα1 expression in nonneuronal cells including hypothalamic oligodendrocytes. In our earlier studies in humans we did not report on oligodendritic expression of TRs (Alkemade et al., 2005b). Interestingly, the absence of a functional MCT8 results a persistent hypomyelination in humans (López-Espíndola et al., 2014). The findings by Wallis et al. fit with the ubiquitous expression of the TH transporter OATP1C1 throughout the human hypothalamus, in both neurons as well as glial cells (Alkemade et al., 2011). In rodents Oatp1C1 does not show neuronal expression in the hypothalamus (Roberts et al., 2008). It is possible that other TH transporters are involved in the transport of TH in and out of TRα1 expressing neurons and glia in rodents. In addition, we have shown that MCT8 is expressed in both neurons and glial cells of the human hypothalamus. Interestingly, in humans MCT10 expression was confined to neurons in the majority of hypothalamic nuclei. The distinct distribution patterns support different roles for the individual TH transporters.

TH SIGNALING IN THE DEVELOPING HUMAN HYPOTHALAMUS

Very few studies have investigated the distribution of protein expression in the developing human hypothalamus, therefore, little is known about its chemoarchitecture. Human brain material obtained is not readily available, and tissue from embryo's, fetuses and children is even scarcer. Koutcherov et al. (2002), studied 33 human hypothalamic specimens ranging in age from 9 weeks of gestation to 3 weeks after term birth. This study describes the development of human hypothalamic zones and individual nuclei and provides a clear schematic representation of the development of the human hypothalamus. Hypothalamic differentiation starts already during the first trimester of pregnancy. The lateral zone is the first zone to differentiate, and gives rise to the lateral hypothalamus (LH), Posterior hypothalamic area (PH), lateral tuberal hypothalamic nucleus (LTu) and perifornical hypothalamic nucleus (PeF). The core zone consists of a heterogeneous collection of nuclei positioned between the LH and midline structure, including medial preoptic nucleus (MPO), ventromedial nucleus (VMH), supramamillary nucleus (SUM) and mammillary bodies (Mb). The midline hypothalamus consists of structures differentiating in close proximity of the ventricular wall, including the suprachiasmatic nucleus (SCN), IFN, PVN and SON. These structures become evident during late gestation.

We have described the developmental expression of proteins involved in TH signaling in 15 fetal and infant human hypothalami obtained at various stages of development (Friesema et al., 2012). To my knowledge comparable studies investigating fetal functional neuroanatomy underlying TH signaling are not available for rodents. In our study on the developing human hypothalamus the first sampling point was at 17 weeks of gestation. Although we did not study TR expression in our human brain specimens, at this time both TRs and the ligand T3 have been reported in the human brain and TR mRNA increases strongly from 10–18 weeks gestation (Iskaros et al., 2000). Interestingly, during development TRα1 is not expressed in the ventricular zone in mice where neurons are born and proliferate (Wallis et al., 2010). These studies showed that TRα1 appears to be expressed in immature neurons, preceding the expression of NeuN. The TRα1 expression increases when cells reach their destination and differentiate. This means that TRα1 acts after cell cycle exit. The specific oligodendrocytic expression of TRα1 fits with data showing that oligodendrocyte precursors differentiate after T3 activation of a transiently expressed TR (Billon et al., 2002). This indicates that in mice TRα1 expression is required only during a specific time window in development (Wallis et al., 2010). Whether a similar pattern is also present in the (human) hypothalamus is unknown.

At 17 weeks of gestation the mamillary bodies become prominent and the LH, SON and IFN can already be distinguished, as well as the fornix and the anlage of the PVN (Koutcherov et al., 2002). In our human studies, we observed some MCT8 expression in blood vessels at 17 weeks, indicating possible presence of TH signaling (Friesema et al., 2012). We only observed few D3 positive neurons in the IFN, whereas D2 did not show any staining. These findings indicate T3 degradation, but not production in the human fetal hypothalamus at this moment in development. This is in line with the prevention of TH exposure during early stages of brain development, which may cause untimely maturation of brain cells as observed in rodents (Obregon et al., 2007). Interestingly, excess TH as a result of deletion of the *Dio3* gene in mice results in premature cerebellar differentiation, as well as a central hypothyroidism associated with defective TRH regulation, which persists throughout life (Hernandez et al., 2006, 2007; Peeters et al., 2013).

At 18 weeks gestation all T3 in the brain is produced via local deiodination (Ferreiro et al., 1988), which fits with D2 activity and T3 content in the cerebral cortex during the second trimester (Kester et al., 2004). At this time TH transporters are also expressed in the cerebral cortex (Chan et al., 2014). It does not appear that at this time point the human hypothalamus is capable of converting T4 into T3. This finding could reflect timing differences between distinct brain areas. At 18–23 weeks of gestation the PVN develops, and the PeF area as well as the LH become discernable. At the end of this period the SCN becomes visible (Koutcherov et al., 2002). At present no data are available on TH signaling at this time-point during development.

At 24–33 weeks the fetal human hypothalamus takes and adult like appearance. At 25 5/7 weeks, we found MCT8 expression in the PVN and IFN, which should now also express Neuropeptide Y (Koutcherov et al., 2002). In addition, MCT8 neurons showed a scattered pattern throughout the hypothalamus, as well as in tanycytes and blood vessels (Friesema et al., 2012). MCT10 showed expression in SON, PVN and IFN. D3 and OATP1C1 were also expressed in the IFN. At this time D2 was still very low and only found surrounding blood vessels. At 27 weeks MCT8 expression in PVN and LH persisted, and MCT10 showed more widespread expression in PVN, LH and SON. OATP1C1 was also present in LH, PVN and IFN. Hardly any D2 was observed, whereas the PVN showed prominent D3 expression.

At 27 2/7 weeks of gestation TH signaling appeared to increase. MCT8 was present in neurons of the PVN, IFN and LH, as well as in tanycytes. MCT10 was strongly expressed in the LH, as well as in neurons of the IFN, PVN and SON. OATP1C1 was present in blood vessels of the organum vasculosum laminae terminalis (OVLT) and in LH, IFN, PVN and SON neurons. D2 at this stage showed expression in tanycytes. In addition D2 staining surrounded blood vessels of the OVLT. Now D3 expression was not observed (Friesema et al., 2012). It is possible that the absence of D3 expression indicates an increased need for TH at this stage of development persisting to late gestation, after which TH signaling appears to decrease again. At 28 3/7 weeks gestation MCT8 staining was present in the IFN, PVN and LH. MCT10 and OATP1C1 also showed expression in the LH. In addition, OATP1C1 was also present in the IFN and in tanycytes, which also expressed D2. Again D3 showed very little expression.

From 34 weeks gestation term gestation, the NTL and TMN can develop further (Koutcherov et al., 2002). At 34 5/7 weeks the expression of all tested TH transporters was low. What is interesting to note, is that during late gestation (35 weeks), D2, MCT8 and OATP1C1 expression was very weak, and MCT10 expression was not observed. This was in contrast to the strong D3 expression observed in the IFN, TMN and LH. These observations led us to speculate that these observations may be related to the TSH surge observed in humans associated with birth, and that the hypothalamus may play a role in giving rise to this TSH surge. Although highly speculative, decreased T3 availability due to decreased outer ring deiodination and TH transport, together with increased inner ring deiodination by D3 could lead to upregulation of TRH, which is negatively regulated by T3. A very similar staining pattern was observed in hypothalami of children that were born at term. Inverse hypothalamic expression levels of D2 and 3 have also been observed in birds and mammals in the context of photoperiod setpoints (Watanabe et al., 2007).

At *2 months of age* staining for MCT8 in SON, PVN, and in the lining of the third ventricle was found in humans. MCT10 immunoreactivity was present in SON and PVN. Sporadic expression was found in the LH. OATP1C1 showed a more scattered pattern and increased staining was observed in SON, PVN, TMN, IFN and the ependymal layer. D2 expression was present in blood vessels. D3 showed expression in PVN as well as other hypothalamic nuclei. In children *aged 20–29 months of age*, we found moderate MCT8 and moderate to strong MCT10 staining in PVN, SON, IFN and weak staining in the LH. OATP1C1 was present in PVN, SON, IFN and in some cells in the ependymal layer of the third ventricle. In addition, scattered OATP1C1 positive cells were present, as well as staining in NTL, TMN, SCN and LH. D2 was expressed in blood vessels especially in the IFN and in tanycytes. At this time point stainings very much resembled our observations in the adult hypothalamus (Alkemade et al., 2005a, 2011; **Figure 2**).

Hypothalamic expression patterns throughout the developmental period studied are summarized in **Figure 3**. This figure indicates that regulation of proteins involved in TH signaling may play an important role in timing of TH availability at different stages of development.

DEFECTIVE HYPOTHALAMIC TH SIGNALING

Defects in proteins involved in hypothalamic TH signaling are potentially reflected in alterations in serum TH and TSH concentrations. A number of mutations in, TRs and TH transporters has been described. These syndromes are described excellently in a recent review (Dumitrescu and Refetoff, 2013), and here only findings relevant for HPT-axis regulation and the brain are recapitulated.

TRs

Complete deletion of all TRs in mice causes serum TSH levels that are 500-fold higher than those of the WT mice, and T4 concentrations 12-fold above the average normal mean (Gauthier et al., 1999). In humans both mutations in the THRA and THRB genes have been reported.

RESISTANCE TO THα

The first subject described suffering from Resistance to THα (RTHα), was diagnosed only recently (Bochukova et al., 2012). RTHα is caused by a mutation in the *THRA* gene, which encodes TRα1 and α2. The mutation caused a truncation of the protein, which lacked the C-terminal α-helix. This 6-year old girl showed low-normal or subnormal levels of total T4 and free T4, high-normal or elevated levels of total T3 and free T3, in addition to normal levels of TSH (Bochukova et al., 2012). Since the description of this young girl, additional patients with RTHα have been described in literature. RTHα patients show cognitive impairment and macrocephaly (Bochukova et al., 2012; van Mullem et al., 2013). In addition, the phenotype observed in a patient with mutations both in TRα1 and α2 was very similar (Moran et al., 2014). Serum TH concentrations do not suggest any major impairment of the classic hypothalamic feedback system. This is corroborated by findings in mice. Mouse models with a mutant TRα1, show a range of phenotypes, dependent on the specific mutation or deletion. Brain changes have been described as well (Wallis et al., 2008; Mittag et al., 2010), and changes resulting from defects in the autonomic nervous system including impaired cardiovascular response to stress, activity and environmental temperature changes. The hypothalamus has only been studied in detail in one of these mouse models, showing the absence of a parvalbumin positive neuronal population in the anterior hypothalamic area with consequences for the regulation of the cardiovascular system

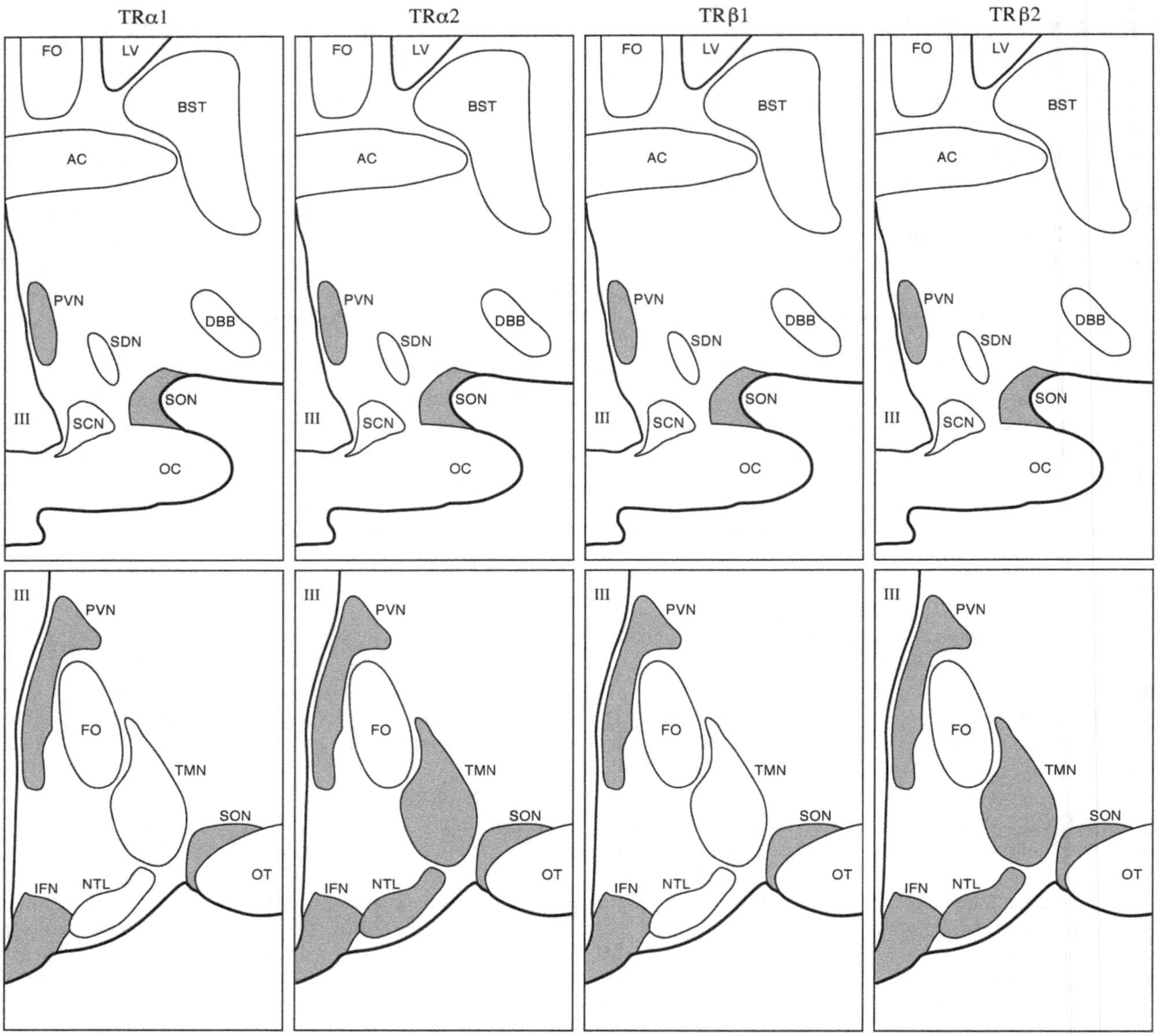

FIGURE 2 | Adult appearance of the human hypothalamus. Gray areas indicate sites of TR isoform expression. Upper panels: rostral level; lower panels: caudal level. III, Third ventricle; AC, anterior commissure; BST, bed nucleus of the stria terminalis; DBB, diagonal band of Broca; FO, fornix; LV, lateral ventricle; NTL, nucleus tuberalis lateralis; OC, optic chiasm; OT, optic tract; SCN, suprachiasmatic nucleus; SDN, sexually dimorphic nucleus; SON, supraoptic nucleus; TMN, tuberomammilary nucleus (Taken from Alkemade et al., 2005b).

(Mittag et al., 2013). The HPA-axis was not affected in these mutant mice as assessed by hypothalamic corticotropin releasing hormone (CRH) and pro-opiomelanocortin (POMC) expression (Mittag et al., 2010).

RESISTANCE TO THβ

Patients harboring mutations in the TRβ1 show more pronounced changes in serum TH concentrations. For the THRB gene number of mutation hotspots have been defined (Dumitrescu and Refetoff, 2013). Characteristic are elevated freeT4 levels, and to a lesser extent T3. In addition, TSH is normal or slightly increased, and responsive to TRH. Patients generally do not display the usual metabolic symptoms associated with hyperthyroidism, although they often present with goiter (Refetoff et al., 1993). TRβ2 knockout mice show a severe disruption of the hypothalamic TH feedback system (Abel et al., 2001).

TH TRANSPORTERS

In MCT8 deficient subjects serum TSH is modestly increased, which fits with the decreased serum T_4 concentration but not with the elevated serum T_3 level. Since MCT8 is expressed in

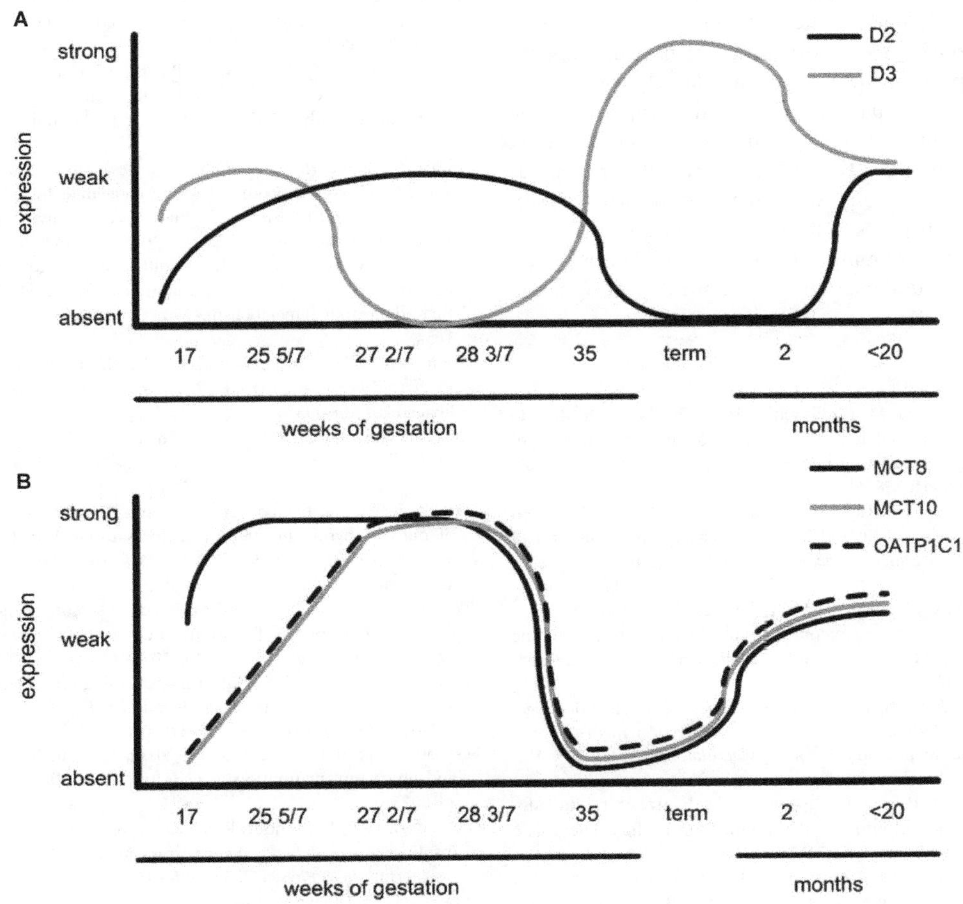

FIGURE 3 | Schematic representation of (A) D2 expression in the human infundibular nucleus/median eminence and periventricular area, D3 expression in the paraventricular nucleus (PVN) and (B) TH transporter expression throughout PVN development. Note the opposite expression pattern of D3 vs. TH transporters and D2 expression (Taken from Friesema et al., 2012).

the hypothalamus and pituitary, it is likely that inactivation of the gene interferes with the negative feedback at the level of the hypothalamus (Fliers et al., 2006). In addition, defects in brain development have been described in patients lacking MCT8 (López-Espíndola et al., 2014). Rodent models for MCT8 mutations do not reproduce the severe psychomotor phenotype observed in humans, but do faithfully reproduce the biochemical phenotype (Trajkovic et al., 2007). In *Mct8*KO mice, hypothalamic TRH expression is markedly increased and high T_3 doses are needed to suppress it. In humans there is clear expression of MCT10 and OATP1C1 already in the second trimester of pregnancy. The presence of these transporters is does compensate for the absence of MCT8 as evidenced by the neurological defects observed in patients lacking MCT8. Wirth et al. suggest that Lat2 might compensate for the Mct8 deletion in mice. This is unlikely in humans, since developing neurons in the human brain only show very low LAT2 expression (Wirth et al., 2009). It is possible that in rodents other transporter variants such as Oatp1a4 and Oatp1a5 may further compensate for MCT8 defects. These transporters appear not to have orthologs in the human brain (Suzuki and Abe, 2008).

TH CONVERSION DEFECTS

Selenocysteine insertion sequence (SECIS) binding protein 2 (SBP2) plays an important role in insertion of selenocysteine into selenoproteins such as deidonases. Defects in the *SBP2* gene therefore interfere with the production of these conversion enzymes, resulting in high T4 and rT3, low T3, normal or slightly elevated TSH concentrations (Dumitrescu et al., 2005). Genetic variants in *DIO2* in humans do not show any clear phenotypic changes (Zevenbergen et al., 2014).

CONCLUSION

TH signaling involves facilitated transport, local conversion and receptor binding. TH signaling is therefore dependent on a number of proteins, each of which can become defective, thereby affecting a plethora of processes modulated by TH. The effects of mutations in TH signaling on the functional neuroanatomy, which underlies the classic negative feedback of TH on the hypothalamus is dependent on the affected gene, the type of mutation, as well as the compensatory mechanisms, which appear to differ between species. These effects are largely assessed by evaluation of biochemical parameters. Detailed studies on the functional neuroanatomy underlying hypothalamic TH signaling are scarce, and are complicated by interspecies differences, as well as the limited availability of human postmortem brain material for research purposes. Future studies on the expression of TR isoforms in the developing (human) hypothalamus would strongly improve our understanding of central TH signaling during development.

REFERENCES

Abel, E. D., Ahima, R. S., Boers, M. E., Elmquist, J. K., and Wondisford, F. E. (2001). Critical role for thyroid hormone receptor $\beta 2$ in the regulation of paraventricular thyrotropin-releasing hormone neurons. *J. Clin. Invest.* 107, 1017–1023. doi: 10.1172/jci10858

Alkemade, A., Friesema, E. C., Kalsbeek, A., Swaab, D. F., Visser, T. J., and Fliers, E. (2011). Expression of thyroid hormone transporters in the human hypothalamus. *J. Clin. Endocrinol. Metab.* 96, E967–E971. doi: 10.1210/jc.2010-2750

Alkemade, A., Friesema, E. C., Unmehopa, U. A., Fabriek, B. O., Kuiper, G. G., Leonard, J. L., et al. (2005a). Neuroanatomical pathways for thyroid hormone feedback in the human hypothalamus. *J. Clin. Endocrinol. Metab.* 90, 4322–4334. doi: 10.1210/jc.2004-2567

Alkemade, A., Vuijst, C. L., Unmehopa, U. A., Bakker, O., Vennström, B., Wiersinga, W. M., et al. (2005b). Thyroid hormone receptor expression in the human hypothalamus and anterior pituitary. *J. Clin. Endocrinol. Metab.* 90, 904–912. doi: 10.1210/jc.2004-0474

Beck-Peccoz, P., Cortelazzi, D., Persani, L., Papandreou, M. J., Asteria, C., Borgato, S., et al. (1992). Maturation of pituitary-thyroid function in the anencephalic fetus. *Acta Med. Austriaca* 19(Suppl. 1), 72–76.

Benbrook, D., and Pfahl, M. (1987). A novel thyroid hormone receptor encoded by a cDNA clone from a human testis library. *Science* 238, 788–791. doi: 10.1126/science.3672126

Bernal, J. (2007). Thyroid hormone receptors in brain development and function. *Nat. Clin. Pract. Endocrinol. Metab.* 3, 249–259. doi: 10.1038/ncpendmet0424

Bianco, A. C., Salvatore, D., Gereben, B., Berry, M. J., and Larsen, P. R. (2002). Biochemistry, cellular and molecular biology and physiological roles of the iodothyronine selenodeiodinases. *Endocr. Rev.* 23, 38–89. doi: 10.1210/er.23.1.38

Billon, N., Jolicoeur, C., Tokumoto, Y., Vennström, B., and Raff, M. (2002). Normal timing of oligodendrocyte development depends on thyroid hormone receptor alpha 1 (TRα1). *EMBO J.* 21, 6452–6460. doi: 10.1093/emboj/cdf662

Bochukova, E., Schoenmakers, N., Agostini, M., Schoenmakers, E., Rajanayagam, O., Keogh, J. M., et al. (2012). A mutation in the thyroid hormone receptor alpha gene. *N. Engl. J. Med.* 366, 243–249. doi: 10.1056/NEJMoa1110296

Bradley, D. J., Young, W. S. 3rd, and Weinberger, C. (1989). Differential expression of alpha and beta thyroid hormone receptor genes in rat brain and pituitary. *Proc. Natl. Acad. Sci. U S A* 86, 7250–7254. doi: 10.1073/pnas.86.18.7250

Chan, S. Y., Hancox, L. A., Martín-Santos, A., Loubière, L. S., Walter, M. N., González, A. M., et al. (2014). MCT8 expression in human fetal cerebral cortex is reduced in severe intrauterine growth restriction. *J. Endocrinol.* 220, 85–95. doi: 10.1530/JOE-13-0400

Cheng, S. Y., Leonard, J. L., and Davis, P. J. (2010). Molecular aspects of thyroid hormone actions. *Endocr. Rev.* 31, 139–170. doi: 10.1210/er.2009-0007

Cook, C. B., Kakucska, I., Lechan, R. M., and Koenig, R. J. (1992). Expression of thyroid hormone receptor beta 2 in rat hypothalamus. *Endocrinology* 130, 1077–1079. doi: 10.1210/en.130.2.1077

Costa-e-Sousa, R. H., and Hollenberg, A. N. (2012). Minireview: the neural regulation of the hypothalamic-pituitary-thyroid axis. *Endocrinology* 153, 4128–4135. doi: 10.1210/en.2012-1467

Davis, P. J., Lin, H. Y., Tang, H. Y., Davis, F. B., and Mousa, S. A. (2013). Adjunctive input to the nuclear thyroid hormone receptor from the cell surface receptor for the hormone. *Thyroid* 23, 1503–1509. doi: 10.1089/thy.2013.0280

Deladoëy, J., Vassart, G., and Van Vliet, G. (2007). Possible non-Mendelian mechanisms of thyroid dysgenesis. *Endocr. Dev.* 10, 29–42. doi: 10.1159/000106818

Diano, S., Leonard, J. L., Meli, R., Esposito, E., and Schiavo, L. (2003). Hypothalamic type II iodothyronine deiodinase: a light and electron microscopic study. *Brain Res.* 976, 130–134. doi: 10.1016/s0006-8993(03)02692-1

Dubuis, J. M., Glorieux, J., Richer, F., Deal, C. L., Dussault, J. H., and Van Vliet, G. (1996). Outcome of severe congenital hypothyroidism: closing the developmental gap with early high dose levothyroxine treatment. *J. Clin. Endocrinol. Metab.* 81, 222–227. doi: 10.1210/jcem.81.1.8550756

Dumitrescu, A. M., Liao, X. H., Abdullah, M. S., Lado-Abeal, J., Majed, F. A., Moeller, L. C., et al. (2005). Mutations in SECISBP2 result in abnormal thyroid hormone metabolism. *Nat. Genet.* 37, 1247–1252. doi: 10.1038/ng1654

Dumitrescu, A. M., and Refetoff, S. (2013). The syndromes of reduced sensitivity to thyroid hormone. *Biochim. Biophys. Acta* 1830, 3987–4003. doi: 10.1016/j.bbagen.2012.08.005

Eayrs, J. T., and Taylor, S. H. (1951). The effecot of thyroid deficiency induced by methylthiouracil on the maturation of the central nervous system. *J. Anat.* 85, 350–358.

Ferreiro, B., Bernal, J., Goodyer, C. G., and Branchard, C. L. (1988). Estimation of nuclear thyroid hormone receptor saturation in human fetal brain and lung during early gestation. *J. Clin. Endocrinol. Metab.* 67, 853–856. doi: 10.1210/jcem-67-4-853

Fliers, E., Unmehopa, U. A., and Alkemade, A. (2006). Functional neuroanatomy of thyroid hormone feedback in the human hypothalamus and pituitary gland. *Mol. Cell. Endocrinol.* 251, 1–8. doi: 10.1016/j.mce.2006.03.042

Ford, G., and LaFranchi, S. H. (2014). Screening for congenital hypothyroidism: a worldwide view of strategies. *Best Pract. Res. Clin. Endocrinol. Metab.* 28, 175–187. doi: 10.1016/j.beem.2013.05.008

Forhead, A. J., and Fowden, A. L. (2014). Thyroid hormones in fetal growth and prepartum maturation. *J. Endocrinol.* 221, R87–R103. doi: 10.1530/JOE-14-0025

Forhead, A. J., Li, J., Gilmour, R. S., and Fowden, A. L. (1998). Control of hepatic insulin-like growth factor II gene expression by thyroid hormones in fetal sheep near term. *Am. J. Physiol.* 275, E149–E156.

Friesema, E. C., Docter, R., Moerings, E. P., Stieger, B., Hagenbuch, B., Meier, P. J., et al. (1999). Identification of thyroid hormone transporters. *Biochem. Biophys. Res. Commun.* 254, 497–501. doi: 10.1006/bbrc.1998.9974

Friesema, E. C., Docter, R., Moerings, E. P., Verrey, F., Krenning, E. P., Hennemann, G., et al. (2001). Thyroid hormone transport by the heterodimeric human system L amino acid transporter. *Endocrinology* 142, 4339–4348. doi: 10.1210/en.142.10.4339

Friesema, E. C., Ganguly, S., Abdalla, A., Manning Fox, J. E., Halestrap, A. P., and Visser, T. J. (2003). Identification of monocarboxylate transporter 8 as a specific thyroid hormone transporter. *J. Biol. Chem.* 278, 40128–40135. doi: 10.1074/jbc.m300909200

Friesema, E. C., Visser, T. J., Borgers, A. J., Kalsbeek, A., Swaab, D. F., Fliers, E., et al. (2012). Thyroid hormone transporters and deiodinases in the developing human hypothalamus. *Eur. J. Endocrinol.* 167, 379–386. doi: 10.1530/EJE-12-0177

Gauthier, K., Chassande, O., Plateroti, M., Roux, J. P., Legrand, C., Pain, B., et al. (1999). Different functions for the thyroid hormone receptors TRα and TRβ in the control of thyroid hormone production and post-natal development. *EMBO J.* 18, 623–631. doi: 10.1093/emboj/18.3.623

Ghaddab-Zroud, R., Seugnet, I., Steffensen, K. R., Demeneix, B. A., and Clerget-Froidevaux, M. S. (2014). Liver X receptor regulation of thyrotropin-releasing hormone transcription in mouse hypothalamus is dependent on thyroid status. *PLoS One* 9:e106983. doi: 10.1371/journal.pone.0106983

Grüters, A., and Krude, H. (2011). Detection and treatment of congenital hypothyroidism. *Nat. Rev. Endocrinol.* 8, 104–113. doi: 10.1038/nrendo.2011.160

Guadaño-Ferraz, A., Obregón, M. J., St Germain, D. L., and Bernal, J. (1997). The type 2 iodothyronine deiodinase is expressed primarily in glial cells in the neonatal rat brain. *Proc. Natl. Acad. Sci. U S A* 94, 10391–10396. doi: 10.1073/pnas.94.19.10391

Guissouma, H., Froidevaux, M. S., Hassani, Z., and Demeneix, B. A. (2006). In vivo siRNA delivery to the mouse hypothalamus confirms distinct roles of TR beta isoforms in regulating TRH transcription. *Neurosci. Lett.* 406, 240–243. doi: 10.1016/j.neulet.2006.07.041

Guissouma, H., Ghaddab-Zroud, R., Seugnet, I., Decherf, S., Demeneix, B., and Clerget-Froidevaux, M. S. (2014). TR alpha 2 exerts dominant negative effects on hypothalamic Trh transcription in vivo. *PLoS One* 9:e95064. doi: 10.1371/journal.pone.0095064

Hennemann, G., Docter, R., Friesema, E. C., de Jong, M., Krenning, E. P., and Visser, T. J. (2001). Plasma membrane transport of thyroid hormones and its role in thyroid hormone metabolism and bioavailability. *Endocr. Rev.* 22, 451–476. doi: 10.1210/er.22.4.451

Hernandez, A., Martinez, M. E., Fiering, S., Galton, V. A., and St Germain, D. (2006). Type 3 deiodinase is critical for the maturation and function of the thyroid axis. *J. Clin. Invest.* 116, 476–484. doi: 10.1172/jci26240

Hernandez, A., Martinez, M. E., Liao, X. H., Van Sande, J., Refetoff, S., Galton, V. A., et al. (2007). Type 3 deiodinase deficiency results in functional abnormalities at multiple levels of the thyroid axis. *Endocrinology* 148, 5680–5687. doi: 10.1210/en.2007-0652

Heuer, H., Maier, M. K., Iden, S., Mittag, J., Friesema, E. C., Visser, T. J., et al. (2005). The monocarboxylate transporter 8 linked to human psychomotor retardation is highly expressed in thyroid hormone-sensitive neuron populations. *Endocrinology* 146, 1701–1706. doi: 10.1210/en.2004-1179

Heuer, H., and Visser, T. J. (2009). Minireview: pathophysiological importance of thyroid hormone transporters. *Endocrinology* 150, 1078–1083. doi: 10.1210/en.2008-1518

Hillman, N. H., Kallapur, S. G., and Jobe, A. H. (2012). Physiology of transition from intrauterine to extrauterine life. *Clin. Perinatol.* 39, 769–783. doi: 10.1016/j.clp.2012.09.009

Iskaros, J., Pickard, M., Evans, I., Sinha, A., Hardiman, P., and Ekins, R. (2000). Thyroid hormone receptor gene expression in first trimester human fetal brain. *J. Clin. Endocrinol. Metab.* 85, 2620–2623. doi: 10.1210/jc.85.7.2620

Kester, M. H., Martinez de Mena, R., Obregon, M. J., Marinkovic, D., Howatson, A., Visser, T. J., et al. (2004). Iodothyronine levels in the human developing brain: major regulatory roles of iodothyronine deiodinases in different areas. *J. Clin. Endocrinol. Metab.* 89, 3117–3128. doi: 10.1210/jc.2003-031832

König, S., and Moura Neto, V. (2002). Thyroid hormone actions on neural cells. *Cell. Mol. Neurobiol.* 22, 517–544. doi: 10.1023/A:1021828218454

Koutcherov, Y., Mai, J. K., Ashwell, K. W., and Paxinos, G. (2002). Organization of human hypothalamus in fetal development. *J. Comp. Neurol.* 446, 301–324. doi: 10.1002/cne.10175

Lechan, R. M., and Fekete, C. (2004). Feedback regulation of thyrotropin-releasing hormone (TRH): mechanisms for the non-thyroidal illness syndrome. *J. Endocrinol. Invest.* 27, 105–119.

Lechan, R. M., Qi, Y., Jackson, I. M., and Mahdavi, V. (1994). Identification of thyroid hormone receptor isoforms in thyrotropin-releasing hormone neurons of the hypothalamic paraventricular nucleus. *Endocrinology* 135, 92–100. doi: 10.1210/en.135.1.92

Legrand, J. (1984). "Effects of thyroid hormones on central nervous system," in *Neurobehavioral Teratology*, ed J. Yanai (Amsterdam: Elsevier), 331–363.

López-Espíndola, D., Morales-Bastos, C., Grijota-Martínez, C., Liao, X. H., Lev, D., Sugo, E., et al. (2014). Mutations of the thyroid hormone transporter MCT8 cause prenatal brain damage and persistent hypomyelination. *J. Clin. Endocrinol. Metab.* 99, E2799–E2804. doi: 10.1210/jc.2014-2162

Mittag, J., Davis, B., Vujovic, M., Arner, A., and Vennström, B. (2010). Adaptations of the autonomous nervous system controlling heart rate are impaired by a mutant thyroid hormone receptor-α1. *Endocrinology* 151, 2388–2395. doi: 10.1210/en.2009-1201

Mittag, J., Lyons, D. J., Sallstrom, J., Vujovic, M., Dudazy-Gralla, S., Warner, A., et al. (2013). Thyroid hormone is required for hypothalamic neurons regulating cardiovascular functions. *J. Clin. Invest.* 123, 509–516. doi: 10.1172/JCI65252

Moran, C., Agostini, M., Visser, W. E., Schoenmakers, E., Schoenmakers, N., Offiah, A. C., et al. (2014). Resistance to thyroid hormone caused by a mutation in thyroid hormone receptor (TR)α1 and TRα: clinical, biochemical and genetic analyses of three related patients. *Lancet Diabetes Endocrinol.* 2, 619–626. doi: 10.1016/s2213-8587(14)70111-1

Morreale de Escobar, G., Escobar del Rey, F., and Ruiz-Marcos, A. (1983). "Thyroid hormone and the developing brain," in *Congenital Hypothyroidism*, eds J. H. Dussault and P. Walker (New York: MArcel Decker Inc.), 85–126.

Morreale de Escobar, G., Obregón, M. J., and Escobar del Rey, F. (2004). Maternal thyroid hormones early in pregnancy and fetal brain development. *Best Pract. Res. Clin. Endocrinol. Metab.* 18, 225–248. doi: 10.1016/s1521-690x(04)00022-3

Morreale de Escobar, G., Obregón, M. J., and Escobar del Rey, F. (2007). Iodine deficiency and brain development in the first half of pregnancy. *Public Health Nutr.* 10, 1554–1570. doi: 10.1017/S1368980007360928

Nilsson, M., and Fagman, H. (2013). Mechanisms of thyroid development and dysgenesis: an analysis based on developmental stages and concurrent embryonic anatomy. *Curr. Top. Dev. Biol.* 106, 123–170. doi: 10.1016/B978-0-12-416021-7.00004-3

Obregon, M. J., Calvo, R. M., Escobar del Rey, F., and Morreale de Escobar, G. (2007). Ontogenesis of thyroid function and interactions with maternal function. *Endocr. Dev.* 10, 86–98. doi: 10.1159/000106821

Peeters, R., Fekete, C., Goncalves, C., Legradi, G., Tu, H. M., Harney, J. W., et al. (2001). Regional physiological adaptation of the central nervous system deiodinases to iodine deficiency. *Am. J. Physiol. Endocrinol. Metab.* 281, E54–E61.

Peeters, R. P., Hernandez, A., Ng L., Ma, M., Sharlin, D. S., Pandey, M., et al. (2013). Cerebellar abnormalities in mice lacking type 3 deiodinase and partial reversal of phenotype by deletion of thyroid hormone receptor α1. *Endocrinology* 154, 550–561. doi: 10.1210/en.2012-1738

Refetoff, S., Weiss, R. E., and Usala, S. J. (1993). The syndromes of resistance to thyroid hormone. *Endocr. Rev.* 14, 348–399. doi: 10.1210/er.14.3.348

Roberts, L. M., Woodford, K., Zhou, M., Black, D. S., Haggerty, J. E., Tate, E. H., et al. (2008). Expression of the thyroid hormone transporters monocarboxylate transporter-8 (SLC16A2) and organic ion transporter-14 (SLCO1C1) at the blood-brain barrier. *Endocrinology* 149, 6251–6261. doi: 10.1210/en.2008-0378

Sap, J., Munoz, A., Damm, K., Goldberg, Y., Ghysdael, J., Leutz, A., et al. (1986). The c-erb-A protein is a high-affinity receptor for thyroid hormone. *Nature* 324, 635–640. doi: 10.1038/324635a0

Sferruzzi-Perri, A. N., Vaughan, O. R., Forhead, A. J., and Fowden, A. L. (2013). Hormonal and nutritional drivers of intrauterine growth. *Curr. Opin. Clin. Nutr. Metab. Care* 16, 298–309. doi: 10.1097/MCO.0b013e32835e3643

Suzuki, T., and Abe, T. (2008). Thyroid hormone transporters in the brain. *Cerebellum* 7, 75–83. doi: 10.1007/s12311-008-0029-9

Szinnai, G. (2014). Clinical genetics of congenital hypothyroidism. *Endocr. Dev.* 26, 60–78. doi: 10.1159/000363156

Trajkovic, M., Visser, T. J., Mittag, J., Horn, S., Lukas, J., Darras, V. M., et al. (2007). Abnormal thyroid hormone metabolism in mice lacking the monocarboxylate transporter 8. *J. Clin. Invest.* 117, 627–635. doi: 10.1172/JCI28253

Tu, H. M., Kim, S. W., Salvatore, D., Bartha, T., Legradi, G., Larsen, P. R., et al. (1997). Regional distribution of type 2 thyroxine deiodinase messenger ribonucleic acid in rat hypothalamus and pituitary and its regulation by thyroid hormone. *Endocrinology* 138, 3359–3368. doi: 10.1210/en.138.8.3359

van Mullem, A. A., Chrysis, D., Eythimiadou, A., Chroni, E., Tsatsoulis, A., de Rijke, Y. B., et al. (2013). Clinical phenotype of a new type of thyroid hormone resistance caused by a mutation of the TRα1 receptor: consequences of LT4 treatment. *J. Clin. Endocrinol. Metab.* 98, 3029–3038. doi: 10.1210/jc.2013-1050

Visser, W. E., Friesema, E. C., Jansen, J., and Visser, T. J. (2008). Thyroid hormone transport in and out of cells. *Trends Endocrinol. Metab.* 19, 50–56. doi: 10.1016/j.tem.2007.11.003

Wallis, K., Dudazy, S., van Hogerlinden, M., Nordström, K., Mittag, J., and Vennström, B. (2010). The thyroid hormone receptor α1 protein is expressed in embryonic postmitotic neurons and persists in most adult neurons. *Mol. Endocrinol.* 24, 1904–1916. doi: 10.1210/me.2010-0175

Wallis, K., Sjögren, M., van Hogerlinden, M., Silberberg, G., Fisahn, A., Nordström, K., et al. (2008). Locomotor deficiencies and aberrant development of subtype-specific GABAergic interneurons caused by an unliganded thyroid hormone receptor α1. *J. Neurosci.* 28, 1904–1915. doi: 10.1523/JNEUROSCI.5163-07.2008

Watanabe, T., Yamamura, T., Watanabe, M., Yasuo, S., Nakao, N., Dawson, A., et al. (2007). Hypothalamic expression of thyroid hormone-activating and -inactivating enzyme genes in relation to photorefractoriness in birds and mammals. *Am. J. Physiol. Regul. Integr. Comp. Physiol.* 292, R568–R572. doi: 10.1152/ajpregu.00521.2006

Weinberger, C., Thompson, C. C., Ong, E. S., Lebo, R., Gruol, D. J., and Evans, R. M. (1986). The c-erb-A gene encodes a thyroid hormone receptor. *Nature* 324, 641–646. doi: 10.1038/324641a0

Wirth, E. K., Roth, S., Blechschmidt, C., Hölter, S. M., Becker, L., Racz, I., et al. (2009). Neuronal 3′,3,5-triiodothyronine (T3) uptake and behavioral phenotype of mice deficient in Mct8, the neuronal T3 transporter mutated in Allan-Herndon-Dudley syndrome. *J. Neurosci.* 29, 9439–9449. doi: 10.1523/JNEUROSCI.6055-08.2009

Wirth, E. K., Schweizer, U., and Köhrle, J. (2014). Transport of thyroid hormone in brain. *Front. Endocrinol. (Lausanne)* 5:98. doi: 10.3389/fendo.2014.00098

Zevenbergen, C., Klootwijk, W., Peeters, R. P., Medici, M., de Rijke, Y. B., Huisman, S. A., et al. (2014). Functional analysis of novel genetic variation in the thyroid hormone activating type 2 deiodinase. *J. Clin. Endocrinol. Metab.* 99, E2429–E2436. doi: 10.1210/jc.2014-2281

11

Anatomical organization of MCH connections with the pallidum and dorsal striatum in the rat

Sandrine Chometton, Vesna Cvetkovic-Lopes, Christophe Houdayer, Gabrielle Franchi, Amandine Mariot, Fabrice Poncet, Dominique Fellmann and Pierre-Yves Risold*

EA3922, SFR FED 4234, UFR Sciences Médicales et Pharmaceutiques, Université de Franche-Comté, Besançon, France

***Correspondence:**
Pierre-Yves Risold, Laboratoire D'histologie, EA3922, SFR FED 4234, UFR Sciences Médicales et Pharmaceutiques, Université de Franche-Comté, 19 rue Ambroise Paré, 25 000 Besançon, France e-mail: pierre-yves.risold@univ-fcomte.fr

Neurons producing the melanin-concentrating hormone (MCH) are distributed in the posterior hypothalamus, but project massively throughout the forebrain. Many aspects regarding the anatomical organization of these projections are still obscure. The present study has two goals: first to characterize the topographical organization of neurons projecting into the cholinergic basal forebrain (globus pallidus, medial septal complex), and second to verify if MCH neurons may indirectly influence the dorsal striatum (caudoputamen) by innervating afferent sources to this structure. In the first series of experiments, the retrograde tracer fluorogold was injected into multiple sites in the pallidal and medial septal regions and the distribution of retrogradely labeled neurons were analyzed in the posterior lateral hypothalamus. In the second series of experiments, fluorogold was injected into the caudoputamen, and the innervation by MCH axons of retrogradely labeled cells was analyzed. Our results revealed that the MCH system is able to interact with the basal nuclei in several different ways. First, MCH neurons provide topographic inputs to the globus pallidus, medial septal complex, and substantia innominata. Second, striatal projecting neurons in the cortex, thalamus, and substantia nigra presumably receive only sparse inputs from MCH neurons. Third, the subthalamic nucleus is heavily innervated by MCH projections, thus, presumably serves as one important intermediate station to mediate MCH influence on other parts of the basal nuclei.

Keywords: neuroanatomy, basal nuclei, subthalamic nucleus, lateral hypothalamus, arousal

INTRODUCTION

Melanin-concentrating hormone (MCH)-containing neurons in the hypothalamus send extensive projections throughout the cerebral cortex (Bittencourt et al., 1992; Risold et al., 1997). In addition, MCH neurons also abundantly innervate several subcortical structures in the basal forebrain that are connected with the cortex. For example, MCH axons innervate cholinergic neurons in the medial septal and diagonal band nuclei and influence memory formation in the hippocampus through this pathway (Chung et al., 2011; Lu et al., 2013). A role for MCH in the motivation of feeding is pointed out in the nucleus accumbens which expresses high levels of the MCH-R1 receptor (Georgescu et al., 2005; Pissios et al., 2008; Guesdon et al., 2009; Sears et al., 2010; Hopf et al., 2013). The nucleus accumbens is heavily connected with the prefrontal cortical areas, ventral pallidum, amygdalar nuclei, and ventral tegmental area. MCH cortical projections also involve the whole isocortex. To date, the general organization of the circuitry that link the MCH system to the isocortical and classical extrapyramidal circuitries is still little investigated. We can found in the literature evidence of MCH projections in the globus pallidus, and more than 10 years ago interactions between the MCH system and the mesostriatal pathway was suspected (Knigge et al., 1996). However, the overall organization of an anatomical circuitry linking the MCH system to the striato-pallido-nigral pathway is unknown at this point.

The aims of the present study was dual: first, to analyze with some details in the rat the topographical organization of MCH neurons projecting into the whole cholinergic basal telencephalon

Abbreviations: AHN, anterior hypothalamic nucleus; AM, anteromedial nucleus thalamus; ARH, arcuate nucleus hypothalamus; BA, bed nucleus accessory olfactory tract; CART, cocaine and amphetamine regulated transcript; ChAT, choline acetyltransferase; Chol, cholinergic; COA, cortical nucleus amygdala; cpd, cerebral peduncle; CP, caudoputamen; da, dopaminergic group in ZI; DGlb, dentate gyrus, lateral blade; DMH, dorsomedial nucleus hypothalamus; FF, fields of Forel; fx, columns of the fornix; GABA, gamma aminobutyric acid; GPe, globus pallidus, external segment; GPi, globus pallidus, internal segment; int, internal capsule; LHA, lateral hypothalamic area; MA, magnocellular preoptic nucleus; ME, median eminence; MEA, medial nucleus amygdala; ml, medial lemniscus; MM, medial mammillary nucleus; MS, medial septal nucleus; mtt, mammillothalamic tract; NDB, nucleus of the diagonal band; opt, optic tract; Parv, parvalbumin; PH, posterior hypothalamic nucleus; PM, premammillary nucleus; PMv, ventral premammillary nucleus; pm, principal mammillary tract; PR, perireuniens nucleus; PV, periventricular nucleus hypothalamus; PVH, paraventricular nucleus hypothalamus; RCH, retrochiasmatic area; REM, rapid eye movement; RE, nucleus reuniens; SBPV, subparaventricular zone hypothalamus; SF, semptofimbrial nucleus; SIc, substantia innominata, caudal part; SIr, substantia innominata, rostral part; SMT, submedial nucleus thalamus; SN, substantia nigra; SNc, substantia nigra, compact part; SNr, substantia nigra, reticular part; SO, supraoptic nucleus; SPF, subparafascicular nucleus thalamus; STN, subthalamic nucleus; SUMl, supramammillary nucleus, lateral part; sup, supraoptic commissures; TM, tuberomammillary nucleus; V3, third ventricle; VM, ventral medial nucleus thalamus; VMH, ventromedial nucleus hypothalamus; VTA, ventral tegmental area; ZI, zona incerta (globus pallidus, substantia innominata and medial septal complex) and second, to identify possible pathways that MCH neurons may use to indirectly influence isocortical output through the dorsal striatum. To achieve our two goals, we performed retrograde tracer injections through the pallidal ventral forebrain of rats and analyzed the expression of MCH in retrogradely labeled cells in the lateral hypothalamic area (LHA). We also made injections in the dorsal striatum and verified whether MCH axons innervate those retrogradely labeled neurons in the other parts of the brain, including the cerebral cortex, thalamus, subthalamus, and substantia nigra.

MATERIALS AND METHODS

ANIMALS

Sprague–Dawley male rats, weighing 280–380 g, were obtained from Janvier (Le Genest-Saint-Isle, France). They were housed under 12 h light: 12 h dark cycle at a constant room temperature and had free access to water and standard laboratory diet. All animal use and care protocols were in accordance with institutional guidelines (all protocols were approved and investigators authorized).

TRACER INJECTIONS

Rats were anesthetized with an intramuscular (IM) injection of a mixture of xylazine and ketamine (Vetokinol, 1 mg/100 g of body weight and 10 mg/100 g, respectively) and placed in a stereotaxic instrument.

Rats received a unilateral iontophoretic injection of 10% Fluorogold (FG, Interchim) solution diluted in 0.9% NaCl. Coordinates were taken according to the Paxinos and Watson stereotaxic atlas (Paxinos and Watson, 2005). Injections were made in different sites of the basal telencephalon (medial septal complex, nucleus of the diagonal band, substantia innominata, globus pallidus, and dorsal striatum). Glass micropipettes (tip diameter: 30–50 μm) were used to inject the FG iontophoretically into these regions using an intermittent current of 5 μA and 7 s on/off time for 5 min. The micropipette was left in place for another 5 min before being removed to avoid FG diffusion along the micropipette track.

After 10 days survival time, rats were deeply anesthetized with intraperitoneal injection (IP) of Pentobarbital (CEVA, 50 mg/kg). Animals were perfused transcardially with 0.9% NaCl followed by ice-cold 4% paraformaldehyde (PFA, Roth) fixative in 0.1 M phosphate buffer saline (PBS) at pH 7.4. Brains were removed, post-fixed in the same fixative for several hours at 4°C, immersed overnight at 4°C in a solution of 15% sucrose in 0.1 M PBS, and then quickly frozen. Brains were cut in four series of 30 μm coronal thick sections, collected in a cryoprotector solution (1:1:2 glycerol/ethylene glycol/PBS), and stored at −40°C.

IMMUNOHISTOCHEMISTRY FG

After rinsing in PBS + 0.3% Triton X100, free-floating sections were incubated with the primary anti-FG antiserum raised in rabbit (polyclonal, Oncogene Research Products) at a dilution of 1:3000 in PBS containing 0.3% Triton X100, 1% bovine serum albumin, 10% lactoproteins, and 0.01% sodium azide, during 65 h at 4°C. Then, free-floating sections were incubated for 24 h at 4°C in a solution of biotinylated goat anti-rabbit IgG antibody (Vector Laboratories) at a dilution of 1:1000 in PBS Triton. Finally, sections were placed in the mixed avidin-biotin horseradish peroxidase (HRP) complex solution (ABC Elite Kit, Vector Laboratories) for 1 h at room temperature. The peroxidase complex was visualized by an exposure to a chromogen solution containing 0.04% 3,3′diaminobenzidine tetrahydrochloride (DAB, Sigma) and 0.006% hydrogen peroxide (Sigma) in PBS at pH 7.4. The reaction was stopped by extensive washing in PBS at pH 7.4. Free-floating sections were mounted on gelatin-coated slides, and then dehydrated and coverslipped with Canada balsam (Roth). An adjacent series was always stained in a solution of 1% toluidine blue (Roth) in water to serve as a reference series for cytoarchitectonic purposes.

TRIPLE STAINING FG/MCH/CART

Sections were incubated with the anti-MCH antibody (rabbit polyclonal, our laboratory, Risold et al., 1992) dissolved in PBS containing 0.3% Triton X100, 1% bovine serum albumin, 10% lactoproteins, and 0.01% sodium azide at 1:1000 for 65 h at 4°C. Tissues were then incubated with Alexa Fluor 488 goat anti-rabbit IgG antibody (Invitrogen) diluted in PBS-T at 1:1000 for 2 h at room temperature.

After the first staining, sections were incubated with the anti-CART antibody (Cocaine and Amphetamine Regulated Transcript, mouse monoclonal, generously provided by Dr J. T. Clausen, Novo Nordisk, Denmark, 1:1000) dissolved in PBS-T for 65 h at 4°C. Tissues were then incubated with Alexa Fluor 555 donkey anti-mouse IgG antibody (Invitrogen) diluted in PBS-T at 1:1000 for 2 h at room temperature. Finally, free-floating sections were mounted on gelatin-coated slides and coverslipped with 60:40 glycerol:PBS-T.

The auto-fluorescence of FG was observed under UV illumination.

DOUBLE STAINING MCH/PARVALBUMIN OR MCH/ChAT

The MCH is revealed by the technique described above. Then, sections were incubated with the anti-parvalbumin (mouse monoclonal, Swant) or anti-ChAT (goat polyclonal, AB144P Chemicon) antibodies dissolved in PBS containing 0.3% Triton X100, 1% bovine serum albumin, 10% lactoproteins and 0.01% sodium azide at 1:1000 for 65 h at 4°C. Tissues were then incubated with Alexa Fluor 555 donkey anti-mouse IgG antibody (Invitrogen) or Cyanine-3 donkey anti-goat IgG antibody (Jackson Immunoresearch) diluted in PBS-T at 1:1000 for 2 h at room temperature. Finally, free-floating sections were mounted on gelatin-coated slides and coverslipped with 60:40 glycerol:PBS-T.

RESULTS

TOPOGRAPHICAL ORGANIZATION OF MCH PROJECTIONS IN THE CHOLINERGIC BASAL TELENCEPHALON

In this work, we mostly employed the nomenclature of Swanson (2004). The magnocellular cholinergic neurons in the basal forebrain are abundant across the borders of the medial septal complex (medial septal nucleus and nucleus of the diagonal band), the magnocellular preoptic nucleus, the substantia innominata and most the internal segment of the globus pallidus. However, in the globus pallidus and the medial septal complex, these cholinergic neurons are segregated within a medial sector (peripheral in the diagonal band nucleus), while an external part (central in the diagonal band nucleus) is rich in parvalbumin-containing neurons (Kiss et al., 1990; Hontanilla et al., 1998; Henderson et al., 2004; Risold, 2004; Croizier et al., 2010; Mallet et al., 2012). Such differentiation of parvalbumin positive vs. cholinergic-rich region is not as clear in the substantia innominata and in the magnocellular preoptic nucleus.

Distribution of MCH axons in the cholinergic-rich pallidal basal telencephalon

MCH projections arising from the medial forebrain bundle are abundant in the cholinergic rich regions of both the *medial septal complex and the globus pallidus*, while the parvalbumin-rich part of the septum received "en passant" inputs as already reported elsewhere (Croizier et al., 2010) (**Figure 1**). This "en passant" input is far less intense in the external segment of the globus pallidus.

Within the *substantia innominata*, MCH axons are especially abundant in the posterior part, compared to the rostral regions and the magnocellular preoptic nucleus that were only diffusely innervated.

Images evocating a direct innervation by MCH axons of cholinergic neurons was observed in all nuclei of the basal forebrain, confirming already recently published information (Lima et al., 2013) and is not further illustrated in the present work. Numerous buttons were observed close to non-ChAT positive cells, clearly suggesting that MCH axons innervate other cell populations than the cholinergic neurons in these structures. As previously reported (Cvetkovic et al., 2004), most of these axons expressed both MCH and CART. MCH/non-CART axons were obviously less numerous.

Origin of the hypothalamic projections into the cholinergic basal telencephalon

The retrograde tracer fluorogold (FG) was injected into the cholinergic basal forebrain. Several injection sites were restricted to the medial septal nucleus, diagonal band nucleus, substantia innominata or internal segment of the globus pallidus (**Table 1**). Their extent through the rostrocaudal basal telencephalon is schematized in **Figure 2**. The distribution of retrogradely labeled cells in the LHA is schematized in **Figure 3**. Retrogradely labeled neurons within the LHA were abundant when injection sites involved the medial septal complex or caudal parts of the substantia innominata, but the number of retrogradely labeled cells was low when injections sites were centered in the magnocellular preoptic nucleus, rostral substantia innominata or globus pallidus.

A clear topographical organization could be recognized with retrogradely labeled neurons being more medial when the injection sites were centered into the medial septal complex. In such cases, retrogradely labeled neurons were abundant in the hypothalamic medial zone. In the LHA proper, the ventral perifornical parts contained the densest condensations of retrogradely labeled neurons. Parts of the medial zona incerta also contained some cells. When injection sites were centered in the caudal substantia innominata, medial zone nuclei as the ventromedial hypothalamic nucleus were labeled, but in the LHA, retrogradely labeled neurons were more laterally observed. When injection sites involved the rostral substantia innominata, very few neurons were found medially in the hypothalamus, only the LHA contained a significant number of FG expressing cells. Finally, after

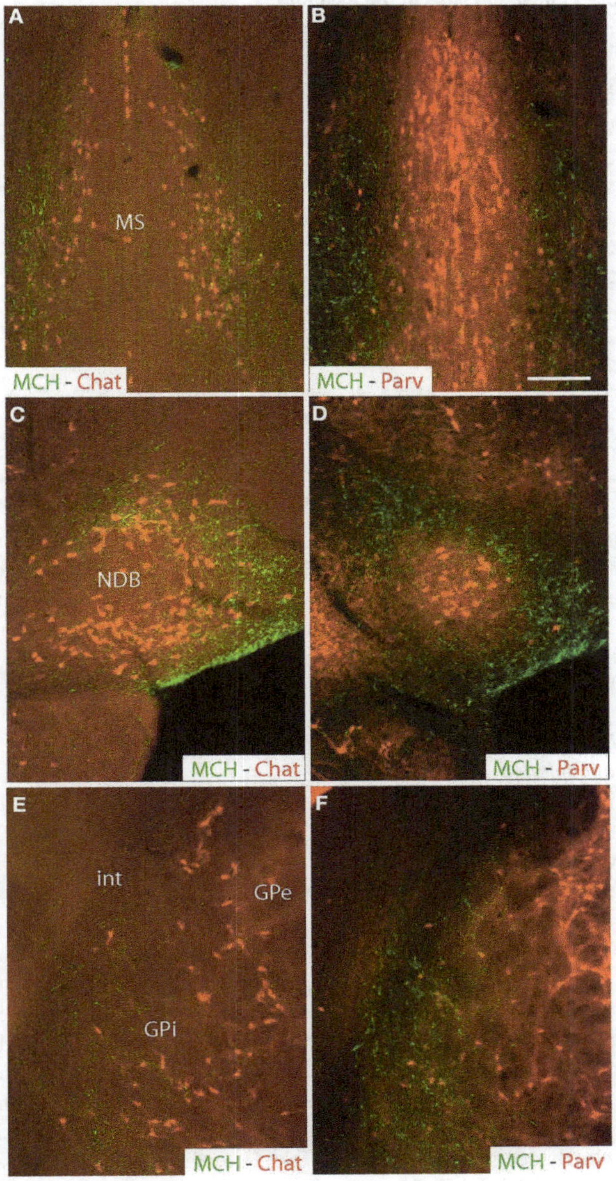

FIGURE 1 | Photomicrographs of coronal sections labeled by double immunohistochemistry to illustrate the distribution of MCH axons (green) in comparison with distributions of cholinergic neurons labeled by an anti-Chat antibody (red), or parvalbumin-expressing neurons (red) in the medial septal nucleus (A,B) the nucleus of the diagonal band (C,D) or the globus pallidus (E,F). Note that in all of these three structures, MCH axons are more abundant in cholinergic-rich parts, but relatively sparse in the parvalbumin-rich parts. Scale bar = 100 μm.

Table 1 | Injection sites in the Pallidum.

Rats no.	FG Injection sites
R3205	Ventral MS/dorsal NDB
R3225	Lateral edge of the MS
R3207	Dorsal NDB
R3211	Caudal MS/septofimbrial nucleus
R3221	NDB/MA
R3209	SIr
R3219	SIr
R3220	MA
R3204	SIc
R3242	SIc
R3238	SIc
R3218	Internal segment of the GP
R3201	Caudal internal segment of the GP

injections in the globus pallidus, retrogradely labeled cells were far less abundant in the hypothalamus, mostly in lateral parts of the LHA close to the cerebral peduncle. The lateral zona incerta contained also some FG expressing cells. By contrast, the adjacent subthalamic nucleus contained a very intense labeling after globus pallidus injections, as expected.

Origin of the MCH projections into the cholinergic basal telencephalon

Using double labeling procedures, many FG-labeled neurons in the hypothalamus proper were also recognized by the MCH-antiserum. The distribution of these cells is reported in the **Figure 4**. Several point retained our attention:

First, similarly to the whole hypothalamic distribution, medial cells, including in the zona incerta, tended to be labeled by the FG when the injection sites involved the medial septal complex (**Figures 4A,B**), while after globus pallidus injections mostly MCH neurons close to the cerebral peduncle contained the retrograde labeling (**Figure 4E**). We did not perform a quantitative analysis as the number of retrogradely labeled cells is clearly dependent of the size of the injection site. Nevertheless, retrogradely labeled MCH neurons appeared to be more abundant when the tracer was injected into the medial septal or posterior regions of the substantia innominata (**Figures 4A–C**) than into the rostral substantia innominata or globus pallidus (**Figures 4D,E**). However, MCH-FG neurons after septal or substantia innominata injections represented only a fraction of the whole number of FG retrogradely labeled cells in the hypothalamus. On the contrary, most FG cells in the LHA after the globus pallidus injections were labeled by the MCH-antiserum.

Second, a caudal perifornical MCH condensation, at caudal levels of the dorsomedial hypothalamic nucleus (**Figures 4A–D** section levels **j–l**), was a major source of MCH projections to the cholinergic medial septal complex, as retrogradely labeled cells were systematically numerous within this condensation in such cases (**Figure 4E**). By contrast, very caudo-medial MCH cell bodies adjacent and in the posterior periventricular nucleus were never retrogradelly labeled in any of the experiments.

Finally, we already reported in the past that most MCH projections in the telencephalon also contained CART. We also confirmed this trend in the present study and as previously mentioned (Cvetkovic et al., 2004), around 80% of MCH-FG neurons were also labeled by CART antibodies (not shown).

INDIRECT MCH PROJECTIONS INTO THE DORSAL STRIATUM

MCH projections are sparse within the dorsal striatum. Fibers labeled for MCH traveled essentially through ventral components of the internal capsule. Only the caudal tail of the caudoputamen nucleus contained some axons providing a very moderate to light innervations of the neuropil.

Four FG injections were aimed at the dorsal striatum, and three were restricted to respectively, dorsal, ventral, or ventrolateral portions of the caudoputamen nucleus (**Figure 5A**). Retrogradely labeled cells were observed in the cerebral cortex, the globus pallidus, intralaminar nuclei of the thalamus, the subthalamic nucleus, the dorsal raphe nucleus, and the substantia nigra. Only one or two per experiment were found within the LHA/zona incerta. These very few cells were labeled by the MCH-antiserum (not shown).

MCH labeled axons were examined in proximity of retrogradely labeled cells in the following regions.

In the cerebral cortex

Many retrogradely labeled neurons were observed dorsally or more laterally in the layer 5 of the isocortex, depending on the location of the injection sites in the striatum. MCH projections are moderately abundant through the isocortex. Although those MCH axons were often seen in the vicinity of these neurons, very few putative contacts were observed. Therefore, it is unlikely that MCH axons provide significant innervation onto those corticostriatal projecting neurons.

In the globus pallidus

Some retrogradely labeled cells were observed in the nucleus. An occasional buttons at immediate proximity of retrogradely labeled cells could be noticed, but most of the retrogradely labeled neurons were not approached by MCH axons.

In the dorsal thalamus

Retrogradely labeled cells were observed in the central lateral and parafascicular nuclei. Again, few MCH axons were seen at the immediate vicinity of retrogradely labeled cells.

In the subthalamic nucleus

Many FG-labeled neurons are distributed in this nucleus. It contains also moderate to intense innervation by MCH axons. Many images evocating synaptic contacts were observed between MCH-labeled axons and FG-expressing perikarya. Almost every FG-expressing perikarya seemed contacted by one or several MCH buttons (**Figures 5B,E**). However, fluorogold containing neurons in the subthalamic nucleus were far more abundant after injections in the globus pallidus.

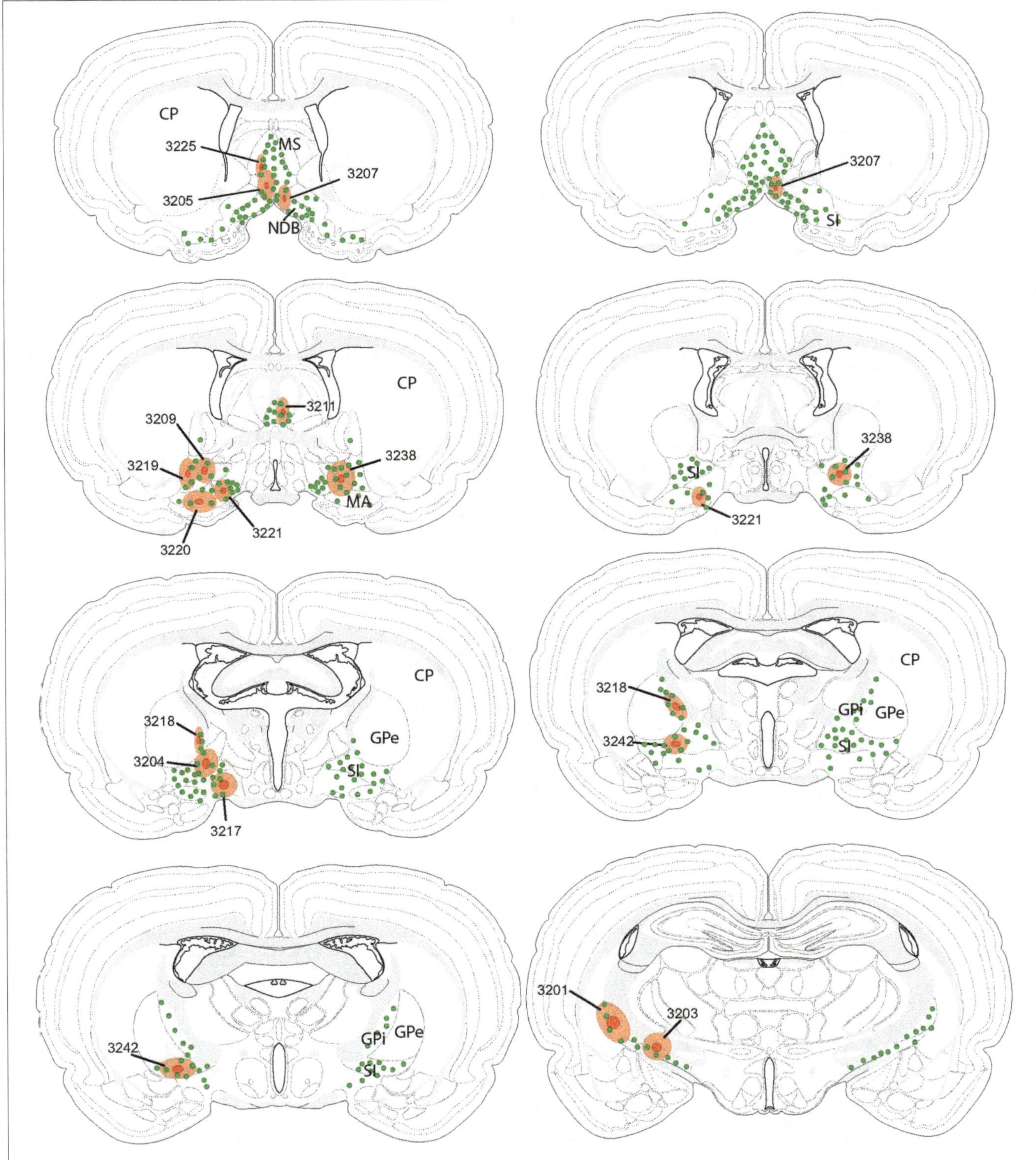

FIGURE 2 | Illustration of all fluorogold injection sites in comparison with the distribution of cholinergic neurons in the basal telencephalon (green dots). In several experiments (individually identified by a four digit number), injection sites were centered (dark red spot) in the medial septal nucleus, nucleus of the diagonal band, substantia innominata or internal segment of the globus pallidus. The hallo around this center (light red area) may slightly extend beyond the borders of targeted nuclei (see also **Table 1**).

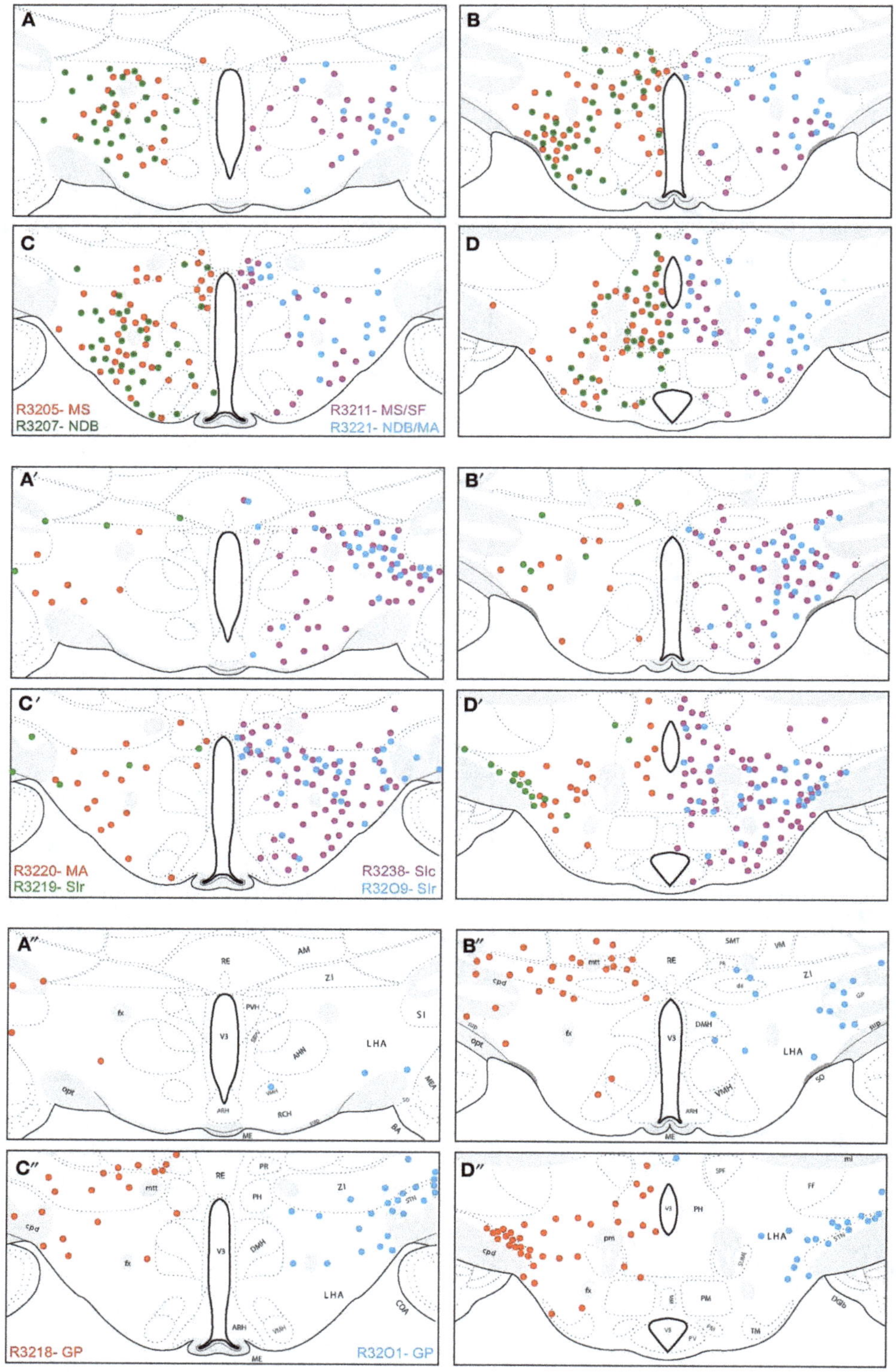

FIGURE 3 | Schematic distribution of neurons retrogradely labeled by the fluorogold after injections in the basal telencephalon (Figure 2 and Table 1 for injection sites). The distribution of these neurons is mapped on four sections in the coronal planes through the posterior hypothalamus. They are organized from rostral **(A)** to caudal **(D)**. Four (upper two panels; 2 on the left and 2 on the right) or two (lower panel) experiments are illustrated per panels. Note the topographical organization of retrogradely labeled cells depending on the location of the injection sites (see text for details).

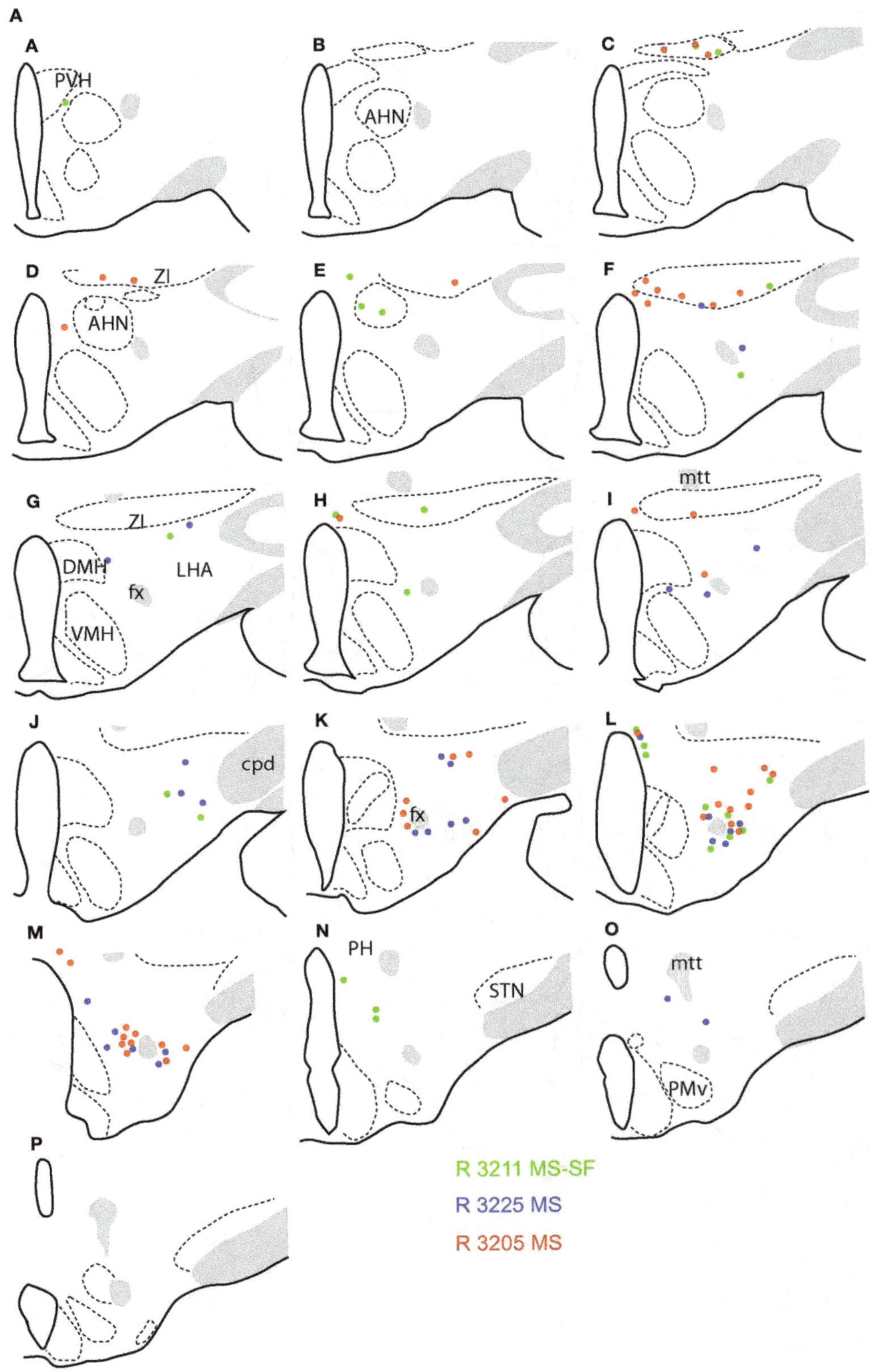

FIGURE 4 | Continued

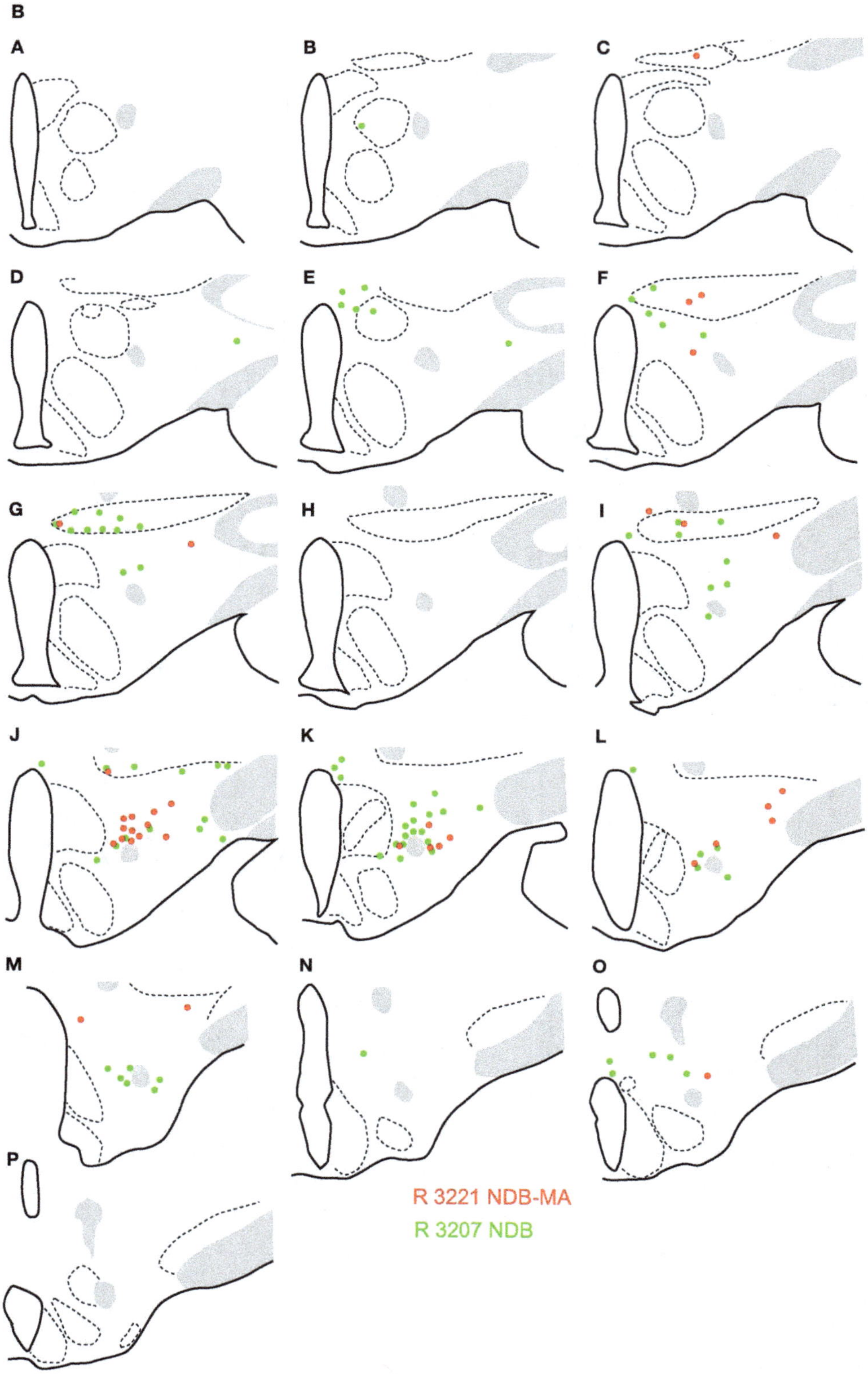

FIGURE 4 | Continued

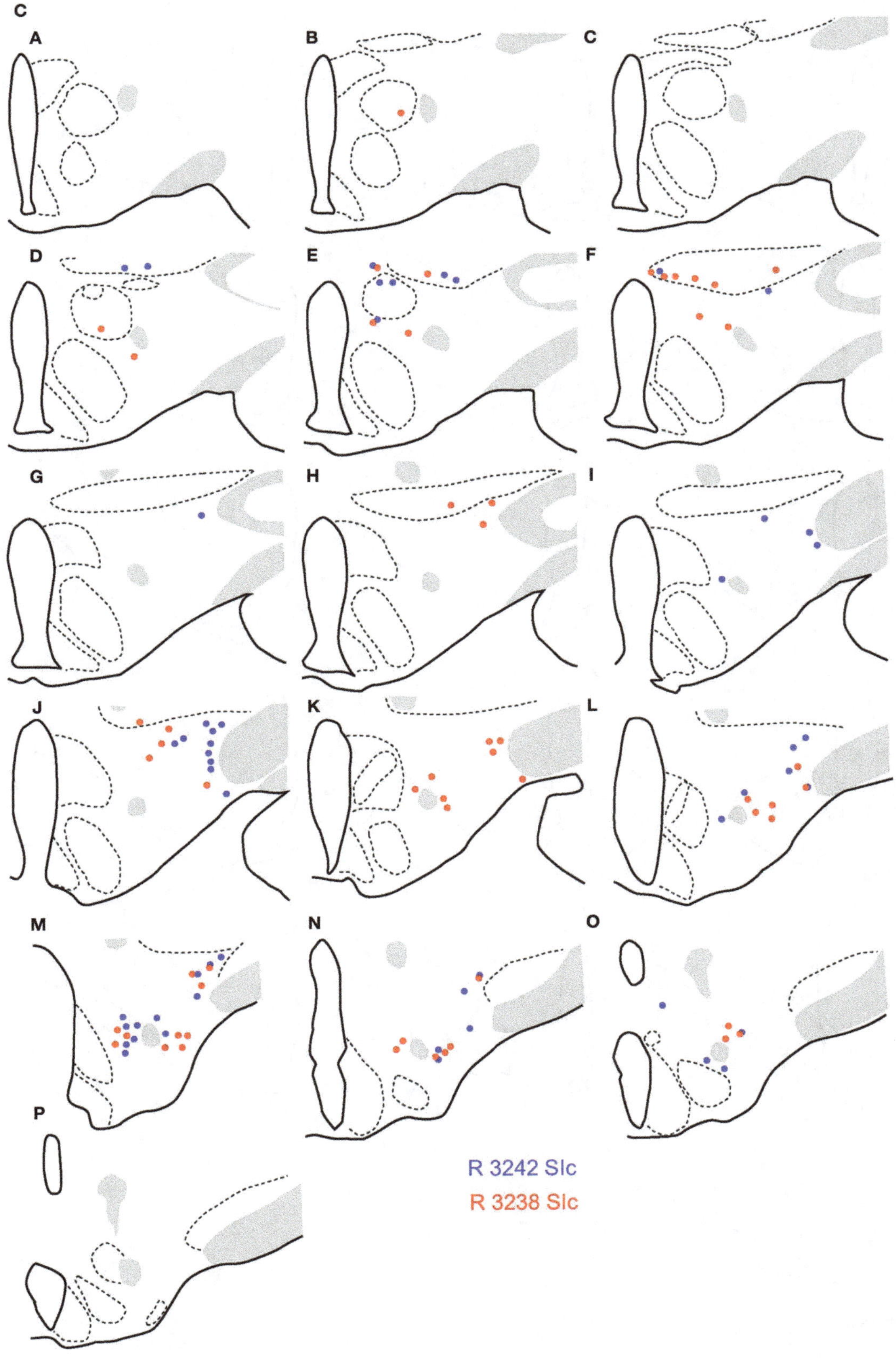

FIGURE 4 | Continued

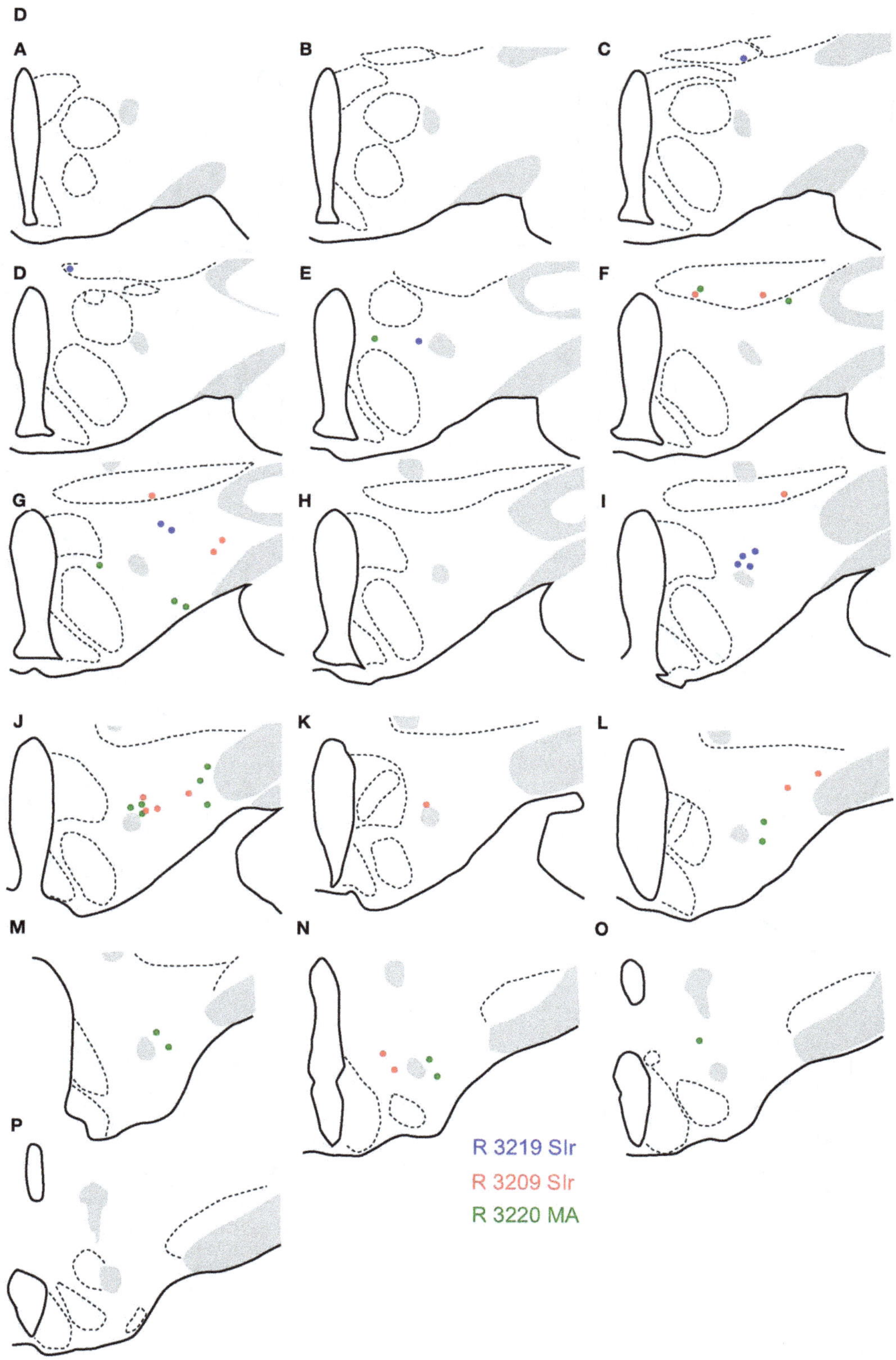

FIGURE 4 | Continued

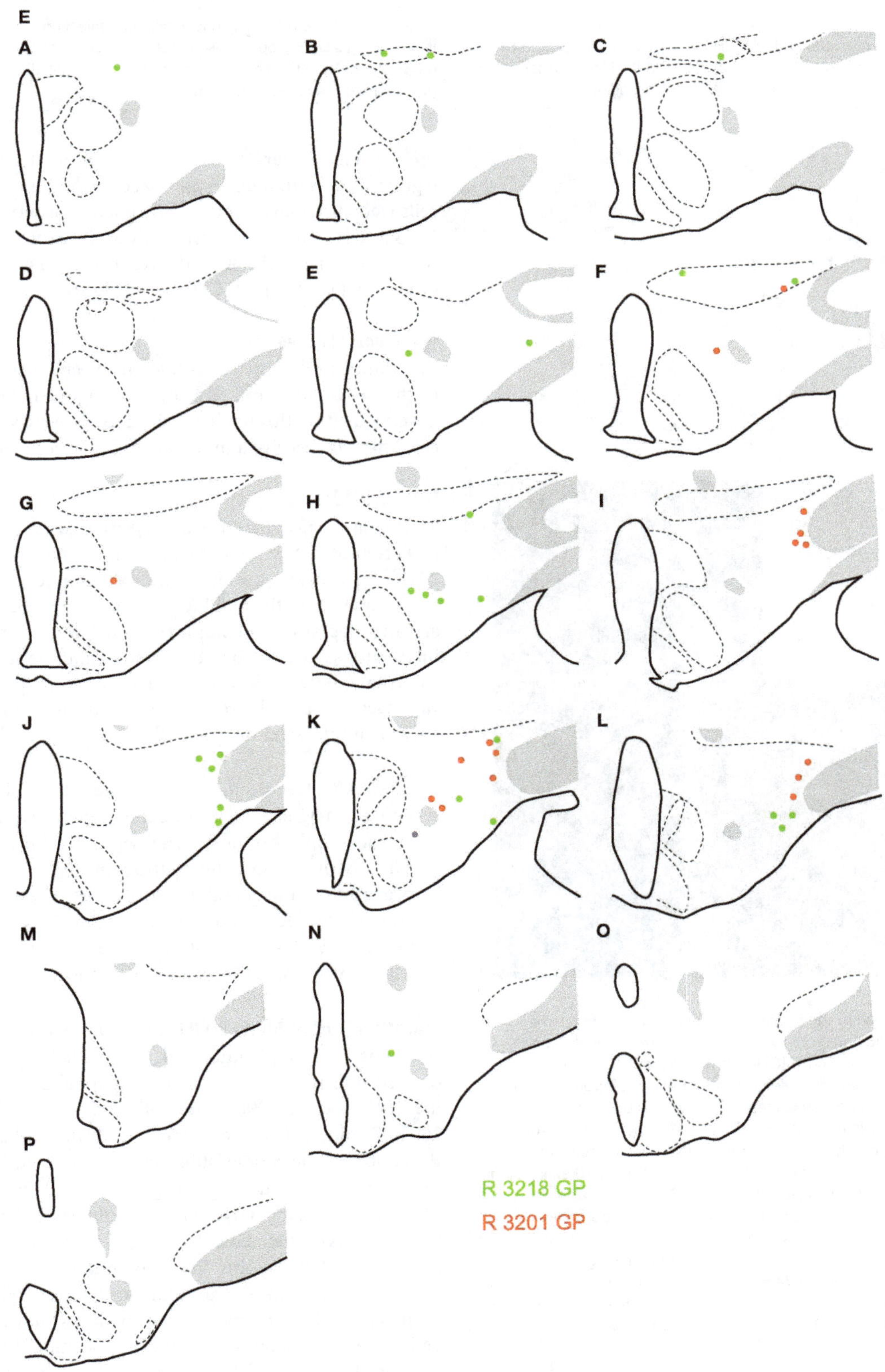

FIGURE 4 | (A–E) Distribution of FG-MCH neurons in the posterior hypothalamus after different FG injections in the basal telencephalon. This distribution is mapped on coronal drawings of the caudal hypothalamus arranged from rostral **(a)** to caudal **(p)**. These drawings were produced from Nissl stained sections and mapping was made with regard to the distribution of MCH cell bodies from an adjacent series of section. Therefore, results of all FG-injected brains were represented on this set of reference drawings and *(Continued)*

FIGURE 4 | Continued
with regard to cytoarchitecture and to MCH distribution. One dot on the drawing corresponds to one MCH cell labeled by the fluorogold observed on the section. After septal injections **(A,B)** retrogradely labeled MCH neurons were medial in the hypothalamus, while after injection in the substantia innominata **(C,D)** or globus pallidus **(E)** retrogradely labeled perikarya were more lateral. Note the dense group of retrogradely labeled cells in the posterior perifornical region **(j–m)**.

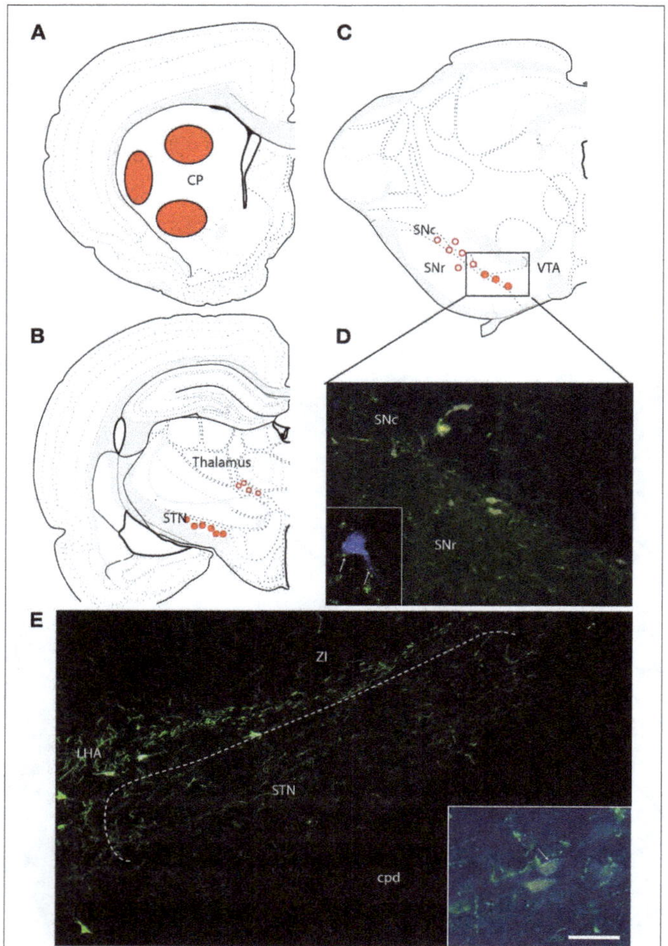

FIGURE 5 | (A) Location of the FG injection sites in the caudoputamen nucleus. **(B,C)** Brief illustration of the distribution of retrogradely labeled cells at thalamic **(B)** and midbrain **(C)** levels after FG injection in the caudoputamen nucleus and represented on schematized coronal sections from Swanson (2004). Open circles represent the distribution of retrogradely labeled cells that were very little innervated by MCH axons. Filled dots represent the distribution of retrogradely labeled cells that were contacted by MCH axons. **(D)** Photomicrographs illustrating FG-expressing cells in the ventral substantia nigra compacta. MCH-labeled axons are observed close to some of these neurons. Framed figure is a confocal micrograph illustrating a MCH axons (in green, arrows) contacting a FG expressing cell (in blue to increase contrast). **(E)** Photomicrographs illustrating the MCH innervations of the subthalamic nucleus. Framed figure is a micrograph illustrating a MCH axons (in green, arrows) contacting a FG labeled neurons. Scale bar = 100 μm (30 μm for framed pictures).

In the substantia nigra

This structure contained the brightest FG neurons after caudoputamen injections. As expected, these cells were mostly observed in the substantia nigra pars compacta, but a few were found in the substantia nigra pars reticulata, or in the adjacent ventral tegmental area. In the pars compacta of the substantia nigra, these cells were distributed in the ventromedial or more dorsal regions. Dorsal cells were not innervated by MCH axons. On the contrary, retrogradely labeled cells in the ventromedial pars compacta were obviously targeted by MCH axons (**Figures 5C,D**).

In the dorsal raphe

The dorsal raphe nucleus is known to send a serotonergic input to the dorsal striatum, and some retrogradely labeled cells were observed within this nucleus. MCH axons were seen close to these cells that may receive a moderate MCH innervation.

DISCUSSION

The basal telencephalon is an essential target of MCH axons in all vertebrates, from agnathians to mammalians (Croizier et al., 2013). In rodents, the literature data implicating MCH in several structures of the basal forebrain, i.e., the nucleus accumbens and the medial septal complex, is now quite abundant. However, interactions between the MCH system and the striatonigral pathways have been little investigated so far. In the present study, we observed several strong anatomical links between the MCH system and the striatonigral pathways:

> First, MCH projections are abundant in all structures that contain magnocellular cholinergic neurons, from the medial septal complex to the internal segment of the globus pallidus. The distribution of the neurons of origin is topographically organized in the lateral hypothalamus. These projections may contact cholinergic but also non-cholinergic cells.
> Second, besides to the internal segment of the globus pallidus, MCH axons innervate the subthalamic nucleus.

ORGANIZATION OF MCH PROJECTIONS INTO THE PALLIDUM

Both the globus pallidus and the medial septal complex are divided into parvalbumin rich and parvalbumin poor compartments (Kiss et al., 1990; Hontanilla et al., 1998; Henderson et al., 2004; Risold, 2004; Croizier et al., 2010; Mallet et al., 2012). By contrast, the whole substantia innominata contains intermixed neuron populations (Lagos et al., 2012; Lu et al., 2013). MCH axons clearly targeted the cholinergic-rich/parvalbumin-poor regions of the medial septal nucleus, nucleus of the diagonal band, and of the globus pallidus, but they are diffuse within the substantia innominata. MCH and cholinergic neurons have been reported to interact in the medial septal complex and to be involved in sleep control and hippocampal functions such as memory formation (Chung et al., 2011; Lagos et al., 2012; Jego et al., 2013; Lu et al., 2013). However, MCH axons may as well-interact with cholinergic neurons in the substantia innominata and globus pallidus. The cholinergic rich basal telencephalon contains other neuronal types such as GABAergic and glutamatergic neurons that are far more abundant than cholinergic cells (Risold, 2004; Gritti et al., 2006), but little attention has been devoted to date to the innervation that MCH axons may provide to these cells. We observed buttons, and putative synaptic contacts targeting ChAT negative and therefore non-cholinergic cells. This is a topic that will clearly need to be investigated in the future to understand the role of the MCH projections into these regions.

Depending on the location of the injection sites, the numbers, and distributions of FG-labeled neurons were markedly different within the hypothalamus. Injection sites within the medial septal complex retrogradely labeled far more neurons in the hypothalamus than injections centered into the globus pallidus. This was expected because the medial forebrain bundle originates in and innervates the septal region and the substantia innominata, while the globus pallidus is associated to the internal capsule and the cerebral peduncle. We also observed a topographical arrangement in the origin of these projections, with neurons projecting to the medial septal complex being more medial than those projecting to the anterior substantia innominata or globus pallidus. Because some of these projections continue farther to reach the pallium, this topographical organization is clearly reminiscent of that described by Saper (1985) after cortical retrograde tracer injections.

Neurons double labeled with MCH and FG display similar distribution patterns in the hypothalamus. There are more MCH neurons projecting into the medial septal complex than into the globus pallidus. However, several points need to be emphasized:

First, although more abundant after the medial septal complex injections, overall these MCH/FG double-labeled neurons were intermixed with many retrogradely labeled non-MCH neurons in the hypothalamus. By contrast, after FG injections into the globus pallidus, most retrogradely labeled neurons in the hypothalamus were MCH positive. This indicates that MCH neurons may have an important and specific role in relaying the results of the hypothalamic (lateral hypothalamic) processing into the striatonigral system.

Second, in none of our experiments ventromedial-most MCH neurons adjacent and in the periventricular nucleus were labeled. These very medial MCH cells may serve different functions than those in the LHA and dorsal hypothalamus. They are suspected to provide an innervation of the arcuate nucleus and are not observed in mice (Croizier et al., 2010). Then, they probably form a specific MCH sub-population in the rat hypothalamus.

SPARSE INDIRECT CONNECTIONS WITH THE DORSAL STRIATUM, INNERVATION OF THE SUBTHALAMIC NUCLEUS

Neurons that were retrogradely labeled after FG injections centered into the caudoputamen nucleus received overall a very modest MCH innervation. Only the very ventromedial sector of the pars compacta of the substantia nigra received a clear MCH input, but this region might very well be also associated to the ventral striatum (nucleus accumbens) (Gerfen and Wilson, 1996).

Only significant putative contacts concerned nuclei for which the dorsal striatum is a secondary target or that have multiple projection sites including the striatum. For example, the dorsal raphe nucleus contained quite abundant MCH buttons, some of which adjacent to FG positive neurons after striatal injections. However, the dorsal raphe nucleus project in multiple telencephalic sites and its neurons often send collaterals in many nuclei or territories (Waselus et al., 2011). Therefore, the MCH input that we observed in this nucleus cannot be interpreted as a strong evidence of exclusive indirect dorsal striatal control.

We noted an intense MCH innervation in the subthalamic nucleus. Some neurons of this nucleus were retrogradely labeled after striatal injections, but its main projections are for the globus pallidus as well as the pars reticulata of the substantia nigra. MCH projections in the subthalamic nucleus have not been investigated so far. MCH-R1 seems not to be abundantly expressed in the rodent subthalamic nucleus (Saito et al., 2001). However, MCH neurons contains other neuropeptides as CART and Nesfatin, but most importantly, they are GABAergic (Sapin et al., 2010; Del Cid-Pellitero and Jones, 2012). Therefore, they may act as inhibitory GABAergic neurons. These projections into the subthalamic nucleus were noted in other species (Croizier et al., 2010; Chometton et al., 2014), and should deserve an increased attention in the future.

MCH NEURONS ARE IMPORTANT ACTORS IN THE BASAL NUCLEI CIRCUITRY THROUGH PALLIDAL AND SUBTHALAMIC NUCLEUS PROJECTIONS

The hypothesis that the MCH system is anatomically associated with the extrapyramidal pathway was advanced by Karl Knigge which unfortunately published too few papers on this topic

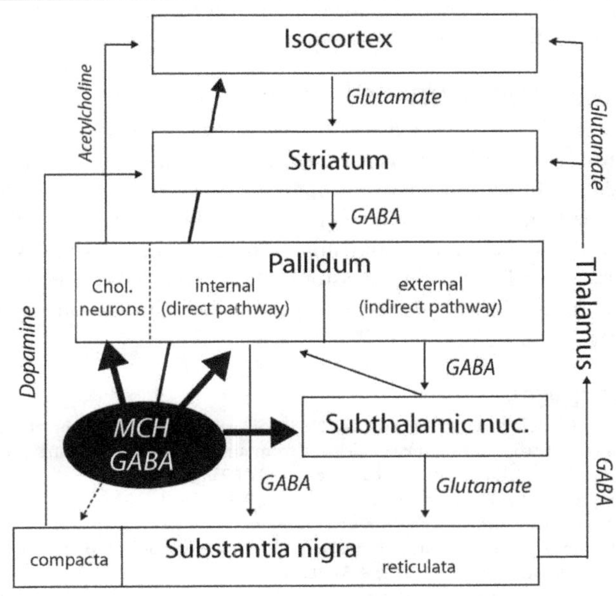

FIGURE 6 | Diagram summarizing interactions of the MCH systems with the cortico-striato-pallido-nigral (extrapyramidal) pathways. Besides direct cortical projections, MCH neurons may indirectly influence the cortex by innervating the cholinopetal projections from the internal segment of the globus pallidus. By projecting into this segment of the globus pallidus and in the subthalamic nucleus, they are also in a good position to influence the extrapyramidal direct, and indirect pathways. Finally, the medial section of the pars compacta of the substantia nigra is also targeted by a modest MCH input.

(Knigge et al., 1996). He advocated quite elegantly that these neurons are in good position to influence the mesostriatal pathway. Since, other authors have convincingly shown that MCH acts on parts of the nucleus accumbens in which a high expression of MCH-R1 is reported (Georgescu et al., 2005; Pissios et al., 2008; Guesdon et al., 2009; Sears et al., 2010; Hopf et al., 2013). Interactions between MCH and mesostriatal pathways have also been reported (Chung et al., 2011). In the present study, we observed that MCH influence on the basal nuclei/extrapyramidal circuitry involved mostly pallidal nuclei as well as the subthalamic nucleus in the rat.

Classically, descending pathways from the striatum take two distinct routes: a direct one that innervates the internal segment of the globus pallidus and the substantia nigra, and an indirect one that involves the external segment of the globus pallidus, subthalamic nucleus, and the substantia nigra (**Figure 6**). Therefore, MCH axons are susceptible to influence both descending routes from the striatum in the rat: into the internal segment of the globus pallidus for the direct pathway, or by innervating the subthalamic nucleus for the indirect pathway. The role of the subthalamic nucleus within this circuitry has been reevaluated in the last decade. From a motor function, it is now admitted that this nucleus has significant cognitive roles as well (Baunez et al., 2011). It is seen now as a central hub controlling important aspects of voluntary motor output. It is an important target for treatment of Parkinson disease by deep brain stimulation approaches. The role of MCH projections into this nucleus is unclear yet, but considering that MCH neurons are active during REM sleep, these projections into the globus pallidus, and subthalamic nucleus may be important to control motor responses as the cerebral cortex is the siege of an intense electrical activity.

AUTHOR CONTRIBUTIONS

Conceived and designed the experiments: Pierre-Yves Risold, Dominique Fellmann. Performed the experiments: Sandrine Chometton, Vesna Cvetkovic-Lopes. Analyzed the data: Sandrine Chometton, Vesna Cvetkovic-Lopes, Pierre-Yves Risold, Dominique Fellmann. Contributed reagents/materials/analysis tools: Gabrielle Franchi, Christophe Houdayer, Fabrice Poncet, Amandine Mariot. Wrote the paper: Sandrine Chometton, Pierre-Yves Risold.

REFERENCES

Baunez, C., Yelnik, J., and Mallet, L. (2011). Six questions on the subthalamic nucleus: lessons from animal models and from stimulated patients. *Neuroscience* 198, 193–204. doi: 10.1016/j.neuroscience.2011.09.059

Bittencourt, J. C., Presse, F., Arias, C., Peto, C., Vaughan, J., Nahon, J. L., et al. (1992). The melanin-concentrating hormone system of the rat brain: an immuno- and hybridization histochemical characterization. *J. Comp. Neurol.* 319, 218–245. doi: 10.1002/cne.903190204

Chometton, S., Franchi, G., Houdayer, C., Mariot, A., Poncet, F., Fellmann, D., et al. (2014). Different distributions of preproMCH and hypocretin/orexin in the forebrain of the pig (Sus scrofa domesticus). *J. Chem. Neuroanat.* 61C–62C, 72–82. doi: 10.1016/j.jchemneu.2014.08.001

Chung, S., Verheij, M. M., Hesseling, P., Van Vugt, R. W., Buell, M., Belluzzi, J. D., et al. (2011). The melanin-concentrating hormone (MCH) system modulates behaviors associated with psychiatric disorders. *PLoS ONE* 6:e19286. doi: 10.1371/journal.pone.0019286

Croizier, S., Cardot, J., Brischoux, F., Fellmann, D., Griffond, B., and Risold, P. Y. (2013). The vertebrate diencephalic MCH system: a versatile neuronal population in an evolving brain. *Front. Neuroendocrinol.* 34, 65–87. doi: 10.1016/j.yfrne.2012.10.001

Croizier, S., Franchi-Bernard, G., Colard, C., Poncet, F., La Roche, A., and Risold, P. Y. (2010). A comparative analysis shows morphofunctional differences between the rat and mouse melanin-concentrating hormone systems. *PLoS ONE* 5:e15471. doi: 10.1371/journal.pone.0015471

Cvetkovic, V., Brischoux, F., Jacquemard, C., Fellmann, D., Griffond, B., and Risold, P. Y. (2004). Characterization of subpopulations of neurons producing melanin-concentrating hormone in the rat ventral diencephalon. *J. Neurochem.* 91, 911–919. doi: 10.1111/j.1471-4159.2004.02776.x

Del Cid-Pellitero, E., and Jones, B. E. (2012). Immunohistochemical evidence for synaptic release of GABA from melanin-concentrating hormone containing varicosities in the locus coeruleus. *Neuroscience* 223, 269–276. doi: 10.1016/j.neuroscience.2012.07.072

Georgescu, D., Sears, R. M., Hommel, J. D., Barrot, M., Bolanos, C. A., Marsh, D. J., et al. (2005). The hypothalamic neuropeptide melanin-concentrating hormone acts in the nucleus accumbens to modulate feeding behavior and forced-swim performance. *J. Neurosci.* 25, 2933–2940. doi: 10.1523/JNEUROSCI.1714-04.2005

Gerfen, C., and Wilson, C. (1996). "The basal ganglia," in *Handbook of Chemical Neuroanatomy: Integrated Systems of the CNS,* eds L. W. Swanson, A. Bjorklund, and T. Hokfelt (Amsterdam: Elsevier), 371–468.

Gritti, I., Henny, P., Galloni, F., Mainville, L., Mariotti, M., and Jones, B. E. (2006). Stereological estimates of the basal forebrain cell population in the rat, including neurons containing choline acetyltransferase, glutamic acid decarboxylase or phosphate-activated glutaminase and colocalizing vesicular glutamate transporters. *Neuroscience* 143, 1051–1064. doi: 10.1016/j.neuroscience.2006.09.024

Guesdon, B., Paradis, E., Samson, P., and Richard, D. (2009). Effects of intracerebroventricular and intra-accumbens melanin-concentrating hormone agonism on food intake and energy expenditure. *Am. J. Physiol. Regul. Integr. Comp. Physiol.* 296, R469–R475. doi: 10.1152/ajpregu.90556.2008

Henderson, Z., Fiddler, G., Saha, S., Boros, A., and Halasy, K. (2004). A parvalbumin-containing, axosomatic synaptic network in the rat medial septum: relevance to rhythmogenesis. *Eur. J. Neurosci.* 19, 2753–2768. doi: 10.1111/j.0953-816X.2004.03399.x

Hontanilla, B., Parent, A., De Las Heras, S., and Gimenez-Amaya, J. M. (1998). Distribution of calbindin D-28k and parvalbumin neurons and fibers in the rat basal ganglia. *Brain Res. Bull.* 47, 107–116. doi: 10.1016/S0361-9230(98)00035-5

Hopf, F. W., Seif, T., Chung, S., and Civelli, O. (2013). MCH and apomorphine in combination enhance action potential firing of nucleus accumbens shell neurons *in vitro*. *PeerJ* 1:e61. doi: 10.7717/peerj.61

Jego, S., Glasgow, S. D., Herrera, C. G., Ekstrand, M., Reed, S. J., Boyce, R., et al. (2013). Optogenetic identification of a rapid eye movement sleep modulatory circuit in the hypothalamus. *Nat. Neurosci.* 16, 1637–1643. doi: 10.1038/nn.3522

Kiss, J., Patel, A. J., and Freund, T. F. (1990). Distribution of septohippocampal neurons containing parvalbumin or choline acetyltransferase in the rat brain. *J. Comp. Neurol.* 298, 362–372. doi: 10.1002/cne.902980308

Knigge, K. M., Baxter-Grillo, D., Speciale, J., and Wagner, J. (1996). Melanotropic peptides in the mammalian brain: the melanin-concentrating hormone. *Peptides* 17, 1063–1073. doi: 10.1016/0196-9781(96)00131-3

Lagos, P., Monti, J. M., Jantos, H., and Torterolo, P. (2012). Microinjection of the melanin-concentrating hormone into the lateral basal forebrain increases REM sleep and reduces wakefulness in the rat. *Life Sci.* 90, 895–899. doi: 10.1016/j.lfs.2012.04.019

Lima, F. F., Sita, L. V., Oliveira, A. R., Costa, H. C., Da Silva, J. M., Mortara, R. A., et al. (2013). Hypothalamic melanin-concentrating hormone projections to the septo-hippocampal complex in the rat. *J. Chem. Neuroanat.* 47, 1–14. doi: 10.1016/j.jchemneu.2012.10.003

Lu, Z. H., Fukuda, S., Minakawa, Y., Yasuda, A., Sakamoto, H., Sawamura, S., et al. (2013). Melanin concentrating hormone induces hippocampal acetylcholine release via the medial septum in rats. *Peptides* 44, 32–39. doi: 10.1016/j.peptides.2013.03.015

Mallet, N., Micklem, B. R., Henny, P., Brown, M. T., Williams, C., Bolam, J. P., et al. (2012). Dichotomous organization of the external globus pallidus. *Neuron* 74, 1075–1086. doi: 10.1016/j.neuron.2012.04.027

Paxinos, G., and Watson, C. (2005). *The Rat Brain in Stereotaxic Coordinates.* Amsterdam: Elsevier.

Pissios, P., Frank, L., Kennedy, A. R., Porter, D. R., Marino, F. E., Liu, F. F., et al. (2008). Dysregulation of the mesolimbic dopamine system and reward in MCH-/- mice. *Biol. Psychiatry* 64, 184–191. doi: 10.1016/j.biopsych.2007.12.011

Risold, P. Y. (2004). "The septal region," in *The Rat Nervous System,* ed G. Paxinos (Elsevier).

Risold, P. Y., Fellmann, D., Rivier, J., Vale, W., and Bugnon, C. (1992). Immunoreactivities for antisera to three putative neuropeptides of the rat melanin-concentrating hormone precursor are coexpressed in neurons of the rat lateral dorsal hypothalamus. *Neurosci. Lett.* 136, 145–149. doi: 10.1016/0304-3940(92)90035-6

Risold, P. Y., Thompson, R. H., and Swanson, L. W. (1997). The structural organization of connections between hypothalamus and cerebral cortex. *Brain Res. Rev.* 24, 197–254. doi: 10.1016/S0165-0173(97)00007-6

Saito, Y., Cheng, M., Leslie, F. M., and Civelli, O. (2001). Expression of the melanin-concentrating hormone (MCH) receptor mRNA in the rat brain. *J. Comp. Neurol.* 435, 26–40. doi: 10.1002/cne.1191

Saper, C. B. (1985). Organization of cerebral cortical afferent systems in the rat. II. Hypothalamocortical projections. *J. Comp. Neurol.* 237, 21–46. doi: 10.1002/cne.902370103

Sapin, E., Berod, A., Leger, L., Herman, P. A., Luppi, P. H., and Peyron, C. (2010). A very large number of GABAergic neurons are activated in the tuberal hypothalamus during paradoxical (REM) sleep hypersomnia. *PLoS ONE* 5:e11766. doi: 10.1371/journal.pone.0011766

Sears, R. M., Liu, R. J., Narayanan, N. S., Sharf, R., Yeckel, M. F., Laubach, M., et al. (2010). Regulation of nucleus accumbens activity by the hypothalamic neuropeptide melanin-concentrating hormone. *J. Neurosci.* 30, 8263–8273. doi: 10.1523/JNEUROSCI.5858-09.2010

Swanson, L. W. (2004). *Brain Maps: Structure of the Rat Brain.* Amsterdam: Elsevier.

Waselus, M., Valentino, R. J., and Van Bockstaele, E. J. (2011). Collateralized dorsal raphe nucleus projections: a mechanism for the integration of diverse functions during stress. *J. Chem. Neuroanat.* 41, 266–280. doi: 10.1016/j.jchemneu.2011.05.011

12

Recent advances in understanding the role of the hypothalamic circuit during aggression

Annegret L. Falkner[1]* and Dayu Lin[1,2]*

[1] *Neuroscience Institute, New York University School of Medicine, New York, NY, USA*
[2] *Department of Psychiatry, New York University School of Medicine, New York, NY, USA*

Correspondence:
Annegret L. Falkner, Neuroscience Institute, New York University School of Medicine, 522 First Avenue, Smilow Research Building, 6th Floor, New York, NY 10016, USA
e-mail: annegret.falkner@nyumc.org;
Dayu Lin, Department of Psychiatry, New York University School of Medicine, 522 First Avenue, Smilow Research Building, Room 611, New York, NY 10016, USA
e-mail: Dayu.Lin@nyumc.org

The hypothalamus was first implicated in the classic "fight or flight" response nearly a century ago, and since then, many important strides have been made in understanding both the circuitry and the neural dynamics underlying the generation of these behaviors. In this review, we will focus on the role of the hypothalamus in aggression, paying particular attention to recent advances in the field that have allowed for functional identification of relevant hypothalamic subnuclei. Recent progress in this field has been aided by the development of new techniques for functional manipulation including optogenetics and pharmacogenetics, as well as advances in technology used for chronic *in vivo* recordings during complex social behaviors. We will examine the role of the hypothalamus through the complimentary lenses of (1) loss of function studies, including pharmacology and pharmacogenetics; (2) gain of function studies, including specific comparisons between results from classic electrical stimulation studies and more recent work using optogenetics; and (3) neural activity, including both immediate early gene and awake-behaving recordings. Lastly, we will outline current approaches to identifying the precise role of the hypothalamus in promoting aggressive motivation and aggressive action.

Keywords: aggression, hypothalmus, VMHvl, optogenetic stimulation, circuits, estrogen receptor alpha, aggressive motivation, optogenetics

Aggression is a primary social behavior used by humans and animals alike to defend territory, secure mates, compete for food, and protect young. The term aggression comes from the Latin word *aggressio*, meaning to attack, but also to approach and initiate action. Specific actions associated with aggression depend on the species, but can include biting, kicking, hitting or pushing. In addition, threatening displays such as hisses, enlarged body size, and changes in facial expression are also parts of the aggressive repertoire of many species. Although humans express aggression in diverse physical and verbal forms (often separated into "reactive" or "instrumental" aggressive behaviors), the underlying goal of human aggression—defense and competition for resources—remains the same. Increases in both human and animal aggression are accompanied by similar autonomic responses including raised heart rate and respiration, and both are influenced by changes in circulating hormones, such as testosterone (Nelson and Trainor, 2007). While the specific actions and musculature used during aggression may differ between humans and animals, the underlying neural mechanisms that drive aggressive behavior are likely to be largely conserved across species.

For nearly a century, neuroscientists have sought to understand the neural basis of aggression by perturbing and monitoring brain activity through a variety of methods. Numerous classic lesion and electric stimulation experiments have established the hypothalamus as a crucial node for the expression of aggressive behavior (Clemente and Chase, 1973; Siegel et al., 1999), but its role in promoting these behaviors has remained elusive. Newly emerging techniques for measuring and manipulating neural circuitry, including optogenetic and pharmacogenetic tools and advances in technology for *in vivo* recording and imaging in the freely moving animal, have opened new avenues for research on aggression and allow study at the level of genetically defined cell type and the single neuron. In this review, we will focus on this recent progress and provide an up-to-date view on the role of the hypothalamus in promoting aggression and compare this to its role in promoting other social interactions such as sexual behavior. Since these novel genetic-based functional manipulation tools are most powerfully applied in the laboratory mouse, this review will focus mainly on advances in understanding the neural substrates of rodent aggression. However, novel contributions to our understanding of aggression circuitry are also currently being done in non-rodent species including humans (Goodson et al., 2012; Franzini et al., 2013; Haller, 2013; Torres et al., 2013).

NOVEL APPROACHES TO FUNCTIONAL MANIPULATION OF HYPOTHALAMIC CIRCUITRY

TARGETED HYPOTHALAMIC INACTIVATION REDUCES NATURAL INTER-MALE AGGRESSION

Many studies have attempted to assess the role of the hypothalamus through inactivation experiments, using diverse surgical, pharmacological, and genetic methods. Some of the earliest experiments on aggression were knife cut experiments performed on cats during the 1920's which demonstrated the importance of hypothalamus in the expression of rage (Bard, 1928). When the forebrain area was dissociated from its posterior structures, leaving the hypothalamus and its downstream connections intact, operated cats showed spontaneous and unprovoked aggressive behaviors (which they termed *sham rage*), such as hissing and paw striking. In contrast, if the cut was made posterior to the caudal hypothalamus, these behaviors were absent, indicating that an intact hypothalamus is indispensable for the generation of these rage behaviors.

Further experiments demonstrated that specific subnuclei within the hypothalamus may be preferentially involved in promoting aggression, though the precise effects remained unclear. Contradictory results were reported regarding the effects of electrolytic lesions of the medial hypothalamus on aggression: while some reports showed decreased aggression after lesioning, others showed the opposite trend (Grossman, 1972; Olivier and Wiepkema, 1974; Oliver, 1977; Albert and Walsh, 1982; Albert et al., 1987). Reasons for these inconsistent results may be the poor spatial control of the lesion site, damage to fibers of passage and/or post-operation compensation. In addition, pharmacological manipulations have provided additional evidence supporting the necessary role for specific hypothalamic subnuclei in natural aggression: blockage of substance P receptor in medial hypothalamus or the destruction of substance P expressing neurons lowers the number of "violent" hard bites in rats (Halasz et al., 2008, 2009) and injection of vasopressin receptor antagonist into the anterior hypothalamic nucleus (AHN) of hamster decreased the number of attacks and increased attack latency (Ferris and Potegal, 1988).

More recent work has focused on a smaller subdivision of the hypothalamus in mouse, the ventromedial hypothalamus, ventrolateral part (VMHvl), and these results have provided the most clear picture to date of the role of the hypothalamus in aggression though its role in mating behavior is less well understood (**Figure 1**). Several novel approaches have been taken to reduce activity in the VMHvl (**Figure 1A**). For example, we reversibly inhibited the VMHvl using virally expressed *Caenorhabditis elegans* ivermectin (IVM)-gated chloride channel (GluCL), which prevents the initiation of action potentials by hyperpolarizing the cells upon ligand binding. We found that attack, but not intermale social investigation, is strongly suppressed by VMHvl inhibition, and this decreased aggression returns to normal levels when VMHvl activity is restored (Lin et al., 2011).

Other studies have capitalized on the fact that the VMHvl is enriched in estrogen receptor alpha (ERα). Since ERα knockout

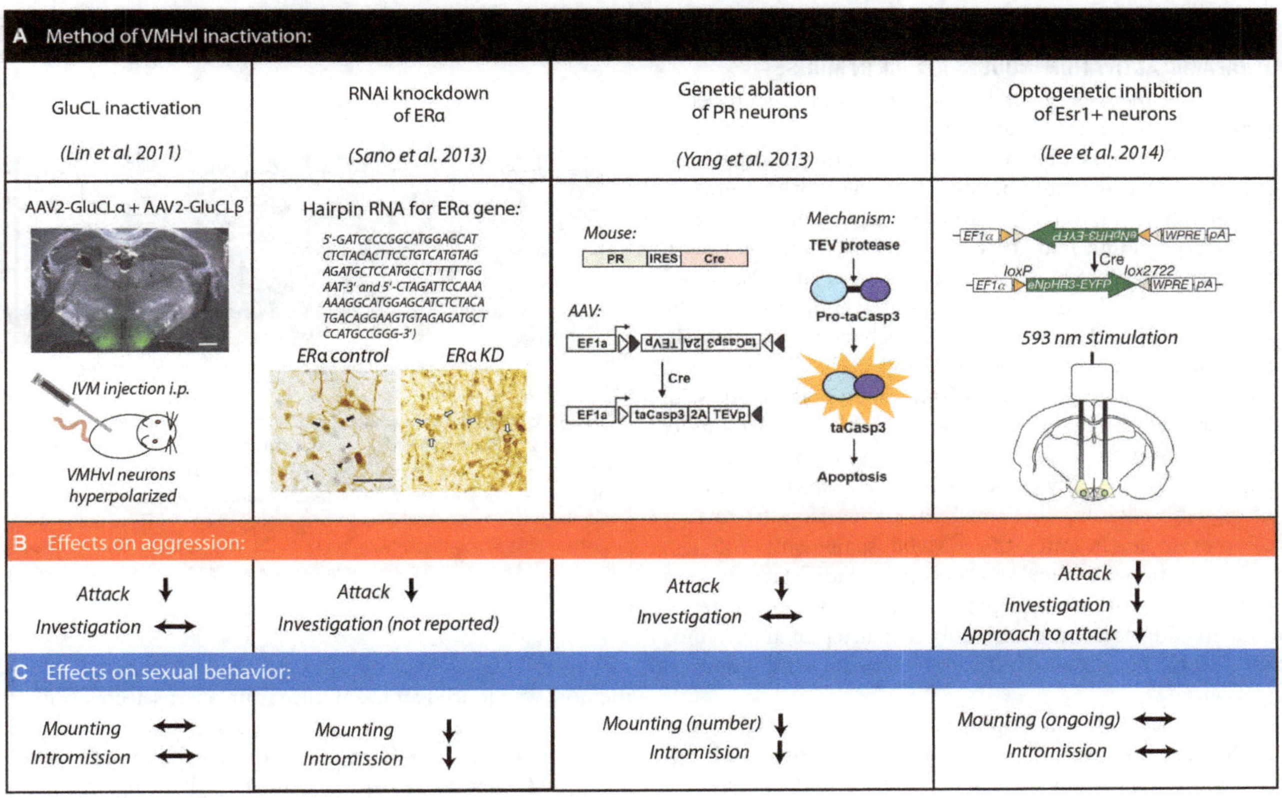

FIGURE 1 | Methods of inactivation of hypothalamic VMHvl neurons to examine fighting and mating behavior. (A) Summary of methods adapted from Lin et al. (2011); Sano et al. (2013); Yang et al. (2013); Lee et al. (2014) with permissions. Effects on aggressive behaviors **(B)** and sexual behaviors **(C)** for each inactivation method.

mice exhibit a severe reduction in aggression, these studies examined the role of ERα cells within the VMHvl on male mouse aggression (Ogawa et al., 1997; Merchenthaler et al., 2004). Both RNAi knockdown of ERα in the VMHvl and ablation of VMHvl cells expressing progesterone receptor (PR), which largely overlaps with the ERα neuronal population, resulted in a dramatic decrease of natural inter-male aggression (Sano et al., 2013; Yang et al., 2013). Most recently, optogenetic inhibition of VMHvl ERα cells during both social approach and attack showed that ongoing activity of VMHvl ERα cells is necessary for both initiation and continuation of attack (Lee et al., 2014).

While the effects of these genetically targeted VMHvl manipulation studies on intermale aggression show clear suppression of attack behaviors, the effects on mating were more varied (**Figure 1C**). When ERα expression is suppressed or PR cells are ablated in the VMHvl, male sexual behavior, like aggression, is reduced. Specifically, manipulated animals spent less time intromitting and achieved fewer ejaculations although the number of mount episodes was not affected (Sano et al., 2013; Yang et al., 2013). In contrast, acute optogenetic inhibition of ERα cells in the VMHvl or pharmacogenetic inhibition of VMHvl in a genetically nonselective manner does not disrupt ongoing sexual behaviors (Lee et al., 2014). These conflicting data suggest that the VMHvl may promote the advance of sexual behaviors but be indispensible for the initiation and execution of attack.

HYPOTHALAMIC ACTIVATION INDUCES ATTACK IN MOUSE

The flipside of the loss-of-function or inactivation study is to artificially activate targeted brain regions and examine the resultant behavioral changes. Electric stimulation of the hypothalamus has been reported to induce attack in a variety of mammalian species including rat, cat and monkey (Lipp, 1978; Lammers et al., 1988; Siegel and Pott, 1988; Siegel et al., 1999). However, electric current activates not only cell bodies but also fibers of passage, thus limiting the control and identification of the neurons responsible for any observed behavioral changes. In comparison, more recent optogenetic approaches have allowed experimenters to target locations within the hypothalamus with higher precision and to identify the targeted cells with more confidence. Advances in location targeting using optogenetic techniques are particularly evident when using mice as a model organism, whose brains are small in comparison to rats or cats. For example, in mice the VMHvl spans only 700 μm along the anterior-posterior axis, 400 μm medial-laterally and 200–400 μm dorsal-ventrally depending on the anterior-posterior position, making this subnuclei only a quarter of the volume of the VMHvl in rats and difficult to isolate with electrical stimulation.

To activate neurons using optogenetic methods, a light gated cation channel, channelrhodopsin (ChR2), often fused with fluorescent protein, is virally or genetically expressed in a specific brain region or a group of molecularly defined cells. Following expression, light pulses delivered through an implanted optic fiber (**Figure 2A**) can control the spiking activity of ChR2 expressing cells with high temporal precision (Boyden et al., 2005). Using this

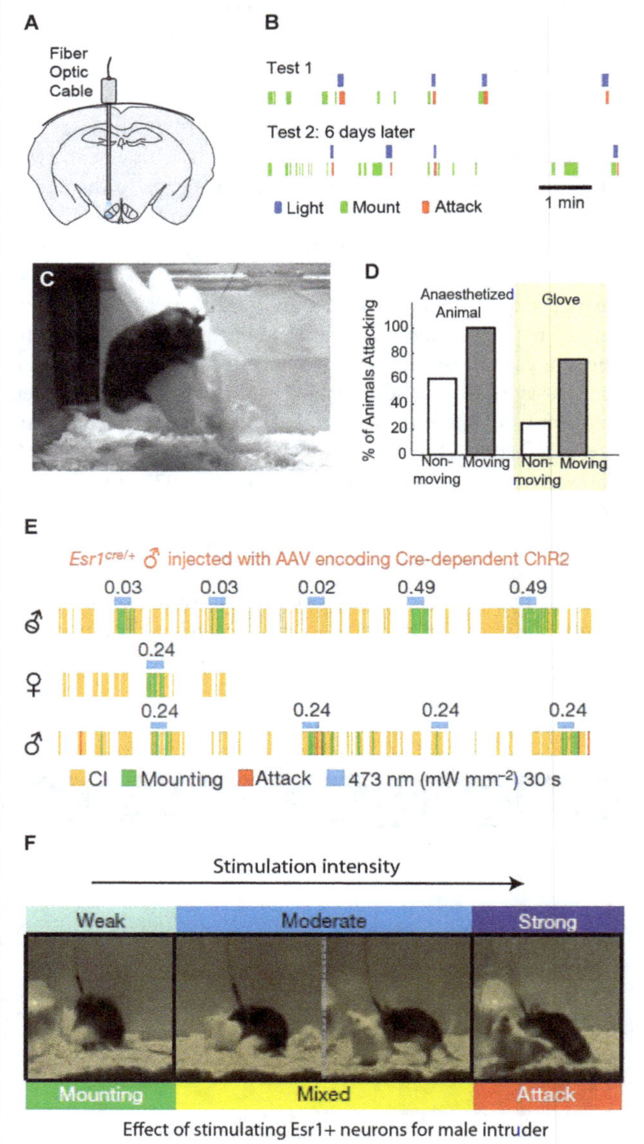

FIGURE 2 | Optogenetic activation of VMHvl neurons evokes attack. Stimulation of wild type VMHvl neurons **(A)** reliably evokes attack to a female or castrated male "intruder" **(B)** and also to either an anesthetized mouse or inanimate object **(C–D)**. **(A–D)** Adapted from Lin et al. (2011) with permissions. Activation of a targeted subpopulation of ERα neurons in the VMHvl evokes mounting at low intensity **(E)**, and attack at high stimulation intensity **(F)** while moderate stimulation evokes a mix of aggressive and sexual behaviors (**E–F** adapted from Lee et al., 2014 with permissions).

method, we induced attack in mice from a nonselectively infected group of cells in VMHvl (**Figures 2B–D**). In contrast, electric stimulation of the VMHvl in mice evoked defensive-like responses and could even cause disengagement during ongoing fighting. These differences in electrically stimulated behaviors are likely due to the activation of axons from the adjacent dorsomedial and central VMH during stimulation which form a part of the defense circuit (Martinez et al., 2008). Although attack can be electrically elicited in rats from a continuous functionally defined "hypothalamic attack area (HAA)" covering VMHvl and its lateral and anterior areas, optogenetic stimulation in mice induces attack only when ChR2 is expressed at least partially in the VMHvl, suggesting that cells in the VMHvl but not its surrounding area are crucial for stimulation-induced attack (Lammers et al., 1988; Lin et al., 2011). This conclusion is further substantiated by restricting ChR2 expression using ERα-CRE transgenic mouse. Activating estrogen receptor-expressing VMHvl cells elicits attack towards males, castrated males, and females (**Figure 2E**), whereas activating estrogen non-expressing cells ("CRE-out") produced no increase in attack (Lee et al., 2014). Taken together, VMHvl has been established as a key hypothalamic node in mediating male mouse aggression. Further experiments which look specifically at the responses of estrogen receptor-expressing neurons during natural behavior, and also at the role of PR expressing neurons will refine our understanding of the role of the VMHvl.

HYPOTHALAMIC NEURAL SUBSTRATES FOR FEMALE AGGRESSION

In most species, males are significantly more aggressive than females, and the vast majority of studies have focused on the role of the VMHvl in intermale aggression. However, although the VMHvl is anatomically sexually dimorphic, with males possessing a larger neural volume, several studies have probed whether there is an analogous hypothalamic substrate for female aggression (Matsumoto and Arai, 1986). Electric stimulation of the hypothalamus in female rats suggests that a functionally defined HAA also exists in the female brain that spans approximately the same area as it does in males (Kruk et al., 1984). More recently, optogenetic activation of the VMHvl ERα subpopulation in female mice failed to elicit attack and instead caused stimulated females to exhibit male-style mounting behaviors (Lee et al., 2014). While these results may suggest that different neural substrates mediate female aggression vs. male aggression in mice, several alternative explanations remain possible. First, in females, aggression may be mediated by non-ERα cells or anatomically distinct neurons. Instead, ERα cells in VMHvl are critical for female sexual behavior: suppressing ERα expression in the VMHvl using RNAi or deleting PR expressing cells in VMHvl significantly reduces receptivity of manipulated animals (Sano et al., 2013; Yang et al., 2013). Second, failure to evoke aggression may be related to the specific animals used in these experiments, since natural aggression levels of female mice or rats differs dramatically between laboratory strains. For instance, the CPB WEzob female rats used for electric stimulation present high level of aggression towards intruders even during non-lactating periods, whereas the genetic background of ERα-CRE mice is C57BL/6 which exhibit little aggression even during lactation (Broida and Svare, 1982; Jones and Brain, 1987). It remains possible that the neural substrates of aggression are abnormally suppressed or degenerated in female C57BL/6 mice, which may make it difficult to elicit attack with artificial activation. Future experiments using mouse strains with higher female aggression levels may help explain the observed behavioral difference in female rats and mice during hypothalamic stimulation.

INTERPRETING STIMULATION-EVOKED ATTACK: INSIGHTS FROM RODENT BEHAVIOR

First asked by Hess (1928) almost a century ago, the question of how we should interpret the effects of stimulation on aggression still remains unresolved. It is tempting to posit the role of the hypothalamus in aggression as a simple "attack generator", but such descriptions do not account for the complexity of stimulation-evoked responses. To start with, both earlier electric stimulation and more recent optogenetic activation experiments demonstrate that hypothalamic evoked attack depends on the presence and reactions of an attack target. When a resident mouse is alone in its home cage (with no target to direct an attack towards), light stimulation induces only slight increases in locomotion, and animals do not exhibit any of the motor patterns typical of aggression (Lin et al., 2011). Similarly, electric stimulation of HAA in rats produces no motor change although it does cause fast adrenocortical stress responses even in the absence of an opponent (Kruk et al., 2004).

In both rats and mice, hypothalamic activation induced attack is also affected by opponents' variable defensive tactics. For instance, if an opponent's back is against the wall, stimulated mice often abort the evoked attack, possibly in part because the preferred biting location is not immediately accessible. In rats, the mode of attack depends critically on the response and location of the opponent: attack jumps arise when the opponents go into an upright position whereas so-called "clinch fights" occur when one of the rats loses balance following an attack jump (Kruk et al., 1983). Because the specific actions evoked by stimulation depend on the context of the fight, the effects of stimulation are unlikely to be that of a stereotyped motor response. Consistent with this conclusion, neither VMHvl nor HAA has direct connection with known voluntary motor coordination structures, such as the basal ganglia (Canteras et al., 1994; Roeling et al., 1994). However, while stimulation-induced attack appears to require a target, the identity of the target may be suboptimal. In both rats and mice, hypothalamic stimulation can elicit quick attack towards anesthetized or dead conspecifics, potential mates, or certain inanimate objects (like an inflated rubber glove), all of which evoke no attack naturally (Koolhaas, 1978; Kruk et al., 1979; Lin et al., 2011). Thus, hypothalamic stimulation induced attack appears to provide a fictive signal that is independent of social context. One possibility is that hypothalamic stimulation increases the animal's predisposition or motivation to attack, while the specific movements that comprise the attack itself are encoded in downstream areas. This is discussed later in this review.

HYPOTHALAMIC CONTROL OF INNATE BEHAVIOR

How are aggression-related neurons organized in relation to neurons mediating other innate behaviors? Answers to this question have evolved over time as activation techniques have become increasingly refined. In previous studies, it was discovered that radically different behaviors could be evoked by electrically stimulating from the same electrode tip if one varied either the stimulation duration, intensity, frequency, or experimental environment (Valenstein et al., 1968; Watson, 1977; Kruk, 2014). The lack of a stable behavioral response from a given anatomical location led researchers to initially conclude that there was no fixed association between specific hypothalamic neural substrates and individual behavioral outputs. As recording and stimulation technologies improved, the size of the stimulation electrodes decreased such that anatomical locations could be targeted with greater precision. Systematic mapping efforts with these electrodes revealed that predictable behaviors could be evoked from specific coordinates, demonstrating that neural substrates underlying behaviors are not diffusively present throughout the hypothalamus (Kruk et al., 1983; Lammers et al., 1988). However, even with these technical refinements, multiple behaviors could often be elicited from the same area across changing stimulation intensity.

Given this overlap of behaviors evoked within a single stimulation site, the question remains whether discrete sets of neurons trigger specific patterns of behavior, or whether behavioral states are encoded by complex patterns of activation in overlapping neural circuits. More directly, do changes in evoked behaviors over stimulation intensity reflect an "intensity coding" in the hypothalamus or a limitation in cell targeting? Recent results using both optogenetics and imaging techniques suggest that the answer appears to be both. For some co-elicited yet distinct behaviors, such as flight and attack, targeted optogenetic stimulation experiments demonstrate that these behaviors likely involve non-overlapping but adjacent hypothalamic areas (Lin et al., 2011). Other behaviors that are commonly co-elicited by electrical stimulation, including social grooming, investigation and attack, can be similarly evoked with optogenetic stimulation: low intensity stimulation induces forceful investigation (sometimes called "close investigation") of the intruder while higher intensity stimulation can elicit attack (Lee et al., 2014), though these behaviors may sometimes be considered part of the aggressive repertoire.

Surprisingly, although mounting has never been reported to be elicited from HAA using electrical stimulation, optogenetic activation in mice has revealed that mounting and fighting can be induced by activating ERα neurons in the VMHvl at different light intensity: low intensity stimulation induces mounting towards both females, males, and castrated males, while higher light intensity evokes mixed attack, with mounting initially and eventually attack exclusively (**Figure 2F**; Lee et al., 2014), Whether the same ERα neurons are involved in mediating both mating and fighting (which would be strong evidence for intensity coding) is not yet known, as ERα neuron activity during mating and/or fighting has not been reported. However, extracellular recordings from non-selective cells in the VMHvl reveals no simple relationship between VMHvl cell responses to males and females (See next section). VMHvl activity escalates as animals switch from male investigation to attack but decreases as animals switch from female investigation to mounting (Lin et al., 2011). Optogenetic activation of a subset of ERα cells at a fixed rate and intensity is unlikely to faithfully recapture the natural activity progression during female or male interaction, and instead, low intensity activation may more closely resemble the female conspecific induced response, while high intensity activation may resemble a more male-like response pattern.

NEURONAL ACTIVITY IN THE HYPOTHALAMUS

A full understanding of hypothalamic functioning during complex social behaviors such as aggression will require a complete description of changing neural activity obtained during well-controlled social environments. However, most of what we know about neural activity during aggression is a crude proxy based on changes in either metabolic level (e.g., 2-deoxyglucose mapping and functional magnetic resonance imaging (fMRI)) or from the expression of immediate early genes (IEGs) such as Fos (Sagar et al., 1988; Kollack-Walker and Newman, 1995; Kollack-Walker et al., 1997; Delville et al., 2000; Gammie and Nelson, 2001; Hasen and Gammie, 2005, 2006; Veening et al., 2005; Haller et al., 2006; Ferris et al., 2008). Across all species and all social behaviors, only a handful of studies have attempted to directly link spiking activity and behaviors by recording populations of hypothalamic neurons in awake behaving animals (Oomura et al., 1983, 1988; Aou et al., 1984, 1988; Horio et al., 1986; Shimura et al., 1994; Lin et al., 2011; Falkner et al., 2014), yet the results from these studies shed considerable light on hypothalamic functioning.

IMMEDIATE EARLY GENES AND THE HYPOTHALAMUS DURING AGGRESSION

The induction of IEGs, in particular Fos, has been of great use throughout the last few decades in mapping brain-wide patterns of activation for both neural and endocrinological signals (Sagar et al., 1988; Bullitt, 1990; Sheng and Greenberg, 1990; Hoffman et al., 1993). Since the time course of IEG induction is relatively slow (5–30 min for IEG mRNA and 1–2 h for IEG protein), it is incapable of reporting detailed correlation between specific behavioral events (e.g., attack) and neural activity. Instead, IEG expression gives a general impression of accumulated brain activation over minutes to hours. Furthermore, the relationship between IEG induction and cell spiking activities remains uncertain. The most popular IEG—Fos, is a transcription factor induced by elevated cAMP levels and is not necessarily associated with action potential increases (Metz and Ziff, 1991). Nevertheless, these experiments are useful in that they provide a comprehensive view of candidate brain regions involved in a behavior. Moreover, examining patterns of co-expression of IEGs and other genetic markers or tracers can provide additional information regarding features of the behaviorally relevant neural population, such as their neurotransmitter type or projection pattern.

A typical IEG induction paradigm for the study of aggression is the "resident-intruder" assay. In this paradigm, a male intruder is introduced into the home cage of a singly housed male conspecific for 5 min to an hour, which typically elicits repeated investigative and attack behaviors from the aggressive resident towards the intruder. Across rodent species, this resident-intruder test induces elevated Fos expression in several hypothalamic nuclei, including the medial preoptic nucleus (MPN), AHN, VMHvl and premammillary nucleus ventral part (PMv; **Figure 3A**; Kollack-Walker and Newman, 1995; Delville et al., 2000; Halasz et al., 2002a; Veening et al., 2005; Haller et al., 2006). The increase in Fos-expressing neurons following induction ranges from 50% to 300% of the baseline activation level. Across many IEG studies, the co-activation of these four

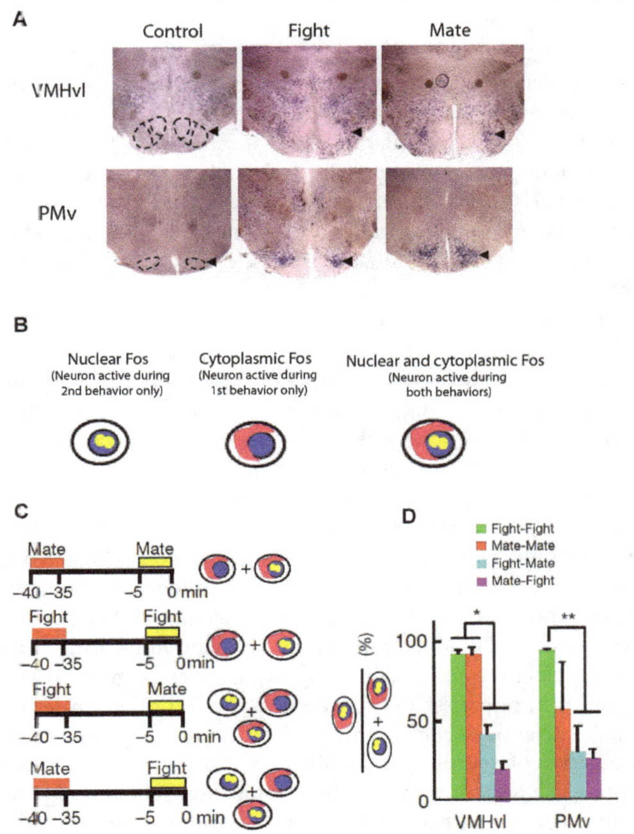

FIGURE 3 | Immediate early gene induction in hypothalamic neurons during fighting and mating behaviors. (A) Traditional Fos induction paradigms show increased activation during fighting and mating in the VMHvl and PMv but do not reveal whether their activation patterns overlap. **(B–C)** Methodology of Fos CatFish paradigm, which allows for localization of neurons involved in both behaviors (fight-mate and mate fight) in comparison to the reliability of a single behavior (mate-mate and fight-fight). **(D)** Fos CatFish induction reveals largely non-overlapping hypothalamic populations activated during fighting and mating. **(A–D** adapted from Lin et al., 2011 with permissions).

hypothalamic nuclei during the resident intruder assay is consistent with their patterns of connectivity. Since the MPN, VMHvl and PMv are reciprocally interconnected and all receive inputs from the medial amygdala subdivision responding to female cues, they have also been proposed as the hypothalamic reproductive circuit (Swanson, 2000). Although AHN is traditionally included in the hypothalamic defense circuit, it receives moderate input from the VMHvl and represents the only major connection between the reproductive and defense hypothalamic circuits and so may place a more specialized role in aggression (Canteras et al., 1994).

Most Fos induction studies also attempt to examine the specificity of the region in mediating aggression by comparing Fos induction after aggression to the Fos activation pattern after a related behavior. For example, Delville et al. (2000) compared Fos expression of hamsters exposed to a woodblock carrying intruder odor and those exposed to an alive intruder and noticed increased Fos in the VMHvl after fighting, supporting a role of VMHvl in consummatory aspect of aggression and not simply that of sensory relay for male social odor cues (Delville et al., 2000). However, comparing activation patterns between two behaviors between different animals cannot reveal whether the same or different cells are involved, making it sometimes difficult to interpret these results. For example, Kollack-Walker et al. reported that PMv and VMHvl are activated similarly after both fighting and mating, though it was unclear whether these activated neurons represented overlapping or non-overlapping populations (Kollack-Walker and Newman, 1995). Similarly, defeated animals who were on the receiving end of attack showed stronger Fos expression in VMHvl than the attackers, even though activating VMHvl induces attack itself (Kollack-Walker et al., 1997). Do these extra neurons in defeated neurons represent a separately activated population of neurons?

These results demonstrate the necessity of comparing IEG activation patterns following two behaviors within the same animal. Since IEGs are first transcribed in the nucleus and then (after ~30 min) translocate to the cytoplasm, the IEG pattern associated with two properly spaced behaviors can be distinguished based on mRNA localization (**Figure 3B**; Guzowski et al., 2001). This method, named Cellular Compartment Analysis of Temporal Activity by Fluorescence *In Situ* Hybridization (CatFish), revealed importantly that mating and fighting induced Fos in male mice is mostly localized in intermingled but non-overlapping cells throughout the hypothalamus (**Figures 3C,D**; Lin et al., 2011). Recently, several other genetic methods that permanently mark IEG expressing cells in a short window have also been described (Reijmers et al., 2007; Guenthner et al., 2013; Kawashima et al., 2013); these methods can be potentially of great use in future studies to address the relationship between neural population(s) involved in aggression and other related behaviors.

NEURAL RECORDING IN THE HYPOTHALAMUS

Perhaps because of its heterogeneity, small size and deep position in the brain, the hypothalamus has long resisted physiological scrutiny. In particular, *in vivo* recordings performed during ethologically relevant behaviors (e.g., fighting) have been difficult because these behaviors often involve brief violent bursts of action that are not ideal for conducting stable recordings, and also because previous recording technologies were too cumbersome for animals to perform complex, quick movement with these devices attached to their heads. Fortunately, recent advances in both the stability and size of chronic extracellular recording technology have allowed us to begin interrogating these nuclei during behaviors of interest.

We performed chronic *in vivo* recordings of populations of VMHvl neurons during fighting and mating (Lin et al., 2011) and compared these responses to a variety of interactions with social and nonsocial stimuli including a castrated male, a source of either male and female urine, and a novel object (Falkner et al., 2014). Consistent with the results of functional manipulation studies, over 40% of VMHvl cells increase their activity when the recorded mice encounter a male intruder (**Figures 4A–C**). VMHvl activity begins to increase several seconds prior to

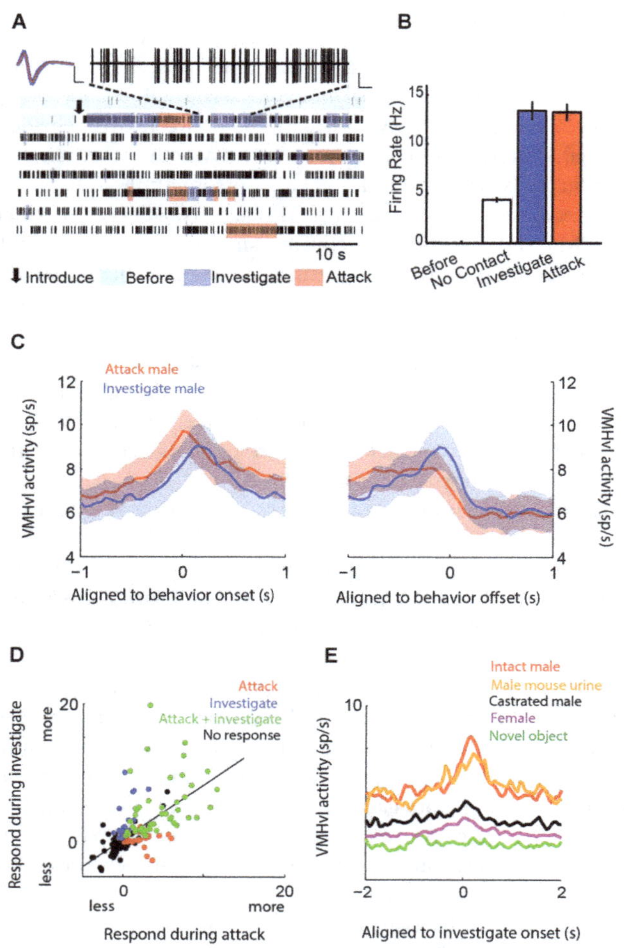

FIGURE 4 | Neural recordings of hypothalamic neurons show activation during attack and investigation of a male intruder. Single neurons **(A–B)** and population average peri-event time histogram **(C)** exhibit acute increases in activity at the onset of both attack and investigation. **(D)** Individual neurons can show selectivity for attack (red), investigation (blue), both behaviors (green), or no increase during either of those behaviors (black). **(E)** VMHvl neurons are activated during the investigation of a source of male mouse urine, but activated little by a castrated male, female, or novel object. **(A–B** adapted from Lin et al., 2011, **C–E** adapted from Falkner et al., 2014 with permissions).

attack initiation and reaches its peak at the onset of attack. Activity then persists at an elevated level for the duration of attack, plummeting when attack ceases (**Figure 4C**). Like attack, neurons also acutely increase in activity during the investigation of a male intruder and these responses are highly correlated: neurons that exhibit increased activity during attack are also likely to increase during investigation (**Figure 4D**). While these responses are correlated across the population, individual neurons may respond selectively during attack (red dots **Figure 4D**), during investigation (blue dots **Figure 4D**), or during both behaviors (green dots **Figure 4D**) such that they may be preferentially active during either the sensory acquisition or the action phase of aggression. Black dots in **Figure 4D** represent neurons that increase neither during attack nor investigation.

Similar to social behaviors, olfactory cues alone appear to be a strong driving force to hypothalamic activity. VMHvl neurons increase their firing rate during the investigation of a source of male mouse urine to similar levels as when the animal investigates a male conspecific (**Figure 4E**). Activity is inversely correlated with either the distance from the male intruder or source of urine. In contrast, investigation of castrated males, who produce reduced levels of social olfactory cues, evoked little increase in VMHvl neuron activity, demonstrating that the odor cue may be more important than the presence of a social stimulus in driving hypothalamic activity (**Figure 4E**).

Neural recordings can begin to directly address how signals for fighting and mating are intermingled within populations of hypothalamic neurons. Unlike IEG studies, which do not have the temporal resolution to address differences between the investigative phase and the action phase (attack or mount), physiological activity in the VMHvl shows clear differences in activity during separable phases of male and female interactions (**Figure 5A**). During interactions with an intruder male, a substantial subpopulation shows an increase during investigation of both a male and a male social odor, and this can be followed by a transition into a greater degree of activation during attack (**Figures 5B–D**). In contrast, responses during the investigation of a female or a female social odor cue are more mixed, engaging a smaller subpopulation of neurons, with a higher portion of them exhibiting suppressive responses during the investigation. The action phase of an encounter with a female (mounting and subsequent mating behaviors) results in a decrease or suppression of overall activity, the opposite of the action phase during intermale encounters (**Figures 5C–E**). This leaves open the critical yet unanswered question of how stimulation (which should increase activity) of ERα neurons in the VMHvl leads to a behavior (mounting) that under natural conditions, is coupled with an overall decrease in activity. Further experiments examining the specific contribution of these neurons during sexual behavior are necessary to resolve this discrepancy.

THE HYPOTHALAMUS AND AGGRESSIVE MOTIVATION

Aggressive motivation can be loosely defined as the internal state that drives animals to seek out opportunities to perform aggressive actions. Signals in the brain that convey information about aggressive motivation should precede and perhaps predict future aggressive actions. Recordings of VMHvl neurons during intermale aggression revealed that VMHvl activity appears to carry information regarding past, current and future attack events (Falkner et al., 2014). First, neurons that respond during the investigation of a male intruder have an increased response if that investigative episode transitions to an attack compared to the response during investigation if the animal turns and walks away without attack (**Figure 6A**). Second, ramping activity prior to the onset of an attack in VMHvl neurons predicts duration of the subsequent attack: higher activity during the pre-attack period correlates with longer attacks (**Figure 6B**). Next, the time elapsed from the previous attack (the inter-attack interval) can predict activity of the onset of the next attack: the longer the wait

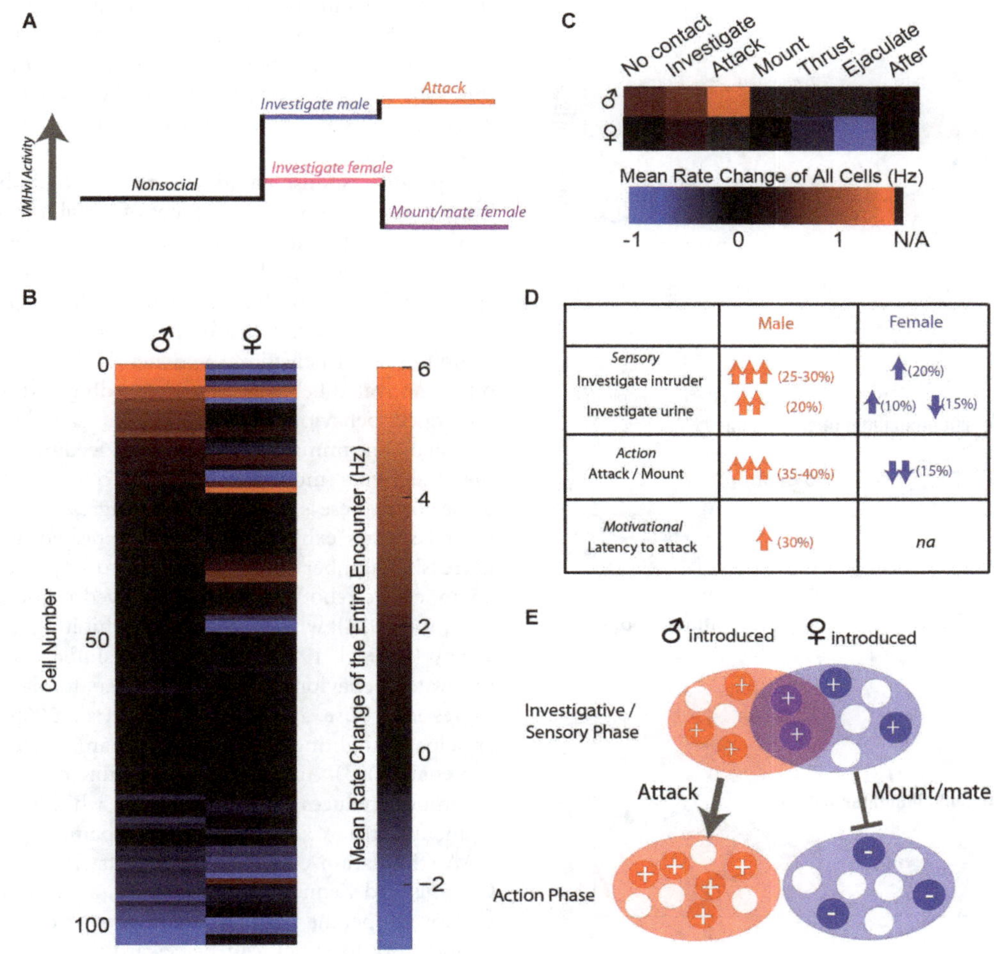

FIGURE 5 | VMHvl activity during male and female interactions reveals opposing response patterns. (A) Average activity during a male interaction increases during investigation and attack, while average activity increases slightly during investigation of a female and is suppressed during subsequent sexual behaviors. **(B)** Response profile across VMHvl neurons during social interactions suggests that neurons that increase activity during male interactions may be suppressed during female interactions but not vice versa. **(C–D)** Summary of VMHvl neurons participating in separable phases of social interactions. **(E)** Schematic illustrating that neurons may increase in activity during the sensory acquisition phase of social behavior to both sexes, while the action phase of the social interaction results in opposing activation patterns in populations with less overlap. **(B–C** adapted from Lin et al., 2011 with permissions).

from the last attack, the larger the attack response is for the next attack (**Figure 6C**). Furthermore, VMHvl activity is negatively correlated with latency to the next attack even when the animal's proximity to odor cues and motion are controlled for. Lastly, increased VMHvl activity towards male intruder or male urine is sustained after the stimulus source is removed (Falkner et al., 2014). Thus, VMHvl neurons convey not only a rich variety of conspecific sensory cues, but also seem to predict aspects of future aggression, consistent with a role for the VMHvl in aggressive motivation.

Stimulation-evoked behaviors can also be interpreted through the lens of aggressive motivation. Early electric stimulation experiments showed that hypothalamic stimulation promotes not only attack but also approach towards a potential attack target (Roberts and Kiess, 1964). A common motivational mechanism that supports seeking behavior for both aggressive and sexual encounters could potentially resolve the apparent conflict between the observation that both sexual and aggressive actions can be evoked by stimulation and evidence from *in vivo* recordings which shows that VMHvl activity increases during aggression and decreases for sexual behaviors. If stimulation acts by increasing levels of motivated approach behavior, the end action may be determined by the sensory information or the specifics of the social interaction.

While these results seems to suggest a hypothalamic substrate for aggressive seeking behavior, it is difficult to assess the relationship between hypothalamic activity, approach behavior, and the social target being approached, because sensory stimuli are constantly changing during approach behavior and these changes may affect ongoing neural activity beyond the effects of the

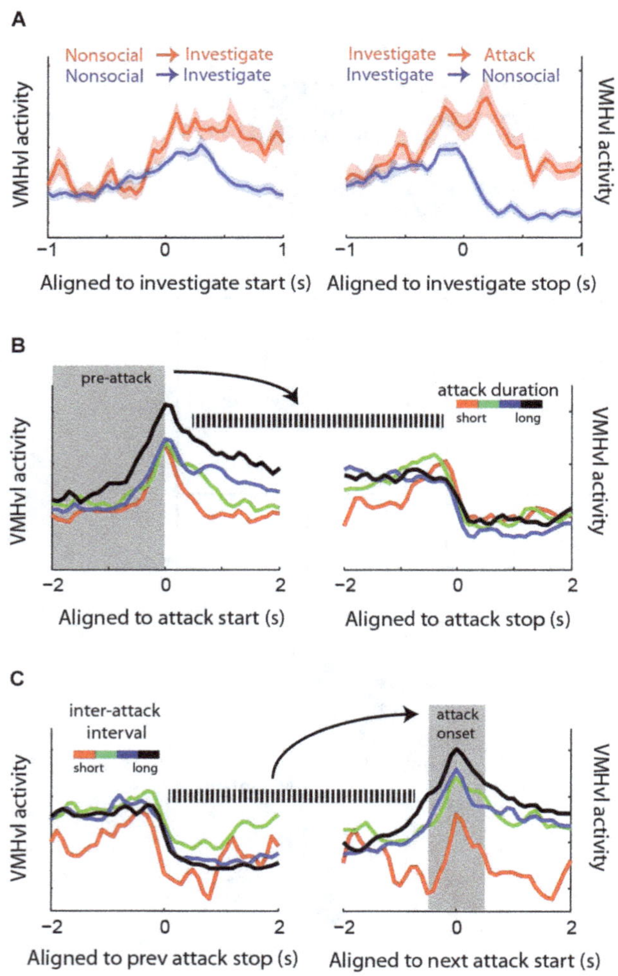

FIGURE 6 | Neuronal activity in the VMHvl is predictive of past and future aggressive events. (A) Activity at the onset of a male investigative episode is increased if that episode leads to attack. **(B)** Activity prior to the start of the attack predicts the duration of the subsequent attack. **(C)** The inter-attack interval (i.e., time elapsed from the last attack) inversely correlates with activity at the onset of the next attack. (adapted from Falkner et al., 2014 with permissions).

stimulation. These confounds necessitate the adoption and adaptation of new methods to assay social motivation. In many classic neuroscience experiments, motivation is assayed using standard operant response paradigms. In these paradigms, a reward (in most cases food or drink) is paired with an initially neutral motor response such as a nosepoke or lever press. By tuning the schedule of the reward delivery, the amount of work an animal is willing to expend to acquire the reward can be assayed, and this "work" reflects the motivation of the animal for the given reward. These paradigms have been commonly adapted to assay the motivation to acquire food, the motivational state that we call "hunger", and several studies have found a clear link between hypothalamic activity and hunger. Most compellingly, optogenetic activation of agouti-related peptide (AGRP) neurons in the arcuate nucleus of the hypothalamus not only induces eating when food is readily available, but also promotes an increase in bar pressing to obtain food that is not immediately present (Krashes et al., 2011). In this way, an operant response can be used to disentangle the motivational state from the sensory cues associated from the reward itself.

Operant response paradigms have been applied thus far in a limited way to assess various types of social motivation including sexual (Everitt and Stacey, 1987) and maternal (Lee et al., 2000) motivation. Is there an equivalent motivational state for aggression? While we have no word in the English language like hunger to encapsulate this motivational state, aggression clearly exhibits several behavioral and neural features associated with other motivated behaviors such as feeding and sex. For example, motivated behaviors typically exhibit satiation, meaning that repeated consummatory actions (e.g., feeding or mating) reduce the underlying motivation to seek out further opportunities to perform these specific actions. Aggressive individuals across several species exhibit satiety after repeated attacks, exhibiting decreasing number of initiated attacks over time, and then exhibit an appetitive rebound after a prolonged non-aggressive interval (Connor, 1974), with some species exhibiting persistent levels of satiety (Potegal, 1984). Additionally, similar to its role in other motivated behaviors, dopamine appears to play a central role in aggression (Wise, 2004; de Almeida et al., 2005). When animals anticipate a fighting opportunity, dopamine levels increase (Ferrari et al., 2003). Antagonizing dopamine receptor in the nucleus accumbens reduces natural aggression, while lesions of the ventral tegmental area (VTA), a harbor for dopaminergic cells, blocks the HAA stimulation-evoked attack in rats (Proshansky et al., 1974; Couppis and Kennedy, 2008). Finally, a handful of studies have employed operant response paradigms to demonstrate that the opportunity to attack can be rewarding for certain individuals (Turnbough and Lloyd, 1973; Fish et al., 2002, 2005; Couppis and Kennedy, 2008; May and Kennedy, 2009). Aggressive mice can readily learn the association between the operant response and the introduction of a weaker intruder that serves as the "reward". In these studies, fixed interval and fixed ratio schedules have been employed to assess the motivation for a single aggressive event. The operationalization of aggressive interaction is a critical next step for assessing the relationship between hypothalamic activity and aggressive motivation, since these paradigms allow for better control of sensory and motor variables and may distinguish the motivated state from the aggressive action.

TOWARDS A COMPUTATIONAL FRAMEWORK FOR HYPOTHALAMIC FUNCTIONING

While new techniques for functional manipulation and recording have deepened our understanding of the role of the hypothalamus in aggression, we are still far from a complete quantitative framework. However, our knowledge about evoked behaviors and types of signals that drive neurons in the VMHvl allows us to speculate about potential models for aggression. One possible model is that the VMHvl acts by performing a sensorimotor transformation, relaying a behaviorally relevant motor command through the transformation of specific sensory signals.

How could this transformation be implemented? Decades of neurophysiological recordings from defined cortical and subcortical circuits provide a useful model for understanding these computations. The oculomotor system is perhaps the canonical circuit described as carrying out a sensorimotor transformation. Sensory information in the form of visual stimuli can be used to guide specific motor sequences, in this case, saccadic eye movements. Neurons at the input level of this circuit can respond to purely sensory (visual) information, and neurons at the output level signal the upcoming movement. In this sensorimotor circuit, sensory information is mapped from visual coordinates into saccade coordinates by neurons in the parietal cortex, superior colliculus, and other key structures that contain neural representations of either the visual stimulus, the saccadic location, or both, and are subject to constant updating by changing environmental factors (Colby and Goldberg, 1999; Optican, 2005). Importantly, neurons in the oculomotor system can signal the location of visual information that is no longer present, and this "persistent" activity can connect sensory representations and motor signals that are separated in time.

Hypothalamic circuitry for aggression shares some broad similarities to other sensorimotor transformation circuits. Neurons in the VMHvl can preferentially signal information about the sensory environment (e.g., olfactory cues from male and female conspecifics) and also can preferentially signal the future actions that are coupled with these cues (e.g., attack or mating). In addition, neurons that signal both sensory and action related information (green dots **Figure 4D**) could serve to bridge sensory and motor representations within the VMHvl. However, since olfactory sensory information is encoded at a different level of complexity relative to the visual system, future computational models will need to account for these fundamental differences. In addition to being supported by current physiological characterizations, the anatomical architecture of the VMHvl could potentially support such a computation. The VMHvl, a densely glutamatergic subnucleus, has a high degree of recurrent connectivity that could support the persistence of a sensory or extrasensory signal (Nishizuka and Pfaff, 1989; Choi et al., 2005). If the role of the VMHvl is to carry out a sensorimotor transformation, one testable hypothesis would be that neurons carrying more action-related information may preferentially project to premotor structures, while neurons carrying more sensory-related information will be preferentially targeted by sensory relays (e.g., medial amygdala) and project more locally, allowing that information to persist within the VMHvl microcircuit. In future studies, this hypothesis and others could be tested by combining projection specific tagging and electrophysiology to compare electrophysiological responses with connectivity (Jennings et al., 2013). Moreover, future studies on aggressive motivation may reveal discrete or overlapping neuronal populations within the hypothalamus that may serve to combine motivational signals with incoming sensory information to drive aggressive actions (**Figure 7**).

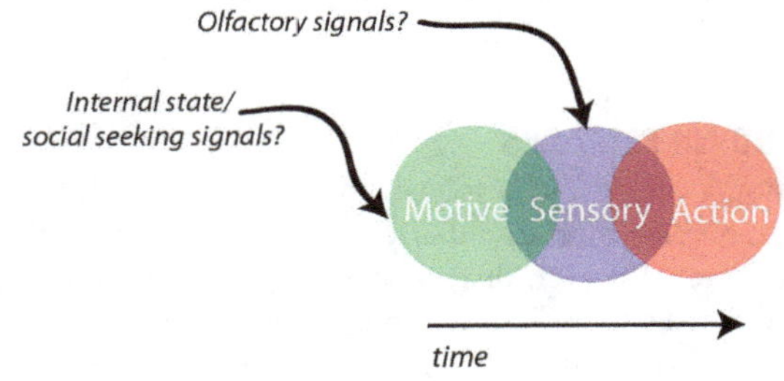

FIGURE 7 | Sensorimotor transformation as a possible model for hypothalamic function. VMHvl neurons have overlapping sensory, action, and sensory-action preferring neurons that may be influenced by social specific olfactory and internal motivational signals.

THE AGGRESSION CIRCUIT BEYOND VMHvl

Of course, the hypothalamus does not act alone to elicit aggression. In rats, the efferent connections from hypothalamic aggression related cells have been examined by comparing anterograde tracing patterns from putative HAA and its adjacent "hypothalamic grooming area (HGA)" and by examining HAA stimulation of induced IEG expression or deoxyglucose uptake pattern (Roeling et al., 1993, 1994; Roberts and Nagel, 1996; Halasz et al., 2002b). These techniques revealed candidate regions that may be recruited during hypothalamic stimulation, many of which were also activated during stimulation of non-attack related areas. This overlap is not surprising, as the HAA covers multiple hypothalamic nuclei with heterogeneous connectivity patterns, and delineations between anatomically and functionally identified subregions of the hypothalamus are unclear.

The recent identification of ERα/PR cells in the VMHvl as a key population for aggression offers an opportunity to track other components in the circuit genetically (Yang et al., 2013; Lee et al., 2014). Yang et al. (2013) used lentivirus to express alkaline phosphatase (PLAP) which labels neuronal processes of PR-expressing cells in the VMHvl and observed a refreshingly simple projection pattern: PLAP+ axons were found in the anteroventral periventricular hypothalamic nucleus (AVPV), preoptic area (POA) and periaqueductal gray (PAG). Interestingly, the PLAP+ axons in AVPV are sexually dimorphic: the fiber density in females is 7-folder greater than the density in males. While unexpected, this difference may be related to the well-known role of VMHvl in lordosis (Pfaff and Sakuma, 1979a,b). Other previously identified VMHvl downstream targets including the medial amygdala (MEA) and bed nucleus of stria terminalis (BNST) didn't appear to be targeted appreciably by the PLAP+ axons (Yang et al., 2013), suggesting that aggression-related cells may selectively project to a subset of VMHvl downstream regions. In rat, stimulation of PAG can also elicit attack although the responses are sometimes accompanied by severe motor disturbance (Mos et al., 1982). Though POA is mostly known for its role in male sexual behaviors, electric lesion of the area suppresses both sexual and aggressive behaviors in rats without affecting animals' predatory mouse killing behavior (Bermond, 1982; Albert et al., 1986a,b). Similar to the VMHvl, both PAG and POA are enriched in hormone receptors such as ERα and androgen receptor (AR), which have profound influence on social behaviors (Murphy et al., 1999; Merchenthaler et al., 2004). Future studies using optogenetic tools to achieve pathway specific functional manipulation will help elucidate the roles of VMHvl → POA and VMHvl → PAG projections in VMHvl evoked aggression (Tye and Deisseroth, 2012).

CONCLUDING REMARKS

Aggression, which has evolved to resolve competition and secure resources, is an essential part of many species' ethological repertoire. However, disregulated or pathological aggression poses huge risks to society. Although aggression studies thrived in the early and middle 20th century, this line of research has substantially declined since then, especially in comparison to other innate and "emotional" behaviors such as fear (Blanchard et al., 2003). The reasons for the decline are complicated and include issues related to both animal and social welfare (Blanchard et al., 2003; Anderson, 2012). Efforts to translate research advances in aggression into clinical use during the 1950s and 1960s have a sordid history, as prominent researchers of the day advocated the use of brain stimulation techniques and psychosurgery on prisoners and as a solution to race-charged problems such as urban rioting and political protest (Mark et al., 1968; Breggin, 1975a,b). At least in part because of this, research on aggression fell out of fashion over the next few decades.

In addition to the political over-interpretation of aggression studies beyond the line of basic research, technical limitations also obstructed advances in the field. As mentioned, classic lesion and stimulation methods lack adequate spatial resolution to pinpoint aggression-relevant cells. However, the recent emergence of genetically based functional manipulation and tracing methods allows one to target neurons with specific functional relevance, projection patterns or molecular features, greatly improving precision in cell manipulation (Lima et al., 2009; Cardin et al., 2010; Yizhar et al., 2011; Madisen et al., 2012; Osakada et al., 2012; Tye and Deisseroth, 2012; Guenthner et al., 2013; Kawashima et al., 2013). Moreover, miniaturized *in vivo* electrophysiological recording devices, wired or wireless, and deep brain optical measuring devices make it possible to follow cell activity reliably over a long period (Fan et al., 2011; Szuts et al., 2011; Cui et al., 2013; Ziv et al., 2013). Using these novel approaches, breakthroughs in research in animals may lead to a greater understanding of pathological violence and potentially to more humane treatment strategies.

REFERENCES

Albert, D. J., Dyson, E. M., Walsh, M. L., and Gorzalka, B. B. (1987). Intermale social aggression in rats: suppression by medial hypothalamic lesions independently of enhanced defensiveness or decreased testicular testosterone. *Physiol. Behav.* 39, 693–698. doi: 10.1016/0031-9384(87)90252-6

Albert, D. J., and Walsh, M. L. (1982). Medial hypothalamic lesions in the rat enhance reactivity and mouse killing but not social aggression. *Physiol. Behav.* 28, 791–795. doi: 10.1016/0031-9384(82)90195-0

Albert, D. J., Walsh, M. L., Gorzalka, B. B., Mendelson, S., and Zalys, C. (1986a). Intermale social aggression—suppression by medial preoptic area lesions. *Physiol. Behav.* 38, 169–173. doi: 10.1016/0031-9384(86)90151-4

Albert, D. J., Walsh, M. L., Gorzalka, B. B., Mendelson, S., and Zalys, C. (1986b). Intermale social aggression: suppression by medial preoptic area lesions. *Physiol. Behav.* 38, 169–173. doi: 10.1016/0031-9384(86)90151-4

Anderson, D. J. (2012). Optogenetics, sex and violence in the brain: implications for psychiatry. *Biol. Psychiatry* 71, 1081–1089. doi: 10.1016/j.biopsych.2011.11.012

Aou, S., Oomura, Y., and Yoshimatsu, H. (1988). Neuron activity of the ventromedial hypothalamus and the medial preoptic area of the female monkey during sexual-behavior. *Brain Res.* 455, 65–71. doi: 10.1016/0006-8993(88)90115-1

Aou, S., Yoshimatsu, H., and Oomura, Y. (1984). Medial preoptic neuronal responses to connatural females in sexually inactive male monkeys (Macaca fuscata). *Neurosci. Lett.* 44, 217–221. doi: 10.1016/0304-3940(84)90084-3

Bard, P. (1928). A diencephalic mechanism for the expression of rage with special reference to the sympathetic nervous system. *Am. J. Physiol.* 84, 490–515.

Bermond, B. (1982). Effects of medial preoptic hypothalamus anterior lesions on 3 kinds of behavior in the rat—intermale aggressive, male-sexual and mouse-killing behavior. *Aggress. Behav.* 8, 335–354. doi: 10.1002/1098-2337(1982)8:4<335::aid-ab2480080403>3.0.co;2-8

Blanchard, R. J., Wall, P. M., and Blanchard, D. C. (2003). Problems in the study of rodent aggression. *Horm. Behav.* 44, 161–170. doi: 10.1016/s0018-506x(03)00127-2

Boyden, E. S., Zhang, F., Bamberg, E., Nagel, G., and Deisseroth, K. (2005). Millisecond-timescale, genetically targeted optical control of neural activity. *Nat. Neurosci.* 8, 1263–1268. doi: 10.1038/nn1525

Breggin, P. R. (1975a). Psychosurgery for political purposes. *Duquesne Law Rev.* 13, 841–862.

Breggin, P. R. (1975b). "Psychosurgery for the control of violence—a critical review," in *Neural Bases of Violence and Aggression*, eds W. S. Fields and W. H. Sweet (St. Louis, MO: Warren H. Green, Inc.), 350–378.

Broida, J., and Svare, B. (1982). Postpartum aggression in C57BL/6J and DBA/2J mice: experiential and environmental influences. *Behav. Neural Biol.* 35, 76–83. doi: 10.1016/s0163-1047(82)91318-8

Bullitt, E. (1990). Expression of C-Fos-like protein as a marker for neuronal-activity following noxious-stimulation in the rat. *J. Comp. Neurol.* 296, 517–530. doi: 10.1002/cne.902960402

Canteras, N. S., Simerly, R. B., and Swanson, L. W. (1994). Organization of projections from the ventromedial nucleus of the hypothalamus: a *Phaseolus vulgaris*-leucoagglutinin study in the rat. *J. Comp. Neurol.* 348, 41–79. doi: 10.1002/cne.903480103

Cardin, J. A., Carlén, M., Meletis, K., Knoblich, U., Zhang, F., Deisseroth, K., et al. (2010). Targeted optogenetic stimulation and recording of neurons in vivo using cell-type-specific expression of Channelrhodopsin-2. *Nat. Protoc.* 5, 247–254. doi: 10.1038/nprot.2009.228

Choi, G. B., Dong, H. W., Murphy, A. J., Valenzuela, D. M., Yancopoulos, G. D., Swanson, L. W., et al. (2005). Lhx6 delineates a pathway mediating innate reproductive behaviors from the amygdala to the hypothalamus. *Neuron* 46, 647–660. doi: 10.1016/j.neuron.2005.04.011

Clemente, C. D., and Chase, M. H. (1973). Neurological substrates of aggressive behavior. *Annu. Rev. Physiol.* 35, 329–356. doi: 10.1146/annurev.ph.35.030173.001553

Colby, C. L., and Goldberg, M. E. (1999). Space and attention in parietal cortex. *Annu. Rev. Neurosci.* 22, 319–349. doi: 10.1146/annurev.neuro.22.1.319

Connor, J. L. (1974). Waning and recovery of conspecific aggression in the house mouse (*Mus musculus* L.). *J. Comp. Physiol. Psychol.* 87, 215–227.

Couppis, M. H., and Kennedy, C. H. (2008). The rewarding effect of aggression is reduced by nucleus accumbens dopamine receptor antagonism in mice. *Psychopharmacology* 197, 449–456. doi: 10.1007/s00213-007-1054-y

Cui, G., Jun, S. B., Jin, X., Pham, M. D., Vogel, S. S., Lovinger, D. M., et al. (2013). Concurrent activation of striatal direct and indirect pathways during action initiation. *Nature* 494, 238–242. doi: 10.1038/nature11846

de Almeida, R. M., Ferrari, P. F., Parmigiani, S., and Miczek, K. A. (2005). Escalated aggressive behavior: dopamine, serotonin and GABA. *Eur. J. Pharmacol.* 526, 51–64. doi: 10.1016/j.ejphar.2005.10.004

Delville, Y., De Vries, G. J., and Ferris, C. F. (2000). Neural connections of the anterior hypothalamus and agonistic behavior in golden hamsters. *Brain Behav. Evol.* 55, 53–76. doi: 10.1159/000006642

Everitt, B. J., and Stacey, P. (1987). Studies of instrumental behavior with sexual reinforcement in male rats (*Rattus norvegicus*): II. Effects of preoptic area lesions, castration and testosterone. *J. Comp. Psychol.* 101, 407–419. doi: 10.1037//0735-7036.101.4.407

Falkner, A. L., Dollar, P., Perona, P., Anderson, D. J., and Lin, D. (2014). Decoding ventromedial hypothalamic neural activity during male mouse aggression. *J. Neurosci.* 34, 5971–5984. doi: 10.1523/jneurosci.5109-13.2014

Fan, D., Rich, D., Holtzman, T., Ruther, P., Dalley, J. W., Lopez, A., et al. (2011). A wireless multi-channel recording system for freely behaving mice and rats. *PLoS One* 6:e22033. doi: 10.1371/journal.pone.0022033

Ferrari, P. F., van Erp, A. M., Tornatzky, W., and Miczek, K. A. (2003). Accumbal dopamine and serotonin in anticipation of the next aggressive episode in rats. *Eur. J. Neurosci.* 17, 371–378. doi: 10.1046/j.1460-9568.2003.02447.x

Ferris, C. F., and Potegal, M. (1988). Vasopressin receptor blockade in the anterior hypothalamus suppresses aggression in hamsters. *Physiol. Behav.* 44, 235–239. doi: 10.1016/0031-9384(88)90144-8

Ferris, C. F., Stolberg, T., Kulkarni, P., Murugavel, M., Blanchard, R., Blanchard, D. C., et al. (2008). Imaging the neural circuitry and chemical control of aggressive motivation. *BMC Neurosci.* 9:111. doi: 10.1186/1471-2202-9-111

Fish, E. W., De Bold, J. F., and Miczek, K. A. (2002). Aggressive behavior as a reinforcer in mice: activation by allopregnanolone. *Psychopharmacology (Berl)* 163, 459–466. doi: 10.1007/s00213-002-1211-2

Fish, E. W., DeBold, J. F., and Miczek, K. A. (2005). Escalated aggression as a reward: corticosterone and GABA(A) receptor positive modulators in mice. *Psychopharmacology (Berl)* 182, 116–127. doi: 10.1007/s00213-005-0064-x

Franzini, A., Broggi, G., Cordella, R., Dones, I., and Messina, G. (2013). Deep-brain stimulation for aggressive and disruptive behavior. *World Neurosurg.* 80, S29.e11–S29.e14. doi: 10.1016/j.wneu.2012.06.038

Gammie, S. C., and Nelson, R. J. (2001). cFOS and pCREB activation and maternal aggression in mice. *Brain Res.* 898, 232–241. doi: 10.1016/s0006-8993(01)02189-8

Goodson, J. L., Kelly, A. M., Kingsbury, M. A., and Thompson, R. R. (2012). An aggression-specific cell type in the anterior hypothalamus of finches. *Proc. Natl. Acad. Sci. U S A* 109, 13847–13852. doi: 10.1073/pnas.1207995109

Grossman, S. P. (1972). The ventromedial hypothalamus and aggressive behaviors. *Physiol. Behav.* 9, 721–725. doi: 10.1016/0031-9384(72)90040-6

Guenthner, C. J., Miyamichi, K., Yang, H. H., Heller, H. C., and Luo, L. (2013). Permanent genetic access to transiently active neurons via TRAP: targeted recombination in active populations. *Neuron* 78, 773–784. doi: 10.1016/j.neuron.2013.03.025

Guzowski, J. F., McNaughton, B. L., Barnes, C. A., and Worley, P. F. (2001). Imaging neural activity with temporal and cellular resolution using FISH. *Curr. Opin. Neurobiol.* 11, 579–584. doi: 10.1016/s0959-4388(00)00252-x

Halasz, J., Liposits, Z., Kruk, M. R., and Haller, J. (2002a). Neural background of glucocorticoid dysfunction-induced abnormal aggression in rats: involvement of fear- and stress-related structures. *Eur. J. Neurosci.* 15, 561–569. doi: 10.1046/j.0953-816x.2001.01883.x

Halasz, J., Liposits, Z., Meelis, W., Kruk, M. R., and Haller, J. (2002b). Hypothalamic attack area-mediated activation of the forebrain in aggression. *Neuroreport* 13, 1267–1270. doi: 10.1097/00001756-200207190-00010

Halasz, J., Toth, M., Mikics, E., Hrabovszky, E., Barsy, B., Barsvari, B., et al. (2008). The effect of neurokinin1 receptor blockade on territorial aggression and in a model of violent aggression. *Biol. Psychiatry* 63, 271–278. doi: 10.1016/j.biopsych.2007.04.022

Halasz, J., Zelena, D., Toth, M., Tulogdi, A., Mikics, E., and Haller, J. (2009). Substance P neurotransmission and violent aggression: the role of tachykinin NK(1) receptors in the hypothalamic attack area. *Eur. J. Pharmacol.* 611, 35–43. doi: 10.1016/j.ejphar.2009.03.050

Haller, J. (2013). The neurobiology of abnormal manifestations of aggression-a review of hypothalamic mechanisms in cats, rodents and humans. *Brain Res. Bull.* 93, 97–109. doi: 10.1016/j.brainresbull.2012.10.003

Haller, J., Toth, M., Halasz, J., and De Boer, S. F. (2006). Patterns of violent aggression-induced brain c-fos expression in male mice selected for aggressiveness. *Physiol. Behav.* 88, 173–182. doi: 10.1016/j.physbeh.2006.03.030

Hasen, N. S., and Gammie, S. C. (2005). Differential fos activation in virgin and lactating mice in response to an intruder. *Physiol. Behav.* 84, 681–695. doi: 10.1016/j.physbeh.2005.02.010

Hasen, N. S., and Gammie, S. C. (2006). Maternal aggression: new insights from Egr-1. *Brain Res.* 1108, 147–156. doi: 10.1016/j.brainres.2006.06.007

Hess, W. R. (1928). Stammganglien-reizversuche. Berichte der gesamten. *Physiologie* 42, 554–555.

Hoffman, G. E., Smith, M. S., and Verbalis, J. G. (1993). C-Fos and related immediate-early gene-products as markers of activity in neuroendocrine systems. *Front. Neuroendocrinol.* 14, 173–213. doi: 10.1006/frne.1993.1006

Horio, T., Shimura, T., Hanada, M., and Shimokochi, M. (1986). Multiple unit activities recorded from the medial preoptic area during copulatory behavior in freely moving male rats. *Neurosci. Res.* 3, 311–320. doi: 10.1016/0168-0102(86)90023-4

Jennings, J. H., Sparta, D. R., Stamatakis, A. M., Ung, R. L., Pleil, K. E., Kash, T. L., et al. (2013). Distinct extended amygdala circuits for divergent motivational states. *Nature* 496, 224–228. doi: 10.1038/nature12041

Jones, S. E., and Brain, P. F. (1987). Performances of inbred and outbred laboratory mice in putative tests of aggression. *Behav. Genet.* 17, 87–96. doi: 10.1007/bf01066013

Kawashima, T., Kitamura, K., Suzuki, K., Nonaka, M., Kamijo, S., Takemoto-Kimura, S., et al. (2013). Functional labeling of neurons and their projections using the synthetic activity-dependent promoter E-SARE. *Nat. Methods* 10, 889–895. doi: 10.1038/nmeth.2559

Kollack-Walker, S., and Newman, S. W. (1995). Mating and agonistic behavior produce different patterns of Fos immunolabeling in the male Syrian hamster brain. *Neuroscience* 66, 721–736. doi: 10.1016/0306-4522(94)00563-k

Kollack-Walker, S., Watson, S. J., and Akil, H. (1997). Social stress in hamsters: defeat activates specific neurocircuits within the brain. *J. Neurosci.* 17, 8842–8855.

Koolhaas, J. M. (1978). Hypothalamically induced intraspecific aggressive behaviour in the rat. *Exp. Brain Res.* 32, 365–375. doi: 10.1007/bf00238708

Krashes, M. J., Koda, S., Ye, C., Rogan, S. C., Adams, A. C., Cusher, D. S., et al. (2011). Rapid, reversible activation of AgRP neurons drives feeding behavior in mice. *J. Clin. Invest.* 121, 1424–1428. doi: 10.1172/JCI46229

Kruk, M. R. (2014). Hypothalamic attack: a wonderful artifact or a useful perspective on escalation and pathology in aggression? A viewpoint. *Curr. Top. Behav. Neurosci.* 17, 143–188. doi: 10.1007/7854_2014_313

Kruk, M. R., Halasz, J., Meelis, W., and Haller, J. (2004). Fast positive feedback between the adrenocortical stress response and a brain mechanism involved in aggressive behavior. *Behav. Neurosci.* 118, 1062–1070. doi: 10.1037/0735-7044.118.5.1062

Kruk, M. R., Van der Laan, C. E., Mos, J., Van der Poel, A. M., Meelis, W., and Olivier, B. (1984). Comparison of aggressive behaviour induced by electrical stimulation in the hypothalamus of male and female rats. *Prog. Brain Res.* 61, 303–314. doi: 10.1016/s0079-6123(08)64443-x

Kruk, M. R., van der Poel, A. M., and de Vos-Frerichs, T. P. (1979). The induction of aggressive behaviour by electrical stimulation in the hypothalamus of male rats. *Behaviour* 70, 292–322. doi: 10.1163/156853979x00106

Kruk, M. R., Vanderpoel, A. M., Meelis, W., Hermans, J., Mostert, P. G., Mos, J., et al. (1983). Discriminant-analysis of the localization of aggression-inducing electrode placements in the hypothalamus of male-rats. *Brain Res.* 260, 61–79. doi: 10.1016/0006-8993(83)90764-3

Lammers, J. H., Kruk, M. R., Meelis, W., and van der Poel, A. M. (1988). Hypothalamic substrates for brain stimulation-induced attack, teeth-chattering and social grooming in the rat. *Brain Res.* 449, 311–327. doi: 10.1016/0006-8993(88)91046-3

Lee, A., Clancy, S., and Fleming, A. S. (2000). Mother rats bar-press for pups: effects of lesions of the mpoa and limbic sites on maternal behavior and operant responding for pup-reinforcement. *Behav. Brain Res.* 108, 215–231. doi: 10.1016/S0166-4328(98)00109-0

Lee, H., Kim, D. W., Remedios, R., Anthony, T. E., Chang, A., Madisen, L., et al. (2014). Scalable control of mounting and attack by Esr1+ neurons in the ventromedial hypothalamus. *Nature* 509, 627–632. doi: 10.1038/nature13169

Lima, S. Q., Hromadka, T., Znamenskiy, P., and Zador, A. M. (2009). PINP: a new method of tagging neuronal populations for identification during in vivo electrophysiological recording. *PLoS One* 4:e6099. doi: 10.1371/journal.pone.0006099

Lin, D., Boyle, M. P., Dollar, P., Lee, H., Lein, E. S., Perona, P., et al. (2011). Functional identification of an aggression locus in the mouse hypothalamus. *Nature* 470, 221–226. doi: 10.1038/nature09736

Lipp, H. P. (1978). Aggression and flight behaviour of the marmoset monkey Callithrix jacchus: an ethogram for brain stimulation studies. *Brain Behav. Evol.* 15, 241–259. doi: 10.1159/000123781

Madisen, L., Mao, T., Koch, H., Zhuo, J. M., Berenyi, A., Fujisawa, S., et al. (2012). A toolbox of Cre-dependent optogenetic transgenic mice for light-induced activation and silencing. *Nat. Neurosci.* 15, 793–802. doi: 10.1038/nn.3078

Mark, V. H., Sweet, W. H., and Ervin, F. R. (1968). Role of brain disease in riots and urban violence. *JAMA* 203, 368–369. doi: 10.1001/jama.1968.03140050052020

Martinez, R. C., Carvalho-Netto, E. F., Amaral, V. C., Nunes-de-Souza, R. L., and Canteras, N. S. (2008). Investigation of the hypothalamic defensive system in the mouse. *Behav. Brain Res.* 192, 185–190. doi: 10.1016/j.bbr.2008.03.042

Matsumoto, A., and Arai, Y. (1986). Male-female difference in synaptic organization of the ventromedial nucleus of the hypothalamus in the rat. *Neuroendocrinology* 42, 232–236. doi: 10.1159/000124445

May, M. E., and Kennedy, C. H. (2009). Aggression as positive reinforcement in mice under various ratio- and time-based reinforcement schedules. *J. Exp. Anal. Behav.* 91, 185–196. doi: 10.1901/jeab.2009.91-185

Merchenthaler, I., Lane, M. V., Numan, S., and Dellovade, T. L. (2004). Distribution of estrogen receptor alpha and beta in the mouse central nervous system: in vivo autoradiographic and immunocytochemical analyses. *J. Comp. Neurol.* 473, 270–291. doi: 10.1002/cne.20128

Metz, R., and Ziff, E. (1991). cAMP stimulates the C/EBP-related transcription factor rNFIL-6 to trans-locate to the nucleus and induce c-fos transcription. *Genes Dev.* 5, 1754–1766. doi: 10.1101/gad.5.10.1754

Mos, J., Kruk, M. R., Vanderpoel, A. M., and Meelis, W. (1982). Aggressive-behavior induced by electrical-stimulation in the midbrain central gray of male-rats. *Aggress. Behav.* 8, 261–284. doi: 10.1002/1098-2337(1982)8:3<261::aid-ab2480080304>3.0.co;2-n

Murphy, A. Z., Shupnik, M. A., and Hoffman, G. E. (1999). Androgen and estrogen (alpha) receptor distribution in the periaqueductal gray of the male rat. *Horm. Behav.* 36, 98–108. doi: 10.1006/hbeh.1999.1528

Nelson, R. J., and Trainor, B. C. (2007). Neural mechanisms of aggression. *Nat. Rev. Neurosci.* 8, 536–546. doi: 10.1038/nrn2174

Nishizuka, M., and Pfaff, D. W. (1989). Intrinsic synapses in the ventromedial nucleus of the hypothalamus: an ultrastructural study. *J. Comp. Neurol.* 286, 260–268. doi: 10.1002/cne.902860210

Ogawa, S., Lubahn, D. B., Korach, K. S., and Pfaff, D. W. (1997). Behavioral effects of estrogen receptor gene disruption in male mice. *Proc. Natl. Acad. Sci. U S A* 94, 1476–1481. doi: 10.1073/pnas.94.4.1476

Oliver, B. (1977). The ventromedial hypothalamus and aggressive behaviour in rats. *Aggress. Behav.* 3, 47–56. doi: 10.1002/1098-2337(1977)3:1<47::aid-ab2480030105>3.0.co;2-h

Olivier, B., and Wiepkema, P. R. (1974). Behaviour changes in mice following electrolytic lesions in the median hypothalamus. *Brain Res.* 65, 521–524. doi: 10.1016/0006-8993(74)90241-8

Oomura, Y., Aou, S., Koyama, Y., Fujita, I., and Yoshimatsu, H. (1988). Central control of sexual behavior. *Brain Res. Bull.* 20, 863–870. doi: 10.1016/0361-9230(88)90103-7

Oomura, Y., Yoshimatsu, H., and Aou, S. (1983). Medial preoptic and hypothalamic neuronal activity during sexual behavior of the male monkey. *Brain Res.* 266, 340–343. doi: 10.1016/0006-8993(83)90666-2

Optican, L. M. (2005). Sensorimotor transformation for visually guided saccades. *Ann. N Y Acad. Sci.* 1039, 132–148. doi: 10.1196/annals.1325.013

Osakada, F., Mori, T., Cetin, A. H., Marshel, J. H., Virgen, B., and Callaway, E. M. (2012). New rabies virus variants for monitoring and manipulating activity and gene expression in defined neural circuits. *Neuron* 71, 617–631. doi: 10.1016/j.neuron.2011.07.005

Pfaff, D. W., and Sakuma, Y. (1979a). Deficit in the lordosis reflex of female rats caused by lesions in the ventromedial nucleus of the hypothalamus. *J. Physiol.* 288, 203–210.

Pfaff, D. W., and Sakuma, Y. (1979b). Facilitation of the lordosis reflex of female rats from the ventromedial nucleus of the hypothalamus. *J. Physiol.* 288, 189–202.

Potegal, M. (1984). The persistence of attack satiation in female golden-hamsters. *Aggress. Behav.* 10, 303–307. doi: 10.1002/1098-2337(1984)10:4<303::aid-ab2480100404>3.0.co;2-d

Proshansky, E., Bandler, R. J., and Flynn, J. P. (1974). Elimination of hypothalamically elicited biting attack by unilateral lesion of the ventral midbrain tegmentum of cats. *Brain Res.* 77, 309–313. doi: 10.1016/0006-8993(74)90793-8

Reijmers, L. G., Perkins, B. L., Matsuo, N., and Mayford, M. (2007). Localization of a stable neural correlate of associative memory. *Science* 317, 1230–1233. doi: 10.1126/science.1143839

Roberts, W. W., and Kiess, H. O. (1964). Motivational properties of hypothalamic aggression in cats. *J. Comp. Physiol. Psychol.* 58, 187–193. doi: 10.1037/h0042377

Roberts, W. W., and Nagel, J. (1996). First-order projections activated by stimulation of hypothalamic sites eliciting attack and flight in rats. *Behav. Neurosci.* 110, 509–527. doi: 10.1037//0735-7044.110.3.509

Roeling, T. A. P., Veening, J. G., Kruk, M. R., Peters, J. P. W., Vermelis, M. E. J., and Nieuwenhuys, R. (1994). Efferent connections of the hypothalamic aggression area in the rat. *Neuroscience* 59, 1001–1024. doi: 10.1016/0306-4522(94)90302-6

Roeling, T. A. P., Veening, J. G., Peters, J. P. W., Vermelis, M. E. J., and Nieuwenhuys, R. (1993). Efferent connections of the hypothalamic grooming area in the rat. *Neuroscience* 56, 199–225. doi: 10.1016/0306-4522(93)90574-y

Sagar, S. M., Sharp, F. R., and Curran, T. (1988). Expression of c-fos protein in brain: metabolic mapping at the cellular level. *Science* 240, 1328–1331. doi: 10.1126/science.3131879

Sano, K., Tsuda, M. C., Musatov, S., Sakamoto, T., and Ogawa, S. (2013). Differential effects of site-specific knockdown of estrogen receptor alpha in the medial amygdala, medial pre-optic area and ventromedial nucleus of the hypothalamus on sexual and aggressive behavior of male mice. *Eur. J. Neurosci.* 37, 1308–1319. doi: 10.1111/ejn.12131

Sheng, M., and Greenberg, M. E. (1990). The regulation and function of c-fos and other immediate early genes in the nervous-system. *Neuron* 4, 477–485. doi: 10.1016/0896-6273(90)90106-p

Shimura, T., Yamamoto, T., and Shimokochi, M. (1994). The medial preoptic area is involved in both sexual arousal and performance in male-rats—reevaluation of neuron activity in freely moving animals. *Brain Res.* 640, 215–222. doi: 10.1016/0006-8993(94)91875-9

Siegel, A., and Pott, C. B. (1988). Neural substrates of aggression and flight in the cat. *Prog. Neurobiol.* 31, 261–283. doi: 10.1016/0301-0082(88)90015-9

Siegel, A., Roeling, T. A. P., Gregg, T. R., and Kruk, M. R. (1999). Neuropharmacology of brain-stimulation-evoked aggression. *Neurosci. Biobehav. Rev.* 23, 359–389. doi: 10.1016/s0149-7634(98)00040-2

Swanson, L. W. (2000). Cerebral hemisphere regulation of motivated behavior. *Brain Res.* 886, 113–164. doi: 10.1016/s0006-8993(00)02905-x

Szuts, T. A., Fadeyev, V., Kachiguine, S., Sher, A., Grivich, M. V., Agrochao, M., et al. (2011). A wireless multi-channel neural amplifier for freely moving animals. *Nat. Neurosci.* 14, 263–269. doi: 10.1038/nn.2730

Torres, C. V., Sola, R. G., Pastor, J., Pedrosa, M., Navas, M., Garcia-Navarrete, E., et al. (2013). Long-term results of posteromedial hypothalamic deep brain stimulation for patients with resistant aggressiveness Clinical article. *J. Neurosurg.* 119, 277–287. doi: 10.3171/2013.4.jns121639

Turnbough, P. D., and Lloyd, K. E. (1973). Operant responding in Siamese fighting fish (*Betta splendens*) as a function of schedule of reinforcement and visual reinforcers. *J. Exp. Anal. Behav.* 20, 355–362. doi: 10.1901/jeab.1973.20-355

Tye, K. M., and Deisseroth, K. (2012). Optogenetic investigation of neural circuits underlying brain disease in animal models. *Nat. Rev. Neurosci.* 13, 251–266. doi: 10.1038/nrn3171

Valenstein, E. S., Cox, V. C., and Kakolewski, J. W. (1968). Modification of motivated behavior elicited by electrical stimulation of the hypothalamus. *Science* 159, 1119–1121. doi: 10.1126/science.159.3819.1119

Veening, J. G., Coolen, L. M., de Jong, T. R., Joosten, H. W., de Boer, S. F., Koolhaas, J. N., et al. (2005). Do similar neural systems subserve aggressive and sexual behaviour in male rats? Insights from c-Fos and pharmacological studies. *Eur. J. Pharmacol.* 526, 226–239. doi: 10.1016/j.ejphar.2005.09.041

Watson, P. J. (1977). Changes in elicited behavior as a function of experience with stimulation and available goal objects. *Physiol. Psychol.* 5, 343–354. doi: 10.3758/bf03335343

Wise, R. A. (2004). Dopamine, learning and motivation. *Nat. Rev. Neurosci.* 5, 483–494. doi: 10.1038/nrn1406

Yang, C. F., Chiang, M. C., Gray, D. C., Prabhakaran, M., Alvarado, M., Juntti, S. A., et al. (2013). Sexually dimorphic neurons in the ventromedial hypothalamus govern mating in both sexes and aggression in males. *Cell* 153, 896–909. doi: 10.1016/j.cell.2013.04.017

Yizhar, O., Fenno, L. E., Davidson, T. J., Mogri, M., and Deisseroth, K. (2011). Optogenetics in neural systems. *Neuron* 71, 9–34. doi: 10.1016/j.neuron.2011.06.004

Ziv, Y., Burns, L. D., Cocker, E. D., Hamel, E. O., Ghosh, K. K., Kitch, L. J., et al. (2013). Long-term dynamics of CA1 hippocampal place codes. *Nat. Neurosci.* 16, 264–266. doi: 10.1038/nn.3329

13

Bariatric surgery in hypothalamic obesity

Nathan C. Bingham[1], Susan R. Rose[1] and Thomas H. Inge[2]*

[1] Division of Endocrinology, Cincinnati Children's Hospital Medical Center, University of Cincinnati College of Medicine, Cincinnati, OH, USA
[2] Division of Pediatric General and Thoracic Surgery, Cincinnati Children's Hospital Medical Center, University of Cincinnati College of Medicine, Cincinnati, OH, USA

***Correspondence:**
Thomas H. Inge, Cincinnati Children's Hospital Medical Center, 3333 Burnet Avenue, Cincinnati, OH 45229, USA.
e-mail: thomas.inge@cchmc.org

Craniopharyngiomas (CP) are epithelial neoplasms generally found in the area of the pituitary and hypothalamus. Despite benign histology, these tumors and/or their treatment often result in significant, debilitating disorders of endocrine, neurological, behavioral, and metabolic systems. Severe obesity is observed in a high percentage of patients with CP resulting in significant comorbidities and negatively impacting quality of life. Obesity occurs as a result of hypothalamic damage and disruption of normal homeostatic mechanisms regulating energy balance. Such pathological weight gain, termed hypothalamic obesity (HyOb), is often severe and refractory to therapy. Unfortunately, neither lifestyle intervention nor pharmacotherapy has proven effective in the treatment of HyOb. Given the limited choices and poor results of these treatments, several groups have examined bariatric surgery as a treatment alternative for patients with CP–HyOb. While a large body of evidence exists supporting the use of bariatric surgery in the treatment of exogenous obesity and its comorbidities, its role in the treatment of HyOb has yet to be defined. To date, the existing literature on bariatric surgery in CP–HyOb is largely limited to case reports and series with short term follow-up. Here we review the current reports on the use of bariatric surgery in the treatment of CP–HyOb. We also compare these results to those reported for other populations of HyOb, including Prader–Willi Syndrome, Bardet–Biedl syndrome, and hypothalamic melanocortin signaling defects. While initial reports of bariatric surgery in CP–HyOb are promising, their limited scope makes it difficult to draw any substantial conclusions as to the long term safety and efficacy of bariatric surgery in CP–HyOb. There continues to be a need for more robust, controlled, prospective studies with long term follow-up in order to better define the role of bariatric surgery in the treatment of HyOb.

Keywords: craniopharyngioma, bariatric surgery, gastric bypass, hypothalamic obesity

INTRODUCTION

Craniopharyngiomas (CP) are generally benign, slow-growing tumors that are thought to arise from rests of embryonic cells residing within the remnants of the craniopharyngeal duct or Rathke's pouch (Abeloff, 2008). Thus, tumors may originate from anywhere along the path of the craniopharyngeal duct, from nasopharynx to tuber cinereum, although most are located in the sellar/parasellar region (Harwood-Nash, 1994; Karavitaki et al., 2005). Although histologically benign, these tumors are often locally aggressive with invasion of adjacent tissues and structures. While mortality is generally low, morbidity as a result of tumor mass effect and/or therapy (resection ± radiotherapy) is substantial and nearly universal (Mortini et al., 2011; Winkfield et al., 2011).

Because of the close proximity to the visual nerve tracts, hypothalamus, pituitary, and ventricular system, CPs predispose patients to a number of adverse endocrine, metabolic, psychologic, and neurologic sequelae. As a primary result of the tumor, the majority of patients present with one or more hypothalamic-pituitary deficits including growth hormone (GH; ~75%), gonadotropins (~60%), adrenocorticotropic hormone (ACTH; ~30%), thyroid-stimulating hormone (TSH; ~25%), and/or antidiuretic hormone (ADH; ~20%; Karavitaki et al., 2006; Muller, 2008). In addition, approximately one-third can develop new or additional endocrinopathies following surgical resection.

HYPOTHALAMIC OBESITY

In addition to pituitary hormone deficiencies, hypothalamic involvement has been shown to result in severe metabolic disturbances and weight gain (Muller et al., 2001; Srinivasan et al., 2004). While a minority (15–20%) of CP patients complain of weight gain as a presenting symptom, more than 50% develop significant obesity following surgical resection (Muller et al., 2004; Ahmet et al., 2006). This number may be as high as 90% in those with demonstrable hypothalamic damage, whether from direct tumor infiltration or as a result of surgical and/or radiation therapy (de Vile et al., 1996; Muller et al., 2004). Such pathological weight gain, termed hypothalamic obesity (HyOb), is often severe, refractory to therapy, and has a significant negative impact on the quality of life for patients with CP (Muller et al., 2005; Eyal et al., 2006; Inge et al., 2007).

Over the last 75 years, experience with animal and human models has shown the basal medial hypothalamus to be a key center of metabolic regulation by the central nervous system (CNS; Hetherington and Ranson, 1940; Sorva, 1988). The hypothalamus receives and integrates a variety of afferent signals communicating the metabolic state of the organism and adjusts autonomic outputs with the ideal physiologic outcome of maintaining adequate energy stores. The afferent arm of the homeostatic loop consists of hormones, such as leptin, insulin, and peptide YY, that target receptor fields within hypothalamic nuclei to convey information on meal size, nutrient composition, and adipose tissue stores. In addition, neurons within the hypothalamus directly sense and respond to nutrients, such as free fatty acids, glucose, and amino acids. Within the hypothalamus, neuropeptides such as neuropeptide Y (NPY), agouti-related protein (AgRP), and alpha-melanocyte stimulating hormone (α-MSH), integrate and convey this information to other brain centers responsible for controlling appetite/satiety, thermogenic, and motor effectors (Schwartz et al., 2000).

A number of monogenetic obesity syndromes have now been shown to involve mutations in such regulatory hypothalamic pathways (Clement et al., 1998; Lubrano-Berthelier et al., 2006; Savastano et al., 2009; Hochberg and Hochberg, 2010). In addition, several complex genetic syndromes, including Prader–Willi (PWS) and Bardet–Biedl syndromes (BBS), are associated with obesity, presumably from hypothalamic dysfunction. PWS results from the loss of paternally imprinted genes on chromosome 15q11-15 and is characterized by an array of multisystemic defects including neonatal hypotonia, short stature, hypogonadism, behavioral and psychiatric phenotypes, aggressive food-seeking behavior, hyperphagia, and obesity (Goldstone et al., 2008). PWS patients have significantly elevated levels of the orexigenic hormone ghrelin, a finding not observed in other causes of HyOb (Cummings et al., 2002a; DelParigi et al., 2002). Interestingly, even young, underweight patients with PWS exhibit higher BMI-adjusted body fat and serum leptin levels, suggesting some intrinsic leptin resistance in PWS (Eiholzer et al., 1999). BBS is a multisystemic disorder characterized by retinal degeneration, hypogonadism, polydactyly, renal dysfunction, mental retardation, and obesity resulting from defects in ciliary function. Hypothalamic dysfunction in these patients is suggested by the study of mice harboring mutations in BBS genes. BBS mutants have been shown to be hyperleptinemic and have defective hypothalamic leptin signaling (Seo et al., 2009; Guo and Rahmouni, 2011).

Thus, damage to, or dysfunction of the hypothalamus results in an inability of the CNS to receive proper feedback. Patients, thus, inappropriately sense a perpetual state of starvation. To correct the perceived negative energy balance, efferent outputs are adjusted to promote caloric intake and decreased caloric expenditure. Decreased sympathetic activation of β_2-, β_3-, and α_2-adrenergic receptors reduce skeletal muscle thermogenesis, reduce adipose tissue lipolysis, and promote pancreatic insulin secretion, respectively. Conversely, increased parasympathetic output through the vagus nerve slows the heart rate reducing myocardial oxygen consumption, promotes gastrointestinal peristalsis and substrate absorption, and accentuates post-prandial insulin secretion (Lustig, 2008). The net result of this reduced sympathetic/parasympathetic ratio is significantly decreased energy expenditure with partitioning of calories away from energy consuming tissue such as muscle and toward energy storage depots such as adipose tissue.

Accumulating evidence supports the hypothesis that CP and its therapies often result in dysfunction of the normal homeostatic mechanisms regulating appetite and metabolism. Leptin, a potent anorexigenic peptide secreted by adipocytes, has been found to be elevated in CP patients compared to obese controls suggesting a defect in the normal feedback inhibition of appetite. In addition, some CP patients have a blunted post-meal increase in the anorexigenic hormone peptide YY. Hypersecretion of the orexigenic gastric hormone ghrelin is thought to contribute to hyperphagia and obesity in PWS, although this does not seem to be the case in CP where pre-meal ghrelin levels are lower than weight-matched controls. Recently, however, Roth et al. found that there may be a reduction in the expected magnitude of post-meal suppression of ghrelin levels in CP patients (Roth et al., 1998, 2011; Holmer et al., 2010).

While there are reports of hyperphagia and obsessive food-seeking behavior after CP (Skorzewska et al., 1989), a number of studies have now shown that caloric expenditure, and not caloric intake, may be the largest contributor to post-CP-HyOb (CP–HyOb). Adults and children with CP–HyOb have been found to have impaired sympathoadrenal activation in response to hypoglycemia, although this defect does not appear to always correlate with development of obesity or hypothalamic involvement (Schofl et al., 2002; Coutant et al., 2003). In a larger study, CP–HyOb patients were found to have lower levels of urine catecholamines than BMI-matched controls (Roth et al., 2007), suggesting decreased sympathetic tone.

As sympathetic tone correlates with spontaneous motor activity, one might also expect lower levels of physical activity in CP patients. Indeed, CP patients consistently report reduced physical activity, even when compared to controls with similar BMI (Roth et al., 2007). Using accelerometric data, Harz et al. demonstrated that obese CP patients had decreased spontaneous motor activity compared with age and BMI-matched controls. Using food diaries, this same group showed that caloric intake was lower in CP patients with hypothalamic damage, despite a significantly increased BMI (Harz et al., 2003). These findings were substantiated by a recent study by Holmer et al. in 42 adult patients with childhood CP, where CP patients were found to have a significantly reduced basal metabolic rate when adjusted for body weight, than age and sex matched controls. Analysis of energy intake showed lower caloric consumption in CP patients which was attributed to cognitive restraint in eating (Holmer et al., 2010). Aside from reduced sympathetic drive, the roadblocks to physical activity are substantial and likely contribute to reduced energy expenditure and risk for obesity. Neurological and visual deficits may contribute to limited movement in some CP patients. In addition, there is evidence that CP patients have disordered sleep patterns secondary to decreased melatonin and/or secondary narcolepsy causing daytime sleepiness (Muller et al., 2002, 2006). Obstructive sleep apnea (OSA) in these patients also likely contributes to poor sleep hygiene.

Under- or overtreatment of hormonal deficiencies may also contribute to poor metabolic parameters and weight gain in CP patients. Glucocorticoid excess is a known cause of significant weight gain, impaired glucose metabolism, sleep disturbance, and defects in bone metabolism and growth (Debono et al., 2009). Most significantly, excess glucocorticoid dosing has been associated with increased mortality from cardiovascular disease. In a large cohort of Scandinavian patients with hypopituitarism, Filipsson et al. (2006) showed that those receiving higher doses of glucocorticoid replacement had significantly higher waist circumference, total cholesterol, serum triglycerides, and HbA1c. Daily cortisol production rates range from 6 to 8 $mg/m^2/day$, much less than previous estimates (Linder et al., 1990; Esteban et al., 1991; Kerrigan et al., 1993; Brandon et al., 1999). Thus, the classic adult dosing of 20 mg of hydrocortisone in the A.M. and 10 mg in the P.M., is likely an excessive dose. Unfortunately, no objective test of adequate glucocorticoid replacement has been shown to be sufficiently consistent to aid in dosing management and patients must be followed closely for clinical signs of glucocorticoid deficiency or excess.

Hypothyroidism also results in poor metabolic health and is associated with fatigue, low basal metabolic rate, increased BMI, and increased cholesterol and triglyceride levels (Kronenberg and Williams, 2008) and adequate replacement has beneficial effects on these parameters (Slawik et al., 2007). Management of thyroid hormone replacement is made more challenging in CP patients by the absence of the patient's own endogenous "thyrostat" as TSH levels cannot be used to judge adequacy of treatment. The significance of this handicap is highlighted in a recent study comparing free T4 (fT4) levels in TSH deficient patients to those in primary hypothyroid patients where TSH levels are used to guide therapy. Nearly 40% of TSH deficient patients were found to have fT4 levels below the 20th centile range compared to 13.4% of primary hypothyroid patients (Koulouri et al., 2011).

Growth hormone deficiency is present in a majority of CP patients and likely contributes to the metabolic derangements seen in this patient population. These metabolic effects are particularly important in adults, where GH replacement results in increased lean body mass and decreased body fat (Kronenberg and Williams, 2008). GH-deficiency has been shown to contribute to increased cardiovascular risk in hypopituitarism (Abs et al., 2006; Verhelst and Abs, 2009). The decision to replace GH in patients with a previous history of CP remains controversial although GH replacement does not appear to have any adverse effect on reoccurrence rates of CP in short term follow-up (Muller et al., 2010; Rohrer et al., 2010).

Hypogonadism and inadequately treated diabetes insipidus (DI) can also potentiate the effects of hypothalamic damage on excessive weight gain. Testosterone replacement, in hypogonadal men has been shown to have beneficial effects on body composition, blood pressure, and glucose homeostasis (Katznelson et al., 1996; Boyanov et al., 2003; Wittert et al., 2003). The effects of estrogen replacement on weight gain and body composition are more mixed and unclear, but premenopausal women who are hypogonadal should be physiologically replaced barring other contraindications (Norman et al., 2000). Inadequate control of DI can lead to excessive drinking of calories, poor sleep quality, and increased appetite (Beccuti and Pannain, 2011).

Altered carbohydrate and insulin dynamics have been shown to occur with CP and its treatment. While fasting glucose levels are generally no different from controls, CP patients have an exaggerated first and second phase insulin response to carbohydrate challenge (Lustig et al., 1999). Hyperinsulinism in hypothalamic damage is a result of both decreased inhibitory tone by sympathetic pathways and augmented vagal parasympathetic signaling to the pancreatic β-cell, and is not primarily a response to insulin resistance. Vagally mediated acetylcholine, acting through M_3 muscarinic receptors, promotes depolarization of the β-cell through increased sodium influx, and mobilization of intracellular calcium stores through activation of the phospholipase C pathway (Miura et al., 1996). In addition, increased vagal activity stimulates release of the intestinal peptide glucagon-like peptide-1, itself a potentiator of insulin secretion (Rocca and Brubaker, 1999; Lustig, 2008). Increased insulin secretion in turn directs calories toward storage within the adipocyte.

Thus, the disruption of hypothalamic centers that occurs as a direct result of CP or its treatment creates a situation in which efferent drives to consume and store energy are disengaged from afferent signals that would otherwise dampen such drives. The obesity that results, driven by neural and biochemical stimuli, is often severe and intractable to therapy. While lifestyle changes such as caloric restriction and increased exercise should be encouraged, these interventions alone are often not successful, leaving patients frustrated with cravings, constant hunger, and lack of progress. Further, in addition to panhypopituitarism, HyOb patients are susceptible to the same metabolic derangements seen in other types of obesity such as diabetes, dyslipidemia, and heart disease (Srinivasan et al., 2004). For patients already facing significant challenges as a result of their primary disease, the negative impact of such comorbidities on quality of life adds insult to injury.

Unfortunately, in the last several years pharmacologic agents available for weight loss treatment have significantly declined, as the most effective agents (i.e., phen–fen, sibutramine) have been withdrawn from the market for unacceptable side-effect profiles. Small studies in CP of stimulants such as modafinil, methylphenidate, and dextroamphetamine have been shown to improve daytime sleepiness, affect, and alertness in HyOb (Mason et al., 2002; Muller et al., 2006), but none have proven truly effective at reversing the severe weight gain seen in this condition. Targeting the hyperinsulinism seen in HyOb, Lustig et al. (2006) demonstrated that octreotide could induce a modest decrease in BMI (0.79 kg/m^2). A recent preliminary trial of diazoxide and metformin combined therapy demonstrated a slowing of weight gain with a stabilization of BMI over the 6-months of therapy (Hamilton et al., 2011). Taken as a whole, the efficacy of pharmacotherapy in treating CP–HyOb is tepid at best. Because CP–HyOb results from damage to the afferent target centers of the hypothalamus, agents targeting the efferent pathways to increase metabolic rate and/or thermogenesis may prove to be more effective (Bays, 2004). Newer agents targeting these efferent pathways are desperately needed.

SURGICAL TREATMENT OF HyOb

Given the limited choices and poor results of pharmacotherapy, combined with emerging data suggesting that gastrointestinal surgical procedures effect weight loss by altering the body's weight regulatory signaling pathways, several groups have looked to bariatric surgery as a viable option for producing sustained weight loss for patients with CP–HyOb. A range of procedures are available and are generally divided into three categories: restrictive, malabsorptive, and hybrid procedures. Restrictive procedures, such as gastric banding (GB) or vertical banded gastroplasty (VBG), aim to reduce stomach volume resulting in early satiety and smaller meal consumption. The natural course that nutrients follow is not altered, however. Pure malabsorptive procedures including jejunoileal and duodenal–jejunal bypass, as well as biliopancreatic diversion (BPD) involve the diversion of ingested food, bypassing one or more sections of intestine. The former two of these procedures have largely fallen out of favor secondary to associated nutritional deficits (Organ et al., 1984). A hybrid procedure, the Roux-en-Y gastric bypass (RYGB) has become the "gold standard" and the most commonly performed bariatric surgery for weight loss. It entails dividing the stomach to create a small gastric pouch which is anastomosed to a roux limb of jejunum. An entero-enterostomy is then made between the excluded biliopancreatic limb and the roux alimentary limb (Karra et al., 2010).

Bariatric surgery remains the most effective treatment for morbid obesity and is indicated for adult patients with a BMI > 40 kg/m^2 or a BMI of >35 kg/m^2 and significant obesity-related comorbidities (Pories et al., 1995). More conservative indications have generally been advocated for weight loss surgery in adolescent patients (see Discussion and Future Directions). An extensive body of research has shown that patients often show measurable improvement in metabolic parameters including glucose homeostasis in the early post-operative period, independent of weight loss. While the exact mechanisms of this phenomenon are still unclear, it appears that gastric bypass alters the secretion of gut hormones that favor improved metabolism and may also counteract certain elements of the orexigenic and energy conserving hypothalamic response to voluntary weight loss. Indeed, a number of studies over the last 30 years have shown that GLP-1, an incretin hormone secreted by enteroendocrine cells of the distal ileum, is increased following bariatric surgery. The evidence is especially consistent for bypass procedures, whereas restrictive procedures have been associated with no change or a decrease in GLP-1 levels (Sarson et al., 1981; Koopmans et al., 1984; Laferrere et al., 2008).

GLP-1 has been shown to have a number of positive effects on glucose metabolism including potentiating glucose-dependent insulin secretion, improving insulin sensitivity, and suppressing glucagon secretion. In addition, it has been shown to slow gastric emptying and promote early satiety. GLP-1 exerts these pleiotropic effect by acting on specific receptors located on pancreatic β-cells, peripheral vagal afferent fibers, as well as centrally located neurons (Baggio and Drucker, 2007). In addition, bariatric surgery has been shown to increase other anorexigenic hormones such as PYY and decrease orexigenic hormones such as ghrelin (Cummings et al., 2002b; le Roux et al., 2006). Human and animal studies appear to indicate that exposure of the distal gut to nutrient-rich, partially digested food results in increased secretion of hormones such as GLP-1 and PYY. This altered hormonal milieu accounts for the greater than 80% remission in diabetes following RYGB, often within days to weeks of surgery, and a combination of malabsorption, gastric restriction, and hormonal changes that accounts for the consistent and durable weight loss seen following such procedures (Buchwald et al., 2004; Karra et al., 2010).

Despite the large body of evidence demonstrating the benefits of bariatric surgery in treating exogenous obesity and its comorbidities, its role in the treatment of HyOb has yet to be defined. To date, the existing literature on bariatric surgery in CP–HyOb is largely limited to case reports and series with short term follow-up. A PubMed search for "craniopharyngioma" and "bariatric surgery" results in four citations with a total of eight patients. Procedures performed include two RYGB, four laparoscopic adjustable band (LAGB), one distal gastric bypass, and one biliopancreatic derivation with duodenal switch.

In the first report of RYGB for CP–HyOb, we reported on an 18-year-old male who underwent a successful RYGB with anterior truncal vagotomy (due to the presumed importance of vagal efferents in CP-related hyperinsulinemia) for massive weight gain following the resection of a CP 3 years previous. At the time of CP diagnosis, his BMI was 25 kg/m^2. During the 2-years following CP resection, he developed hyperphagia and significant weight gain (70 kg/year) despite outpatient and inpatient dietary and physical activity interventions. Significant hyperinsulinism was noted and the patient was started on octreotide therapy with significant deceleration in weight gain but no weight loss. At the time of his bariatric surgery consultation, he had developed severe OSA, left ventricular hypertrophy, and hypertriglyceridemia. The post-operative course was significant for a 49-kg weight loss over 2.5 years, although weight appeared to stabilize thereafter (BMI ~50 kg/m^2). Further, serum triglycerides and left ventricular hypertrophy normalized. Hyperphagia decreased and food cravings (as measured by a Food Craving Inventory) diminished for all food types. Ten days following RYGB surgery, there was a fivefold decrease in fasting insulin, with normalization of fasting levels by 7 months. His post-prandial insulin excursion completely normalized by 14 months. As well, measurements of the orexigenic hormone ghrelin revealed a moderate decrease over the same time period.

In a different approach, Schultes et al. describe their approach to bypass surgery in a 29-year-old male with childhood CP. Following CP resection 21 years previous, the patient had experienced continuous weight gain, developed type 2 diabetes, and OSA requiring continuous positive airway pressure therapy at night. At the time of HyOb surgical consultation, this patient was on hormone replacement for panhypopituitarism as well as metformin and nateglinide for diabetes treatment. To promote preoperative weight loss, he was started on 15 mg sibutramine and enrolled in a rigorous supervised diet and exercise regimen which resulted in 9 kg weight loss over 9 months. Because bypass-induced hormonal alterations may exert their influence via hypothalamic mechanisms, it was felt that this patient, with complete hypothalamic atrophy, may not benefit. Therefore, a distal gastric bypass, producing a significantly shorter common channel of 80 cm, was performed with the goal of inducing a strong malabsorption component. Following surgery, the patient experienced a precipitous weight loss, losing over 50 kg (~30% of preoperative weight) over 18 months. In addition, the patient exhibited complete resolution of his diabetes and OSA and distinct reduction feelings of hunger and disinhibition on the three factor eating questionnaire (Schultes et al., 2009). The post-operative course was largely uneventful, although the patient did develop mild nutritional deficiencies despite standardized supplementation. These included anemia, deficiencies in vitamin D, B12, and zinc as well as hypoproteinemia.

In a series of four adolescent patients with childhood CP and obesity, Muller et al. found significant weight loss in all patients after LAGB. Patients participated in the German multicenter surveillance study on childhood CP termed "HIT-Endo-Kraniopharyngeom." The age of the patients ranged from 13 to

24 years of age and BMI–SDS scores ranged from +7.3 to +13.9. Following surgery, BMI–SDS scores improved on average by −0.7 per year of follow-up, with follow-up ranging from 1.5 to 4.5 years. Patients also reported significant changes in eating behavior, with reduced food cravings especially for sweets. Quality of life and functional capacity, measured by a standardized and validated scale, remained stable following surgery. Of the four patients, two experienced dislocation of the LAGB resulting in temporary weight gain and requiring laparoscopic revision. No other side-effects were reported (Muller et al., 2007).

Rottembourg et al. (2009) reported on two adolescents with post-CP–HyOb who underwent bariatric surgery as treatment for morbid obesity associated with significant comorbidities. The first was a 12-year-old female diagnosed with CP at age of 6 years. After gross total resection she developed panhypopituitarism and exhibited a rapid weight gain of 20 kg in the first 6 months. At the time of RYGB her BMI was 65 kg/m^2 and she had developed dyslipidemia, hepatosteatosis, frequent respiratory tract infections, and evidence of hypoventilation. Postoperatively, she demonstrated sustained weight loss over 4 years (BMI 43 kg/m^2 at last follow-up). In addition, dyslipidemia normalized, sleep patterns improved, and she had no further respiratory infections. She was subsequently diagnosed with fibromyalgia and symptomatic hyperuricemia, which were treated with regular analgesia and allopurinol. She also required ongoing treatment for depression. In addition, she developed a dumping-type syndrome (pallor, diaphoresis, and shakiness following meals) without associated hypoglycemia. The second patient was a 15-year-old male, diagnosed with CP at age of 4 years, also with panhypopituitarism and rapid weight gain following gross total resection. Comorbidities included dyslipidemia, hepatosteatosis, and hyperinsulinism. At the age of 14 years, a trial of octreotide led to no reduction of weight gain. At the time of bariatric surgery, his BMI was 42 kg/m^2. Given that the underlying cause of obesity was biological and would be present life-long, the surgeons involved felt that a diversionary surgical procedure would be a better option than LAGB. Following a BPD with duodenal switch, his BMI decreased to 32 kg/m^2 over the 2-year follow-up. The post-operative course was complicated by bradycardia requiring pacemaker placement, and stenosis of the distal surgical anastomosis requiring several laparoscopic repairs. Overall, both patients exhibited robust, sustained weight loss with resolution of metabolic comorbidities.

The efficacy of bariatric surgery for weight loss has also been examined in other HyOb patient populations. Scheimann et al. recently reported a retrospective critical analysis of bariatric procedures in PWS. PWS is a complex genetic disorder that results in marked hyperphagia and obesity felt to be secondary to hypothalamic dysfunction. The critical analysis revealed that a number of procedures, including BPD, RYGB, VBG, and endoscopic intragastric balloon placement have been used in this population. A review of 60 PWS patients highlighted the limited effectiveness and concerning safety profile of operations for weight loss in this unique population (Scheimann et al., 2008). In the short term, there appears to be some limited weight loss that is variable across different procedures. For RYGB, average weight loss was 4.2% for PWS patients after 6 months. Twelve month and 24 month follow-up revealed 6.5 and 2% weight loss, respectively. This weight loss is far less than the 35% reduction in BMI we see 1 year after RYGB for adolescents who do not have PWS. Five year follow-up, while limited, showed only a 2.4% weight loss in PWS patients after RYGB ($n = 9$). Long term weight loss was worse with VBG, with PWS patients experiencing a 3.5% weight gain after 5 years ($n = 2$). Patients undergoing BPD had higher weight loss of 27.6% at 12-months, but nearly half regained weight within 2–5 years. In addition, the report highlights what appears to be a high post-operative complication rate, with 47% requiring surgical revision after RYGB and 27% experiencing acute gastric dilation (Scheimann et al., 2008).

Bariatric surgery has also been reported in an adolescent patient with BBS. Patients with BBS demonstrate hyperphagia and obesity which have been linked to disruption of primary cilia in POMC neurons in the hypothalamus and possibly to altered leptin receptor functioning. In this 16-year-old with a BMI of 53 kg/m^2, RYGB resulted in a 33% reduction in BMI 3 years following surgery (Daskalakis et al., 2010). Improvement in hypertension and hyperuricemia was also observed.

Finally, as melanocortin 4 receptor (MC4R) variants represent the most common monogenetic form of HyOb in humans, it is relevant to assess the outcome of bariatric surgery in individuals with documented MC4R mutations. Surgical experience in this special group of HyOb patients is very limited. A group of investigators at the University of California San Francisco (UCSF) described surgical outcomes in an adolescent patient with a complete loss of function mutation at MC4R. This 18-year-old male presented with a preoperative weight of 166 kg and BMI of 54 kg/m^2 and underwent bilateral truncal vagotomy and laparoscopic adjustable GB. In this patient, the surgical intervention did not result in successful weight loss. Indeed, after an initial modest weight reduction of 12 kg over the first 4 months, the patient regained weight and by 1 year was 6.5 kg over his preoperative weight. Several features of the case however are relevant to interpretation of the outcome. First, the patient had moved away to college 4 months prior to the operation, and had in that time experienced a 66-kg weight gain. Also, the patient returned for only two band adjustments in the 1-year period of time, which is markedly less than the typically recommended post-operative adjustment schedule. Finally, the authors described an insatiable hunger 1 year after the operation, which was almost certainly a factor contributing to weight gain (Aslan et al., 2011b).

In a more recent publication from the same group at UCSF, the first report of an experience with gastric bypass in the setting of mutant MC4R contrasts with the results obtained after GB. Aslan et al. analyzed 1 year outcomes of four adults with heterozygous MC4R mutations in comparison to matched controls with normal MC4R gene sequences. Excess weight loss (EWL) in these four subjects was identical to the 60–70% EWL seen in matched controls. There was no mention of changes in post-operative appetite in these patients, nor any changes in metabolic features in this cohort (Aslan et al., 2011a).

DISCUSSION AND FUTURE DIRECTIONS

Hypothalamic obesity is observed in a high percentage of patients with CP, resulting in significant comorbidities and negatively impacting quality of life. Unfortunately, few treatments have proven effective in this patient population. First line therapy for HyOb should include aggressive lifestyle modification including appropriate caloric intake and activity. Pituitary hormone deficiencies, if any, should be replaced and doses optimized. As mentioned previously, glucocorticoid replacement should be targeted at replacement doses (8–10 mg/m^2/day hydrocortisone equivalent) and patients should be given the lowest dose possible that is adequate to avoid symptoms of adrenal insufficiency. Thyroid replacement should generally target the fT4 at the upper third of the normal range and patients should be clinically and biochemically monitored for signs/symptoms of hyper- and hypothyroidism (Rose, 2010). The decision to replace GH should be made in consultation with the patient, family, and other team members such as their oncologist and neurosurgeon. If done, GH doses should be titrated to keep IGF-1 levels within the median range. Ideally, other medical treatments aimed specifically at ameliorating weight should be pursued through approved protocols at centers capable of collecting outcomes data on a sufficiently large number of patients so that risks and benefits of treatment can be more precisely defined. This is especially important with respect to bariatric surgery in this population.

Here, we have reviewed the current body of published research on bariatric surgery in CP–HyOb. We have also included several published reports of bariatric surgery in other populations of HyOb, including PWS, BBS, and patients with MC4R mutations. While the limited scope of these reports makes comparison difficult, the experience in PWS patients demonstrates that all cases of HyOb should not be treated equally. Likely as a result of the multisystemic nature of their disorder, PWS patients have a significantly increased incidence of complications following bariatric surgery without the benefits of sustained weight loss. In addition, it appears that early dietary interventions are able to partially abrogate weight gain this population (Schmidt et al., 2008). Thus, the risk–benefit ratio of bariatric surgery in PWS does not appear to be favorable.

The initial reports of bariatric surgery in CP–HyOb and patients with MC4Rappear more promising, but again, their limited scope makes it difficult to draw any substantial conclusions as to the long term safety and efficacy of these procedures in this population. The limited number of cases inhibits comparison among various procedures. For instance, how does RYGB compare to LAGB with regard to long term, sustained weight loss, or with regard to safety and side-effects? In addition, more work is needed to understand the hormonal alterations that occur in CP–HyOb following bariatric surgery. Are such alterations similar to those seen in diet-induced obesity? If not, why? If so, do CP–HyOb patients derive the same benefits given their underlying hypothalamic damage? If hyperinsulinism is an underlying factor in the development of HyOb, will patients benefit or be harmed from increased levels of the insulin secretagogues such as GLP-1. Will potentiating insulin secretion place these patients at higher risk of hypoglycemia secondary to the mismatch of insulin secretion and carbohydrate absorption? These and other questions remain unanswered by the current body of research in this population and should be the subject of future work.

In addition, as 50% of patients diagnosed with CP are children, there are serious medical, psychological, and ethical concerns regarding bariatric surgery that must be considered in this population (Inge et al., 2004). Generally, adolescent candidates for bariatric surgery must meet more conservative patient selection criteria than are acceptable in adults. However, exact criteria are still of some debate. In 2008, the Endocrine Society, in conjunction with the Pediatric Endocrine Society, published a Clinical Practice Guideline on the Prevention and Treatment of Pediatric Obesity, wherein the task force recommended limiting bariatric surgery to adolescents with a BMI $\geq$ 50 kg/m^2 or a BMI $\geq$ 40 kg/m^2 with significant, severe comorbidities. In addition, the task force recommended that candidates have attained Tanner 4 or 5 pubertal development and near-final adult height, experienced continued weight gain despite following a formal program of lifestyle modification, and belong to a stable, medically competent family unit. The patient and family should understand that bariatric surgery is not a cure for obesity, but rather an adjunct to a continued commitment to lifestyle modifications in diet and activity. The surgery should be performed by an experienced surgeon in a medical center employing a team capable of long term follow-up and participating in a study of bariatric surgery outcomes. These recommendations largely agree with guidelines previously published and advocate the priority of avoiding unforeseen complications associated with life-long exposure to anatomical and functional alterations above the value of weight loss and amelioration of obesity-related complications provided by bariatric surgery (August et al., 2008).

More recently, Pratt et al. (2009) suggest that adolescents with a BMI $\geq$ 35 kg/m^2 and serious comorbidities including Type 2 diabetes, moderate to severe OSA, and/or pseudotumor cerebri or those with BMI $\geq$ 40 kg/m^2 with less serious comorbid conditions such as hypertension, dyslipidemia, gastroesophageal reflux disease, and/or psychosocial stress should be considered as candidates for bariatric surgery. While concurring with the other physical, lifestyle, and psychosocial criteria previously published, they use several lines of evidence to defend the lower BMI criteria. First, they cite data to indicate that patient safety and weight loss outcomes for extremely obese adolescents who undergo bariatric surgery are comparable to, or better than, those seen in adults. Second, even with the lower BMI criteria of 35 kg/m^2, candidates under the age of 18 would still be above the 99th BMI percentile and be at substantially increased risk for short and long term medical comorbidities. Third, they stress that selection for bariatric surgery during adolescence should be closely linked to obesity-related comorbidities. The less severe comorbidities and/or fewer risk factors for long term disease, the higher the BMI cut point should be before considering bariatric surgery. Finally, some have suggested that because younger patients will generally have fewer advanced comorbidities, early bariatric surgery may decrease the risk of future perioperative mortality, assuming the needed surgery is delayed until adulthood (Garcia and DeMaria, 2006).

Importantly, none of the guidelines for bariatric surgery directly addresses the use of bariatric surgery in HyOb generally or CP–HyOb in particular. In general, we believe that most criteria from the published guidelines can be applied to the HyOb patients, especially in adults. Whether one or more of the published criteria should be modified in the context of children and adolescents is subject to ongoing debate. Given what is known about the natural history of HyOb, its resistance to diet and lifestyle modification, and the extreme and progressive weight gain involved, some may consider bariatric surgery appropriate at ages currently considered too young in patients with exogenous obesity. However, in general, the younger the patient the more compelling and serious the comorbidities must be to justify surgical intervention. Because of the need for life-long medical support, optimal care of HyOb patients will be best met in the setting of tertiary care centers where they can receive treatment in a coordinated, multidisciplinary fashion. Team members should include the primary care physician and as needed subspecialists in neurosurgery, neurology, oncology, endocrinology, bariatric surgery, and mental health. Ideally, ancillary support by nutrition, physical therapy, nursing, and social work should also be available. Patients and families choosing to undergo bariatric surgery should be properly informed regarding specific risks and benefits associated with surgical weight loss and age appropriate consent or assent obtained. To facilitate needed research in this area, patients should be encouraged to enroll in available databases and research protocols.

These early reports of outcome of surgical weight loss treatment of HyOb are limited in scope and number, but give us a glimpse of the possible role of surgery in treatment of these conditions. They also make evident the need for more robust, controlled, prospective studies with long term follow-up in order to better define the role of medical as well as surgical therapies in the treatment of HyOb. In order to ultimately understand the outcome of surgical therapy for HyOb, sufficiently long follow-up of sufficient numbers of similar patients who undergo surgery as well as non-surgical controls will be required. Non-human surgical models might also in the future permit a better understanding of the mechanisms of obesity, and the importance of tailoring specific operative elements to each unique population.

Research in this important area is hampered by the difficulty of assembling a sufficiently large cohort of CP–HyOb patients. Given the relative rarity of the condition, it would take a single institution many years to put together a study large enough to reach valid, persuasive conclusions regarding the treatment of HyOb – surgical or otherwise. In order to increase public awareness of HyOb, facilitate future research and ultimately improve the management of HyOb, the International Registry for HyOb Disorders (www.IRHOD.org) has been established. The web-based interface will permit both healthcare providers and patient/families to easily enter basic information regarding their HyOb case. The systematic accumulation of a large world-wide cohort of patients with HyOb will facilitate recognition of individuals eligible for participation in studies of HyOb and its treatment. This registry, therefore, has potential to fill many of the numerous knowledge gaps around pathogenesis, coexisting disease, and treatment outcomes for this debilitating form of obesity.

REFERENCES

Abeloff, M. D. (2008). *Abeloff's Clinical Oncology*. Philadelphia: Churchill Livingstone/Elsevier.

Abs, R., Feldt-Rasmussen, U., Mattsson, A. F., Monson, J. P., Bengtsson, B. A., Goth, M. I., Wilton, P., and Koltowska-Haggstrom, M. (2006). Determinants of cardiovascular risk in 2589 hypopituitary GH-deficient adults – a KIMS database analysis. *Eur. J. Endocrinol.* 155, 79–90.

Ahmet, A., Blaser, S., Stephens, D., Guger, S., Rutkas, J. T., and Hamilton, J. (2006). Weight gain in craniopharyngioma – a model for hypothalamic obesity. *J. Pediatr. Endocrinol. Metab.* 19, 121–127.

Aslan, I. R., Campos, G. M., Calton, M. A., Evans, D. S., Merriman, R. B., and Vaisse, C. (2011a). Weight loss after Roux-en-Y gastric bypass in obese patients heterozygous for MC4R mutations. *Obes. Surg.* 21, 930–934.

Aslan, I. R., Ranadive, S. A., Ersoy, B. A., Rogers, S. J., Lustig, R. H., and Vaisse, C. (2011b). Bariatric surgery in a patient with complete MC4R deficiency. *Int. J. Obes. (Lond.)* 35, 457–461.

August, G. P., Caprio, S., Fennoy, I., Freemark, M., Kaufman, F. R., Lustig, R. H., Silverstein, J. H., Speiser, P. W., Styne, D. M., and Montori, V. M. (2008). Prevention and treatment of pediatric obesity: an endocrine society clinical practice guideline based on expert opinion. *J. Clin. Endocrinol. Metab.* 93, 4576–4599.

Baggio, L. L., and Drucker, D. J. (2007). Biology of incretins: GLP-1 and GIP. *Gastroenterology* 132, 2131–2157.

Bays, H. E. (2004). Current and investigational antiobesity agents and obesity therapeutic treatment targets. *Obes. Res.* 12, 1197–1211.

Beccuti, G., and Pannain, S. (2011). Sleep and obesity. *Curr. Opin. Clin. Nutr. Metab. Care* 14, 402–412.

Boyanov, M. A., Boneva, Z., and Christov, V. G. (2003). Testosterone supplementation in men with type 2 diabetes, visceral obesity and partial androgen deficiency. *Aging Male* 6, 1–7.

Brandon, D. D., Isabelle, L. M., Samuels, M. H., Kendall, J. W., and Loriaux, D. L. (1999). Cortisol production rate measurement by stable isotope dilution using gas chromatography-negative ion chemical ionization mass spectrometry. *Steroids* 64, 372–378.

Buchwald, H., Avidor, Y., Braunwald, E., Jensen, M. D., Pories, W., Fahrbach, K., and Schoelles, K. (2004). Bariatric surgery: a systematic review and meta-analysis. *JAMA* 292, 1724–1737.

Clement, K., Vaisse, C., Lahlou, N., Cabrol, S., Pelloux, V., Cassuto, D., Gourmelen, M., Dina, C., Chambaz, J., Lacorte, J. M., Basdevant, A., Bougneres, P., Lebouc, Y., Froguel, P., and Guy-Grand, B. (1998). A mutation in the human leptin receptor gene causes obesity and pituitary dysfunction. *Nature* 392, 398–401.

Coutant, R., Maurey, H., Rouleau, S., Mathieu, E., Mercier, P., Limal, J. M., and Le Bouil, A. (2003). Defect in epinephrine production in children with craniopharyngioma: functional or organic origin? *J. Clin. Endocrinol. Metab.* 88, 5969–5975.

Cummings, D. E., Clement, K., Purnell, J. Q., Vaisse, C., Foster, K. E., Frayo, R. S., Schwartz, M. W., Basdevant, A., and Weigle, D. S. (2002a). Elevated plasma ghrelin levels in Prader Willi syndrome. *Nat. Med.* 8, 643–644.

Cummings, D. E., Weigle, D. S., Frayo, R. S., Breen, P. A., Ma, M. K., Dellinger, E. P., and Purnell, J. Q. (2002b). Plasma ghrelin levels after diet-induced weight loss or gastric bypass surgery. *N. Engl. J. Med.* 346, 1623–1630.

Daskalakis, M., Till, H., Kiess, W., and Weiner, R. A. (2010). Roux-en-Y gastric bypass in an adolescent patient with Bardet-Biedl syndrome, a monogenic obesity disorder. *Obes. Surg.* 20, 121–125.

de Vile, C. J., Grant, D. B., Hayward, D., Kendall, B. E., Neville, B. G., and Stanhope, R. (1996). Obesity in childhood craniopharyngioma: relation to post-operative hypothalamic damage shown by magnetic resonance imaging. *J. Clin. Endocrinol. Metab.* 81, 2734–2737.

Debono, M., Ross, R. J., and Newell-Price, J. (2009). Inadequacies of glucocorticoid replacement and improvements by physiological circadian therapy. *Eur. J. Endocrinol.* 160, 719–729.

DelParigi, A., Tschop, M., Heiman, M. L., Salbe, A. D., Vozarova, B., Sell, M., Bunt, J. C., and Tataranni, P. A. (2002). High circulating ghrelin: a potential cause for hyperphagia and obesity in Prader-Willi syndrome. *J. Clin. Endocrinol. Metab.* 87, 5461–5464.

Eiholzer, U., Blum, W. F., and Molinari, L. (1999). Body fat determined by skinfold measurements is elevated despite underweight in infants with Prader-Labhart-Willi syndrome. *J. Pediatr.* 134, 222–225.

Esteban, N. V., Loughlin, T., Yergey, A. L., Zawadzki, J. K., Booth, J. D., Winterer, J. C., and Loriaux, D. L. (1991). Daily cortisol production rate in man determined by stable isotope dilution/mass spectrometry. *J. Clin. Endocrinol. Metab.* 72, 39–45.

Eyal, O., Sundararajan, S., Inge, T. H., and Rose, S. R. (2006). Obesity in patients with craniopharyngioma. *Endocrinologist* 16, 286–293.

Filipsson, H., Monson, J. P., Koltowska-Haggstrom, M., Mattsson, A., and Johannsson, G. (2006). The impact of glucocorticoid replacement regimens on metabolic outcome and comorbidity in hypopituitary patients. *J. Clin. Endocrinol. Metab.* 91, 3954–3961.

Garcia, V. F., and DeMaria, E. J. (2006). Adolescent bariatric surgery: treatment delayed, treatment denied, a crisis invited. *Obes. Surg.* 16, 1–4.

Goldstone, A. P., Holland, A. J., Hauffa, B. P., Hokken-Koelega, A. C., and Tauber, M. (2008). Recommendations for the diagnosis and management of Prader-Willi syndrome. *J. Clin. Endocrinol. Metab.* 93, 4183–4197.

Guo, D. F., and Rahmouni, K. (2011). Molecular basis of the obesity associated with Bardet-Biedl syndrome. *Trends Endocrinol. Metab.* 22, 286–293.

Hamilton, J. K., Conwell, L. S., Syme, C., Ahmet, A., Jeffery, A., and Daneman, D. (2011). Hypothalamic obesity following craniopharyngioma surgery: results of a pilot trial of combined diazoxide and metformin therapy. *Int. J. Pediatr. Endocrinol.* 2011, 417949.

Harwood-Nash, D. C. (1994). Neuroimaging of childhood craniopharyngioma. *Pediatr. Neurosurg.* 21(Suppl. 1), 2–10.

Harz, K. J., Muller, H. L., Waldeck, E., Pudel, V., and Roth, C. (2003). Obesity in patients with craniopharyngioma: assessment of food intake and movement counts indicating physical activity. *J. Clin. Endocrinol. Metab.* 88, 5227–5231.

Hetherington, A. W., and Ranson, S. W. (1940). Hypothalamic lesions and adiposity in the rat. *Anat. Rec.* 78, 149–172.

Hochberg, I., and Hochberg, Z. (2010). Expanding the definition of hypothalamic obesity. *Obes. Rev.* 11, 709–721.

Holmer, H., Pozarek, G., Wirfalt, E., Popovic, V., Ekman, B., Bjork, J., and Erfurth, E. M. (2010). Reduced energy expenditure and impaired feeding-related signals but not high energy intake reinforces hypothalamic obesity in adults with childhood onset craniopharyngioma. *J. Clin. Endocrinol. Metab.* 95, 5395–5402.

Inge, T. H., Krebs, N. F., Garcia, V. F., Skelton, J. A., Guice, K. S., Strauss, R. S., Albanese, C. T., Brandt, M. L., Hammer, L. D., Harmon, C. M., Kane, T. D., Klish, W. J., Oldham, K. T., Rudolph, C. D., Helmrath, M. A., Donovan, E., and Daniels, S. R. (2004). Bariatric surgery for severely overweight adolescents: concerns and recommendations. *Pediatrics* 114, 217–223.

Inge, T. H., Pfluger, P., Zeller, M., Rose, S. R., Burget, L., Sundararajan, S., Daniels, S. R., and Tschop, M. H. (2007). Gastric bypass surgery for treatment of hypothalamic obesity after craniopharyngioma therapy. *Nat. Clin. Pract. Endocrinol. Metab.* 3, 606–609.

Karavitaki, N., Brufani, C., Warner, J. T., Adams, C. B., Richards, P., Ansorge, O., Shine, B., Turner, H. E., and Wass, J. A. (2005). Craniopharyngiomas in children and adults: systematic analysis of 121 cases with long-term follow-up. *Clin. Endocrinol. (Oxf.)* 62, 397–409.

Karavitaki, N., Cudlip, S., Adams, C. B., and Wass, J. A. (2006). Craniopharyngiomas. *Endocr. Rev.* 27, 371–397.

Karra, E., Yousseif, A., and Batterham, R. L. (2010). Mechanisms facilitating weight loss and resolution of type 2 diabetes following bariatric surgery. *Trends Endocrinol. Metab.* 21, 337–344.

Katznelson, L., Finkelstein, J. S., Schoenfeld, D. A., Rosenthal, D. I., Anderson, E. J., and Klibanski, A. (1996). Increase in bone density and lean body mass during testosterone administration in men with acquired hypogonadism. *J. Clin. Endocrinol. Metab.* 81, 4358–4365.

Kerrigan, J. R., Veldhuis, J. D., Leyo, S. A., Iranmanesh, A., and Rogol, A. D. (1993). Estimation of daily cortisol production and clearance rates in normal pubertal males by deconvolution analysis. *J. Clin. Endocrinol. Metab.* 76, 1505–1510.

Koopmans, H. S., Ferri, G. L., Sarson, D. L., Polak, J. M., and Bloom, S. R. (1984). The effects of ileal transposition and jejunoileal bypass on food intake and GI hormone levels in rats. *Physiol. Behav.* 33, 601–609.

Koulouri, O., Auldin, M. A., Agarwal, R., Kieffer, V., Robertson, C., Falconer Smith, J., Levy, M. J., and Howlett, T. A. (2011). Diagnosis and treatment of hypothyroidism in TSH deficiency compared to primary thyroid disease: pituitary patients are at risk of under-replacement with levothyroxine. *Clin. Endocrinol. (Oxf.)* 74, 744–749.

Kronenberg, H., and Williams, R. H. (2008). *Williams Textbook of Endocrinology*. Philadelphia: Saunders/Elsevier.

Laferrere, B., Teixeira, J., Mcginty, J., Tran, H., Egger, J. R., Colarusso, A., Kovack, B., Bawa, B., Koshy, N., Lee, H., Yapp, K., and Olivan, B. (2008).

Effect of weight loss by gastric bypass surgery versus hypocaloric diet on glucose and incretin levels in patients with type 2 diabetes. *J. Clin. Endocrinol. Metab.* 93, 2479–2485.

le Roux, C. W., Aylwin, S. J., Batterham, R. L., Borg, C. M., Coyle, F., Prasad, V., Shurey, S., Ghatei, M. A., Patel, A. G., and Bloom, S. R. (2006). Gut hormone profiles following bariatric surgery favor an anorectic state, facilitate weight loss, and improve metabolic parameters. *Ann. Surg.* 243, 108–114.

Linder, B. L., Esteban, N. V., Yergey, A. L., Winterer, J. C., Loriaux, D. L., and Cassorla, F. (1990). Cortisol production rate in childhood and adolescence. *J. Pediatr.* 117, 892–896.

Lubrano-Berthelier, C., Dubern, B., Lacorte, J. M., Picard, F., Shapiro, A., Zhang, S., Bertrais, S., Hercberg, S., Basdevant, A., Clement, K., and Vaisse, C. (2006). Melanocortin 4 receptor mutations in a large cohort of severely obese adults: prevalence, functional classification, genotypephenotype relationship, and lack of association with binge eating. *J. Clin. Endocrinol. Metab.* 91, 1811–1818.

Lustig, R. H. (2008). Hypothalamic obesity: causes, consequences, treatment. *Pediatr. Endocrinol. Rev.* 6, 220–227.

Lustig, R. H., Greenway, F., Velasquez-Mieyer, P., Heimburger, D., Schumacher, D., Smith, D., Smith, W., Soler, N., Warsi, G., Berg, W., Maloney, J., Benedetto, J., Zhu, W., and Hohneker, J. (2006). A multicenter, randomized, double-blind, placebo-controlled, dose-finding trial of a long-acting formulation of octreotide in promoting weight loss in obese adults with insulin hypersecretion. *Int. J. Obes. (Lond.)* 30, 331–341.

Lustig, R. H., Rose, S. R., Burghen, G. A., Velasquez-Mieyer, P., Broome, D. C., Smith, K., Li, H., Hudson, M. M., Heideman, R. L., and Kun, L. E. (1999). Hypothalamic obesity caused by cranial insult in children: altered glucose and insulin dynamics and reversal by a somatostatin agonist. *J. Pediatr.* 135, 162–168.

Mason, P. W., Krawiecki, N., and Meacham, L. R. (2002). The use of dextroamphetamine to treat obesity and hyperphagia in children treated for craniopharyngioma. *Arch. Pediatr. Adolesc. Med.* 156, 887–892.

Miura, Y., Gilon, P., and Henquin, J. C. (1996). Muscarinic stimulation increases Na+ entry in pancreatic B-cells by a mechanism other than the emptying of intracellular Ca2+pools. *Biochem. Biophys. Res. Commun.* 224, 67–73.

Mortini, P., Losa, M., Pozzobon, G., Barzaghi, R., Riva, M., Acerno, S., Angius, D., Weber, G., Chiumello, G., and Giovanelli, M. (2011). Neurosurgical treatment of craniopharyngioma in adults and children: early and long-term results in a large case series. *J. Neurosurg.* 114, 1350–1359.

Muller, H. L. (2008). Childhood craniopharyngioma. Recent advances in diagnosis, treatment and follow-up. *Horm. Res.* 69, 193–202.

Muller, H. L., Bruhnken, G., Emser, A., Faldum, A., Etavard-Gorris, N., Gebhardt, U., Kolb, R., and Sorensen, N. (2005). Longitudinal study on quality of life in 102 survivors of childhood craniopharyngioma. *Childs Nerv. Syst.* 21, 975–980.

Muller, H. L., Bueb, K., Bartels, U., Roth, C., Harz, K., Graf, N., Korinthenberg, R., Bettendorf, M., Kuhl, J., Gutjahr, P., Sorensen, N., and Calaminus, G. (2001). Obesity after childhood craniopharyngioma – German multicenter study on pre-operative risk factors and quality of life. *Klin. Padiatr.* 213, 244–249.

Muller, H. L., Emser, A., Faldum, A., Bruhnken, G., Etavard-Gorris, N., Gebhardt, U., Oeverink, R., Kolb, R., and Sorensen, N. (2004). Longitudinal study on growth and body mass index before and after diagnosis of childhood craniopharyngioma. *J. Clin. Endocrinol. Metab.* 89, 3298–3305.

Muller, H. L., Gebhardt, U., Schroder, S., Pohl, F., Kortmann, R. D., Faldum, A., Zwiener, I., Warmuth-Metz, M., Pietsch, T., Calaminus, G., Kolb, R., Wiegand, C., and Sorensen, N. (2010). Analyses of treatment variables for patients with childhood craniopharyngioma – results of the multicenter prospective trial KRAN-IOPHARYNGEOM 2000 after three years of follow-up. *Horm. Res. Paediatr.* 73, 175–180.

Muller, H. L., Gebhardt, U., Wessel, V., Schroder, S., Kolb, R., Sorensen, N., Maroske, J., and Hanisch, E. (2007). First experiences with laparoscopic adjustable gastric banding (LAGB) in the treatment of patients with childhood craniopharyngioma and morbid obesity. *Klin. Padiatr.* 219, 323–325.

Muller, H. L., Handwerker, G., Wollny, B., Faldum, A., and Sorensen, N. (2002). Melatonin secretion and increased daytime sleepiness in childhood craniopharyngioma patients. *J. Clin. Endocrinol. Metab.* 87, 3993–3996.

Muller, H. L., Muller-Stover, S., Gebhardt, U., Kolb, R., Sorensen, N., and Handwerker, G. (2006). Secondary narcolepsy may be a causative factor of increased daytime sleepiness in obese childhood craniopharyngioma patients. *J. Pediatr. Endocrinol. Metab.* 19(Suppl. 1), 423–429.

Norman, R. J., Flight, I. H., and Rees, M. C. (2000). Oestrogen and progestogen hormone replacement therapy for peri-menopausal and post-menopausal women: weight and body fat distribution. *Cochrane Database Syst. Rev.* 2, CD001018.

Organ, C. H. Jr., Kessler, E., and Lane, M. (1984). Long-term results of jejunoileal bypass in the young. *Am. Surg.* 50, 589–593.

Pories, W. J., Swanson, M. S., Macdonald, K. G., Long, S. B., Morris, P. G., Brown, B. M., Barakat, H. A., deRamon, R. A., Israel, G., Dolezal, J. M., and Dohm, L. (1995). Who would have thought it? An operation proves to be the most effective therapy for adult-onset diabetes mellitus. *Ann. Surg.* 222, 339–350; discussion 350–332.

Pratt, J. S., Lenders, C. M., Dionne, E. A., Hoppin, A. G., Hsu, G. L., Inge, T. H., Lawlor, D. F., Marino, M. F., Meyers, A. F., Rosenblum, J. L., and Sanchez, V. M. (2009). Best practice updates for pediatric/adolescent weight loss surgery. *Obesity (Silver Spring)* 17, 901–910.

Rocca, A. S., and Brubaker, P. L. (1999). Role of the vagus nerve in mediating proximal nutrient-induced glucagon-like peptide-1 secretion. *Endocrinology* 140, 1687–1694.

Rohrer, T. R., Langer, T., Grabenbauer, G. G., Buchfelder, M., Glowatzki, M., and Dorr, H. G. (2010). Growth hormone therapy and the risk of tumor recurrence after brain tumor treatment in children. *J. Pediatr. Endocrinol. Metab.* 23, 935–942.

Rose, S. R. (2010). Improved diagnosis of mild hypothyroidism using time-of-day normal ranges for thyrotropin. *J. Pediatr.* 157, 662–667.

Roth, C., Wilken, B., Hanefeld, F., Schroter, W., and Leonhardt, U. (1998). Hyperphagia in children with craniopharyngioma is associated with hyperleptinaemia and a failure in the downregulation of appetite. *Eur. J. Endocrinol.* 138, 89–91.

Roth, C. L., Gebhardt, U., and Muller, H. L. (2011). Appetite-regulating hormone changes in patients with craniopharyngioma. *Obesity (Silver Spring)* 19, 36–42.

Roth, C. L., Hunneman, D. H., Gebhardt, U., Stoffel-Wagner, B., Reinehr, T., and Muller, H. L. (2007). Reduced sympathetic metabolites in urine of obese patients with craniopharyngioma. *Pediatr. Res.* 61, 496–501.

Rottembourg, D., O'gorman, C. S., Urbach, S., Garneau, P. Y., Langer, J. C., Van Vliet, G., Hamilton, J., and Huot, C. (2009). Outcome after bariatric surgery in two adolescents with hypothalamic obesity following treatment of craniopharyngioma. *J. Pediatr. Endocrinol. Metab.* 22, 867–872.

Sarson, D. L., Scopinaro, N., and Bloom, S. R. (1981). Gut hormone changes after jejunoileal (JIB) or biliopancreatic (BPB) bypass surgery for morbid obesity. *Int. J. Obes.* 5, 471–480. Savastano, D. M., Tanofsky-Kraff, M., Han, J. C., Ning, C., Sorg, R. A., Roza, C. A., Wolkoff, L. E., Anandalingam, K., Jefferson-George, K.

S., Figueroa, R. E., Sanford, E. L., Brady, S., Kozlosky, M., Schoeller, D. A., and Yanovski, J. A. (2009). Energy intake and energy expenditure among children with polymorphisms of the melanocortin-3 receptor. *Am. J. Clin. Nutr.* 90, 912–920.

Scheimann, A. O., Butler, M. G., Gourash, L., Cuffari, C., and Klish, W. (2008). Critical analysis of bariatric procedures in Prader-Willi syndrome. *J. Pediatr. Gastroenterol. Nutr.* 46, 80–83.

Schmidt, H., Pozza, S. B., Bonfig, W., Schwarz, H. P., and Dokoupil, K. (2008). Successful early dietary intervention avoids obesity in patients with Prader-Willi syndrome: a ten-year follow-up. *J. Pediatr. Endocrinol. Metab.* 21, 651–655.

Schofl, C., Schleth, A., Berger, D., Terkamp, C., Von Zur Muhlen, A., and Brabant, G. (2002). Sympathoadrenal counterregulation in patients with hypothalamic craniopharyngioma. *J. Clin. Endocrinol. Metab.* 87, 624–629.

Schultes, B., Ernst, B., Schmid, F., and Thurnheer, M. (2009). Distal gastric bypass surgery for the treatment of hypothalamic obesity after childhood craniopharyngioma. *Eur. J. Endocrinol.* 161, 201–206.

Schwartz, M. W., Woods, S. C., Porte, D. Jr., Seeley, R. J., and Baskin, D. G. (2000). Central nervous system control of food intake. *Nature* 404, 661–671.

Seo, S., Guo, D. F., Bugge, K., Morgan, D. A., Rahmouni, K., and Sheffield, V. C. (2009). Requirement of Bardet-Biedl syndrome proteins for leptin receptor signaling. *Hum. Mol. Genet.* 18, 1323–1331.

Skorzewska, A., Lal, S., Waserman, J., and Guyda, H. (1989). Abnormal food-seeking behavior after surgery for craniopharyngioma. *Neuropsychobiology* 21, 17–20.

Slawik, M., Klawitter, B., Meiser, E., Schories, M., Zwermann, O., Borm, K., Peper, M., Lubrich, B., Hug, M. J., Nauck, M., Olschewski, M., Beuschlein, F., and Reincke, M. (2007). Thyroid hormone replacement for central hypothyroidism: a randomized controlled trial comparing two doses of thyroxine (T4) with a combination of T4 and triiodothyronine. *J. Clin. Endocrinol. Metab.* 92, 4115–4122.

Sorva, R. (1988). Children with craniopharyngioma. Early growth failure and rapid postoperative weight gain. *Acta Paediatr. Scand.* 77, 587–592.

Srinivasan, S., Ogle, G. D., Garnett, S. P., Briody, J. N., Lee, J. W., and Cowell, C. T. (2004). Features of the metabolic syndrome after childhood craniopharyngioma. *J. Clin. Endocrinol. Metab.* 89, 81–86.

Verhelst, J., and Abs, R. (2009). Cardiovascular risk factors in hypopituitary GH-deficient adults. *Eur. J. Endocrinol.* 161(Suppl. 1), S41–S49.

Winkfield, K. M., Tsai, H. K., Yao, X., Larson, E., Neuberg, D., Pomeroy, S. L., Ullrich, N. J., Cohen, L. E., Kieran, M. W., Scott, R. M., Goumnerova, C., and Marcus, K. J. (2011). Long-term clinical outcomes following treatment of childhood craniopharyngioma. *Pediatr. Blood Cancer* 56, 1120–1126.

Wittert, G. A., Chapman, I. M., Haren, T., Mackintosh, S., Coates, P., and Morley, J. E. (2003). Oral testosterone supplementation increases muscle and decreases fat mass in healthy elderly males with lownormal gonadal status. *J. Gerontol. A Biol. Sci. Med. Sci.* 58, 618–625.

14

Hypothalamic response to the chemo-signal androstadienone in gender dysphoric children and adolescents

Sarah M. Burke[1,2]*, Peggy T. Cohen-Kettenis[1], Dick J. Veltman[3], Daniel T. Klink[4] and Julie Bakker[1,2,5]

[1] Center of Expertise on Gender Dysphoria, Neuroscience Campus Amsterdam, Department of Medical Psychology, VU University Medical Center, Amsterdam, Netherlands

[2] Neuroendocrinology Group, Netherlands Institute for Neuroscience, Amsterdam, Netherlands

[3] Department of Psychiatry, Neuroscience Campus Amsterdam, VU University Medical Center, Amsterdam, Netherlands

[4] Center of Expertise on Gender Dysphoria, Department of Pediatric Endocrinology, VU University Medical Center, Amsterdam, Netherlands

[5] GIGA Neuroscience, University of Liege, Liege, Belgium

***Correspondence:**
Sarah M. Burke, Center of Expertise on Gender Dysphoria, Neuroscience Campus Amsterdam, Department of Medical Psychology, VU University Medical Center, De Boelelaan 1131, Amsterdam 1081 HX, Netherlands
e-mail: s.burke@vumc.nl

The odorous steroid androstadienone, a putative male chemo-signal, was previously reported to evoke sex differences in hypothalamic activation in adult heterosexual men and women. In order to investigate whether puberty modulated this sex difference in response to androstadienone, we measured the hypothalamic responsiveness to this chemo-signal in 39 pre-pubertal and 41 adolescent boys and girls by means of functional magnetic resonance imaging. We then investigated whether 36 pre-pubertal children and 38 adolescents diagnosed with gender dysphoria (GD; DSM-5) exhibited sex-atypical (in accordance with their experienced gender), rather than sex-typical (in accordance with their natal sex) hypothalamic activations during olfactory stimulation with androstadienone. We found that the sex difference in responsiveness to androstadienone was already present in pre-pubertal control children and thus likely developed during early perinatal development instead of during sexual maturation. Adolescent girls and boys with GD both responded remarkably like their experienced gender, thus sex-atypical. In contrast, pre-pubertal girls with GD showed neither a typically male nor female hypothalamic activation pattern and pre-pubertal boys with GD had hypothalamic activations in response to androstadienone that were similar to control boys, thus sex-typical. We present here a unique data set of boys and girls diagnosed with GD at two different developmental stages, showing that these children possess certain sex-atypical functional brain characteristics and may have undergone atypical sexual differentiation of the brain.

Keywords: androstadienone, chemo-signal, fMRI, gender dysphoria, hypothalamus, puberty, sex difference

INTRODUCTION

In humans, the odorous steroid 4,16-androstadien-3-one (androstadienone) has been studied intensively as a putative male modulator chemo-signal. Androstadienone, probably synthesized in the gonads (1), is secreted by the apocrine glands and can be found on the skin surface and axillary hairs (2), as well as in several body fluids including sweat and semen (3, 4). Higher concentrations of androstadienone in sweat have been found in men compared to women (5, 6). Exposure to androstadienone has been shown to affect women's mental state (7–10), and to elicit physiological responses in a sex-dependent manner (7, 9, 11–15). Moreover, smelling androstadienone had an impact on women's hormone levels (16) and affected their behavioral responses dependent on the phase of the menstrual cycle (17).

In line with the effects androstadienone had on the autonomic nervous system and on behavior, studies conducted by Savic et al. (18), using positron emission tomography (PET), showed that smelling androstadienone induced a response in the hypothalamus of heterosexual women but not in heterosexual men. The latter only showed an activation in brain areas belonging to the main olfactory system, such as the piriform cortex and amygdala (18). Thus, olfactory stimulation with androstadienone offers a relatively simple and objective experimental procedure for investigating functional sex differences in the human brain. Using functional magnetic resonance imaging (fMRI), we recently replicated the finding of women showing a stronger hypothalamic activation than men, after smelling the highest (10 mM) out of three concentrations tested (19).

Secretion of androstadienone increases substantially during puberty. As a result, sex-related changes in olfactory sensitivity to androstenes have been reported during adolescence (20–23) with male adolescents exhibiting more anosmia to androstadienone, and an increase of odor threshold with age, compared to female adolescents. It may be inferred that the decrease in sensitivity to odorous steroids in pubescent boys is related to their increased production of endogenous androgens during puberty, probably reflecting adaptation toward (male) body odors.

Sisk and colleagues (24, 25) proposed a two-stage model of sexual differentiation of brain and behavior, in which early perinatal organizational effects of steroid hormones are followed by a second steroid-dependent sensitive phase of neurodevelopment during adolescence. Thus, puberty may be considered an organizational period in itself, in which sex differences in brain morphology and function are established or consolidated. Therefore, our first aim was to investigate whether the hypothalamic response to androstadienone develops during puberty, as part of sexual maturation, or whether it would already be present in pre-pubertal children and thus established during early brain development. Thus, we tested whether the response to androstadienone varied as a function of sex and pubertal status in four groups of pre-pubertal and adolescent boys and girls.

Of note, further studies by Savic et al. (26–28) showed that hypothalamic activation upon exposure to androstadienone also depended on sexual orientation (27, 28) and gender identity. Adult men diagnosed with gender dysphoria (GD) [DSM-5, Ref. (29)], and thus having a female gender identity showed a sex-atypical hypothalamic response, which reflected more on their experienced gender than their natal sex (26). This is in line with the hypothesis that individuals, diagnosed with GD might have undergone a sex-atypical programing of the nervous system (30, 31). The etiology of GD is currently unknown, however, a multitude of factors, ranging from adverse psycho-dynamic parent–child interactions (32), an anxious personality predisposition (33), genetic risk factors (34), and exposure to atypical levels of perinatal sex steroids during a critical period of sexual differentiation of the brain (35) have all been proposed to facilitate the development of GD.

At the Center of Expertise on Gender Dysphoria in Amsterdam, the current treatment protocol allows adolescents diagnosed with GD that persisted from childhood into adolescence to start treatment with gonadotropin-releasing hormone analogs (GnRHa) from the age of 12 years, to suppress endogenous gonadal stimulation and thus the development of irreversible sex characteristics of the natal sex (36). From the age of 16 years on, as a first step in sex reassignment they receive cross-sex hormone treatment, i.e., biological boys receive estrogens and biological girls receive androgens (37, 38).

A second aim of the current study was therefore to explore whether children and adolescents, diagnosed with GD, would show brain responses that reflect their expressed/experienced gender rather than their natal sex, and whether these would vary as a function of their developmental phase. Four groups of subjects, all diagnosed with GD, participated in the current study: girls and boys that were pre-pubertal and treatment-naïve, and girls and boys that were adolescent in age (though in hypogonadal state due to GnRHa treatment). None of our participants received cross-sex hormones at the time of data acquisition.

MATERIALS AND METHODS

SUBJECTS

The initial study sample consisted of a total of 158 participants. Four subjects were excluded from further analysis, because of anatomical anomalies (one adolescent), technical errors during data collection (one child), or because the diagnosis GD had been revised since their participation in the study (two boys with GD in remission). All participants diagnosed with GD, were recruited via the Center of Expertise on Gender Dysphoria at the VU University Medical Center in Amsterdam. The control participants were recruited via several primary and secondary schools in the Netherlands and by inviting friends and relatives of the participants with GD.

The children sample consisted of 19 control girls [mean years of age (M) = 9.7, standard deviation (SD) = 0.9], 20 control boys (M = 9.5, SD = 1.1), 17 girls with GD (M = 9.6, SD = 1.1), and 19 boys with GD (M = 10.4, SD = 0.9). All children underwent a short physical examination by a pediatric endocrinologist (Daniel T. Klink) in order to ascertain their pre-pubertal status (Tanner stage 1) (39, 40).

The adolescent groups consisted of 21 control girls (M = 16.3, SD = 0.9), 20 control boys (M = 15.0, SD = 0.6), 21 girls with GD (M = 16.1, SD = 0.8), and 17 boys with GD (M = 15.3, SD = 1.2). The adolescent participants, diagnosed with GD, had been treated monthly with 3.75 mg of Triptorelin (Decapeptyl-CR®, Ferring, Hoofddorp, the Netherlands) by injection for on average 24 months (range 2-48 months), resulting in complete suppression of gonadal hormone production. Female adolescent controls were tested randomly according to their menstrual cycle and 11 out of 21 control girls reported using hormonal contraception.

ASSESSMENTS AND SUBJECT CHARACTERISTIC

Sexual orientation was difficult to assess, especially in the pre-pubertal sample, because most children were simply too young to be able to report their sexual orientation. Therefore, current or presumed future sexual attraction was assessed by asking whether the participant had ever been in love with somebody, and if yes, whether that person was a boy or a girl. Normal olfactory function was ascertained by means of an extended version of the "Sniffin' Sticks" test battery (32-item odor identification test and olfactory threshold measurement) (41–43). Furthermore, participants were asked to report the perceived intensity of a 10 mM androstadienone solution (on a scale from 0 to 10). Separately, for the adolescent and the children samples, one-way analyses of variance (ANOVA) were conducted, using the Statistical Package for the Social Sciences, version 20 (SPSS Inc., Chicago, IL, USA), testing whether the four gender groups differed on any of these measures. Bonferroni correction for multiple comparisons was applied for *post hoc* tests, considering a threshold of $p < 0.05$ as statistically significant. All subjects and their legal guardians gave their informed consent according to the Declaration of Helsinki, and the study was approved by the Ethics Committee of the VU University Medical Center Amsterdam (application number NL31283.029.10).

OLFACTORY STIMULATION

Androstadienone (Steraloids Inc., Newport, RI 02840, USA) was diluted in propylene glycol (Sigma) to a concentration of 10 mM, according to the "high" concentration used in our previous study (19). The volume of the solution used during the fMRI experiments was 20 ml. Olfactory stimuli were delivered through a tubing system to the subjects' nostrils by means of a custom-built air-dilution olfactometer [for details of the olfactometer set-up and procedure see Ref. (19)]. With a total air flow of about 1 L/min, during "ON" periods every 2 s, the odor was delivered during 1 s, while during "OFF" periods subjects received odorless air.

IMAGE ACQUISITION

Scans were performed on a 3.0-T GE Signa HDxt scanner (General Electric, Milwaukee, WI, USA). A gradient echo, echo planar imaging sequence was used for functional imaging (19.2 cm^2 field of view, TR of 1950 ms, TE of 25 ms, an 80° flip angle, isotropic voxels of 3 mm, and 36 slices). Before each imaging session, a local high-order shimming technique was used to reduce susceptibility artifacts. A scanning session consisted of six alternating ON-OFF cycles over 108 volumes in a classical block design (one block consisted of nine volumes), lasting 3.6 min. For co-registration with the functional images, a T1-weighted scan was obtained (3D FSPGR sequence, 25 cm^2 field of view, TR of 7.8 ms, TE of 3.0 ms; slice thickness of 1 mm, and 176 slices).

IMAGE PROCESSING

Data analysis was performed with SPM8 software (Statistical Parametric Mapping; Wellcome Department of Imaging Neuroscience, Institute of Neurology at the University College London, UK) implemented in Matlab R2009b (Math Works Inc., Natick, MA, USA). Functional images were slice-timed and realigned to the mean image, followed by unwarp. Applying the "New Segment" and "Create Template" options of the DARTEL (Diffeomorphic Anatomical Registration Through Exponentiated Lie Algebra) toolbox, structural images were segmented. Then, gray matter and white matter images were used for creating age-group specific templates (one for the children and the adolescents sample each), registered in Montreal neurological institute (MNI) space. Functional images were spatially normalized to their respective group-template, applying each individual's DARTEL flow field, and finally, images were smoothed by means of a 5-mm full width half maximum (FWHM) isotropic Gaussian kernel.

Individual image data were analyzed using boxcar regressors convolved with a synthetic hemodynamic response function and a first-order time-modulation (TM) regressor to test for possible effects of adaptation/sensitization to androstadienone. In order to account for assumed late "wash-out" effects during OFF blocks and an early peak response to the odor stimulation during ON blocks, first-level contrast images were built by subtracting the second half (b) of the OFF blocks (four volumes) from the first part (a) of the ON blocks (four volumes). Accordingly, this was done with the associated TM regressor blocks. Further, based on the image realignment process, individual head jerks were identified (>1 mm displacement) (44). Together with the six motion parameters, these so-called scan nulling regressors were included in every first-level design matrix to account for the effects of excessive head motion.

STATISTICAL ANALYSES

First, in order to test whether the sex difference in response to androstadienone was present in both developmental control groups, and whether that sex difference in responsiveness varied as a function of adaptation/sensitization to the odor, we conducted a *sex* (control boys, control girls) by *odor stimulation* ANOVA, for both the pre-pubertal and the adolescent control groups. The factor *odor stimulation* consisted of two levels, a regressor modeling the condition ON_a-OFF_b effect, thus the hypothesized hypothalamic response to the odor, and a first-order parametric modulation TM ON_a-TM OFF_b regressor, which signifies how well the hypothalamic response correlates with changes over time, thus modeling possible effects of adaptation or sensitization.

Second, by means of four *gender* by *odor stimulation* ANOVAs separately for the pre-pubertal and the adolescent groups, we tested whether boys and girls diagnosed with GD differed significantly in response to the steroid odor in comparison to their respective natal sex or their experienced gender control group.

Analyses were restricted to the hypothalamus area as region of interest (ROI), defined [with Marsbar (45)] as a sphere (centered at MNI coordinates $x = 0$, $y = -10$, $z = -7$; with a 7-mm radius), and based on anatomical demarcations following (46) and (47). The threshold for statistical significance was set at $p < 0.05$ family-wise error (FWE)-corrected for the extent of the hypothalamus ROI.

RESULTS

PSYCHOPHYSICS AND SUBJECT CHARACTERISTICS

Demographic, self-report, and subject characteristics are presented in **Table 1**. The adolescent boys with GD were significantly younger and less physically mature than the three other adolescent groups. The pre-pubertal boys with GD were significantly older than the pre-pubertal control boys. Therefore, in all group comparisons involving boys with GD, age was included as covariate. As expected, both adolescent control groups differed significantly from the boys and girls diagnosed with GD with respect to reported sexual orientation. There were no group differences in olfactory performance and on ratings of the perceived intensity of androstadienone.

SEX DIFFERENCES IN HYPOTHALAMIC ACTIVATION – EFFECTS OF PUBERTY

In order to determine whether hypothalamic activation upon smelling androstadienone is dependent on puberty, we conducted separate ANOVAs in the pre-pubertal and the adolescent groups, and compared hypothalamic activation in control girls to that of control boys during exposure to androstadienone. Results are displayed in **Table 2**.

Pre-pubertal girls and boys did not differ in terms of general hypothalamic responsiveness (condition effect ON > OFF) to androstadienone, but directional t-tests showed that the sex difference (girls > boys) was significantly modulated by the effect of the TM regressor ($t = 3.3$; $p = 0.033$), indicating that hypothalamic activation in boys differed from that of the girls during the course of the scanning session, thus suggesting differences in adaptation and/or sensitization to the odor between groups (see **Figures 1A** and **2A,C**).

Accordingly, similar comparisons were done in the adolescent groups. Again, the sex difference in hypothalamic activation (girls > boys) was significantly dependent on the factor time ($t = 3.5$; $p = 0.019$) (see **Figures 1B** and **3A,D**). Visual inspection of the data (see **Figure 1**) revealed that control girls' activation increased with repeated exposure to androstadienone (sensitization), particularly toward the end of the session, whereas control boys' responsiveness to the steroid odor seemed relatively stable, showing a slight decrease in activation during the course of the stimulation session.

Table 1 | Subject characteristics and psychophysiological data.

			Pre-pubertal children						Adolescents					
			Ctrl girls	**Ctrl boys**	**Girls with GD**	**Boys with GD**	***F*(df)**	***p*-Value**	**Ctrl girls**	**Ctrl boys**	**Girls with GD**	**Boys with GD**	***F*(df)**	***p*-Value**
Group size	*N*		19	20	17	19			21	20	21	17		
Age in years	Mean (SD)		9.7 (0.9)	9.5 (1.1)	9.6 (1.1)	10.4 (0.9)	3.1 (3.71)	**0.033**	16.3 (0.9)	15.9 (0.6)	16.1 (0.8)	15.3 (1.2)	4.6 (3.75)	**0.005**
Pubertal stage	Mean (SD)	P	1	1	1	1	–	–	4.2 (0.7)	4.7 (0.7)	4.7 (0.6)	3.1 (1.1)	17.4 (3.74)	**<0.001**
		G/M[a]	1	1	1	1	–	–	4.1 (0.8)	4.1 (0.8)	4.1 (1.1)	3.1 (0.8)	5.1 (3.74)	**0.003**
Sexual orientation	% (*N*)	Gynephilic	–	66.0 (13)	17.6 (5)	21.1 (4)			–	100 (20)	100 (21)	–		
		Androphilic	89.5 (17)	–	29.4 (3)	42.1 (8)			100 (21)	–	–	70.6 (12)		
		Ambiphilic	–	–	5.9 (1)	–	1.1 (3.71)	0.364	–	–	–	5.9 (1)	33.3 (3.74)	**<0.001**
		Don't know	10.5 (2)	35.0 (7)	47.1 (8)	36.8 (7)			–	–	–	17.6 (3)		
		Missing	–	–	–	–			–	–	–	5.9 (1)		
Androstadienone[b]	Mean (SD)		6.1 (2.4)	6.9 (1.5)	6.2 (2.7)	5.7 (2.6)	0.7 (3.55)	0.548	5.7 (2.3)	4.8 (1.9)	5.5 (1.9)	4.6 (2.0)	1.1 (3.63)	0.351
Sniffin' sticks	Mean (SD)	Threshold	7.3 (3.9)	6.2 (4.1)	8.5 (3.4)	8.6 (3.4)	1.6 (3.58)	0.212	9.9 (3.3)	8.5 (3.4)	8.1 (2.9)	9.1 (3.4)	1.1 (3.68)	0.356
		Identification	21.5 (3.6)	18.5 (3.8)	19.1 (4.0)	19.9 (5.3)	1.8 (3.66)	0.162	25.2 (3.8)	23.9 (2.8)	23.5 (3.9)	23.7 (2.8)	1.0 (3.71)	0.419

Ctrl, control; GD, gender dysphoria; N, group size; SD, standard deviation; P, pubic hair growth; G, genital development; M, breast development.

[a] *G applies for natal boys and M for natal girls; pubertal stages were assessed by means of the five-point (1 = pre-pubertal, 5 = post-pubertal) Tanner Maturation Scale.*

[b] *Androstadienone was rated for perceived intensity on a scale from 0 to 10; scores on the Sniffin' sticks threshold test range from 1 (low sensitivity) to 16 (high sensitivity); scores on the odor identification test range from 1 to 32. Bold font indicates statistically significant effects.*

Table 2 | ANOVA results showing sex differences in hypothalamus activations in the control groups, and *sex-atypical* hypothalamic activations, reflecting their experienced gender, in individuals with GD.

	Effect	Z_{max}	x	y	z	N	P_{FWE}
CTRL GIRLS > CTRL BOYS							
Children	Gender	2.5	-6	-12	-5	30	0.202
	Odor	2.4	-2	-15	-2	39	0.244
	ON-OFF	1.8	0	-10	-14	1	0.456
	ON_{TM}-OFF_{TM}	3.2	-6	-12	-5	92	**0.033**
		2.9	6	-7	-8		
Adolescents	Gender	1.7	-3	-7	-2	17	0.091
	Odor	1.7	6	-7	-6	8	0.655
	ON-OFF	3.4	6	-7	-8	1	0.522
	ON_{TM}-OFF_{TM}	2.5	-6	-12	-5	115	**0.019**
CTRL GIRLS > GIRLS WITH GD							
Children	No effects						
Adolescents	Gender	3.5	6	-7	-9	76	**0.016**
	Odor	1.7	-6	-7	-6	1	0.627
	ON-OFF	–	–	–	–	–	–
	ON_{TM}-OFF_{TM}	4.1	6	-7	-9	214	**0.002**
BOYS WITH GD > CTRL BOYS							
Children	Gender	1.8	2	-14	-2	4	0.447
	Odor	1.9	0	-10	0	3	0.436
	ON-OFF	1.7	-4	-6	-4	12	0.437
	ON_{TM}-OFF_{TM}	1.9	0	-10	-12	31	0.329
		2.4	0	-14	-12		
Adolescents	Gender	2.2	6	-8	-6	11	0.237
	Odor	3.0	0	-14	-12	1	0.341
	ON-OFF	1.8	2	-14	-2	36	**0.046**
	ON_{TM}-OFF_{TM}	–	–	–	–	–	–
BOYS WITH GD > GIRLS WITH GD							
Children	No effects						
Adolescents	Gender	–	–	–	–	–	–
	Odor	1.9	3	-12	-9	12	0.535
	ON-OFF	–	–	–	–	–	–
	ON_{TM}-OFF_{TM}	2.1	3	-10	-2	26	0.323

Ctrl, control; GD, gender dysphoria; Z_{max}, z-value of peak activation voxel; x y z, coordinates in Montreal Neurological Institute (MNI) space; N, number of clustering voxels (cluster size); FEW, family-wise error; the effects "Gender" and "Odor" indicate omnibus F-contrasts for the factors gender and odor stimulation; "ON-OFF" and "ON_{TM}-OFF_{TM}" indicate directional t-contrasts for the condition effect and the first-order time-modulation regressor, respectively. Bold font indicates statistically significant effects.

GENDER IDENTITY AND HYPOTHALAMIC ACTIVATION

In order to test whether individuals diagnosed with GD would show a hypothalamic activation that reflected their experienced gender, and whether this brain response would be different for pre-pubertal and adolescent subjects, four ANOVAs were conducted, in which control girls were compared to girls with GD, and control boys were compared to boys with GD (see **Table 2**). In addition, we investigated the reverse effects, i.e., whether individuals with GD showed sex-typical activations, and thus deviated from their experienced gender by comparing girls with GD to control boys, and boys with GD to control girls (see **Table 3**). Comparing girls with GD to boys with GD revealed no significant differences, thus the sex difference in response to androstadienone observed in the control groups was absent in the groups diagnosed with GD.

Girls diagnosed with GD

None of the comparisons between pre-pubertal control girls and pre-pubertal girls with GD revealed any differences in hypothalamic activation upon smelling androstadienone. However, no sex-typical effects (i.e., a female-typical hypothalamus response), when compared to control boys, could be confirmed. Thus, pre-pubertal girls with GD neither differed significantly from their experienced (control boys) nor from their natal sex (control girls) in terms of hypothalamic activation when smelling androstadienone.

In contrast, the comparison of adolescent control girls to girls diagnosed with GD revealed a significant effect of *gender* (control girls > girls with GD), which was mainly explained by the effect of the TM regressor ($t = 4.3$; $p = 0.002$) (see **Table 2; Figures 3B,E**). Thus, control girls showed a significantly stronger hypothalamic response to androstadienone over time as described earlier, whereas the activation in girls with GD, similar to adolescent control boys, remained stable throughout the scanning session. The reverse group comparisons (girls with GD > control boys) revealed no significant effects (see **Figure 3F**), indicating that adolescent girls with GD showed no hypothalamic activation upon smelling androstadienone as was observed in adolescent control boys.

Boys diagnosed with GD

No significant effects were revealed when comparing pre-pubertal boys with GD with control boys. In contrast, a significant effect of *gender*, driven by the TM regressor ($t = 3.5$; $p = 0.013$ FWE-corrected) was revealed when comparing pre-pubertal boys with GD to control girls, indicating that pre-pubertal boys with GD showed a pattern of hypothalamic activation that was similar to that of the pre-pubertal control boys (see **Table 3; Figures 2B,D,E**).

When adolescent boys with GD were compared to adolescent control boys we observed a significant effect of condition (ON > OFF) ($t = 1.8$; $p = 0.046$) (see **Table 2; Figures 3C,G,H**). Thus, adolescent boys with GD showed a significantly stronger, thus sex-atypical response to androstadienone compared to control boys, irrespective of the factor time. The reverse contrast (control girls > adolescent boys with GD), i.e., testing whether adolescent boys with GD would show an activation according to their natal sex, revealed no significant activations. Thus, adolescent boys with GD showed female-typical hypothalamic responses upon smelling androstadienone without, however, any effects due to sensitization.

DISCUSSION

SEX DIFFERENCES IN HYPOTHALAMIC ACTIVATION – EFFECTS OF PUBERTY

The present study is, to our knowledge, the first to demonstrate that sex differences in hypothalamic activation upon smelling androstadienone are already present before puberty, and thus may be considered as a sex difference established during early brain development. We found that pre-pubertal as well as

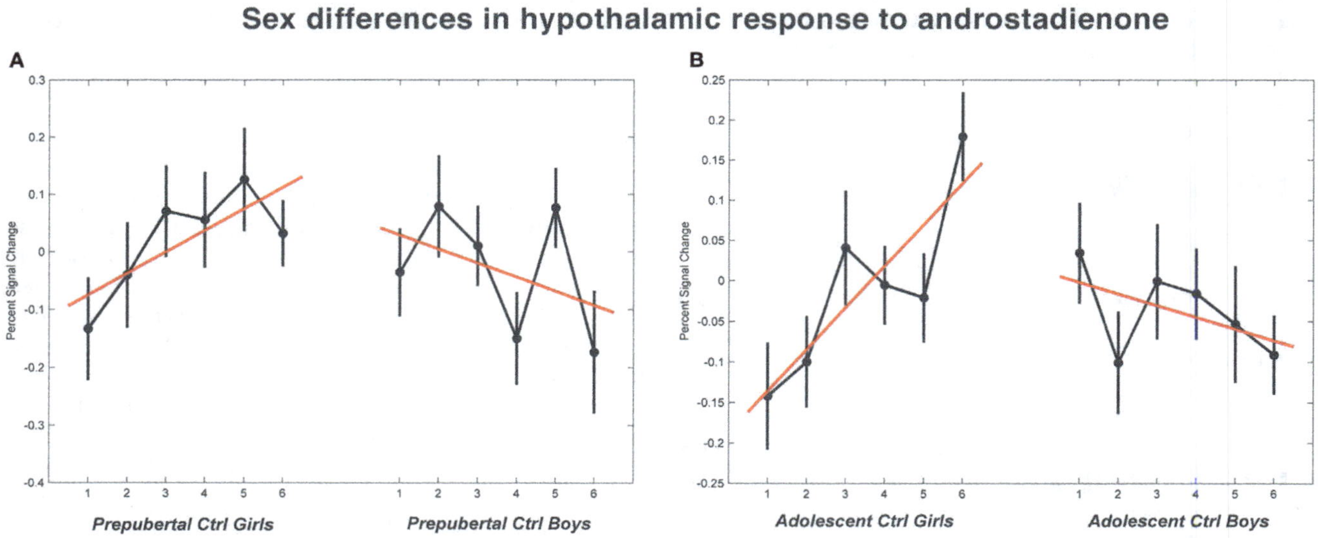

FIGURE 1 | The mean percent signal change for the hypothalamic region of interest during the course of the scanning session in the control groups. **(A)** Shows the responses in the pre-pubertal boys and girls; **(B)** shows the changes in activation over time in the adolescent control groups. Numbers 1–6 indicate the six time bins of the odor stimulation block design. Irrespective of pubertal status, both female age groups showed a significant increase ($p = 0.033$ in the pre-pubertal girls; $p = 0.019$ in the adolescent girls) in activation with repeated exposure to androstadienone, whereas hypothalamic activations tended to decrease in boys toward the end of the odor stimulation. The data for this figure was visualized using the toolbox rfxplot by Gläscher (55).

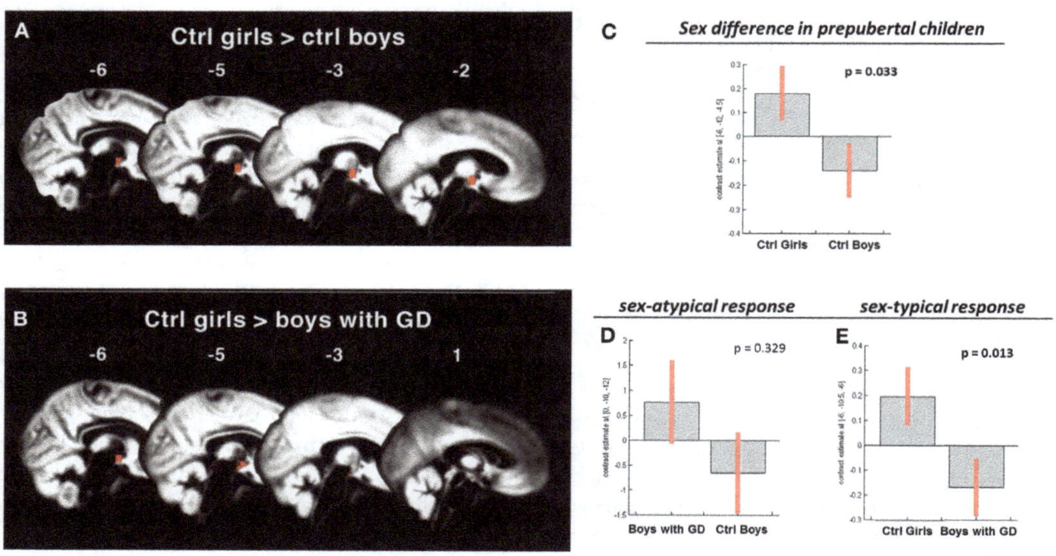

FIGURE 2 | (A,B) Show the anatomic locations of the significant hypothalamic activations, indicated in red, in response to the chemo-signal androstadienone in the pre-pubertal age groups. The numbers above each sagittal plane represent the *x*-axis coordinates in Montreal Neurological Institute space. All voxels within the hypothalamic region of interest, surviving the statistical threshold of $p < 0.05$ (FWE-corrected) are shown. **(C–E)** Show the bar graphs of the corresponding group contrasts for the first-order time-modulation regressor, indicating group differences in sensitization to the steroid odor. **(C)** Displays the sex difference, i.e., between control girls and boys; **(D)** shows the non-significant sex-atypical (i.e., female-like) and **(E)** indicates the significant sex-typical (i.e., male-like) response of boys with gender dysphoria.

adolescent control girls showed a stronger hypothalamic activation compared to boys (at both developmental stages), and that this sex difference was crucially modulated by effects of sensitization to androstadienone.

Previous psychophysiological studies in children and adolescents have shown that olfactory sensitivity to androgenic odors differed between boys and girls during development, due to the increased production of endogenous androgens by boys

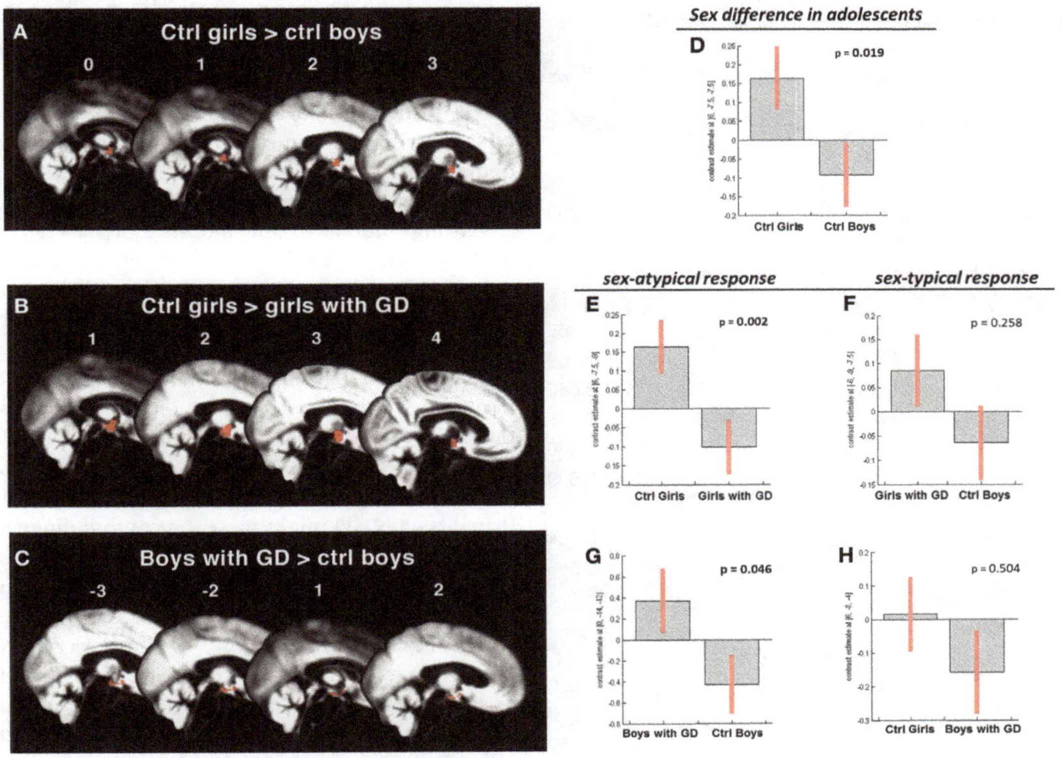

FIGURE 3 | (A–C) Show the anatomic locations of the significant hypothalamic activations, indicated in red, in response to the chemo-signal androstadienone in the adolescent age groups. The numbers above each sagittal plane represent the *x*-axis coordinates in Montreal Neurological Institute space. All voxels within the hypothalamic region of interest, surviving the statistical threshold of $p < 0.05$ (FWE-corrected) are shown. **(D–H)** Show the bar graphs of the corresponding group contrasts. **(D–E)** Show the significant group contrasts of the first-order time-modulation regressor, indicating sensitization to the steroid odor in control girls compared with **(A)** control boys and **(E)** girls with gender dysphoria. **(F)** Shows the non-significant sex-typical (female-like) response of girls with gender dysphoria. **(G)** Displays the significant female-typical response of the boys with gender dysphoria for the contrast of the condition ON > OFF, irrespective of any effects of time; **(H)** shows the non-significant male-typical response of boys with gender dysphoria.

during puberty and the assumed resulting adaptation to their own body odors (20–23). These findings suggested that puberty plays an important role in the development of sex differences in the olfactory sensitivity to androstadienone (48). Therefore, we hypothesized that the hypothalamic response in males, in contrast to that in females, would similarly be subject to neuronal adaptation after repeated exposure to the steroid odor. However, our results suggested only slight neuronal adaptation effects in boys, their activation remained relatively stable throughout the scanning session; instead, we found that girls showed an increase in hypothalamic responsiveness during the course of the odor stimulation. In line with the idea that androstadienone may function as a male modulator chemo-signal, our findings thus suggest that androstadienone indeed affects brain functions in females. Moreover, we showed that the sex difference in hypothalamic activation was not related to any hormonal or sexual maturation-related changes during puberty. Therefore, sex differences in neural responsiveness are probably not associated with differences in olfactory sensitivity to androstadienone and thus, its subjectively perceived intensity. Accordingly, we did not find any significant sex differences in the reported intensity ratings of androstadienone in both the pre-pubertal and adolescent groups.

GENDER IDENTITY AND HYPOTHALAMIC ACTIVATION

Gender dysphoria has been hypothesized to develop due to an altered sexual differentiation of the body and the brain during early development (30, 31). Here, we investigated a unique data set of individuals with GD at two different developmental stages, in order to determine whether they would respond to androstadienone in accordance with their natal sex, rather than their experienced gender. We found that both, adolescent girls and boys with GD showed hypothalamic activations that reflected their experienced gender. The sex difference that we observed in the control groups, was absent in both age groups of boys and girls diagnosed with GD. However, pre-pubertal girls with GD showed no differences in hypothalamic activation compared to both control boys and girls, whereas pre-pubertal boys with GD showed significant sex-typical hypothalamic activations and thus, in accordance with their natal sex. These findings thus suggest that individuals with GD possess certain functional brain characteristics, i.e., hypothalamic activation to androstadienone, of their experienced gender and thus that they may have undergone atypical neuronal sexual differentiation. However, this can only be observed reliably in adolescents with GD.

Table 3 | ANOVA results showing *sex-typical* hypothalamic activations, reflecting their natal sex, in individuals with GD.

	Effect	Z_{max}	x	y	z	N	P_{FWE}
GIRLS WITH GD > CTRL BOYS							
Children	No effects						
Adolescents	Gender	–	–	–	–	–	–
	Odor	2.5	6	-9	-5	25	0.203
	ON-OFF	1.7	-6	-7	-5	2	0.512
	ON_{TM}-OFF_{TM}	2.3	-6	-9	-8	25	0.258
CTRL GIRLS > BOYS WITH GD							
Children	Gender	3.0	-6	-10	-6	35	0.065
	Odor	2.6	3	-16	-9	27	0.168
	ON-OFF	1.6	-2	-16	-6	4	0.550
	ON_{TM}-OFF_{TM}	3.5	-6	-10	-6	126	**0.013**
Adolescents	Gender	2.2	-2	-4	-10	5	0.336
	Odor	1.5	2	-14	-12	4	0.699
	ON-OFF	–	–	–	–	–	–
	ON_{TM}-OFF_{TM}	1.7	6	-8	-4	7	0.504
		1.6	-6	-12	-8	16	0.553
GIRLS WITH GD > BOYS WITH GD							
Children	No effects						
Adolescents	Gender	–	–	–	–	–	–
	Odor	1.9	3	-12	-9	12	0.535
	ON-OFF	–	–	–	–	–	–
	ON_{TM}-OFF_{TM}	1.9	-6	-7	-11	1	0.459

Ctrl, control; GD, gender dysphoria; Z_{max}, z-value of peak activation voxel; x y z, coordinates in Montreal Neurological Institute (MNI) space; N, number of clustering voxels (cluster size); FWE, family-wise error; the effects "Gender" and "Odor" indicate omnibus F-contrasts for the factors gender and odor stimulation; "ON-OFF" and "ON_{TM}-OFF_{TM}" indicate directional t-contrasts for the condition effect and the first-order time-modulation regressor, respectively. Bold font indicates statistically significant effects.

Girls diagnosed with GD

Pre-pubertal girls with GD did not differ in hypothalamic activation from control girls indicating that they did not show a male-typical response. However, they also did not show a female-typical hypothalamic activation, when compared to control boys, indicating that they did not differ from either of the control groups. It is possible that pre-pubertal girls with GD constitute a rather heterogeneous group with respect to future persisting GD. It has been shown that only about 15.8% of the childhood GD cases will eventually lead to adult GD (49). However, women present more often early-onset cases (50) and girls have overall higher persistency rates of GD into adolescence compared to boys (51). Thus, our finding that pre-pubertal girls with GD did not show a clear-cut female- or male-typical response to androstadienone awaits further confirmation in the future, when it will be known who of our participants showed persisting GD into adolescence and adulthood.

The comparison of adolescent female controls versus adolescent girls with GD revealed very similar results as the control group comparisons, i.e., stronger hypothalamic activations in those subjects experiencing a female gender identity, and this effect was mainly driven by effects over time, reflecting sensitization. Thus, adolescent girls with GD responded remarkably like their experienced gender (control boys). While speculative, these findings fit with the idea that this group of girls with GD (who are more homogenous in terms of future persisting GD compared to the pre-pubertal groups) may have had a more male-typical perinatal hormonal environment, resulting in the development of certain typically male functional sex characteristics of the brain. The hypogonadal state of adolescent girls with GD using GnRHa at the moment of data acquisition is not likely to account for these findings, since our results in the pre-pubertal control groups suggest that hypothalamic responsiveness to androstadienone is probably independent of puberty, and thus not affected by circulating sex hormones. Furthermore, animal studies showed that sexually dimorphic responses to volatile urinary odors were not dependent on circulating sex steroids, but rather developed under the influence of organizational effects of sex hormones (52, 53).

It should be noted, though, that sexual orientation of the participants with GD might present a confounding factor. Berglund et al. (27) showed that hypothalamic responsiveness to androstadienone in lesbian women was comparable to that of heterosexual men. In the literature, the majority of natal females with GD are reported to be gynephilic (50, 54), which was true as well for our group of adolescent gender dysphoric girls. Therefore, it cannot be ruled out that the resemblance in hypothalamic activation with the control boys might be due to their shared sexual orientation rather than their shared gender identity.

Boys diagnosed with GD

The hypothalamic response to androstadienone in the pre-pubertal boys with GD was not significantly stronger than that shown by the pre-pubertal control boys. Moreover, the reverse contrast (control girls > boys with GD) revealed that pre-pubertal control girls showed significantly stronger hypothalamic activation, implying that boys with GD responded according to their natal sex. Again, it is likely that the younger, pre-pubertal sample of boys with GD constitutes a rather heterogeneous group in terms of future persistence of their gender dysphoric feelings (49, 51). Therefore, they may show more variability in hypothalamic responsiveness to androstadienone.

Adolescent boys with GD showed significantly stronger, thus sex-atypical hypothalamic activations, compared to control boys, although this effect was not modulated by any effects of time, thus sensitization to androstadienone, as we did observe in the control girls. Accordingly, the reverse comparison (control girls > boys with GD) revealed no significant effects. The female-typical activation in adolescent boys with GD is in line with a previous study by Berglund et al. (26), who reported that adult men with GD differed significantly from a group of male controls in terms of hypothalamic activation during exposure to androstadienone. Their adult participants with GD were matched to control men with regard to hormonal status and gynephilic sexual orientation, whereas in our study adolescent boys with GD received GnRHa at the moment of data acquisition and the majority of our participants reported to have an androphilic sexual orientation. Thus, despite differences with regard to the participants' age, hormonal status, and sexual orientation, the findings of both studies suggest that males with GD possess certain female-typical brain functions, and may therefore have undergone sex-atypical early brain development.

Some limitations of the present study should be mentioned and may be addressed in future research. In most comparisons, the gender differences in hypothalamic response to androstadienone showed relatively small effect sizes. These effect sizes, in combination with relatively small group sizes (especially that of the pre-pubertal girls with GD with $N = 17$), suggest that a lack of statistical power may be related to our failure in finding any significant effects for particularly this group. Therefore, additional analyses in other functional and structural (e.g., gray and white matter volumes or diffusion tensor imaging data) MRI measures, which are in preparation, should corroborate the present preliminary findings. Sexual orientation was difficult to assess in our young groups of participants. We therefore estimated their (future) sexual orientation by asking whether he/she had ever been in love. However, any relationship between sexual orientation and the response to androstadienone could not reliably be investigated in our groups.

In summary, the present study is the first to demonstrate that sex differences in hypothalamic activation upon smelling the chemo-signal androstadienone are not acquired during sexual maturation, under the influence of gonadal hormones during puberty, but may be considered hard-wired responses, which already can be observed in pre-pubertal children. Moreover, the current study is the first to explore sex-atypical hypothalamic responses to androstadienone in male and female individuals with GD at two different developmental stages. Our results indeed suggest that individuals with GD possess certain functional brain characteristics of their experienced gender and may have undergone atypical neuronal sexual differentiation.

AUTHOR CONTRIBUTIONS

Julie Bakker and Sarah M. Burke designed the study set-up. Sarah M. Burke performed the neuroimaging experiments, conducted the data analyses with advice of Dick J. Veltman, and wrote the manuscript. Daniel T. Klink performed the clinical assessments. Peggy T. Cohen-Kettenis, Dick J. Veltman, and Julie Bakker supervised the project. All authors contributed to interpretation of the data and revisions of the manuscript.

ACKNOWLEDGMENTS

We thank Prof. Thomas Hummel and his Smell and Taste lab at the University Medical School in Dresden (Germany) for his hospitality and the kind introduction into the field of olfactory fMRI. We thank Paul Groot from the Academic Medical Centre Amsterdam for his help with the data analyses, and we thank Prof Michael Baum from Boston University for his helpful comments on earlier versions of this manuscript. Last but not least, we are especially thankful to Dipl.-Ing. Johannes Burke, who developed and built the olfactometer equipment and programed the application software. This study was funded by a VICI grant (453-08-003) from the Dutch Science Foundation (Nederlandse Organisatie voor Wetenschappelijk Onderzoek) to Dr. Julie Bakker. Dr. Julie Bakker is a senior research associate of the Belgian Fonds National de la Recherche Scientifique.

REFERENCES

Kwan TK, Kraevskaya MA, Makin HL, Trafford DJ, Gower DB. Use of gas chromatographic-mass spectrometric techniques in studies of androst-16-ene and androgen biosynthesis in human testis; cytosolic specific binding of 5alpha-androst-16-en-3-one. *J Steroid Biochem Mol Biol* (1997) **60**:137–46. doi:10.1016/S0960-0760(96)00162-8

Nixon A, Mallet AI, Gower DB. Simultaneous quantification of five odorous steroids (16-androstenes) in the axillary hair of men. *J Steroid Biochem* (1988) **29**:505–10. doi:10.1016/0022-4731(88)90185-9

Brooksbank BW, Cunningham AE, Wilson DA. The detection of androsta-4,16-dien-3-one in peripheral plasma of adult men. *Steroids* (1969) **13**:29–50. doi:10.1016/S0039-128X(69)80058-9

Kwan TK, Trafford DJ, Makin HL, Mallet AI, Gower DB. GC-MS studies of 16-androstenes and other C19 steroids in human semen. *J Steroid Biochem Mol Biol* (1992) **43**:549–56. doi:10.1016/0960-0760(92)90243-C

Brooksbank BW, Wilson DA, MacSweeney DA. Fate of androsta-4,16-dien-3-one and the origin of 3-hydroxy-5-androst-16-ene in man. *J Endocrinol* (1972) **52**:239–51. doi:10.1677/joe.0.0520239

Gower DB, Ruparelia BA. Olfaction in humans with special reference to odorous 16-androstenes: their occurrence, perception and possible social, psychological and sexual impact. *J Endocrinol* (1993) **137**:167–87. doi:10.1677/joe.0.1370167

Bensafi M, Brown WM, Khan R, Levenson B, Sobel N. Sniffing human sex-steroid derived compounds modulates mood, memory and autonomic nervous system function in specific behavioral contexts. *Behav Brain Res* (2004) **152**:11–22. doi:10.1016/j.bbr.2003.09.009

Jacob S, McClintock MK. Psychological state and mood effects of steroidal chemosignals in women and men. *Horm Behav* (2000) **37**:57–78. doi:10.1006/ hbeh.1999.1559

Jacob S, Hayreh DJ, McClintock MK. Context-dependent effects of steroid chemosignals on human physiology and mood. *Physiol Behav* (2001) **74**:15–27. doi:10.1016/S0031-9384(01)00537-6

Villemure C, Bushnell MC. The effects of the steroid androstadienone and pleasant odorants on the mood and pain perception of men and women. *Eur J Pain* (2007) **11**:181–91. doi:10.1016/j.ejpain.2006.02.005

Bensafi M, Tsutsui T, Khan R, Levenson RW, Sobel N. Sniffing a human sexsteroid derived compound affects mood and autonomic arousal in a dose-dependent manner. *Psychoneuroendocrinology* (2004) **29**:1290–9. doi:10.1016/j. psyneuen.2004.03.007

Bensafi M, Brown WM, Tsutsui T, Mainland JD, Johnson BN, Bremner EA, et al. Sex-steroid derived compounds induce sex-specific effects on autonomic nervous system function in humans. *Behav Neurosci* (2003) **117**:1125–34. doi:10.1037/0735-7044.117.6.1125

Grosser BI, Monti-Bloch L, Jennings-White C, Berliner DL. Behavioral and electrophysiological effects of androstadienone, a human pheromone. *Psychoneuroendocrinology* (2000) **25**:289–99. doi:10.1016/S0306-4530(99)00056-6

Lundstöm J, Lundström JN, Gonçalves M, Esteves F, Olsson MJ. Psychological effects of subthreshold exposure to the putative human pheromone 4,16-androstadien-3-one. *Horm Behav* (2003) **44**:395–401. doi:10.1016/j. yhbeh. 2003.06.004

Lundström JN, Olsson MJ. Subthreshold amounts of social odorant affect mood, but not behavior, in heterosexual women when tested by a male, but not a female, experimenter. *Biol Psychol* (2005) **70**:197–204. doi:10.1016/j. biopsycho. 2005.01.008

Wyart C, Webster WW, Chen JH, Wilson SR, McClary A, Khan RM, et al. Smelling a single component of male sweat alters levels of cortisol in women. *J Neurosci* (2007) **27**:1261–5. doi:10.1523/JNEUROSCI.4430-06.2007

Parma V, Tirindelli R, Bisazza A, Massaccesi S, Castiello U. Subliminally perceived odours modulate female intrasexual competition: an eye movement study. *PLoS One* (2012) **7**:e30645. doi:10.1371/journal.pone.0030645

Savic I, Berglund H, Gulyas B, Roland P. Smelling of odorous sex hormone-like compounds causes sex-differentiated hypothalamic activations in humans. *Neuron* (2001) **31**:661–8. doi:10.1016/S0896-6273(01)00390-7

Burke SM, Veltman DJ, Gerber J, Hummel T, Bakker J. Heterosexual men and women both show a hypothalamic response to the chemo-signal androstadienone. *PLoS One* (2012) **7**:e40993. doi:10.1371/journal.pone.0040993

Chopra A, Baur A, Hummel T. Thresholds and chemosensory event-related potentials to malodors before, during, and after puberty: differences related to sex and age. *Neuroimage* (2008) **40**:1257–63. doi:10.1016/j.neuroimage.2008. 01.015

Dorries KM, Schmidt HJ, Beauchamp GK, Wysocki CJ. Changes in sensitivity to the odor of androstenone during adolescence. *Dev Psychobiol* (1989) **22**:423–35. doi:10.1002/dev.420220502

Hummel T, Krone F, Lundström JN, Bartsch O. Androstadienone odor thresholds in adolescents. *Horm Behav* (2005) **47**:306–10. doi:10.1016/j.yhbeh.2004. 10.007

Koelega HS, Köster EP. Some experiments on sex differences in odor perception. *Ann N Y Acad Sci* (1974) **237**:234–46. doi:10.1111/j.1749-6632.1974.tb49859.x

Schulz KM, Molenda-Figueira H, Sisk CL. Back to the future: the organizational-activational hypothesis adapted to puberty and adolescence. *Horm Behav* (2009) **55**:597–604. doi:10.1016/j.yhbeh.2009.03.010

Sisk CL, Zehr JL. Pubertal hormones organize the adolescent brain and behavior. *Front Neuroendocrinol* (2005) **26**:163–74. doi:10.1016/j.yfrne.2005.10.003

Berglund H, Lindström P, Dhejne-Helmy C, Savic I. Male-to-female transsexuals show sex-atypical hypothalamus activation when smelling odorous steroids. *Cereb Cortex* (2008) **18**:1900–8. doi:10.1093/cercor/bhm216

Berglund H, Lindström P, Savic I. Brain response to putative pheromones in lesbian women. *Proc Natl Acad Sci U S A* (2006) **103**:8269–74. doi:10.1073/pnas. 0600331103

Savic I, Berglund H, Lindström P. Brain response to putative pheromones in homosexual men. *Proc Natl Acad Sci U S A* (2005) **102**:7356–61. doi:10.1073/pnas.0407998102

American Psychiatric Association. *Diagnostic and Statistical Manual of Mental Disorders, Fifth Edition (DSM-5).* Arlington, VA: American Psychiatric Association (2013).

Swaab DF, Garcia-Falgueras A. Sexual differentiation of the human brain in relation to gender identity and sexual orientation. *Funct Neurol* (2009) **24**:17–28.

van Goozen SH, Gooren LJG, Sanders G, Cohen-Kettenis PT, Slabbekoorn D. Organizing and activating effects of sex hormones in homosexual transsexuals. *Behav Neurosci* (2002) **116**:982–8. doi:10.1037/0735-7044.116.6.982

Marantz S, Coates S. Mothers of boys with gender identity disorder: a comparison of matched controls. *J Am Acad Child Adolesc Psychiatry* (1991) **30**:310–5. doi:10.1097/00004583-199103000-00022

Zucker KJ, Bradley SJ. *Gender Identity Disorder and Psychosexual Problems in Children and Adolescents.* New York, NY: The Guilford Press (1995).

Coolidge FL, Thede LL, Young SE. The heritability of gender identity disorder in a child and adolescent twin sample. *Behav Genet* (2002) **32**:251–7. doi:10.1023/A:1019724712983

Gooren L. The biology of human psychosexual differentiation. *Horm Behav* (2006) **50**:589–601. doi:10.1016/j.yhbeh.2006.06.011

Kreukels BPC, Cohen-Kettenis PT. Puberty suppression in gender identity disorder: the Amsterdam experience. *Nat Rev Endocrinol* (2011) **7**:466–72. doi:10.1038/nrendo.2011.78

Delemarre-van de Waal HA, Cohen-Kettenis PT. Clinical management of gender identity disorder in adolescents: a protocol on psychological and paediatric endocrinology aspects. *Eur J Endocrinol* (2006) **155**:S131–7. doi:10.1530/eje.1. 02231

Hembree WC, Cohen-Kettenis P, Delemarre-van de Waal HA, Gooren LJ, Meyer WJ, Spack NP, et al. Endocrine treatment of transsexual persons: an Endocrine Society clinical practice guideline. *J Clin Endocrinol Metab* (2009) **94**:3132–54. doi:10.1210/jc.2009-0345

Marshall WA, Tanner JM. Variations in the pattern of pubertal changes in boys. *Arch Dis Child* (1970) **45**:13–23. doi:10.1136/adc.45.239.13

Marshall WA, Tanner JM. Variations in pattern of pubertal changes in girls. *Arch Dis Child* (1969) **44**:291–303. doi:10.1136/adc.44.235.291

Hummel T, Kobal G, Gudziol H, Mackay-Sim A. Normative data for the "Sniffin'sticks" including tests of odor identification, odor discrimination, and olfactory thresholds: an upgrade based on a group of more than 3,000 subjects. *Eur Arch Otorhinolaryngol* (2007) **264**:237–43. doi:10.1007/s00405-006-0173-0

Kobal G, Klimek L, Wolfensberger M, Gudziol H, Temmel A, Owen CM, et al. Multicenter investigation of 1,036 subjects using a standardized method for the assessment of olfactory function combining tests of odor identification, odor discrimination, and olfactory thresholds. *Eur Arch Otorhinolaryngol* (2000) **257**:205–11. doi:10.1007/s004050050223

Kobal G, Hummel T, Sekinger B, Barz S, Roscher S, Wolf S. "Sniffin' sticks": screening of olfactory performance. *Rhinology* (1996) **34**:222–6.

Lemieux L, Salek-Haddadi A, Lund TE, Laufs H, Carmichael D. Modelling large motion events in fMRI studies of patients with epilepsy. *Magn Reson Imaging* (2007) **25**:894–901. doi:10.1016/j.mri.2007.03.009

Brett M, Anton J, Valabregue R, Poline J-B. Region of interest analysis using an SPM toolbox [abstract]. *Presented at the 8th International Conference on Functional Mapping of the Human Brain.* Sendai (2002).

Makris N, Swaab DF, van der Kouwe A, Abbs B, Boriel D, Handa RJ, et al. Volumetric parcellation methodology of the human hypothalamus in neuroimaging: normative data and sex differences. *Neuroimage* (2013) **69**:1–10. doi:10.1016/j.neuroimage.2012.12.008

Baroncini M, Jissendi P, Balland E, Besson P, Pruvo J-P, Francke J-P, et al. MRI atlas of the human hypothalamus. *Neuroimage* (2012) **59**:168–80. doi:10.1016/ j.neuroimage.2011.07.013

Lundström JN, Hummel T, Olsson MJ. Individual differences in sensitivity to the odor of 4,16-androstadien-3-one. *Chem Senses* (2003) **28**:643–50. doi:10.1093/chemse/bjg057

Steensma TD, Biemond R, de Boer F, Cohen-Kettenis PT. Desisting and persisting gender dysphoria after childhood: a qualitative follow-up study. *Clin Child Psychol Psychiatry* (2011) **16**:499–516. doi:10.1177/1359104510378303

Nieder TO, Herff M, Cerwenka S, Preuss WF, Cohen-Kettenis PT, De Cuypere G, et al. Age of onset and sexual orientation in transsexual males and females. *J Sex Med* (2011) **8**:783–91. doi:10.1111/j.1743-6109.2010.02142.x

Steensma TD, McGuire JK, Kreukels BPC, Beekman AJ, Cohen-Kettenis PT. Factors associated with desistence and persistence of childhood gender dysphoria: a quantitative follow-up study. *J Am Acad Child Adolesc Psychiatry* (2013) **52**:582–90. doi:10.1016/j.jaac.2013.03.016

Baum MJ, Keverne EB. Sex difference in attraction thresholds for volatile odors from male and estrous female mouse urine. *Horm Behav* (2002) **41**:213–9. doi:10.1006/hbeh.2001.1749

Pierman S, Douhard Q, Balthazart J, Baum MJ, Bakker J. Attraction thresholds and sex discrimination of urinary odorants in male and female aromatase knockout (ArKO) mice. *Horm Behav* (2006) **49**:96–104. doi:10.1016/j.yhbeh. 2005.05.007

Lawrence AA. Sexual orientation versus age of onset as bases for typologies (sub-types) for gender identity disorder in adolescents and adults. *Arch Sex Behav* (2010) **39**:514–45. doi:10.1007/s10508-009-9594-3

Gläscher, J. Visualization of group inference data in functional neuroimaging *Neuroinformatics* (2009) **7**:73–82. doi:10.1007/s12021-008-9042-x

15

Role of estrogen receptors and G protein-coupled estrogen receptor in regulation of hypothalamus–pituitary–testis axis and spermatogenesis

Adele Chimento, Rosa Sirianni, Ivan Casaburi and Vincenzo Pezzi* *

Laboratory of Applied Biology, Department of Pharmacy, Health and Nutrition Sciences, University of Calabria, Cosenza, Italy

***Correspondence:**
Vincenzo Pezzi, Laboratory of Applied Biology, Department of Pharmacy, Health and Nutrition Sciences, University of Calabria, Edificio Polifunzionale, Arcavacata di Rende, Cosenza 87036, Italy
e-mail: v.pezzi@unical.it

Male reproductive function is under the control of both gonadotropins and androgens through a negative feedback loop that involves the hypothalamus, pituitary, and testis known as hypothalamus–pituitary–gonadal axis (HPG). Indeed, estrogens also play an important role in regulating HPG axis but the study on relative contribution to the inhibition of gonadotropins secretion exerted by the amount of estrogens produced within the hypothalamus and/or the pituitary or by the amount of circulating estrogens is still ongoing. Moreover, it is known that the maintenance of spermatogenesis is controlled by gonadotropins and testosterone, the effects of which are modulated by a complex network of locally produced factors, including estrogens. Physiological effects of estrogens are mediated by the classical nuclear estrogen receptor alpha and estrogen receptor beta, which mediate both genomic and rapid signaling events. In addition, estrogens induce rapid non-genomic responses through a membrane-associated G protein-coupled estrogen receptor (GPER). Ours and other studies reported that, in the testis, GPER is expressed in both normal germ cells and somatic cells and it is involved in mediating the estrogen action in spermatogenesis controlling proliferative and/or apoptotic events. Interestingly, GPER expression has been revealed also in the hypothalamus and pituitary. However, its role in mediating estrogen rapid actions in this context is under investigation. Recent studies indicate that GPER is involved in modulating gonadotropin-releasing hormone (GnRH) release as well as gonadotropins secretion. In this review, we will summarize the current knowledge concerning the role of estrogen/estrogen receptors molecular pathways in regulating GnRH, follicle-stimulating hormone, and luteinizing hormone release at the hypothalamic and pituitary levels in males as well as in controlling specific testicular functions such as spermatogenesis, focusing our attention mainly on estrogen signaling mediated by GPER.

Keywords: ESR1, ESR2, GPER, gonadotropins, HPG axis, spermatogenesis

INTRODUCTION

Male fertility and hence its reproductive potential is a result of a complex and intricate as a fine neuroendocrine control. Traditionally the adult male reproductive function was considered to be controlled by both gonadotropins and androgens through a negative feedback loop that involves the hypothalamus, pituitary, and testis known as the hypothalamus–pituitary–gonadal axis (HPG). As such, spermatogenesis is regulated by the pulsatile release of gonadotropin-releasing hormone (GnRH) from the arcuate nucleus of the hypothalamus, which stimulates the anterior pituitary to release follicle-stimulating hormone (FSH) and luteinizing hormone (LH) (1). Accordingly, at the testicular level, LH stimulates the Leydig cells to produce testosterone, which has a local effect on the interstitium and seminiferous tubules and results in sperm production and maturation while FSH exerts its effect directly on the Sertoli cells that in turn promote and sustain spermatogenesis (1). Both GnRH and gonadotropin secretion could be modulated by testosterone and more surprisingly, estradiol (E2) acting on the hypothalamus or on the pituitary via a feedback regulating mechanisms (2). However, the specific role of each sex steroid in the regulation of gonadotropin negative feedback is still not completely clarified.

In males, the major source of circulating estrogens is the aromatization of androgens as a consequence of the action of the enzyme complex known as aromatase that is widely expressed in a number of male tissues including the testis and brain (3, 4).

Cellular effects of estrogens occur via classical estrogen receptor alpha (ESR1) and estrogen receptor beta (ESR2) located in the nucleus and cytoplasm of the target cells and belong to the nuclear receptor superfamily members that act as nuclear transcription factors, binding to estrogen response elements (EREs) within specific genes to alter their rate of transcription (5). However, it has become clear that estrogens also exert rapid, non-genomic effects by altering different signaling pathways both in central and nervous system peripheral tissues (6).

These "non-genomic effects" could be mediated by extranuclear estrogen receptors (ERs) or by non-classical membrane bound receptors such as G protein-coupled estrogen receptor also named GPR30/GPER that has been identified as a novel ER (7). Estradiol through GPER rapidly activates different pathways including the stimulation of adenylyl cyclase, mobilization of intracellular calcium (Ca^{2+}) stores, and activation of mitogen-activated protein kinase (MAPK) and phosphoinositide 3-kinase (PI3K) signaling pathways (8, 9).

In this review, we will summarize the current knowledge concerning the role of estrogen/ERs signaling in regulating GnRH, FSH, and LH release at the hypothalamic and pituitary levels in males as well as in controlling specific testicular functions such as spermatogenesis, focusing our attention mainly on estrogen signaling mediated by GPER.

ROLE OF ESTROGEN AND ESTROGENS RECEPTORS IN GnRH, LH, AND FSH SECRETION IN MALES

ESTROGEN FUNCTIONS AT THE HYPOTHALAMIC LEVEL

Gonadotropins and gonadal steroids, being involved in the regulation of secondary sex characteristics, gametogenesis, cellular functions, and also behavior, are the main driving force for reproductive function. The hypothalamic GnRH neurons that control LH and FSH release from the pituitary represent the final common pathway for neuronally derived endogenous as well as exogenous stimuli (10). In both males and females, gonadal steroid hormones exert negative feedback regulation on HPG axis activity at both the hypothalamus and pituitary levels. In females, the feedback mechanism is more complex since estrogen and progesterone induce both negative and positive feedback responsible for generating the pre-ovulatory GnRH and LH surge (10). Thus, the neuroendocrine mechanism underlying the ovulatory LH and FSH surge, characteristic of the mature female reproductive system, is usually extinguished in males by neonatal androgen imprinting (10).

Several evidences indicate that testicular steroids, androgens, and estrogens could mediate the feedback actions on gonadotropin secretion interacting with their receptors, ERs or androgen receptors (ARs) that were found in the male hypothalamus (11). However, there is no clear consensus on the role of ER versus AR signaling in males (12, 13). Aromatization of testosterone to estradiol and reduction to 5α-dihydrotestosterone (DHT) is mandatory for normal male reproduction and occurs in peripheral (14) and central tissues (15, 16). Sharma and co-workers have demonstrated that aromatase inhibitor administration into the third cerebral ventricle of intact rams resulted in an increased frequency of LH pulses without affecting estradiol plasma concentrations (17). In addition, existence of these feedback actions is further clearly illustrated in a range of species by an increased secretion of the gonadotropins following castration (18–20). Accordingly, an increased LH secretion was found also in intact or castrated rams passively or actively immunized against estradiol (18). However, how testosterone and/or its primary metabolites act within the brain to suppress the synthesis and/or secretion of GnRH need more investigation.

In humans, androgen aromatization for normal gonadotropins feedback function (21) has been discovered by the use of testosterone or estradiol infusion in men affected by idiopathic hypothalamic hypogonadism (IHH). On the other hand, the authors did not record any change in LH and FSH secretion when pure androgen DHT was administered. These data indirectly suggest that the peripheral 5α-reduction of testosterone to DHT plays a minor role in the control of the secretion of gonadotropins (21). Thus, the inhibitory effect on gonadotropin secretion is mediated mainly by estradiol from endogenous conversion of testosterone rather than direct androgen action, at least in the pituitary gland (21). Indeed, other studies suggested that *in situ* aromatization of testosterone is required both at the hypothalamic and pituitary levels to insure a complete feedback mechanism of gonadotropins (22, 23). Moreover, the results coming from basal, GnRH-stimulated, and pulsatile evaluation of LH and FSH secretion in two aromatase-deficient men have provided direct evidence that circulating estrogens exert an inhibitory control in LH feedback at both the hypothalamic and pituitary levels (24).

It is universally accepted that estradiol actions were mediated by its interaction with ERs ESR1 and ESR2 that act as hormone-inducible transcription factors determining estrogen-dependent gene transactivation (1). Several studies, involving a range of species and both sexes, have demonstrated that GnRH neurons do not express ESR1 (25–27), even though a small number of GnRH neurons containing ESR1 were found in female rats (28). Indeed, accumulating evidence suggests that estrogen could act in GnRH neurons through ESR2. In fact, ESR2 immunoreactivity was detected first in rodents (29, 30) and later in humans (31). However, studies performed in *Esr1* knock-out mice suggest that in males, ESR1 is the predominant receptor involved in mediating estradiol suppression of GnRH content (12). Moreover, it was also demonstrated that in mouse LHRH neurons (29) ESR2 may mediate the rapid estradiol effects because mouse LHRH neurons expressed only ESR2, and the nuclear ER antagonist, ICI 182,780, suppressed the effect of estradiol on Ca^{2+} oscillations. However, in primate LHRH neurons, estradiol appears to cause its action through a different mechanism, because ICI 182,780 failed to block the estradiol-induced changes in Ca^{2+} oscillations and synchronization (32). This finding could be explained by the study of Noel and co-workers (33) suggesting a GPER involvement in the rapid action of estradiol in hypothalamic neurons. In fact these authors demonstrated that GPER is expressed in olfactory placode cultured cells and in a subset of LHRH neurons and that GPER gene knockdown in LHRH neurons completely abrogate both estradiol- and estrogen-dendrimer conjugate-induced changes in Ca^{2+} oscillations. Furthermore, using a selective specific GPER-agonist, they obtained changes in Ca^{2+} oscillations similar to those observed upon estradiol treatment confirming that estradiol rapid action appears to be mediated, at least partially, through GPER (33). However, further investigation is needed to better clarify what the specific target cells for estrogens action at the hypothalamic level are and what receptors are involved.

ESTROGEN FUNCTIONS AT THE PITUITARY LEVEL

In male vertebrates, LH and FSH plasma levels are largely regulated by GnRH and activins as stimulators and steroids and inhibins as inhibitors (34, 35). The negative feedback action of testicular androgens on serum LH and FSH was first demonstrated utilizing castrated animal models evidencing a substantial increase in LH and FSH levels that were prevented by the administration of physiological levels of testosterone (36). Later studies have pointed out the hypothalamus and pituitary as targets for such feedback. Although there are conflicting data concerning the effects of testosterone on GnRH synthesis and secretion, studies have demonstrated that castration and steroid replacement alter levels of GnRH messenger RNA (mRNA) (37), processing of GnRH prohormone (38), hypothalamic GnRH contents (39), and patterns of pulsatile GnRH release (39, 40). Besides examining hypothalamic sites of action, a number of investigators have also examined feedback directly on the pituitary. Testosterone, DHT, or estradiol is able to suppress GnRH-stimulated LH secretion from pituitary cultures (41), whereas T treatments increase basal FSH secretion and intrapituitary FSH levels (42). Furthermore, molecular analyses of the promoter regions of the gonadotropin genes such as α-gonadotropin subunit (αGSU), FSHβ, and LHβ subunits (43) have revealed the presence of responsive elements through which AR or ER mediated the feedback effects exerted by testosterone or estradiol, respectively.

It is worth noting that estrogen responsiveness of the pituitary gland requires the presence of ERs, including the classical ESR1 and ESR2 (44). The ER expression and distribution patterns in pituitary glands have been studied in rats (45), sheep (46), and humans (47). The localization of ARs in the pituitary is also well-established since AR expression has been reported in the anterior pituitary gland of humans (48), rhesus monkeys, rats (49), Brazilian opossums (50), and mice (51).

Although these data support pituitary sites of steroid action, mainly in feedback regulation, it is unclear whether the effects of T are primarily mediated directly through the AR or indirectly via aromatization and activation of ERs. Experiments performed with a non-aromatizable androgen DHT has been demonstrated to suppress serum LH and basal levels of αGSU and LHβ mRNA in rats (52), confirming AR-mediated feedback. As such, antiandrogen flutamide induced up-regulates of LH serum concentrations (53). At the molecular levels it was also demonstrated that the enhancer elements of the αGSU gene is a target of AR-mediated suppression (43).

In addition, other studies have demonstrated that exogenous estradiol treatment (34) reduced LH and FSH concentrations and gonadotropin mRNAs content, while treatment with aromatase inhibitors determines an increase of LH serum levels (54). The roles of estrogens/ESR1 signaling are further supported clinically by the elevated serum FSH levels in an estrogen-resistant patient (55) as well as in aromatase-deficient humans (24). The unsolved debate focusing on what steroid receptor, AR and/or ESR1, is able to mediate negative feedback on serum gonadotropins is further complicated by the presence of ESR2 (56). Although ESR2 mRNA levels are very low in adult mouse pituitaries (57), there are studies, as already above mentioned, reporting that the hypothalamic nuclei of both rats and mice express ESR2 at both transcriptional and post-transcriptional levels (57, 58). Thus, it is reasonable to hypothesize that testicular steroids could modulate hypothalamic-pituitary activity directly through AR or indirectly through aromatization and activation of either ESR1 or ESR2 signaling pathways.

Estradiol effects in the pituitary gland occur mainly through genomic mechanisms (59) as evidenced in a mouse gonadotroph cell line (LβT2) where estradiol administration increased LHβ mRNA levels (60) due to the presence of EREs within the promoter region of LHβ gene (61). It is noteworthy that there is also experimental evidence for estrogen-independent ESR1 transcriptional activation in gonadotrope cells most probably through GnRH receptor and signaling via protein kinase C (PKC) and MAPK pathways (62). Recent studies indicate that GPER is involved in suppressing GnRH-stimulated LH release in primary pituitary cell culture derived from ovariectomized ewes (63). However, to date there are no studies showing GPER-mediated non-genomic signaling events in the male pituitary. Since GPER has been identified in the plasma membrane of a variety of target tissues, including anterior pituitary (64, 65), we can speculate that GPER could have a role in mediating the non-genomic effects of estradiol in the male pituitary.

ESTROGEN AND HPG AXIS IN MALES: LESSONS FROM ANIMAL MODELS

The development of knock-out or transgenic mice with targeted disruptions of ERs and/or aromatase has increased our understanding of estrogen function in reproduction (66).

Controversy aspect regarding the male hypothalamic and pituitary feedback regulation by steroids has been partially resolved by the observation of data coming from the castration and steroids replacement experiments in *Esr1* knock-out (ERKO) mouse (67) model. Lindzey and co-workers demonstrated that in males, ESR1 is the predominant receptor involved in mediating estradiol suppression of gonadotropin release and gonadotropin subunit mRNA expression (12). The role of an activated AR by testosterone is, of course, not secondary, as demonstrated by the ability of testosterone administration to suppress serum LH in ERKO male mice but its aromatization seems to produce a more functional inhibitory effect on the hypothalamic-pituitary feedback and this is also true for FSH production (12).

Other *in vivo* studies confirmed that estrogens have important roles in the regulation of spermatogenesis. The hypogonadal (*hpg*) mouse (68) that does not produce mature GnRH decapeptide due to a truncation in the GnRH gene is widely used as an animal model to investigate the endocrine regulation of spermatogenesis (69). *Hpg* mice are infertile because they do not produce gonadotropins and hence the testis failed to develop (70). By the *hpg* mice model it was demonstrated that treatment with LH stimulate steroidogenesis (71) and a combined treatment with FSH and androgens induce normal spermatogenesis (72, 73). More interestingly, later research demonstrated that chronic estradiol treatment of this animal model was able to restore spermatogenesis (69, 74, 75), via a mechanism involving a weak neuroendocrine activation of FSH secretion. These latter results raised the question about the site specific action of estrogen in *hpg* mouse model. Further studies based on traditional pharmacological approaches using selective ER agonists in engineered *hpg* animals knocked-out for ERs (*hpg*/ESR1 and *hpg*/ESR2) revealed that estradiol-mediated spermatogenesis takes place in *hpg* animals through the involvement of ESR1, but not ESR2, dependent mechanism responsible for the increase of FSH and testis (mainly Sertoli cells) function.

Spermatogenesis as a target for estrogen/ER signaling has been documented by the use of knock-out mice model for all three ERs (ESR1, ESR2, and GPER) as well as for the aromatase gene. *Esr1* KO animals have reduced fertility because of abnormal fluid reabsorption in the efferent ductules (76), whereas initially spermatogenesis, steroidogenesis, and fertility were found unaffected in *Esr2* KO animals (66). However, all these *Esr2* mutants displayed alternative splicing transcripts that could compensate for the lack of full-length receptor isoform. An interesting study showed that a new *Esr2*$^{-/-}$ mutant mouse, in which exon 3 of *Esr2* was deleted by Cre/LoxP-mediated excision, completely avoiding any downstream transcripts, produced sterile males (77). The cause for the sterility of these male mice is still unknown, because their gonads and internal genital organs appear *histologically* normal and the mobility of their spermatozoa appears normal too (77). In aromatase knock-out (ArKO) mice the lack of estrogen production results in an alteration of a complex hormonal balance controlling meiosis progression, leading to a significant decrease in spermatocytes and round and elongated spermatids number associated with apoptotic features (78, 79). The more severe testicular phenotype observed in ArKO mice compared to ERKO mice (66) supports the hypothesis that an alternative receptor (i.e., GPER) and alternative pathways could be involved in mediating the effects of estrogen on spermatogenesis.

A study with *Gper* deficient mice (80) claimed that Gper was not involved in estrogenic responses of reproductive organs. However, even though male and female *Gper* KO mice were found fertile, it is noteworthy that the study did not show data on the spermatogenetic process, while a careful examination of estrogenic response was carried out only on the uterus and mammary glands.

A mouse model harboring a two amino-acid mutation of the DNA-binding domain (E207A, G208A) that precludes direct binding of ESR1 to an ERE has allowed discrimination between estrogen action through ERE versus non-ERE pathways (81). The loss of non-classical ESR1 signaling pathways is responsible for most of the reproductive tract defects observed in male ERKO mice (81). These data do not, however, distinguish between the various non-classical pathways (e.g., tethering versus membrane signaling) but support strongly the hypothesis that rapid estrogen signaling could play a crucial role in spermatogenesis.

An original study using estrogen non-responsive *Esr1* knock-in (ENERK1) mice, which have a point mutation in the LBD of *Esr1* that significantly reduces interaction with and response to endogenous estrogens, but does not affect activation of Esr1 by growth factors, showed that estrogen-dependent Esr1 signaling is required for germ cell viability (82).

New information on the role of ESR1 signaling in the regulation of chromatin remodeling during spermiogenesis were obtained from recent works on Type 1 Cannabinoid Receptor Knock-out Mice (*Cnr1*$^{-/-}$) model by Cacciola et al. (83, 84). The characterization of the reproductive *Cnr1*$^{-/-}$ Mice phenotype [reviewed in Ref. (85)] revealed that estrogen through its receptor is able to preserve chromatin condensation and DNA integrity of spermatozoa by promoting histone displacement in spermatids.

In summary, the studies *in vivo* support the findings that estrogen and its major receptor, ESR1, have important roles in the regulation of spermatogenesis, particularly with aging (86) and that this activity occurs through both rapid non-classical membrane-associated/growth factor receptors as well as classical transcriptional mediated pathways. Future studies are required to better understand the separation of these pathways and their potential interactions with other steroid receptors that coexist in the same cell types.

ESTROGEN AND ESTROGEN RECEPTORS IN SPERMATOGENESIS

Spermatogenesis, which takes place in the seminiferous epithelium, can be divided into three major steps: spermatogonia proliferation by mitosis, formation of preleptotene spermatocytes which then gives birth to round spermatids (RSs) via meiosis, and spermiogenesis that allows the maturation of spermatids into mature spermatozoa. This complex and coordinated process is regulated by numerous endocrine, paracrine, or autocrine factors (87, 88) including gonadotropins LH and FSH, androgens, and estrogens (86, 89, 90).

It is known that estrogen action mediated by its specific receptors, such as ESR1, ESR2, and GPER, has different localization and expression through the entire mammalian male reproductive tract (86, 91) with major differences between species, as well as between individuals belonging to the same species (86). In mouse testis, ESR1 was found in Leydig cells, in some peritubular myoid cells (92, 93), and in Sertoli cells (94), whereas ESR2 was found in Leydig cells, Sertoli cells, and some germ cells, particularly spermatocytes (92, 93). In the rat, ESR1 immunodetection was restricted to the Leydig cells (95), in immature rat Sertoli cells (94, 96), in the seminiferous compartment (97), and in purified germ cells (98, 99). Regarding ESR2, there is a general consensus concerning its localization in seminiferous tubules but conflicting data regarding its presence in germ cells (86, 100) although Bois and co-workers detected the presence of ESR2 in pachytene spermatocytes (PS) and RSs (101). The presence of ERs in testicular cells of humans is well documented (90, 102). The two types of ERs, 1 and 2, have been identified in isolated immature germ cells in men, the full-length protein ESR1 (66 kDa) and one isoform lacking the exon 1 (46 kDa). In mature spermatozoa, only the 46-kDa band was observed. For ESR2, two proteins that correspond to the long (60 kDa) and short (50 kDa) forms have been detected in germ cells (102). However, the presence of ESR1 and ESR2 in the human ejaculated spermatozoa has been demonstrated (90, 103).

Recently, ours and other studies have demonstrated the presence of a functional GPER in both normal (98, 99, 104, 105) and malignant testicular cell lines (106).

The important role of estrogens in spermatogonial cell proliferation has been evidenced by works of Chieffi et al. where the authors demonstrated at the molecular level the involvement of ERK/c-fos signaling (107, 108). Accordingly, studies with the mouse spermatogonial GC-1 cell line showed that estradiol rapidly activates EGFR/ERK/fos/cyclin D1 pathway through a functional cross-talk between GPER and ESR1 responsible for cell proliferation (104). Conversely, estradiol-mediated rapid ESR1 and/or GPER/EGFR/ERK/c-jun pathway activation in primary cultures of rat PS (98) and in GC-2 cells (105), an immortalized mouse pachytene spermatocyte-derived cell line, induces an apoptotic mechanism. In particular, in PS cells GPER activation is related to a reduction of cyclin A1 and B1 expression concomitantly with an increase of bax protein expression (98), while in GC-2 cells GPER signaling is associated with the phosphorylation of all MAPK family members initiating the intrinsic apoptotic pathway (105). Similarly, a functional cross-talk between ESR1 and GPER in mediating apoptotic effects was observed also in primary cultures of adult rat RSs (99). It is noteworthy that in this cellular context, the contribution of ESR2 seems to be related to anti-apoptotic events (99).

G protein-coupled estrogen receptor expression and signaling was also investigated in cultured immature rat Sertoli cells (109, 110) where it has been observed that ERs are able to regulate gene expression involved in both cell proliferation and apoptosis. Indeed, ESR1 activated by its ligand rapidly induces EGFR/ERK1/2 and PI3K pathways that in turn increase cyclin D1 expression responsible for Sertoli cell proliferation (111). Interestingly, through the same molecular pathways the activation of GPER determines anti-apoptotic events by upregulating BCL2 and BCL2L2 proteins. Alternatively, the anti-apoptotic effects could be mediated by estradiol or G-1-GPER/EGFR/ERK1/2/pCREB dependent pathway driving a decrease of bax expression (111).

All these data evidenced that ERs and GPER through different molecular signaling may mediate estradiol action important for the function and maintenance of testicular cells where the complex balance between cellular maturation and cell death drive spermatogenesis and male (in)fertility.

Regarding GPER role in malignant testicular cell lines it has been shown that it is highly expressed in testicular germ cell cancer (TGCC) (112) as well as in Leydig and Sertoli cell tumors (113–115). However, also in this context, GPER activity appears to be cell type specific. In fact, in human testicular seminoma cell line, GPER activation is associated with increased cell proliferation (116), while in rat tumor, Leydig cell line is related to cell growth inhibition and apoptosis (106).

CONCLUDING REMARKS

The reproductive hormonal axis in males normally functions in a tightly regulated manner to produce concentrations of circulating steroids required for normal male sexual development, sexual function, and fertility. The testis has the ability to also produce significant amounts of estrogenic hormones and a regulated balance between androgens and estrogens seems to be essential for normal testicular physiology and reproduction acting both within the testis as well as in regulating HPG axis.

Studies discussed in this review have suggested that estradiol is the main hormone that provides negative feedback at the hypothalamic level, whereas the pituitary requires both estradiol and DHT for a complete negative feedback effect. However, further investigation is necessary to better understand how testosterone and/or its primary metabolites act within the brain to suppress the synthesis and/or secretion of GnRH. Accumulating evidence suggests that estrogen could act in the hypothalamus through rapid action mediated by ESR2, and at least partially, through GPER (33). However, it remains to establish: (i) the specific target cells (GnRH neurons, glia cells, etc.) for estrogen action at the hypothalamic level; (ii) the ER isoforms involved; (iii) the signal transduction activated by estrogen in the different cell types. An unsolved debate is focused on clarifying what steroid (DHT and/or E2) and consequently what steroid receptors (AR and/or ESR1, ESR2) are able to induce and mediate negative feedback at the pituitary level. Interesting studies using engineered *hpg* animals knocked-out for ERs (*hpg*/ESR1 and *hpg*/ESR2), revealed that estradiol-mediated spermatogenesis takes place in *hpg* animals through the involvement of ESR1, but not ESR2, which increases FSH release and testis (mainly Sertoli cells) functions. However, the debate on negative feedback at the pituitary level is further complicated by recent observations that GPER could be involved in suppressing GnRH-stimulated LH release in primary pituitary cell culture derived from ovariectomized ewes (63). However, to date, there are no studies showing GPER-mediated non-genomic signaling events in the male pituitary.

Another important finding is that estrogen plays a direct role in modulating spermatogenesis influencing, in a cell specific manner, germ cells proliferation, differentiation, as well as germ cell survival and apoptosis. The widespread presence of ESR1 and ESR2 in all testicular cells supports this finding and the discovery of GPER in the testis has opened new perspectives to better understand the rapid membrane pathways induced by estrogens. In fact, estrogenic activity in the testis as well as at the hypothalamic level appears to involve not only the classical genomic pathway, but also rapid membrane receptor initiated pathways. Studies discussed in this review indicate the ability of ERs to trigger rapid and converging pathways controlling proliferation (i.e., proliferation through ESR1 and GPER in spermatogonia or apoptosis through the same receptors in spermatids); or trigger, independently from each other, pathways controlling the same cell function (i.e., apoptosis through ESR1 and/or GPER in spermatocytes). Moreover, these studies support the hypothesis that in the testis, as in other tissues, estrogen effects are a result of the combination of different ER mediated activities, including the classic genomic as well as rapid actions at the membrane receptors via a functional cross-talk with growth factor receptors.

Another interesting aspect is that genomic and rapid pathways can work independently from each other but at same time cooperate to reach a common goal (i.e., in Sertoli cells E2-genomic action on cyclin D1 induces proliferation and estradiol rapid action through GPER activates anti-apoptotic signals).

Further studies are necessary to clarify the role of estrogen/ERs signaling in regulating GnRH, FSH, and LH release at the male hypothalamic and pituitary levels as well as in controlling spermatogenesis. Such studies could be helpful to better understand the impact of environmental endocrine disruptors' exposure, such as xenoestrogens, on male reproduction. In addition, more investigation is required to clarify the molecular mechanisms related to estrogen-dependent testicular tumorigenesis as well as to also provide a potential target for the development of a non-androgen male contraceptive.

ACKNOWLEDGMENTS

This work was supported by grants from Associazione Italiana per la Ricerca sul Cancro (AIRC) project no. IG14433.

REFERENCES

Akingbemi BT. Estrogen regulation of testicular function. *Reprod Biol Endocrinol* (2005) **3**:51. doi:10.1186/1477-7827-3-51

Tilbrook AJ, Clarke IJ. Negative feedback regulation of the secretion and actions of gonadotropin-releasing hormone in males. *Biol Reprod* (2001) **64**(3):735–42. doi:10.1095/biolreprod64.3.735

Simpson ER, Mahendroo MS, Means GD, Kilgore MW, Hinshelwood MM, Graham-Lorence S, et al. Aromatase cytochrome P450, the enzyme responsible for estrogen biosynthesis. *Endocr Rev* (1994) **15**(3):342–55. doi:10.1210/er. 15.3.342

Boon WC, Chow JD, Simpson ER. The multiple roles of estrogens and the enzyme aromatase. *Prog Brain Res* (2010) **181**:209–32. doi:10.1016/S0079-6123(08)81012-6

Mangelsdorf DJ, Thummel C, Beato M, Herrlich P, Schutz G, Umesono K, et al. The nuclear receptor superfamily: the second decade. *Cell* (1995) **83**(6):835–9. doi:10.1016/0092-8674(95)90199-X

Kelly MJ, Wagner EJ. Estrogen modulation of G-protein-coupled receptors. *Trends Endocrinol Metab* (1999) **10**(9):369–74. doi:10.1016/S1043-2760(99)00190-3

Prossnitz ER, Maggiolini M. Mechanisms of estrogen signaling and gene expression via GPR30. *Mol Cell Endocrinol* (2009) **308**(1–2):32–8. doi:10.1016/ j.mce.2009.03.026

Lappano R, De Marco P, De Francesco EM, Chimento A, Pezzi V, Maggiolini M. Cross-talk between GPER and growth factor signaling. *J Steroid Biochem Mol Biol* (2013) **137**:50–6. doi:10.1016/j.jsbmb.2013.03.005

Prossnitz ER, Arterburn JB, Smith HO, Oprea TI, Sklar LA, Hathaway HJ. Estrogen signaling through the transmembrane G protein-coupled receptor GPR30. *Annu Rev Physiol* (2008) **70**:165–90. doi:10.1146/annurev.physiol.70.113006. 100518

Herbison AE. Physiology of the GnRH neuronal network. In: Neill JD, editor. *Knobil and Neill's Physiology of Reproduction*, 3rd edn. San Diego: Academic Press (2006). p. 1415–82.

Scott CJ, Tilbrook AJ, Rawson JA, Clarke IJ. Gonadal steroid receptors in the regulation of GnRH secretion in farm animals. *Anim Reprod Sci* (2000) **60-61**:313–26. doi:10.1016/S0378-4320(00)00103-2

Lindzey J, Wetsel WC, Couse JF, Stoker T, Cooper R, Korach KS. Effects of castration and chronic steroid treatments on hypothalamic gonadotropin-releasing hormone content and pituitary gonadotropins in male wild-type and estrogen receptor-alpha knockout mice. *Endocrinology* (1998) **139**(10):4092–101. doi:10.1210/en.139.10.4092

Wersinger SR, Haisenleder DJ, Lubahn DB, Rissman EF. Steroid feedback on gonadotropin release and pituitary gonadotropin subunit mRNA in mice lacking a functional estrogen receptor alpha. *Endocrine* (1999) **11**(2):137–43. doi:10.1385/ENDO:11:2:137

Hileman SM, Lubbers LS, Kuehl DE, Schaeffer DJ, Rhodes L, Jackson GL. Effect of inhibiting 5 alpha-reductase activity on the ability of testosterone to inhibit luteinizing hormone release in male sheep. *Biol Reprod* (1994) **50**(6):1244–50. doi:10.1095/biolreprod50.6.1244

Naftolin F, Ryan KJ, Davies IJ, Petro Z, Kuhn M. The formation and metabolism of estrogens in brain tissues. *Adv Biosci* (1975) **15**:105–21.

Selmanoff MK, Brodkin LD, Weiner RI, Siiteri PK. Aromatization and 5alpha-reduction of androgens in discrete hypothalamic and limbic regions of the male and female rat. *Endocrinology* (1977) **101**(3):841–8. doi:10.1210/endo-101-3-841

Sharma TP, Blache D, Blackberry MA, Martin GB. Role of peripheral and central aromatization in the control of gonadotrophin secretion in the male sheep. *Reprod Fertil Dev* (1999) **11**(4–5):293–302. doi:10.1071/RD99084

Tilbrook AJ, Clarke IJ. Negative feedback regulation of the secretion and actions of GnRH in male ruminants. *J Reprod Fertil Suppl* (1995) **49**:297–306.

Plant TM. Effects of orchidectomy and testosterone replacement treatment on pulsatile luteinizing hormone secretion in the adult rhesus monkey (*Macaca mulatta*). *Endocrinology* (1982) **110**(6):1905–13. doi:10.1210/endo-110-6-1905

Damassa DA, Kobashigawa D, Smith ER, Davidson JM. Negative feedback control of LH by testosterone: a quantitative study in male rats. *Endocrinology* (1976) **99**(3):736–42. doi:10.1210/endo-99-3-736

Bagatell CJ, Dahl KD, Bremner WJ. The direct pituitary effect of testosterone to inhibit gonadotropin secretion in men is partially mediated by aromatization to estradiol. *J Androl* (1994) **15**(1):15–21.

Schnorr JA, Bray MJ, Veldhuis JD. Aromatization mediates testosterone's shortterm feedback restraint of 24-hour endogenously driven and acute exogenous gonadotropin-releasing hormone-stimulated luteinizing hormone and follicle-stimulating hormone secretion in young men. *J Clin Endocrinol Metab* (2001) **86**(6):2600–6. doi:10.1210/jc.86.6.2600

Veldhuis JD, Dufau ML. Estradiol modulates the pulsatile secretion of biologically active luteinizing hormone in man. *J Clin Invest* (1987) **80**(3):631–8. doi:10.1172/JCI113115

Rochira V, Zirilli L, Genazzani AD, Balestrieri A, Aranda C, Fabre B, et al. Hypothalamic-pituitary-gonadal axis in two men with aromatase deficiency: evidence that circulating estrogens are required at the hypothalamic level for the integrity of gonadotropin negative feedback. *Eur J Endocrinol* (2006) **155**(4):513–22. doi:10.1530/eje.1.02254

Herbison AE, Robinson JE, Skinner DC. Distribution of estrogen receptor-immunoreactive cells in the preoptic area of the ewe: co-localization with glutamic acid decarboxylase but not luteinizing hormone-releasing hormone. *Neuroendocrinology* (1993) **57**(4):751–9. doi:10.1159/000126433

Shivers BD, Harlan RE, Morrell JI, Pfaff DW. Absence of oestradiol concentration in cell nuclei of LHRH-immunoreactive neurones. *Nature* (1983) **304**(5924):345–7. doi:10.1038/304345a0

Laflamme N, Nappi RE, Drolet G, Labrie C, Rivest S. Expression and neuropeptidergic characterization of estrogen receptors (ERalpha and ERbeta) throughout the rat brain: anatomical evidence of distinct roles of each subtype. *J Neurobiol* (1998) **36**(3):357–78. doi:10.1002/(SICI)1097-4695(19980905)36: 3<357::AID-NEU5>3.0.CO;2-V

Butler JA, Sjoberg M, Coen CW. Evidence for oestrogen receptor alpha-immunoreactivity in gonadotrophin-releasing hormone-expressing neurones. *J Neuroendocrinol* (1999) **11**(5):331–5. doi:10.1046/j.1365-2826.1999.00347.x

Temple JL, Laing E, Sunder A, Wray S. Direct action of estradiol on gonadotropin-releasing hormone-1 neuronal activity via a transcription-dependent mechanism. *J Neurosci* (2004) **24**(28):6326–33. doi:10.1523/JNEUROSCI.1006-04.2004

Hrabovszky E, Steinhauser A, Barabas K, Shughrue PJ, Petersen SL, Merchenthaler I, et al. Estrogen receptor-beta immunoreactivity in luteinizing hormone-releasing hormone neurons of the rat brain. *Endocrinology* (2001) **142**(7):3261–4. doi:10.1210/en.142.7.3261

Hrabovszky E, Kallo I, Szlavik N, Keller E, Merchenthaler I, Liposits Z. Gonadotropin-releasing hormone neurons express estrogen receptor-beta. *J Clin Endocrinol Metab* (2007) **92**(7):2827–30. doi:10.1210/jc.2006-2819

Abe H, Keen KL, Terasawa E. Rapid action of estrogens on intracellular calcium oscillations in primate luteinizing hormone-releasing hormone-1 neurons. *Endocrinology* (2008) **149**(3):1155–62. doi:10.1210/en.2007-0942

Noel SD, Keen KL, Baumann DI, Filardo EJ, Terasawa E. Involvement of G protein-coupled receptor 30 (GPR30) in rapid action of estrogen in primate LHRH neurons. *Mol Endocrinol* (2009) **23**(3):349–59. doi:10.1210/me.2008-0299

Gharib SD, Wierman ME, Shupnik MA, Chin WW. Molecular biology of the pituitary gonadotropins. *Endocr Rev* (1990) **11**(1):177–99. doi:10.1210/edrv- 11-1-177

Gregory SJ, Kaiser UB. Regulation of gonadotropins by inhibin and activin. *Semin Reprod Med* (2004) **22**(3):253–67. doi:10.1055/s-2004-831901

Ramirez VD, McCann SM. Inhibitory effect of testosterone on luteinizing hormone secretion in immature and adult rats. *Endocrinology* (1965) **76**:412–7. doi:10.1210/endo-76-3-412

Selmanoff M, Shu C, Petersen SL, Barraclough CA, Zoeller RT. Single cell levels of hypothalamic messenger ribonucleic acid encoding luteinizing hormone-releasing hormone in intact, castrated, and hyperprolactinemic male rats. *Endocrinology* (1991) **128**(1):459–66. doi:10.1210/endo-128-1-459

Roselli CE, Kelly MJ, Ronnekleiv OK. Testosterone regulates progonadotropin-releasing hormone levels in the preoptic area and basal hypothalamus of the male rat. *Endocrinology* (1990) **126**(2):1080–6. doi:10.1210/endo-126-2-1080

Giri M, Kaufman JM. Effects of long-term orchidectomy on in vitro pulsatile gonadotropin-releasing hormone release from the medial basal hypothalamus of the adult guinea pig. *Endocrinology* (1994) **134**(4):1621–6. doi:10.1210/en. 134.4.1621

Levine JE, Duffy MT. Simultaneous measurement of luteinizing hormone (LH)-releasing hormone, LH, and follicle-stimulating hormone release in intact and short-term castrate rats. *Endocrinology* (1988) **122**(5):2211–21. doi:10.1210/endo-122-5-2211

Frawley LS, Neill JD. Biphasic effects of estrogen on gonadotropin-releasing hormone-induced luteinizing hormone release in monolayer cultures of rat and monkey pituitary cells. *Endocrinology* (1984) **114**(2):659–63. doi:10.1210/ endo-114-2-659

Kennedy J, Chappel S. Direct pituitary effects of testosterone and luteinizing hormone-releasing hormone upon follicle-stimulating hormone: analysis by radioimmuno- and radioreceptor assay. *Endocrinology* (1985) **116**(2):741–8. doi:10.1210/endo-116-2-741

Heckert LL, Wilson EM, Nilson JH. Transcriptional repression of the alpha-subunit gene by androgen receptor occurs independently of DNA binding but requires the DNA-binding and ligand-binding domains of the receptor. *Mol Endocrinol* (1997) **11**(10):1497–506. doi:10.1210/me.11.10.1497

Demay F, Tiffoche C, Thieulant ML. Sex- and cell-specific expression of an estrogen receptor isoform in the pituitary gland. *Neuroendocrinology* (1996) **63**(6):522–9. doi:10.1159/000127081

Mitchner NA, Garlick C, Ben-Jonathan N. Cellular distribution and gene regulation of estrogen receptors alpha and beta in the rat pituitary gland. *Endocrinology* (1998) **139**(9):3976–83. doi:10.1210/en.139.9.3976

Sheng C, McNeilly AS, Brooks AN. Immunohistochemical distribution of oestrogen receptor and luteinizing hormone B subunit in the ovine pituitary gland during foetal development. *J Neuroendocrinol* (1998) **10**(9):713–8. doi:10.1046/j.1365-2826.1998.00255.x

Brandenberger AW, Tee MK, Lee JY, Chao V, Jaffe RB. Tissue distribution of estrogen receptors alpha (ER-alpha) and beta (ER-beta) mRNA in the midgestational human fetus. *J Clin Endocrinol Metab* (1997) **82**(10):3509–12. doi:10.1210/jc.82.10.3509

Kimura N, Mizokami A, Oonuma T, Sasano H, Nagura H. Immunocytochemical localization of androgen receptor with polyclonal antibody in paraffin-embedded human tissues. *J Histochem Cytochem* (1993) **41**(5):671–8. doi:10.1177/41.5.8468448

Okada Y, Fujii Y, Moore JP Jr, Winters SJ. Androgen receptors in gonadotrophs in pituitary cultures from adult male monkeys and rats. *Endocrinology* (2003) **144**(1):267–73. doi:10.1210/en.2002-220770

Iqbal J, Swanson JJ, Prins GS, Jacobson CD. Androgen receptor-like immunoreactivity in the Brazilian opossum brain and pituitary: distribution and effects of castration and testosterone replacement in the adult male. *Brain Res* (1995) **703**(1–2):1–18. doi:10.1016/0165-3806(96)83481-X

Crocoll A, Zhu CC, Cato AC, Blum M. Expression of androgen receptor mRNA during mouse embryogenesis. *Mech Dev* (1998) **72**(1–2):175–8. doi:10.1016/S0925-4773(98)00007-0

Wierman ME, Gharib SD, LaRovere JM, Badger TM, Chin WW. Selective failure of androgens to regulate follicle stimulating hormone beta messenger ribonucleic acid levels in the male rat. *Mol Endocrinol* (1988) **2**(6):492–8. doi:10.1210/mend-2-6-492

Urban RJ, Davis MR, Rogol AD, Johnson ML, Veldhuis JD. Acute androgen receptor blockade increases luteinizing hormone secretory activity in men. *J Clin Endocrinol Metab* (1988) **67**(6):1149–55. doi:10.1210/jcem-67-6-1149

Juniewicz PE, Oesterling JE, Walters JR, Steele RE, Niswender GD, Coffey DS, et al. Aromatase inhibition in the dog. I. Effect on serum LH, serum testosterone concentrations, testicular secretions and spermatogenesis. *J Urol* (1988) **139**(4):827–31.

Smith EP, Boyd J, Frank GR, Takahashi H, Cohen RM, Specker B, et al. Estrogen resistance caused by a mutation in the estrogen-receptor gene in a man. *N Engl J Med* (1994) **331**(16):1056–61. doi:10.1056/NEJM199410203311604

Tremblay GB, Tremblay A, Copeland NG, Gilbert DJ, Jenkins NA, Labrie F, et al. Cloning, chromosomal localization, and functional analysis of the murine estrogen receptor beta. *Mol Endocrinol* (1997) **11**(3):353–65. doi:10.1210/me. 11.3.353

Couse JF, Lindzey J, Grandien K, Gustafsson JA, Korach KS. Tissue distribution and quantitative analysis of estrogen receptor-alpha (ERalpha) and estrogen receptor-beta (ERbeta) messenger ribonucleic acid in the wildtype and ERalpha-knockout mouse. *Endocrinology* (1997) **138**(11):4613–21. doi:10.1210/en.138.11.4613

Shughrue PJ, Komm B, Merchenthaler I. The distribution of estrogen receptorbeta mRNA in the rat hypothalamus. *Steroids* (1996) **61**(12):678–81. doi:10. 1016/S0039-128X(96)00222-X

Hewitt SC, Korach KS. Oestrogen receptor knockout mice: roles for oestrogen receptors alpha and beta in reproductive tissues. *Reproduction* (2003) **125**(2):143–9. doi:10.1530/rep.0.1250143

Nicol L, McNeilly JR, Stridsberg M, Crawford JL, McNeilly AS. Influence of steroids and GnRH on biosynthesis and secretion of secretogranin II and chromogranin A in relation to LH release in LbetaT2 gonadotroph cells. *J Endocrinol* (2002) **174**(3):473–83. doi:10.1677/joe.0.1740473

Shupnik MA, Rosenzweig BA. Identification of an estrogen-responsive element in the rat LH beta gene. DNA-estrogen receptor interactions and functional analysis. *J Biol Chem* (1991) **266**(26):17084–91.

Demay F, De Monti M, Tiffoche C, Vaillant C, Thieulant ML. Steroid-independent activation of ER by GnRH in gonadotrope pituitary cells. *Endocrinology* (2001) **142**(8):3340–7. doi:10.1210/en.142.8.3340

Rudolf FO, Kadokawa H. Expression of estradiol receptor, GPR30, in bovine anterior pituitary and effects of GPR30 agonist on GnRH-induced LH secretion. *Anim Reprod Sci* (2013) **139**(1–4):9–17. doi:10.1016/j.anireprosci.2013. 04.003

Brailoiu E, Dun SL, Brailoiu GC, Mizuo K, Sklar LA, Oprea TI, et al. Distribution and characterization of estrogen receptor G protein-coupled receptor 30 in the rat central nervous system. *J Endocrinol* (2007) **193**(2):311–21. doi:10.1677/JOE-07-0017

Hazell GG, Yao ST, Roper JA, Prossnitz ER, O'Carroll AM, Lolait SJ. Localisation of GPR30, a novel G protein-coupled oestrogen receptor, suggests multiple functions in rodent brain and peripheral tissues. *J Endocrinol* (2009) **202**(2):223–36. doi:10.1677/JOE-09-0066

Hewitt SC, Harrell JC, Korach KS. Lessons in estrogen biology from knockout and transgenic animals. *Annu Rev Physiol* (2005) **67**:285–308. doi:10.1146/annurev.physiol.67.040403.115914

Lubahn DB, Moyer JS, Golding TS, Couse JF, Korach KS, Smithies O. Alteration of reproductive function but not prenatal sexual development after insertional disruption of the mouse estrogen receptor gene. *Proc Natl Acad Sci U S A* (1993) **90**(23):11162–6. doi:10.1073/pnas.90.23.11162

Cattanach BM, Iddon CA, Charlton HM, Chiappa SA, Fink G. Gonadotrophin-releasing hormone deficiency in a mutant mouse with hypogonadism. *Nature* (1977) **269**(5626):338–40. doi:10.1038/269338a0

Ebling FJ, Brooks AN, Cronin AS, Ford H, Kerr JB. Estrogenic induction of spermatogenesis in the hypogonadal mouse. *Endocrinology* (2000) **141**(8):2861–9. doi:10.1210/en.141.8.2861

Myers M, Ebling FJ, Nwagwu M, Boulton R, Wadhwa K, Stewart J, et al. Atypical development of Sertoli cells and impairment of spermatogenesis in the hypogonadal (hpg) mouse. *J Anat* (2005) **207**(6):797–811. doi:10.1111/j.1469-7580. 2005.00493.x

Scott IS, Charlton HM, Cox BS, Grocock CA, Sheffield JW, O'Shaughnessy PJ. Effect of LH injections on testicular steroidogenesis, cholesterol side-chain cleavage P450 mRNA content and Leydig cell morphology in hypogonadal mice. *J Endocrinol* (1990) **125**(1):131–8. doi:10.1677/joe.0.1250131

Singh J, O'Neill C, Handelsman DJ. Induction of spermatogenesis by androgens in gonadotropin-deficient (hpg) mice. *Endocrinology* (1995) **136**(12):5311–21. doi:10.1210/en.136.12.5311

Singh J, Handelsman DJ. The effects of recombinant FSH on testosterone-induced spermatogenesis in gonadotrophin-deficient (hpg) mice. *J Androl* (1996) **17**(4):382–93.

Baines H, Nwagwu MO, Furneaux EC, Stewart J, Kerr JB, Mayhew TM, et al. Estrogenic induction of spermatogenesis in the hypogonadal (hpg) mouse: role of androgens. *Reproduction* (2005) **130**(5):643–54. doi:10.1530/rep.1.00693

Nwagwu MO, Baines H, Kerr JB, Ebling FJ. Neonatal androgenization of hypogonadal (hpg) male mice does not abolish estradiol-induced FSH production and spermatogenesis. *Reprod Biol Endocrinol* (2005) **3**:48. doi:10.1186/1477- 7827-3-48

Hess RA, Bunick D, Lee KH, Bahr J, Taylor JA, Korach KS, et al. A role for oestrogens in the male reproductive system. *Nature* (1997) **390**(6659):509–12. doi:10.1038/37352

Antal MC, Krust A, Chambon P, Mark M. Sterility and absence of histopathological defects in nonreproductive organs of a mouse ERbeta-null mutant. *Proc Natl Acad Sci U S A* (2008) **105**(7):2433–8. doi:10.1073/pnas.0712029105

Robertson KM, O'Donnell L, Jones ME, Meachem SJ, Boon WC, Fisher CR, et al. Impairment of spermatogenesis in mice lacking a functional aromatase (cyp 19) gene. *Proc Natl Acad Sci U S A* (1999) **96**(14):7986–91. doi:10.1073/pnas.96.14.7986

Robertson KM, O'Donnell L, Simpson ER, Jones ME. The phenotype of the aromatase knockout mouse reveals dietary phytoestrogens impact significantly on testis function. *Endocrinology* (2002) **143**(8):2913–21. doi:10.1210/en.143. 8.2913

Otto C, Fuchs I, Kauselmann G, Kern H, Zevnik B, Andreasen P, et al. GPR30 does not mediate estrogenic responses in reproductive organs in mice. *Biol Reprod* (2009) **80**(1):34–41. doi:10.1095/biolreprod.108.071175

Weiss J, Bernhardt ML, Laronda MM, Hurley LA, Glidewell-Kenney C, Pillai S, et al. Estrogen actions in the male reproductive system involve estrogen response element-independent pathways. *Endocrinology* (2008) **149**(12):6198–206. doi:10.1210/en.2008-0122

Sinkevicius KW, Woloszyn K, Laine M, Jackson KS, Greene GL, Woodruff TK, et al. Characterization of the ovarian and reproductive abnormalities in prepubertal and adult estrogen non-responsive estrogen receptor alpha knock-in (ENERKI) mice. *Steroids* (2009) **74**(12):913–9. doi:10.1016/j.steroids. 2009.06.012

Cacciola G, Chioccarelli T, Altucci L, Ledent C, Mason JI, Fasano S, et al. Low 17beta-estradiol levels in CNR1 knock-out mice affect spermatid chromatin remodeling by interfering with chromatin reorganization. *Biol Reprod* (2013) **88**(6):152. doi:10.1095/biolreprod.112.105726

Cacciola G, Chioccarelli T, Altucci L, Viggiano A, Fasano S, Pierantoni R, et al. Nuclear size as estrogen-responsive chromatin quality parameter of mouse spermatozoa. *Gen Comp Endocrinol* (2013) **193**:201–9. doi:10.1016/j.ygcen.2013.07.018

Cacciola G, Chioccarelli T, Fasano S, Pierantoni R, Cobellis G. Estrogens and spermiogenesis: new insights from type 1 cannabinoid receptor knockout mice. *Int J Endocrinol* (2013) **2013**:501350. doi:10.1155/2013/501350

Carreau S, Hess RA. Oestrogens and spermatogenesis. *Philos Trans R Soc Lond B Biol Sci* (2010) **365**(1546):1517–35. doi:10.1098/rstb.2009.0235

Franca LR, Parreira GG, Gates RJ, Russell LD. Hormonal regulation of spermatogenesis in the hypophysectomized rat: quantitation of germ-cell population and effect of elimination of residual testosterone after long-term hypophy-sectomy. *J Androl* (1998) **19**(3):335–40 discussion 41–2.

Handelsman DJ. Hormonal regulation of spermatogenesis: insights from constructing genetic models. *Reprod Fertil Dev* (2011) **23**(4):507–19. doi:10.1071/ RD10308

O'Donnell L, Robertson KM, Jones ME, Simpson ER. Estrogen and spermatogenesis. *Endocr Rev* (2001) **22**(3):289–318. doi:10.1210/er.22.3.289

Carreau S, Wolczynski S, Galeraud-Denis I. Aromatase, oestrogens and human male reproduction. *Philos Trans R Soc Lond B Biol Sci* (2010) **365**(1546):1571–9. doi:10.1098/rstb.2009.0113

Rochira V, Granata AR, Madeo B, Zirilli L, Rossi G, Carani C. Estrogens in males: what have we learned in the last 10 years? *Asian J Androl* (2005) **7**(1):3–20. doi:10.1111/j.1745-7262.2005.00018.x

Zhou Q, Nie R, Prins GS, Saunders PT, Katzenellenbogen BS, Hess RA. Localization of androgen and estrogen receptors in adult male mouse reproductive tract. *J Androl* (2002) **23**(6):870–81. doi:10.1002/j.1939-4640.2002.tb02345.x

Kotula-Balak M, Gancarczyk M, Sadowska J, Bilinskai B. The expression of aromatase, estrogen receptor alpha and estrogen receptor beta in mouse Leydig cells in vitro that derived from cryptorchid males. *Eur J Histochem* (2005) **49**(1):59–62.

Lucas TF, Siu ER, Esteves CA, Monteiro HP, Oliveira CA, Porto CS, et al. 17Beta-estradiol induces the translocation of the estrogen receptors ESR1 and ESR2 to the cell membrane, MAPK3/1 phosphorylation and proliferation of cultured immature rat Sertoli cells. *Biol Reprod* (2008) **78**(1):101–14. doi:10.1095/biolreprod.107.063909

Fisher JS, Millar MR, Majdic G, Saunders PT, Fraser HM, Sharpe RM. Immunolocalisation of oestrogen receptor-alpha within the testis and excurrent ducts of the rat and marmoset monkey from perinatal life to adulthood. *J Endocrinol* (1997) **153**(3):485–95. doi:10.1677/joe.0.1530485

van Pelt AM, de Rooij DG, van der Burg B, van der Saag PT, Gustafsson JA, Kuiper GG. Ontogeny of estrogen receptor-beta expression in rat testis. *Endocrinology* (1999) **140**(1):478–83. doi:10.1210/en.140.1.478

Pelletier G, El-Alfy M. Immunocytochemical localization of estrogen receptors alpha and beta in the human reproductive organs. *J Clin Endocrinol Metab* (2000) **85**(12):4835–40. doi:10.1210/jc.85.12.4835

Chimento A, Sirianni R, Delalande C, Silandre D, Bois C, Ando S, et al. 17 Betaestradiol activates rapid signaling pathways involved in rat pachytene spermatocytes apoptosis through GPR30 and ER alpha. *Mol Cell Endocrinol* (2010) **320**(1–2):136–44. doi:10.1016/j.mce.2010.01.035

Chimento A, Sirianni R, Zolea F, Bois C, Delalande C, Ando S, et al. Gper and ESRs are expressed in rat round spermatids and mediate oestrogen-dependent rapid pathways modulating expression of cyclin B1 and Bax. *Int J Androl* (2011) **34**(5 Pt 1):420–9. doi:10.1111/j.1365-2605.2010.01100.x

Yamada-Mouri N, Hirata S, Kato J. Existence and expression of the untranslated first exon of aromatase mRNA in the rat brain. *J Steroid Biochem Mol Biol* (1996) **58**(2):163–6. doi:10.1016/0960-0760(96)00022-2

Bois C, Delalande C, Nurmio M, Parvinen M, Zanatta L, Toppari J, et al. Age-and cell-related gene expression of aromatase and estrogen receptors in the rat testis. *J Mol Endocrinol* (2010) **45**(3):147–59. doi:10.1677/JME-10-0041

Lambard S, Galeraud-Denis I, Saunders PT, Carreau S. Human immature germ cells and ejaculated spermatozoa contain aromatase and oestrogen receptors. *J Mol Endocrinol* (2004) **32**(1):279–89. doi:10.1677/jme.0.0320279

Aquila S, Sisci D, Gentile M, Middea E, Siciliano L, Ando S. Human ejaculated spermatozoa contain active P450 aromatase. *J Clin Endocrinol Metab* (2002) **87**(7):3385–90. doi:10.1210/jc.87.7.3385

Sirianni R, Chimento A, Ruggiero C, De Luca A, Lappano R, Ando S, et al. The novel estrogen receptor, G protein-coupled receptor 30, mediates the proliferative effects induced by 17beta-estradiol on mouse spermatogonial GC-1 cell line. *Endocrinology* (2008) **149**(10):5043–51. doi:10.1210/en.2007-1593

Chimento A, Sirianni R, Casaburi I, Ruggiero C, Maggiolini M, Ando S, et al. 17Beta-estradiol activates GPER- and ESR1-dependent pathways inducing apoptosis in GC-2 cells, a mouse spermatocyte-derived cell line. *Mol Cell Endocrinol* (2012) **355**(1):49–59. doi:10.1016/j.mce.2012.01.017

Chimento A, Casaburi I, Bartucci M, Patrizii M, Dattilo R, Avena P, et al. Selective GPER activation decreases proliferation and activates apoptosis in tumor Leydig cells. *Cell Death Dis* (2013) **4**:e747. doi:10.1038/cddis.2013.275

Chieffi P, Colucci-D'Amato GL, Staibano S, Franco R, Tramontano D. Estradiol-induced mitogen-activated protein kinase (extracellular signalregulated kinase 1 and 2) activity in the frog (*Rana esculenta*) testis. *J Endocrinol* (2000) **167**(1):77–84. doi:10.1677/joe.0.1670077

Chieffi P, Colucci D'Amato L, Guarino F, Salvatore G, Angelini F. 17 Betaestradiol induces spermatogonial proliferation through mitogen-activated protein kinase (extracellular signal-regulated kinase 1/2) activity in the lizard (*Podarcis s. sicula*). *Mol Reprod Dev* (2002) **61**(2):218–25. doi:10.1002/mrd.1151

Lucas TF, Royer C, Siu ER, Lazari MF, Porto CS. Expression and signaling of G protein-coupled estrogen receptor 1 (GPER) in rat Sertoli cells. *Biol Reprod* (2010) **83**(2):307–17. doi:10.1095/biolreprod.110.084160

Lucas TF, Pimenta MT, Pisolato R, Lazari MF, Porto CS. 17Beta-estradiol signaling and regulation of Sertoli cell function. *Spermatogenesis* (2011) **1**(4):318–24. doi:10.4161/spmg.1.4.18903

Royer C, Lucas TF, Lazari MF, Porto CS. 17Beta-estradiol signaling and regulation of proliferation and apoptosis of rat Sertoli cells. *Biol Reprod* (2012) **86**(4):108. doi:10.1095/biolreprod.111.096891

Franco R, Boscia F, Gigantino V, Marra L, Esposito F, Ferrara D, et al. GPR30 is overexpressed in post-puberal testicular germ cell tumors. *Cancer Biol Ther* (2011) **11**(6):609–13. doi:10.4161/cbt.11.6.14672

Rago V, Romeo F, Giordano F, Maggiolini M, Carpino A. Identification of the estrogen receptor GPER in neoplastic and non-neoplastic human testes. *Reprod Biol Endocrinol* (2011) **9**:135. doi:10.1186/1477-7827-9-135

Rago V, Romeo F, Giordano F, Ferraro A, Ando S, Carpino A. Identification of ERbeta1 and ERbeta2 in human seminoma, in embryonal carcinoma and in their adjacent intratubular germ cell neoplasia. *Reprod Biol Endocrinol* (2009) **7**:56. doi:10.1186/1477-7827-7-56

Carpino A, Rago V, Pezzi V, Carani C, Ando S. Detection of aromatase and estrogen receptors (ERalpha, ERbeta1, ERbeta2) in human Leydig cell tumor. *Eur J Endocrinol* (2007) **157**(2):239–44. doi:10.1530/EJE-07-0029

Chevalier N, Bouskine A, Fenichel P. Role of GPER/GPR30 in tumoral testicular germ cells proliferation. *Cancer Biol Ther* (2011) **12**(1):2–3. doi:10.4161/cbt.12.1.15726

16

Impact of hypothalamic reactive oxygen species in the regulation of energy metabolism and food intake

Anne Drougard *, Audren Fournel, Philippe Valet and Claude Knauf *

NeuroMicrobiota, European Associated Laboratory, INSERM/UCL, Institut National de la Santé et de la Recherche Médicale, U1048, Institut des Maladies Métaboliques et Cardiovasculaires (I2MC), CHU Rangueil, Université Paul Sabatier, Toulouse, France

Correspondence:
Anne Drougard and Claude Knauf, NeuroMicrobiota, European Associated Laboratory, INSERM/UCL, Institut National de la Santé et de la Recherche Médicale, U1048, Institut des Maladies Métaboliques et Cardiovasculaires (I2MC), CHU Rangueil, Université Paul Sabatier, 1 Avenue du Professeur Jean Poulhès, Bâtiment L4 - BP 84225, 31432 Toulouse Cedex 4, France
e-mail: anne.drougard@inserm.fr; claude.knauf@inserm.fr

Hypothalamus is a key area involved in the control of metabolism and food intake via the integrations of numerous signals (hormones, neurotransmitters, metabolites) from various origins. These factors modify hypothalamic neurons activity and generate adequate molecular and behavioral responses to control energy balance. In this complex integrative system, a new concept has been developed in recent years, that includes reactive oxygen species (ROS) as a critical player in energy balance. ROS are known to act in many signaling pathways in different peripheral organs, but also in hypothalamus where they regulate food intake and metabolism by acting on different types of neurons, including proopiomelanocortin (POMC) and agouti-related protein (AgRP)/neuropeptide Y (NPY) neurons. Hypothalamic ROS release is under the influence of different factors such as pancreatic and gut hormones, adipokines (leptin, apelin,...), neurotransmitters and nutrients (glucose, lipids,...). The sources of ROS production are multiple including NADPH oxidase, but also the mitochondria which is considered as the main ROS producer in the brain. ROS are considered as signaling molecules, but conversely impairment of this neuronal signaling ROS pathway contributes to alterations of autonomic nervous system and neuroendocrine function, leading to metabolic diseases such as obesity and type 2 diabetes. In this review we focus our attention on factors that are able to modulate hypothalamic ROS release in order to control food intake and energy metabolism, and whose deregulations could participate to the development of pathological conditions. This novel insight reveals an original mechanism in the hypothalamus that controls energy balance and identify hypothalamic ROS signaling as a potential therapeutic strategy to treat metabolic disorders.

Keywords: ROS, hypothalamus, food intake, metabolism, diabetes, obesity

INTRODUCTION

The role of the brain in the control of energy homeostasis has been suggested at the middle of the nineteenth century by Claude Bernard who was the first to evoke its importance with the famous experiment "la piqûre diabétique" (Bernard, 1849). Indeed, he observed an important rise of glycemia after a stimulation of the floor of the fourth ventricle. In 1953, Gordon Kennedy identified the precise brain area involved in this phenomenon. He has demonstrated that circulating factors released by the adipose tissue could reach the hypothalamus in order to modulate food intake and energy expenditure, and thus regulate body weight (Kennedy, 1953). Moreover, the medio-basal hypothalamus is a privileged central area which directly senses various factors (hormones, metabolites). In fact, at the close proximity of the arcuate nucleus (ARC), the median eminence is a circumventricular organ that presents a blood-brain barrier-free area that allows peripheral factors to inform hypothalamic structures about the energy status (Rodriguez et al., 2010). Since 1940, the development of stereotaxic methods in animals has offered researchers the opportunity to practice stimulation or localized destructions of various hypothalamic nuclei, and then identified their precise role (Brobeck, 1946).

The first neurons in contact with peripheral signals are called "neurons of first order." These neurons are only present in the ARC (Cone et al., 2001) and a lesion of this hypothalamic region induces hyperphagia and obesity (Olney, 1969). It is largely well described in the literature that the ARC presents two subsets of neurons that have opposite effects on feeding. One of these group of neurons express pro-opiomelanocortin (POMC) and cocaine-amphetamine-regulated transcript (CART), and upon stimulation, these neurons produce anorectic effects (Cone, 2005). The POMC precursor is cleaved into α-melanocyte-stimulating hormones (α-MSH) which reduces food intake, body weight and increases energy expenditure (Kim et al., 2000; Yasuda et al., 2004). The second group of neurons in the ARC leads to orexigenic responses upon activation. These neurons express neuropeptide Y (NPY) and the agouti-gene-related transcript (AgRP) (Clark et al., 1984; Rossi et al., 1998) which stimulate food intake and reduce energy expenditure (Fekete et al., 2002). In genetically-modified obese rodents, as well as in fasted normal animals, NPY mRNA expression and protein content are elevated in ARC (Sanacora et al., 1990; Wilding et al., 1993; Park et al., 2004). Collectively, this suggests that (1) over-activation or dysfunction of NPY neurons is involved in the emergence of metabolic diseases, but also that (2) NPY neurons can inhibit melanocortin system. Interestingly, subsets of POMC neurons contain both gamma amino butyric acid (GABA) and glutamate (Dicken et al., 2012). Subsets of NPY neurons also contain GABA (Horvath et al., 1997) and GABA from NPY neurons participates to inhibition of POMC neurons. This unidirectional input from the NPY to POMC cells brings to light one anatomical basis of energy regulation. This neuronal interaction seems to favor the tonic inhibition of satiety signal, and also promotes feeding or over-feeding when food is available in excess. This finding reinforces the key role of an intact melanocortin system in the control of energy balance.

The POMC and NPY/AgRP neurons of the ARC interact with various brain regions that include hypothalamic areas such as ventromedial hypothalamus (VMH), dorsomedial hypothalamus (DMH), paraventricular nucleus (PVN) and lateral hypothalamus (LH) (Wynne et al., 2005). Lesion studies in rodent have shown that ablation of VMH, DMH or PVN results in hyperphagia and obesity (Leibowitz et al., 1981; Shimizu et al., 1987; Bellinger and Bernardis, 2002) whereas lesions in the LH lead to hypophagia (Bernardis and Bellinger, 1993). To summarize, a proposal of dual-center model has been proposed that identifies the VMH as the "satiety center" and the LH as the "hunger center" (Stellar, 1994).

These hypothalamic nuclei have the ability to sense the level of available fuel energy in the body. This detection of peripheral signals involves various molecular actors such as classical neurotransmitters but also "non-classical" diffusible molecules such as reactive nitrogen species (RNS) and reactive oxygen species (ROS). To this aim, nitric oxide (NO) is an atypical molecular actor which belongs to RNS family, but could also be associated to ROS family since it is a radical gas derived from nitric and oxygen. NO has a very short half-life and can largely diffuse in cells (Palmer et al., 1987). It has a single electron, allowing numerous interactions with cellular components. In the brain, chemical properties of NO permits its diffusion across hypothalamic cells to control neurotransmitter release (Ohkuma and Katsura, 2001), but also synaptic plasticity (Shibuki and Okada, 1991), that leads to the modulation of food intake (Morley and Flood, 1991) and glucose metabolism (Duparc et al., 2011a). In addition to RNS, recent data argue that differential fuel utilization in response to nutrients is linked to ROS formation. This ROS generation is not merely a "byproduct" of substrate oxidation, but has a crucial role in regulating neuronal response in a substrate-dependent manner.

In this review, we will describe the molecular mechanisms generating ROS in response to metabolic signals, in order to control metabolism and food intake. In physiological conditions, ROS production is considered as a signaling actor produced at low level and in a transient manner. On the other hand, over-production of ROS, associated to a dysfunction of ROS buffering systems, can lead to the development of chronic diseases. Thus, central chronic ROS release participates in the establishment of numerous diseases such as type 2 diabetes (T2D), but also in cancer and neurodegenerative disorders (as Parkinson and Alzheimer disease).

ROS PRODUCTION: FOCUS ON NEURONAL CELLS

INTRODUCTION

ROS are radical species derived from oxygen of which the most known are the superoxide anion (O_2^-), the hydrogen peroxide (H_2O_2) and the hydroxyl radical (OH^-). These "free-radical" ROS have unpaired electrons on an oxygen atom. This property makes ROS very unstable as they react quickly with others surrounding chemical molecules in order to pair their electrons. These radical reactions often lead to a new radical formation generating a chain reaction, and thus activate numerous signaling pathways (Gutteridge and Halliwell, 2000).

Within the cell, all processes using oxygen may produce ROS. However, the mitochondrial transport electron chain is a major source of ROS generation in physiological conditions (Bashan et al., 2009). ROS are also produced by the NADPH oxidases (NOX) which are membrane-bound enzymatic complexes able to transfer electrons from cytosolic NADPH to oxygen (Lambeth, 2004; Hordijk, 2006). Finally, another source of ROS is the endoplasmic reticulum (ER) (Cross and Jones, 1991) and the peroxisome (Schrader and Fahimi, 2006).

In order to limit ROS concentration, cells are equipped with various enzymatic and non-enzymatic antioxidant systems. Several enzymes directly degrade ROS such as the superoxide dismutase (SOD), the catalase and the glutathione peroxidase (Turrens, 2003). Various non-enzymatic scavengers can also support detoxification of free radicals. The majority are lipophilic (vitamin E, ubiquinone or coenzyme Q, and carotenoids) or hydrophilic (vitamin C, glutathione) (Clark, 2002).

When ROS are moderately and transiently produced, they are able to reversibly modify some surrounding targets and act as "signal" molecules (Droge, 2002). However, when oxidants-antioxidants balance is altered, due to an excessive production of ROS and/or a decrease in antioxidant systems, and is associated to the expansion of oxidative stress (Droge, 2002), ROS become toxic to the cell, and could be involved in the development of specific diseases markers such as insulin resistance and type 2 diabetes (Bashan et al., 2009).

ROS AND NEURONS

ROS are also strongly present in the brain. The large majority of ROS produced by neurons have a mitochondrial origin (Bao et al., 2009). However, localization of NOX in different regions of the central nervous system have been determined by immunohistochemical approaches in rats (Kim et al., 2005) and mice (Serrano et al., 2003). Indeed, NOX are present in hippocampus, cortex, amygdala, striatum, thalamus and hypothalamus.

ROS can act directly on the brain to control many central functions. Neurons can sense, transmit and convert ROS signals into appropriate intracellular responses, including synaptic plasticity. For example, NOX activity in the hippocampus is required to induce normal cellular process in these neurons, such as long-term potentiation (a form of activity-dependent synaptic plasticity) and hippocampus-dependent memory (Infanger et al., 2006). ROS production by mitochondria also occurs in the hypothalamus, and NOX subunits are also present in the ARC, VMN, and PVN (Infanger et al., 2006). Hypothalamus is a key area involved in control of glucose homeostasis (Knauf et al., 2013). Indeed, a population of specialized hypothalamic neurons is identified as gluco-sensors (Oomura et al., 1964). These neurons are classified into two categories, which differ both by their mode of action and by their precise localization, i.e., neurons excited by glucose (named glucose-excited or GE) and neurons inhibited by glucose (named glucose-inhibited or GI). Raising plasma glucose level after a large meal results in an increased brain level to 4,5 mM and an increase in brain glucose activates GE neurons, while GI remain inactive (Routh, 2002). At the opposite, during a period of fasting, reduction in the concentration of brain glucose inhibits GE neurons and activates GI ones (Routh, 2010). Although K_{ATP} channels seem to be essential for the function of gluco-sensors, several studies show a depolarization of these neurons via K_{ATP} channels independent mechanisms (Ainscow et al., 2002; Fioramonti et al., 2004). Among these mechanisms, mitochondrial ROS (mROS) are clearly involved in hypothalamic glucose sensing (Leloup et al., 2006). Indeed, a transient increase of glucose stimulates mROS generation on hypothalamic slices *ex vivo*. In addition, intra-carotid glucose load (therefore only detectable by the hypothalamus) in rats triggers a significant increase of ARC neuronal activity (Leloup et al., 2006) which is abolished by a co-injection of the antioxidant enzyme catalase. These results demonstrate that hypothalamic glucose sensing requires the acute generation of ROS as signaling molecules to induce a neuronal response.

Strong evidences demonstrate that ROS action in the brain can affect most of the peripheral tissues via the Autonomous Nervous System (ANS). For example, Zimmerman et al., observed that O_2^- was necessary to elicit vasopressor and bradycardiac responses produced by intracerebroventricular (icv) administration of Angiotensin-II (Ang-II) in mice. Indeed, scavenging O_2^- in brain completely abolished cardiovascular actions of Ang-II (Zimmerman et al., 2002). Moreover, central administration of a SOD mimetic attenuates the increase in renal sympathetic nerve activity, norepinephrine release and blood pressure induced by icv injection of Ang-II (Campese et al., 2004, 2005; Lu et al., 2004). Therefore, ROS in the brain are of crucial importance to provide signals in periphery via autonomous nervous system.

Thus, ROS have a strong role as signaling molecules in the central nervous system, and more particularly in the hypothalamus. Since hypothalamus is a key area involved in the control of energy homeostasis, we are now going to focus on the role of hypothalamic ROS in the regulation of energy metabolism and food intake.

INVOLVEMENT OF HYPOTHALAMIC ROS IN THE CONTROL OF METABOLISM AND FOOD INTAKE

We have previously discussed that a physiological increase of ROS levels has a signaling role in the hypothalamus. This brain area receives signals from the periphery such as nutrients (glucose and lipids) and hormones, which in turn are able to modulate the activity of hypothalamic neurons. This effect on hypothalamic neurons, including POMC and NPY/AgRP neurons, further impact peripheral fuel metabolism via the ANS or neuroendocrine mediators. Here, we will describe the effect of nutrient action (such as glucose and lipids) and hormones on hypothalamic ROS release, associated with peripheral metabolic regulation and food intake.

NUTRIENTS

Glucose and lipids are directly detected by hypothalamic neurons in order to implement the adaptive response for the metabolism. An intracarotid injection of glucose, which targets specifically the hypothalamus, generates a transient release of hypothalamic ROS (Leloup et al., 2006). This release of hypothalamic ROS induces, via the parasympathetic nervous system outflow, a peak of insulin 1–3 min later with no change in peripheral blood glucose. Scavenging ROS generation in the brain by the use of antioxidant molecules significantly disturbs insulin secretion induced by the cerebral glucose load, demonstrating the key role of hypothalamic ROS in the control of energy metabolism. In this experimental model, ROS production involved in glucose sensing has a mitochondrial origin. In fact, glucose co-injected with the mitochondrial uncoupler CCCP decreases significantly the peak of insulin (Leloup et al., 2006). If we focus on food intake, a VMH glucose infusion attenuates the increase of food intake after refeeding following an overnight fast, via a mechanism dependent on hypothalamic mROS production (Carneiro et al., 2012).

Concerning lipids, the literature also showed that these circulating nutrients can directly act as signaling molecules in the hypothalamus (Lam et al., 2005). A provoked acute hypertriglyceridemia in rats generates an acute ROS production in the VMH 30 min after an intraperitoneal injection of lipids (Benani et al., 2007). This hypothalamic ROS release is local, rapid and transient since it returns to basal levels within 4 h after injection. Therefore, this hypothalamic ROS modulation is able to inhibit food intake only 1 h after lipid injection. This anorectic effect is directly attributable to hypothalamic ROS release since icv infusion of antioxidant drugs, such as glutathion and trolox (an analog of vitamin E), abolishes the decrease of food intake. Similarly to glucose, lipids generate hypothalamic mitochondrial ROS production concomitant to an increase in mitochondrial respiration (Benani et al., 2007).

We described above that glucose and lipids generate hypothalamic ROS release through an action on mitochondria. Mitochondrial morphology is associated with mROS production and energy status (Yoon et al., 2011). Mitochondria are dynamic organelles that continuously change their structures under the control of different sets of proteins through fission and fusion mechanisms. A recent study has demonstrated that, in AgRP neurons, changes of mitochondrial morphology (size and number) are associated with the metabolic state of these neurons (Dietrich et al., 2013). Indeed, food deprivation during 24 h leads to an increase in mitochondria density and a decrease in mitochondria size in AgRP neurons, which are characteristic of changes in mitochondria dynamic toward fission, while neighboring anorexic POMC neurons display a decrease in mitochondria density. Conversely, high-fat-diet feeding (HFD) (i.e., positive energy balance) leads to mitochondrial fusion in AgRP neurons. These changes were cell-type specific because this phenomenon did not occur in POMC neurons. The fission machinery involves dynamin-related protein 1 (DRP1), which is translocated to the mitochondrial membrane where it forms a contractile "ring" involved in the division of mitochondria. Under basal conditions, DRP1 is cytoplasmic. In response to an intracarotid glucose bolus injection, DRP1 level is increased in mitochondria from VMH extract 1 min post-injection, and correlates with hypothalamic mROS production (Carneiro et al., 2012). These results indicate that mitochondrial fission is necessary for the induction of hypothalamic mROS release in response to glucose. Inhibition of DRP1 recruitment in the VMH mitochondria using siRNA is deleterious by the loss of hypothalamic mROS signaling, insulin release and the satiating effect of glucose. On the other hand, fusion machinery involves mitofusins (Mfn 1 and Mfn2). AgRP-specific Mfn1 or Mfn2 knock-out mice gain less weight when fed with a HFD (Dietrich et al., 2013). Interestingly, these changes in fusion-like mitochondrial dynamics are neuron-type specific because POMC-specific Mfn2 knockout mice exhibit hyperphagia, an increase in body weight and a decrease in energy expenditure (Schneeberger et al., 2013). In this mouse model, it is noteworthy that the number of mitochondria-ER contacts was significantly reduced in POMC neurons. This result indicates a synergy of action between hypothalamic RE and mitochondria in metabolic control. The change in mitochondrial dynamics in hypothalamic neurons directly affects distal metabolic organs and suggests a key role of mROS.

Other key molecular actors of mitochondrial function are uncoupling proteins (UCP) which are mitochondrial inner membrane proteins promoting proton leak (Aquila et al., 1985). These proteins control mROS release and specifically UCP2 which was described as a negative regulator of mitochondrial hydrogen peroxide production (Negre-Salvayre et al., 1997). Besides allowing protons to transit from the matrix to the inter-membrane space of the mitochondria, it has been suggested that UCP2 allows the transport of metabolites such as aspartate, malate and oxaloacetate. As such, UCP2 could reduce substrates of Krebs cycle, decrease electrons transport chain activity and also attenuates ROS production (Vozza et al., 2014). UCP2 is highly expressed in the hypothalamus (Richard et al., 1998), and more precisely in both POMC and NPY/AgRP neurons. This mitochondrial protein is strongly linked to nutritional status because the hypothalamic mRNA and protein expression of UCP2 is increased during the fasted state (Coppola et al., 2007). A hypothesis developed by Andrews et al., suggests that during negative energy balance (such as fasting or before a meal), NPY/AgRP neurons are activated via a decrease in basal mROS production, probably because of the activation of UCP2 (Andrews et al., 2008). Conversely, mROS levels in POMC neurons are also reduced, but these neurons are silent. In contrast, during positive energy balance, mROS are able to accumulate in POMC neurons to inhibit food intake. As expected, genetic inactivation of UCP2 attenuates the refeeding signal, due to an uncontrolled increase of ROS in NPY/AgRP neurons that lead to decrease their activities. These results underscore the importance of the level of ROS released, depending on the type of neurons.

As previously described, changes in glucose levels are sensed in the brain by GE and GI neurons. Arcuate nucleus POMC neurons are considered as GE while AgRP/NPY neurons are GI. Parton et al., have demonstrated the essential role of glucose sensing by POMC neurons in the overall physiological control of blood glucose (Parton et al., 2007). Specific genetic deletion of Kir6.2 subunit in K_{ATP} channels, required for glucose detection in POMC neurons, impairs the whole-body response to a systemic glucose load. In the same study, the authors demonstrated that UCP2 negatively regulates glucose sensing in POMC neurons. By using genipin (an UCP2 inhibitor) or UCP2 knock-out mice, they have induced an increase in POMC neurons firing rate. Glucose sensing by POMC neurons became defective in obese mice fed a HFD, suggesting that loss of glucose sensing has a causal role in the development of type 2 diabetes.

Thus, it appears that NPY/AgRP neurons activation is mediated by a decrease in ROS levels while POMC neurons activation is driven by ROS (Andrews et al., 2008). Indeed, icv administration of ROS scavengers induces significantly lower c-Fos expression in POMC neurons and increases food intake during light cycle, observed via an increase of c-Fos expression in AgRP/NPY neurons (Diano et al., 2011). Similarly, addition of H_2O_2 depolarizes POMC neurons, increases the firing rate, and an icv injection of H_2O_2 causes significantly less feeding of mice after an overnight fast.

From a molecular perspective, POMC neurons seem to use glucose as their main fuel since their firing rate vary as a function of in glucose concentrations (Ibrahim et al., 2003). On the other hand, NPY/AgRP neurons are inhibited by high levels of glucose and may use free fatty acids as their main fuel (Mountjoy et al., 2007; Andrews et al., 2008). This differential fuel utilization underlies the presence of two distinct and competitive mechanisms in these neuronal populations: glycolysis and β-oxidation. When glycolysis is elevated, end-product derived from this reaction inhibit β-oxidation, and conversely, when β-oxidation is increased, glycolysis is inhibited. Both systems are opposite and produce ROS. An increase in the activity of NPY/AgRP neurons is followed by Ca^{2+} influx, which was demonstrated to elevate ROS production in neurons (Hernandez-Fonseca et al., 2008). However, NPY/AgRP neurons do not produce considerable amount of ROS, indicating that these neurons have cellular properties associated with low capacity for ROS production and/or high capacity to buffer ROS. These opposite effects of ROS release in POMC and NPY/AgRP neurons, that contribute to nutrient sensing and appetite regulation, have been demonstrated by the work of Kuo et al., By using an appetite-suppressing sympathomimetic agent, phenylpropranolamine (PPA), authors have shown the involvement of Protein Kinase C (PKC) in the generation of hypothalamic ROS which stimulates POMC neurons activity and inhibits NPY neurons (Kuo et al., 2011). Central inhibition of ROS production by icv infusion of glutathione attenuates PPA anorectic effect together with the icv injection of PKC oligonucleotide antisense. In a similar study, the same authors demonstrated that hypothalamic NF-kB signaling is also involved in decrease of food intake by PPA treatment. This anorectic effect is mediated by the decrease of NPY expression and the rise of the expression of endogenous antioxidants such as SOD or glutathione peroxidase, demonstrating the impact of ROS (Kuo et al., 2012). Another essential actor which participate to the regulation of ROS production is Ca^{2+}. Voltage-gated Ca^{2+} channels are expressed throughout the entire hypothalamus contributing to the increase of cytoplasmic Ca^{2+} levels in sensitive neurons (Marques-Da-Silva and Gutierrez-Merino, 2012). The maintenance of intracellular Ca^{2+} homeostasis depends on (1) the precise control of Ca^{2+}-ATPases activity in the plasma membrane, (2) the Ca^{2+} uptake into intracellular compartments, (3) the influx through voltage-operated channels and 4) the effectiveness of Ca^{2+} buffering via Calcium Binding Proteins (CBPs) (Strehler et al., 2007; Nicholls, 2009). Excessive intracellular Ca^{2+} accumulation causes mitochondrial ROS production (Weber et al., 2010) and hypothalamic CBPs such as Secretagogin (Scgn) modulate this ROS release by buffering Ca^{2+}(Gyengesi et al., 2012). Thus, Scgn which is widely expressed in the NPY/AgRP neurons (Gyengesi et al., 2013) from the ARC but not in POMC neurons, could explain the lower production of ROS by these neurons. There seems to be a direct requirement to buffer Ca^{2+} in NPY but not in POMC neurons, to maintain cellular firing rate. Thus, buffering Ca^{2+} controls ROS production and allows the modulation of neurons as a function of the nutritional state (**Figure 1**).

All these actors involved in transient ROS production in response to nutrients, clearly demonstrate a key role of ROS signaling as a real gauge of energy status, which induces a fine tuning control of energy metabolism and food intake.

HORMONES

Like nutrients, hormones which are key signals of the metabolic state of organs, must be detected by the hypothalamus to control energy homeostasis. We will now discuss the role of the orexigenic hormone ghrelin and of two anorectic hormones leptin and insulin. These hormones reach the hypothalamus, have their receptors on hypothalamic POMC and NPY/AgRP neurons and are clearly involved in the control of food intake and energy metabolism via signaling pathways involving ROS release.

Ghrelin

Ghrelin is a gut-derived hormone secreted into the bloodstream which activates NPY/AgRP neurons and increases food intake (Andrews, 2011). Levels of this hormone rise during the fasting state, making a signal of starvation for neurons. Ghrelin receptor (GHSR), a seven trans-membrane G-coupled protein linked to Gq, is predominantly expressed in NPY/AgRP neurons (Willesen et al., 1999). In response to intraperitoneal injection of ghrelin, the number of mitochondria in NPY neuronal perikarya is increased in a UCP2-dependent manner while POMC perikarya remains unaffected (Andrews et al., 2008). In the same way, ghrelin induces symmetric, putatively inhibitory synapses on POMC neurons correlated with recruitment of miniature inhibitory post-synaptic currents (mIPSCs) on these cells. Conversely, ghrelin significantly reduces the number of asymmetric, putatively excitatory synapses on POMC neurons. This synaptic plasticity demonstrates how ghrelin hyperpolarizes POMC neurons by activating inhibitory NPY/AgRP (especially GABAergic) inputs. In parallel, ghrelin increases UCP2 expression, which scavenges free radicals in NPY neurons without affecting ROS production in POMC neurons. All these effects previously described are linked to the decrease in ROS levels in NPY/AgRP via UCP2 since the effect of ghrelin is totally lost in UCP2 knock-out mice. The scavenging of ROS by icv infusion of a cocktail of antioxidants in UCP2 knock-out mice restores the action of ghrelin demonstrating the key role of hypothalamic ROS in ghrelin effects (Andrews et al., 2008).

From a molecular perspective, ghrelin activates AMPK in NPY neurons, which importantly raises mitochondrial respiration and ROS production (Andrews et al., 2008). Via the activation of GHSR on NPY neurons, ghrelin generates an increase in intracellular Ca^{2+} levels. Indeed, ghrelin induces a presynaptic signaling pathway that induces direct Ca^{2+} release from internal stores in NPY/AGRP neurons (Yang et al., 2011) and also activates Calmodulin-dependent protein Kinase Kinase (CaMKK) (Cummings et al., 2005). Activated CaMKK induces AMPK activation which generates ATP and fatty acid oxidation that might contribute to the neuron-specific activation of fatty acid oxidation and the resulting buffering of ROS (Horvath et al., 2009). CaMKK is particularly involved in the hypothalamic control of appetite because its deletion in NPY/AgRP neurons reduces food intake and body weight, while deleting CaMKK in POMC neurons does not affect energy homeostasis (Anderson et al., 2008; Gyengesi et al., 2012). Systemic injection of ghrelin fails to induce food intake in CamKK knock-out mice, demonstrating that CaMKK is also involved in the effect of ghrelin (Anderson et al., 2008). This synergy of effects between ROS and Ca^{2+} is necessary to generate signaling pathways in NPY/AgRP neurons which is involved in the action of ghrelin on food intake. Precise mechanisms need to be determined.

Finally, it is also known that motivation is an essential part of food intake, involving reward system and memory, which are regulated by dopamine neurons. Ghrelin has been shown to play a role for incentive value of food cue by controlling the activity of dopamine neurons (Abizaid et al., 2006; Andrews et al., 2006). Similar to its effect on NPY/AgRP neurons, ghrelin activates dopamine neurons in an UCP2-dependent manner and via a decrease of ROS production. Indeed, UCP2 knock-out mice exhibit a reduced dopamine turnover (Andrews et al., 2006). Besides its direct effect on the dopamine reward system, ghrelin regulates dopamine neurons directly via activation of AgRP neurons and inhibition of PVN, which induces food seeking behavior (Krashes et al., 2011; Atasoy et al., 2012).

Leptin

Leptin is an adipose tissue derived hormone (i.e., adipokine) which plays a central role in the regulation of energy homeostasis. Leptin acts on both NPY/AgRP and POMC neurons through its receptor LepRb (Morton and Schwartz, 2011). Leptin reaches hypothalamus and increases the activity of POMC neurons. This effect on POMC neurons induces a decrease in food intake and a rise in energy expenditure via the action of sympathetic nervous system on Brown Adipose Tissue (BAT) and muscles. Unlike ghrelin which modulates ROS levels in NPY/AgRP neurons, leptin seems to induce ROS levels in POMC neurons (Diano et al., 2011). Indeed, by using dihydroethidium (DHE; a substrate for fluorimetric detection of peroxidase as a readout of ROS), Diano et al., have demonstrated the lowest level of ROS in POMC neurons of leptin knock-out mice (ob/ob). In contrast, a 48 h leptin

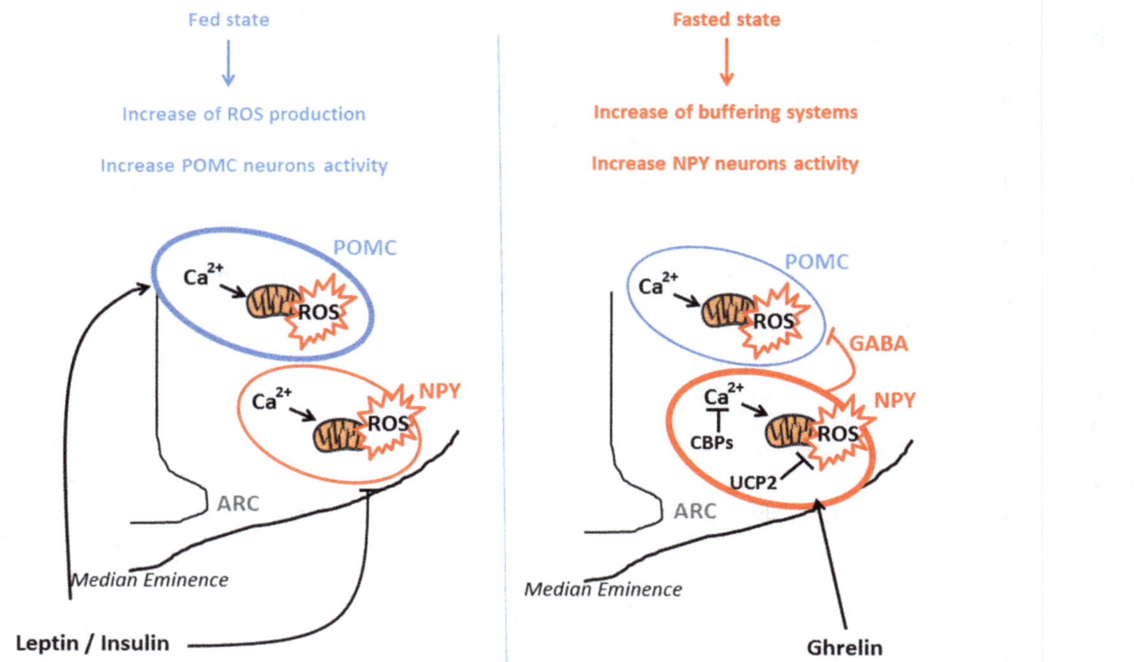

FIGURE 1 | POMC and NPY/AgRP activation via ROS release in function of nutritional state. POMC and NPY/AgRP neurons generate opposing effects on food intake and metabolism. In the fed state, glucose, lipids, insulin, and leptin actions lead to ROS release in both type of neurons, for instance via a rise of Ca^{2+} concentration and mitochondrial dynamics. This transient increase in intracellular ROS stimulates POMC neurons activity and inhibits NPY/AgRP neurons, engendering decrease in food intake and increased energy expenditure. In the fasted state, NPY/AgRP neurons become more active, via an increase in Calcium Binding Proteins (CBPs) and UCP2 expression that respectively buffer excessive intracellular Ca^{2+} and prevent ROS release. This NPY/Agrp activation is mediated via ghrelin and stimulates food intake. In parallel, these neurons present GABAergic inhibitory synapses around POMC neurons, amplifying the orexigenic signal.

treatment in ob/ob mice results in elevated DHE expression in POMC neurons. This increase in DHE expression is also found in POMC neurons of fed wild-type mice compared with fasted mice, demonstrating a key role of ROS signaling in POMC neurons on the nutritional state. Moreover, the level of ROS in POMC neurons is correlated with those of leptin in wild-type and ob/ob mice, but this correlation is lost in HFD-fed mice. In parallel, the authors noted the presence of peroxisomes in POMC neurons (Diano et al., 2011). Indeed, in POMC neurons from ob/ob mice, the number of mitochondria and peroxisomes is very low while it is increased in lean mice. More particularly, mitochondria are outnumbered in lean fed mice compared with lean fasted mice, without differences in peroxisomes number. On the other hand, peroxisomes were almost three-fold higher in POMC neurons of HFD fed mice, suggesting a role of this organelle in leptin resistance and specifically in the disruption of ROS release in POMC neurons. Hydrogen peroxide icv injection in HFD-fed mice resulted in increased c-Fos expression in POMC neurons and decreased feeding in response to peripheral leptin injection. This spectacular experiment has proved that ROS alone could reverse POMC function and mediate leptin actions.

Leptin was also shown to be a key molecular actor involved in synaptic plasticity around POMC neurons (Pinto et al., 2004). In ob/ob mice, a significantly greater number of excitatory synapses (EPSCs) on NPY neurons was observed, while the number of inhibitory synapses (IPSCs) is higher on POMC neurons. After 2 days of intraperitoneal injection of leptin, NPY neurons display an 85% reduction of the number of EPSCs and an almost 70% increase in the number of IPSCs. At the same time, there is also a doubling of the synapses number on POMC neurons, with an almost 300% increase in the number of EPSCs. This regulation resembles those of ghrelin on synaptic plasticity (Andrews et al., 2008), suggesting again an involvement of ROS. Similarly, the effect of leptin are potentiated by intracellular Ca^{2+} like ghrelin (Qiu et al., 2010).

Insulin

In addition to its peripheral effect on glucose storage, insulin acts on the hypothalamus to modulate energy metabolism and food intake (Abraham et al., 2014). In particular, insulin inhibits food intake in the hypothalamus through ROS production. A first study has demonstrated the key role of the mitochondrial respiratory chain in the phosphorylation of insulin receptor on neuronal cells (Storozhevykh et al., 2007). This study suggests that insulin might trigger ROS production within the hypothalamus, which, in turn, inhibit food intake. Indeed, insulin injection in the third ventricle generates a transient ROS release 15 min post-injection and induces food intake (Jaillard et al., 2009). This insulin-induced ROS increase is transient because no ROS are observed at either 5 or 30 min post-injection. Moreover, this insulin-induced

ROS increase is dependent on the nutritional state, because a decrease of food intake is not observed in fasted mice. The antioxidant trolox delivery by icv injection 30 min prior to insulin completely prevents insulin-stimulated ROS increase and suppresses insulin-induced food intake inhibition. Interestingly, the mROS seems to be not involved in this insulin effect. Indeed, icv injection of an inhibitor of NADPH oxidase (DPI) 30 min before insulin treatment inhibits the effect of insulin on ROS production and food intake.

CONSEQUENCES OF THE ALTERATION OF HYPOTHALAMIC ROS RELEASE IN PATHOLOGICAL STATE

The short-term hypothalamic ROS peak generated by metabolic signals (nutrients and hormones) appears to be fundamental to elicit a proper behavioral, endocrine and autonomic response to nutrient intake. A pathology characterized by a disruption in nutrient sensing and by an inability to maintain energy homeostasis is type 2 diabetes (T2D) (Schwartz and Porte, 2005). T2D is especially characterized by impaired metabolic and hormonal hypothalamic sensing, and by a chronic whole-body low-grade inflammatory background (Purkayastha and Cai, 2013). An important part of this low-grade inflammation is due to oxidative stress. As previously described, transient ROS release is now considered as a molecular signal. When ROS production is chronically elevated, the over-abundance of radical species triggers activation of inflammatory kinases, leading to alterations of tissue functions. This phenomenon is exacerbated by a decrease in the expression of antioxidant enzymes (Gonzalez-Chavez et al., 2011). In particular in the brain, this pathological ROS release induces over-activation of the sympathetic nervous system (Hirooka et al., 2011). This rise of sympathetic excitation is responsible for disorders associated with obesity and T2D such as hypertension, cardiovascular and renal dysfunctions (Campese et al., 2004), and antioxidant icv injection improves this deleterious phenotype. Oxidative stress and inflammation are also develop in the hypothalamus during T2D (Purkayastha and Cai, 2013).

In this review, transgenic models of obesity or nutritional models (HFD) mice will be considered as type 2 diabetic mice.

OXIDATIVE STRESS IN THE HYPOTHALAMUS DURING T2D

The different characteristics of T2D suggest an alteration of redox signaling and ROS release in the hypothalamus. Zücker rats are obese and insulin resistant with dramatic autonomic disturbances including modification of sympathovagal balance (York et al., 1985). In this model, a hypothalamic hypersensitivity to glucose has been demonstrated (Colombani et al., 2009). In lean rats, intracarotid injection of low-dose of glucose (3 mg/kg) does not generate ROS release nor a peak of insulin secretion, while a most important dose of glucose (9 mg/kg) induces insulin release 1–3 min later associated with hypothalamic mROS production. This same low-dose of glucose (3 mg/kg) is sufficient to produce a rapid and transient increase in plasma insulin in Zücker rats. Similarly, low-dose of glucose increases hypothalamic ROS in Zücker rats. These diabetic rats present an altered redox state, together with an increase of hypothalamic mitochondrial activity in response to substrates, and a decrease in antioxidant enzymes activity. In rats, icv infusion of glutathione for 3 days restores a normal hypothalamic glucose sensing.

In association with these data, our group has observed that ROS, and more particularly H_2O_2 release, is exacerbated in hypothalamus of HFD-fed mice compared with normal mice (Duparc et al., 2011a; Drougard et al., 2014). In this study, we demonstrated that icv injection of high levels of apelin, similar to that observed in the hypothalamus of obese/diabetic mice (Reaux-Le Goazigo et al., 2011), in normal mice, induces a diabetic phenotype with fasting hyperglycemia, fasting hyperinsulinemia and glucose intolerance. In fact, these disturbance of glucose homeostasis via hypothalamic apelin are due to an over-activation of sympathetic nervous system that triggers hepatic glucose production. Central apelin effects are directly linked to hypothalamic over-production of H_2O_2, since an icv injection of trolox 30 min before apelin icv injection inhibits the establishment of T2D characteristics. Production of hypothalamic H_2O_2 seems to have a mitochondrial origin, since icv injection of DPI 30 min before apelin treatment does not inhibit fasting hyperglycemia. This high level of hypothalamic H_2O_2 release reflects an oxidative stress. Indeed, this release is exacerbated in hypothalamus of HFD-fed mice in response to apelin, and is inhibited by trolox pretreatment. Moreover, over-expression of apelin by lentivectors in the VMH promotes an increase of pro-inflammatory cytokines expression (Drougard et al., 2014), which are known to alter the control of metabolism (De Souza et al., 2005).

ALTERATIONS OF ROS SIGNALING IN POMC AND NPY/AgRP NEURONS DURING T2D

POMC neurons

Neuronal alterations observed in genetic diabetic mice in response to glucose are also found in HFD-fed mice (Parton et al., 2007). Approximately 46% of POMC neurons from lean mice significantly increase their firing rate after a rise in glucose concentration from 3 to 5 mM compared with HFD-fed mice, in which only 10% of POMC neurons respond. Moreover, glucose fails to enhance the release of α-MSH in POMC neurons of HFD-fed mice. We have previously described that POMC neurons need to release ROS to be effective in response to glucose, and UCP2 inhibits ROS production. As expected, UCP2 expression is increased in hypothalamus of HFD-fed mice and genipin treatment restores α-MSH release in response to glucose in POMC neurons of HFD-fed mice. These results are confirmed by the protection from obesity, T2D and alteration of glucose sensing in POMC neurons from UCP2 knock-out mice.

An increase in ROS production in POMC neurons compared to NPY neurons under "basal" conditions has been observed, suggesting that POMC neurons might be prone to free radical-induced degeneration (Andrews et al., 2008). The decline in functional POMC neurons may promote increased orexigenic NPY tone, hyperphagia and weight gain. Indeed, ROS levels are significantly higher in POMC neurons of HFD-fed mice compared to chow-fed mice (Diano et al., 2011). The lack of difference in ROS levels in POMC neurons between chow-fed mice and HFD-fed mice is associated with the loss of correlation between leptin and ROS levels in HFD-fed mice. Indeed, the absence of a positive correlation between elevated leptin levels and ROS release in HFD-fed mice, could be explained by the important rise of peroxisomes in POMC neurons of these mice. This proliferation of peroxisome is governed by the nuclear receptor peroxisome proliferator-activated receptor-γ (PPAR-γ) (Green, 1995) which is associated with brain inflammation, gliosis (Bernardo and Minghetti, 2006) and ROS production (Yu et al., 2008). PPAR-γ expression is increased in hypothalamic POMC and NPY/AgRP neurons of HFD-fed mice (Diano et al., 2011). These peroxisome in POMC neurons interfere clearly with ROS signaling, since icv treatment with a PPAR-γ agonist in normal mice elevates peroxisome number, decreases ROS production and increases food intake. Conversely, icv treatment with a PPAR-γ antagonist in HFD-fed mice decreases peroxisome number, increases ROS in POMC neurons and reduces daily food intake. Consistent with these results, icv treatment with a PPAR-γ antagonist in HFD-fed mice increases c-Fos staining and firing rate in POMC neurons, and decreases NPY/AgRP neurons excitation compared with HFD control mice. As expected, PPAR-γ knock-out mice fed with a HFD are protected from obesity and T2D (Long et al., 2014). These mice present a decrease in peroxisomes density in POMC neurons, which allows ROS signaling and firing rate in these neurons. On a metabolic standpoint, these mice are protected from hyperphagia, body weight gain, decrease of energy expenditure and leptin resistance. As previously described, this ROS signaling is overriding in POMC neurons, and icv injection of H_2O_2 in HFD-fed mice induces c-Fos expression in POMC neurons, decreases feeding and improves leptin sensitivity in response to peripheral leptin injection (Diano et al., 2011). It has been shown that only 3% of POMC neurons from HFD-fed mice are sensitive to leptin, and that H_2O_2 treatment leads to an 18% increase of POMC neurons, demonstrating the key role of ROS signaling from POMC neurons for leptin sensitivity.

NPY/AgRP neurons

NPY/AgRP neurons also seem affected, because if ROS generation is uncontrolled in these cells, neuronal firing is impaired. To this aim, emerging concept indicates that T2D is also characterized by ghrelin resistance, since ghrelin fails to induce AgRP or NPY secretion in hypothalamic explants from HFD-fed mice (Andrews et al., 2008; Briggs et al., 2010). This global hypothalamic oxidative stress disrupts all the redox balance in POMC, but also in NPY/AgRP neurons, which alters nutrient sensing and energy balance. Indeed, insulin, an anorectic hormone, fails to induce a decrease of food intake in HFD-fed mice, demonstrating a lack of responsiveness of hypothalamus to peripheral signals (Storozhevykh et al., 2007).

Mitochondrial dynamics

From the viewpoint of the mitochondrial dynamics, VMH mitochondrial fission via DRP1 is essential to respond to glucose load (Carneiro et al., 2012). Moreover, mitochondrial density in POMC neurons from HFD-fed mice was increased (Diano et al., 2011). These mitochondria present a significant reduction in the number of contacts with ER, indicating that both mitochondrial network complexity and their association to ER in POMC neurons are altered in HFD-fed mice (Schneeberger et al., 2013). The protein involved in mitochondrial fusion protein Mfn2 seems to be the most crucial protein implicated in the HFD-fed mice phenotype, since its hypothalamic expression is decreased in HFD-fed mice when compared to other mitochondrial fusion/fission proteins such as DRP1 and Mfn1. Indeed, Mfn2 over-expression in ARC neurons decreases food intake and body weight, while Mfn2 knock-out mice demonstrate an increase in food intake and body weight, a decrease of energy expenditure and a resistance to leptin. These mice also present an alteration of the mitochondrial respiratory capacity and an increase in ROS production. This over-production of ROS appears to be a consequence of hypothalamic ER stress. In fact, injection of ROS scavenger does not improve the phenotype of these mice, whereas inhibition of ER stress restores a normal phenotype.

TREATMENTS AGAINST TYPE 2 DIABETES IN CONNECTION WITH THE HYPOTHALAMIC ROS

T2D is a worldwide expanding disease that is difficult to treat because of multiple organ dysfunction. So far, therapies have targeted insulin-sensitive organs such as muscles, liver and adipose tissue to improve hyperglycemia, hyperinsulinemia and resistance to insulin (Altaf et al., 2014). However, considerable progress that have been made in the field of neurophysiology have demonstrated a key role of the brain, and more particularly the hypothalamus, in the control of energy homeostasis. It is now established that ROS release in hypothalamic neurons is necessary to generate the "periphery-hypothalamus-periphery" regulation loop in response to the nutritional state. This hypothalamic ROS balance finely regulated could be altered and generate oxidative stress, which is a disruption of the balance between oxidant and antioxidant molecules in favor of oxidant molecules, masking beneficial effects of ROS (Sies and Cadenas, 1985). The best treatment against T2D is calorie restriction (Bantle, 1988) to avoid abundance of substrates for mitochondria, and reduce the ROS overproduction. This change in lifestyle is efficient in humans in the prediabetic state, however patient's adherence is poor. Regarding direct targeting of oxidative stress, treatments with antioxidants could have the potential to prevent or delay the development of diabetic complications. Despite the preponderance of evidence from animal studies supporting this hypothesis, large scale prospective studies using antioxidant treatments in humans have been disappointingly inconclusive, probably because of issues with dosage and bioavailability of these molecules (Johansen et al., 2005; Pazdro and Burgess, 2010).

OXIDATIVE STRESS, A LINK BETWEEN T2D AND OTHERS DISEASES

Over-production of ROS (arising either from mitochondrial electron-transport chain or excessive stimulation of NADPH oxidase) results in oxidative stress, a deleterious process that can be an important mediator of cell damage. Indeed, hypothalamic oxidative stress during T2D is a risk factor for many chronic diseases such as neurodegenerative disorders (Valko et al., 2007). It has been clearly demonstrated that T2D increases the risk of the development of Alzheimer and Parkinson diseases via brain oxidative stress (Butterfield et al., 2014; Santiago and Potashkin, 2014). It is particularly interesting to underlie that both neuronal pathologies are characterized by mitochondrial dysfunctions inducing alteration of brain ROS release.

Given the failure of care therapies against T2D coupled to the massive expansion of the disease and the associated-pathologies; it is critical to elaborate integrated therapeutics. Indeed, we have shown in this review the key role of ROS production in hypothalamus with a different pattern of release between POMC and NPY/AgRP neurons. ROS signaling is largely altered in T2D, and the hypothalamus has an "open-access" to bloodstream signals via the median eminence. Via this anatomical characteristic, it is now primordial to evaluate the consequences of new therapies on this hypothalamic balance sensing. Therefore, it will be interesting to elaborate non-invasive treatments to normalize this hypothalamic ROS production via targeting all molecular actors involved in this ROS release control. To this aim, a study of our group has demonstrated the alteration of hypothalamic NO release via the dysfunction of gut-brain axis in response to glucose in db/db mice (Duparc et al., 2011b). Modulation of this gut-brain axis could be an attractive therapeutic strategy to normalize hypothalamic ROS production.

CONCLUSION

Energy metabolism and food intake are complex processes that involve homeostatic mechanisms driven by hypothalamic network signaling pathways. This review brings light to the fact that hypothalamic ROS levels, controlled by various molecules and fuel signals, play an important role in this hypothalamic control of energy balance. The control of hypothalamic ROS release involves many molecular actors such as mitochondrial dynamics, NADPH oxidase activity, synaptic plasticity, peroxisomes, endoplasmic reticulum,... At high levels that saturate buffering mechanisms, ROS may initiate cellular degeneration in either NPY/AgRP or POMC neurons, and impair energy homeostasis, resulting in pathologies such as obesity and type 2 diabetes. In addition to the brain, future therapeutic strategies have to take into account the large part played by ROS signaling in other structures (including pancreas, adipose tissue, intestine, liver and heart).

REFERENCES

Abizaid, A., Liu, Z. W., Andrews, Z. B., Shanabrough, M., Borok, E., Elsworth, J. D., et al. (2006). Ghrelin modulates the activity and synaptic input organization of midbrain dopamine neurons while promoting appetite. *J. Clin. Invest.* 116, 3229–3239. doi: 10.1172/JCI29867

Abraham, M. A., Filippi, B. M., Kang, G. M., Kim, M. S., and Lam, T. K. (2014). Insulin action in the hypothalamus and dorsal vagal complex. *Exp. Physiol.* 99, 1104–1109. doi: 10.1113/expphysiol.2014.079962

Ainscow, E. K., Mirshamsi, S., Tang, T., Ashford, M. L., and Rutter, G. A. (2002). Dynamic imaging of free cytosolic ATP concentration during fuel sensing by rat hypothalamic neurones: evidence for ATP-independent control of ATP-sensitive $K^{(+)}$ channels. *J. Physiol.* 544, 429–445. doi: 10.1113/jphysiol.2002.022434

Altaf, Q. A., Barnett, A. H., and Tahrani, A. A. (2014). Novel therapeutics for type 2 diabetes: insulin resistance. *Diabetes Obes. Metab.* doi: 10.1111/dom.12400. [Epub ahead of print].

Anderson, K. A., Ribar, T. J., Lin, F., Noeldner, P. K., Green, M. F., Muehlbauer, M. J., et al. (2008). Hypothalamic CaMKK2 contributes to the regulation of energy balance. *Cell Metab.* 7, 377–388. doi: 10.1016/j.cmet.2008.02.011

Andrews, Z. B. (2011). Central mechanisms involved in the orexigenic actions of ghrelin. *Peptides* 32, 2248–2255. doi: 10.1016/j.peptides.2011.05.014

Andrews, Z. B., Liu, Z. W., Walllingford, N., Erion, D. M., Borok, E., Friedman, J. M., et al. (2008). UCP2 mediates ghrelin's action on NPY/AgRP neurons by lowering free radicals. *Nature* 454, 846–851. doi: 10.1038/nature07181

Andrews, Z. B., Rivera, A., Elsworth, J. D., Roth, R. H., Agnati, L., Gago, B., et al. (2006). Uncoupling protein-2 promotes nigrostriatal dopamine neuronal function. *Eur. J. Neurosci.* 24, 32–36. doi: 10.1111/j.1460-9568.2006.04906.x

Aquila, H., Link, T. A., and Klingenberg, M. (1985). The uncoupling protein from brown fat mitochondria is related to the mitochondrial ADP/ATP carrier. Analysis of sequence homologies and of folding of the protein in the membrane. *EMBO J.* 4, 2369–2376.

Atasoy, D., Betley, J. N., Su, H. H., and Sternson, S. M. (2012). Deconstruction of a neural circuit for hunger. *Nature* 488, 172–177. doi: 10.1038/nature11270

Bantle, J. P. (1988). The dietary treatment of diabetes mellitus. *Med. Clin. North Am.* 72, 1285–1299.

Bao, L., Avshalumov, M. V., Patel, J. C., Lee, C. R., Miller, E. W., Chang, C. J., et al. (2009). Mitochondria are the source of hydrogen peroxide for dynamic brain-cell signaling. *J. Neurosci.* 29, 9002–9010. doi: 10.1523/JNEUROSCI.1706-09.2009

Bashan, N., Kovsan, J., Kachko, I., Ovadia, H., and Rudich, A. (2009). Positive and negative regulation of insulin signaling by reactive oxygen and nitrogen species. *Physiol. Rev.* 89, 27–71. doi: 10.1152/physrev.00014.2008

Bellinger, L. L., and Bernardis, L. L. (2002). The dorsomedial hypothalamic nucleus and its role in ingestive behavior and body weight regulation: lessons learned from lesioning studies. *Physiol. Behav.* 76, 431–442. doi: 10.1016/S0031-9384(02)00756-4

Benani, A., Troy, S., Carmona, M. C., Fioramonti, X., Lorsignol, A., Leloup, C., et al. (2007). Role for mitochondrial reactive oxygen species in brain lipid sensing: redox regulation of food intake. *Diabetes* 56, 152–160. doi: 10.2337/db06-0440

Bernard, C. (1849). "Cooperation between brain and islet in glucose homeostasis and diabetes," in *Leçons de Physiologie Experimentale Appliquées á la Médecine* (Paris: J.-B. Bailliére).

Bernardis, L. L., and Bellinger, L. L. (1993). The lateral hypothalamic area revisited: neuroanatomy, body weight regulation, neuroendocrinology and metabolism. *Neurosci. Biobehav. Rev.* 17, 141–193. doi: 10.1016/S0149-7634(05)80149-6

Bernardo, A., and Minghetti, L. (2006). PPAR-gamma agonists as regulators of microglial activation and brain inflammation. *Curr. Pharm. Des.* 12, 93–109. doi: 10.2174/138161206780574579

Briggs, D. I., Enriori, P. J., Lemus, M. B., Cowley, M. A., and Andrews, Z. B. (2010). Diet-induced obesity causes ghrelin resistance in arcuate NPY/AgRP neurons. *Endocrinology* 151, 4745–4755. doi: 10.1210/en.2010-0556

Brobeck, J. R. (1946). Mechanism of the development of obesity in animals with hypothalamic lesions. *Physiol. Rev.* 26, 541–559.

Butterfield, D. A., Di Domenico, F., and Barone, E. (2014). Elevated risk of type 2 diabetes for development of Alzheimer disease: a key role for oxidative stress in brain. *Biochim. Biophys. Acta* 1842, 1693–1706. doi: 10.1016/j.bbadis.2014.06.010

Campese, V. M., Shaohua, Y., and Huiquin, Z. (2005). Oxidative stress mediates angiotensin II-dependent stimulation of sympathetic nerve activity. *Hypertension* 46, 533–539. doi: 10.1161/01.HYP.0000179088.57586.26

Campese, V. M., Ye, S., Zhong, H., Yanamadala, V., Ye, Z., and Chiu, J. (2004). Reactive oxygen species stimulate central and peripheral sympathetic nervous system activity. *Am. J. Physiol. Heart Circ. Physiol.* 287, H695–H703. doi: 10.1152/ajpheart.00619.2003

Carneiro, L., Allard, C., Guissard, C., Fioramonti, X., Tourrel-Cuzin, C., Bailbe, D., et al. (2012). Importance of mitochondrial dynamin-related protein 1 in hypothalamic glucose sensitivity in rats. *Antioxid. Redox Signal.* 17, 433–444. doi: 10.1089/ars.2011.4254

Clark, J. T., Kalra, P. S., Crowley, W. R., and Kalra, S. P. (1984). Neuropeptide Y and human pancreatic polypeptide stimulate feeding behavior in rats. *Endocrinology* 115, 427–429. doi: 10.1210/endo-115-1-427

Clark, S. F. (2002). The biochemistry of antioxidants revisited. *Nutr. Clin. Pract.* 17, 5–17. doi: 10.1177/011542650201700105

Colombani, A. L., Carneiro, L., Benani, A., Galinier, A., Jaillard, T., Duparc, T., et al. (2009). Enhanced hypothalamic glucose sensing in obesity: alteration of redox signaling. *Diabetes* 58, 2189–2197. doi: 10.2337/db09-0110

Cone, R. D. (2005). Anatomy and regulation of the central melanocortin system. *Nat. Neurosci.* 8, 571–578. doi: 10.1038/nn1455

Cone, R. D., Cowley, M. A., Butler, A. A., Fan, W., Marks, D. L., and Low, M. J. (2001). The arcuate nucleus as a conduit for diverse signals relevant to energy homeostasis. *Int. J. Obes. Relat. Metab. Disord.* 25(Suppl. 5), S63–S67. doi: 10.1038/sj.ijo.0801913

Coppola, A., Liu, Z. W., Andrews, Z. B., Paradis, E., Roy, M. C., Friedman, J. M., et al. (2007). A central thermogenic-like mechanism in feeding regulation: an interplay between arcuate nucleus T3 and UCP2. *Cell Metab.* 5, 21–33. doi: 10.1016/j.cmet.2006.12.002

Cross, A. R., and Jones, O. T. (1991). Enzymic mechanisms of superoxide production. *Biochim. Biophys. Acta* 1057, 281–298. doi: 10.1016/S0005-2728(05)80140-9

Cummings, D. E., Overduin, J., Shannon, M. H., and Foster-Schubert, K. E. (2005). Hormonal mechanisms of weight loss and diabetes resolution after bariatric surgery. *Surg. Obes. Relat. Dis.* 1, 358–368. doi: 10.1016/j.soard.2005.03.208

De Souza, C. T., Araujo, E. P., Bordin, S., Ashimine, R., Zollner, R. L., Boschero, A. C., et al. (2005). Consumption of a fat-rich diet activates a proinflammatory response and induces insulin resistance in the hypothalamus. *Endocrinology* 146, 4192–4199. doi: 10.1210/en.2004-1520

Diano, S., Liu, Z. W., Jeong, J. K., Dietrich, M. O., Ruan, H. B., Kim, E., et al. (2011). Peroxisome proliferation-associated control of reactive oxygen species sets melanocortin tone and feeding in diet-induced obesity. *Nat. Med.* 17, 1121–1127. doi: 10.1038/nm.2421

Dicken, M. S., Tooker, R. E., and Hentges, S. T. (2012). Regulation of GABA and glutamate release from proopiomelanocortin neuron terminals in intact hypothalamic networks. *J. Neurosci.* 32, 4042–4048. doi: 10.1523/JNEUROSCI.6032-11.2012

Dietrich, M. O., Liu, Z. W., and Horvath, T. L. (2013). Mitochondrial dynamics controlled by mitofusins regulate Agrp neuronal activity and diet-induced obesity. *Cell* 155, 188–199. doi: 10.1016/j.cell.2013.09.004

Droge, W. (2002). Free radicals in the physiological control of cell function. *Physiol. Rev.* 82, 47–95. doi: 10.1152/physrev.00018.2001

Drougard, A., Duparc, T., Brenachot, X., Carneiro, L., Gouaze, A., Fournel, A., et al. (2014). Hypothalamic apelin/reactive oxygen species signaling controls hepatic glucose metabolism in the onset of diabetes. *Antioxid. Redox Signal.* 20, 557–573. doi: 10.1089/ars.2013.5182

Duparc, T., Colom, A., Cani, P. D., Massaly, N., Rastrelli, S., Drougard, A., et al. (2011a). Central apelin controls glucose homeostasis via a nitric oxide-dependent pathway in mice. *Antioxid. Redox Signal.* 15, 1477–1496. doi: 10.1089/ars.2010.3454

Duparc, T., Naslain, D., Colom, A., Muccioli, G. G., Massaly, N., Delzenne, N. M., et al. (2011b). Jejunum inflammation in obese and diabetic mice impairs enteric glucose detection and modifies nitric oxide release in the hypothalamus. *Antioxid. Redox Signal.* 14, 415–423. doi: 10.1089/ars.2010.3330

Fekete, C., Sarkar, S., Rand, W. M., Harney, J. W., Emerson, C. H., Bianco, A. C., et al. (2002). Agouti-related protein (AGRP) has a central inhibitory action on the hypothalamic-pituitary-thyroid (HPT) axis; comparisons between the effect of AGRP and neuropeptide Y on energy homeostasis and the HPT axis. *Endocrinology* 143, 3846–3853. doi: 10.1210/en.2002-220338

Fioramonti, X., Lorsignol, A., Taupignon, A., and Penicaud, L. (2004). A new ATP-sensitive K+ channel-independent mechanism is involved in glucose-excited neurons of mouse arcuate nucleus. *Diabetes* 53, 2767–2775. doi: 10.2337/diabetes.53.11.2767

Gonzalez-Chavez, A., Elizondo-Argueta, S., Gutierrez-Reyes, G., and Leon-Pedroza, J. I. (2011). Pathophysiological implications between chronic inflammation and the development of diabetes and obesity. *Cir. Cir.* 79, 209–216.

Green, S. (1995). PPAR: a mediator of peroxisome proliferator action. *Mutat. Res.* 333, 101–109. doi: 10.1016/0027-5107(95)00136-0

Gutteridge, J. M., and Halliwell, B. (2000). Free radicals and antioxidants in the year 2000. A historical look to the future. *Ann. N.Y. Acad. Sci.* 899, 136–147. doi: 10.1111/j.1749-6632.2000.tb06182.x

Gyengesi, E., Andrews, Z. B., Paxinos, G., and Zaborszky, L. (2013). Distribution of secretagogin-containing neurons in the basal forebrain of mice, with special reference to the cholinergic corticopetal system. *Brain Res. Bull.* 94, 1–8. doi: 10.1016/j.brainresbull.2013.01.009

Gyengesi, E., Paxinos, G., and Andrews, Z. B. (2012). Oxidative Stress in the Hypothalamus: the Importance of Calcium Signaling and Mitochondrial ROS in Body Weight Regulation. *Curr. Neuropharmacol.* 10, 344–353. doi: 10.2174/157015912804499438

Hernandez-Fonseca, K., Cardenas-Rodriguez, N., Pedraza-Chaverri, J., and Massieu, L. (2008). Calcium-dependent production of reactive oxygen species is involved in neuronal damage induced during glycolysis inhibition in cultured hippocampal neurons. *J. Neurosci. Res.* 86, 1768–1780. doi: 10.1002/jnr.21634

Hirooka, Y., Kishi, T., Sakai, K., Takeshita, A., and Sunagawa, K. (2011). Imbalance of central nitric oxide and reactive oxygen species in the regulation of sympathetic activity and neural mechanisms of hypertension. *Am. J. Physiol. Regul. Integr. Comp. Physiol.* 300, R818–R826. doi: 10.1152/ajpregu.00426.2010

Hordijk, P. L. (2006). Regulation of NADPH oxidases: the role of Rac proteins. *Circ Res.* 98, 453–462. doi: 10.1161/01.RES.0000204727.46710.5e

Horvath, T. L., Andrews, Z. B., and Diano, S. (2009). Fuel utilization by hypothalamic neurons: roles for ROS. *Trends Endocrinol. Metab.* 20, 78–87. doi: 10.1016/j.tem.2008.10.003

Horvath, T. L., Bechmann, I., Naftolin, F., Kalra, S. P., and Leranth, C. (1997). Heterogeneity in the neuropeptide Y-containing neurons of the rat arcuate nucleus: GABAergic and non-GABAergic subpopulations. *Brain Res.* 756, 283–286. doi: 10.1016/S0006-8993(97)00184-4

Ibrahim, N., Bosch, M. A., Smart, J. L., Qiu, J., Rubinstein, M., Ronnekleiv, O. K., et al. (2003). Hypothalamic proopiomelanocortin neurons are glucose responsive and express K(ATP) channels. *Endocrinology* 144, 1331–1340. doi: 10.1210/en.2002-221033

Infanger, D. W., Sharma, R. V., and Davisson, R. L. (2006). NADPH oxidases of the brain: distribution, regulation, and function. *Antioxid. Redox Signal.* 8, 1583–1596. doi: 10.1089/ars.2006.8.1583

Jaillard, T., Roger, M., Galinier, A., Guillou, P., Benani, A., Leloup, C., et al. (2009). Hypothalamic reactive oxygen species are required for insulin-induced food intake inhibition: an NADPH oxidase-dependent mechanism. *Diabetes* 58, 1544–1549. doi: 10.2337/db08-1039

Johansen, J. S., Harris, A. K., Rychly, D. J., and Ergul, A. (2005). Oxidative stress and the use of antioxidants in diabetes: linking basic science to clinical practice. *Cardiovasc. Diabetol.* 4:5. doi: 10.1186/1475-2840-4-5

Kennedy, G. C. (1953). The role of depot fat in the hypothalamic control of food intake in the rat. *Proc. R. Soc. Lond. B Biol. Sci.* 140, 578–596. doi: 10.1098/rspb.1953.0009

Kim, M. J., Shin, K. S., Chung, Y. B., Jung, K. W., Cha, C. I., and Shin, D. H (2005). Immunohistochemical study of p47Phox and gp91Phox distributions in rat brain. *Brain Res.* 1040, 178–186. doi: 10.1016/j.brainres.2005.01.066

Kim, M. S., Small, C. J., Stanley, S. A., Morgan, D. G., Seal, L. J., Kong, W. M., et al. (2000). The central melanocortin system affects the hypothalamo-pituitary thyroid axis and may mediate the effect of leptin. *J. Clin. Invest.* 105, 1005–1011 doi: 10.1172/JCI8857

Knauf, C., Drougard, A., Fournel, A., Duparc, T., and Valet, P. (2013). Hypothalamic actions of apelin on energy metabolism: new insight on glucose homeostasis and metabolic disorders. *Horm. Metab. Res.* 45, 928–934. doi 10.1055/s-0033-1351321

Krashes, M. J., Koda, S., Ye, C., Rogan, S. C., Adams, A. C., Cusher, D. S., et al (2011). Rapid, reversible activation of AgRP neurons drives feeding behavior in mice. *J. Clin. Invest.* 121, 1424–1428. doi: 10.1172/JCI46229

Kuo, D. Y., Chen, P. N., Chu, S. C., and Hsieh, Y. S. (2012). Knocking down the transcript of NF-kappaB modulates the reciprocal regulation of endogenous antioxidants and feeding behavior in phenylpropanolamine-treated rats. *Arch. Toxicol.* 86, 453–463. doi: 10.1007/s00204-011-0761-7

Kuo, D. Y., Chen, P. N., Yang, S. F., Chu, S. C., Chen, C. H., Kuo, M. H., et al. (2011). Role of reactive oxygen species-related enzymes in neuropeptide y and proopiomelanocortin-mediated appetite control: a study using atypical protein kinase C knockdown. *Antioxid. Redox Signal.* 15, 2147–2159. doi: 10.1089/ars.2010.3738

Lam, T. K., Schwartz, G. J., and Rossetti, L. (2005). Hypothalamic sensing of fatty acids. *Nat. Neurosci.* 8, 579–584. doi: 10.1038/nn1456

Lambeth, J. D. (2004). NOX enzymes and the biology of reactive oxygen. *Nat. Rev. Immunol.* 4, 181–189. doi: 10.1038/nri1312

Leibowitz, S. F., Hammer, N. J., and Chang, K. (1981). Hypothalamic paraventricular nucleus lesions produce overeating and obesity in the rat. *Physiol. Behav.* 27, 1031–1040. doi: 10.1016/0031-9384(81)90366-8

Leloup, C., Magnan, C., Benani, A., Bonnet, E., Alquier, T., Offer, G., et al. (2006). Mitochondrial reactive oxygen species are required for hypothalamic glucose sensing. *Diabetes* 55, 2084–2090. doi: 10.2337/db06-0086

Long, L., Toda, C., Jeong, J. K., Horvath, T. L., and Diano, S. (2014). PPARgamma ablation sensitizes proopiomelanocortin neurons to leptin during high-fat feeding. *J. Clin. Invest.* 124, 4017–4027. doi: 10.1172/JCI76220

Lu, N., Helwig, B. G., Fels, R. J., Parimi, S., and Kenney, M. J. (2004). Central Tempol alters basal sympathetic nerve discharge and attenuates sympathetic excitation to central ANG II. *Am. J. Physiol. Heart Circ. Physiol.* 287, H2626–H2633. doi: 10.1152/ajpheart.00030.2004

Marques-Da-Silva, D., and Gutierrez-Merino, C. (2012). L-type voltage-operated calcium channels, N-methyl-D-aspartate receptors and neuronal nitric-oxide synthase form a calcium/redox nano-transducer within lipid rafts. *Biochem. Biophys. Res. Commun.* 420, 257–262. doi: 10.1016/j.bbrc.2012.02.145

Morley, J. E., and Flood, J. F. (1991). Evidence that nitric oxide modulates food intake in mice. *Life Sci.* 49, 707–711. doi: 10.1016/0024-3205(91)90102-H

Morton, G. J., and Schwartz, M. W. (2011). Leptin and the central nervous system control of glucose metabolism. *Physiol. Rev.* 91, 389–411. doi: 10.1152/physrev.00007.2010

Mountjoy, P. D., Bailey, S. J., and Rutter, G. A. (2007). Inhibition by glucose or leptin of hypothalamic neurons expressing neuropeptide Y requires changes in AMP-activated protein kinase activity. *Diabetologia* 50, 168–177. doi: 10.1007/s00125-006-0473-3

Negre-Salvayre, A., Hirtz, C., Carrera, G., Cazenave, R., Troly, M., Salvayre, R., et al. (1997). A role for uncoupling protein-2 as a regulator of mitochondrial hydrogen peroxide generation. *FASEB J.* 11, 809–815.

Nicholls, D. G. (2009). Mitochondrial calcium function and dysfunction in the central nervous system. *Biochim. Biophys. Acta* 1787, 1416–1424. doi: 10.1016/j.bbabio.2009.03.010

Ohkuma, S., and Katsura, M. (2001). Nitric oxide and peroxynitrite as factors to stimulate neurotransmitter release in the CNS. *Prog. Neurobiol.* 64, 97–108. doi: 10.1016/S0301-0082(00)00041-1

Olney, J. W. (1969). Brain lesions, obesity, and other disturbances in mice treated with monosodium glutamate. *Science* 164, 719–721. doi: 10.1126/science.164.3880.719

Oomura, Y., Kimura, K., Ooyama, H., Maeno, T., Iki, M., and Kuniyoshi, M. (1964). Reciprocal activities of the ventromedial and lateral hypothalamic areas of cats. *Science* 143, 484–485. doi: 10.1126/science.143.3605.484

Palmer, R. M., Ferrige, A. G., and Moncada, S. (1987). Nitric oxide release accounts for the biological activity of endothelium-derived relaxing factor. *Nature* 327, 524–526. doi: 10.1038/327524a0

Park, E. S., Yi, S. J., Kim, J. S., Lee, H. S., Lee, I. S., Seong, J. K., et al. (2004). Changes in orexin-A and neuropeptide Y expression in the hypothalamus of the fasted and high-fat diet fed rats. *J. Vet. Sci.* 5, 295–302.

Parton, L. E., Ye, C. P., Coppari, R., Enriori, P. J., Choi, B., Zhang, C. Y., et al. (2007). Glucose sensing by POMC neurons regulates glucose homeostasis and is impaired in obesity. *Nature* 449, 228–232. doi: 10.1038/nature06098

Pazdro, R., and Burgess, J. R. (2010). The role of vitamin E and oxidative stress in diabetes complications. *Mech. Ageing Dev.* 131, 276–286. doi: 10.1016/j.mad.2010.03.005

Pinto, S., Roseberry, A. G., Liu, H., Diano, S., Shanabrough, M., Cai, X., et al. (2004). Rapid rewiring of arcuate nucleus feeding circuits by leptin. *Science* 304, 110–115. doi: 10.1126/science.1089459

Purkayastha, S., and Cai, D. (2013). Neuroinflammatory basis of metabolic syndrome. *Mol. Metab.* 2, 356–363. doi: 10.1016/j.molmet.2013.09.005

Qiu, J., Fang, Y., Ronnekleiv, O. K., and Kelly, M. J. (2010). Leptin excites proopiomelanocortin neurons via activation of TRPC channels. *J. Neurosci.* 30, 1560–1565. doi: 10.1523/JNEUROSCI.4816-09.2010

Reaux-Le Goazigo, A., Bodineau, L., De Mota, N., Jeandel, L., Chartrel, N., Knauf, C., et al. (2011). Apelin and the proopiomelanocortin system: a new regulatory pathway of hypothalamic alpha-MSH release. *Am. J. Physiol. Endocrinol. Metab.* 301, E955–E966. doi: 10.1152/ajpendo.00090.2011

Richard, D., Rivest, R., Huang, Q., Bouillaud, F., Sanchis, D., Champigny, O., et al. (1998). Distribution of the uncoupling protein 2 mRNA in the mouse brain. *J. Comp. Neurol.* 397, 549–560.

Rodriguez, E. M., Blazquez, J. L., and Guerra, M. (2010). The design of barriers in the hypothalamus allows the median eminence and the arcuate nucleus to enjoy private milieus: the former opens to the portal blood and the latter to the cerebrospinal fluid. *Peptides* 31, 757–776. doi: 10.1016/j.peptides.2010.01.003

Rossi, M., Kim, M. S., Morgan, D. G., Small, C. J., Edwards, C. M., Sunter, D., et al. (1998). A C-terminal fragment of Agouti-related protein increases feeding and antagonizes the effect of alpha-melanocyte stimulating hormone *in vivo*. *Endocrinology* 139, 4428–4431. doi: 10.1210/endo.139.10.6332

Routh, V. H. (2002). Glucose-sensing neurons: are they physiologically relevant? *Physiol. Behav.* 76, 403–413. doi: 10.1016/S0031-9384(02)00761-8

Routh, V. H. (2010). Glucose sensing neurons in the ventromedial hypothalamus. *Sensors (Basel).* 10, 9002–9025. doi: 10.3390/s101009002

Sanacora, G., Kershaw, M., Finkelstein, J. A., and White, J. D. (1990). Increased hypothalamic content of preproneuropeptide Y messenger ribonucleic acid in genetically obese Zucker rats and its regulation by food deprivation. *Endocrinology* 127, 730–737. doi: 10.1210/endo-127-2-730

Santiago, J. A., and Potashkin, J. A. (2014). System-based approaches to decode the molecular links in Parkinson's disease and diabetes. *Neurobiol. Dis.* 72(Pt A), 84–91. doi: 10.1016/j.nbd.2014.03.019

Schneeberger, M., Dietrich, M. O., Sebastian, D., Imbernon, M., Castano, C., Garcia, A., et al. (2013). Mitofusin 2 in POMC neurons connects ER stress with leptin resistance and energy imbalance. *Cell* 155, 172–187. doi: 10.1016/j.cell.2013.09.003

Schrader, M., and Fahimi, H. D. (2006). Peroxisomes and oxidative stress. *Biochim. Biophys. Acta* 1763, 1755–1766. doi: 10.1016/j.bbamcr.2006.09.006

Schwartz, M. W., and Porte, D. Jr. (2005). Diabetes, obesity, and the brain. *Science* 307, 375–379. doi: 10.1126/science.1104344

Serrano, F., Kolluri, N. S., Wientjes, F. B., Card, J. P., and Klann, E. (2003). NADPH oxidase immunoreactivity in the mouse brain. *Brain Res.* 988, 193–198. doi: 10.1016/S0006-8993(03)03364-X

Shibuki, K., and Okada, D. (1991). Endogenous nitric oxide release required for long-term synaptic depression in the cerebellum. *Nature* 349, 326–328. doi: 10.1038/349326a0

Shimizu, N., Oomura, Y., Plata-Salaman, C. R., and Morimoto, M. (1987). Hyperphagia and obesity in rats with bilateral ibotenic acid-induced lesions of the ventromedial hypothalamic nucleus. *Brain Res.* 416, 153–156. doi: 10.1016/0006-8993(87)91503-3

Sies, H., and Cadenas, E. (1985). Oxidative stress: damage to intact cells and organs. *Philos. Trans. R. Soc. Lond. B Biol. Sci.* 311, 617–631. doi: 10.1098/rstb.1985.0168

Stellar, E. (1994). The physiology of motivation. 1954. *Psychol. Rev.* 101, 301–311. doi: 10.1037/0033-295X.101 2.301

Storozhevykh, T. P., Senilova, Y. E., Persiyantseva, N. A., Pinelis, V. G., and Pomytkin, I. A. (2007). Mitochondrial respiratory chain is involved in insulin-stimulated hydrogen peroxide production and plays an integral role in insulin receptor autophosphorylation in neurons. *BMC Neurosci.* 8:84. doi: 10.1186/1471-2202-8-84

Strehler, E. E., Caride, A. J., Filoteo, A. G., Xiong, Y., Penniston, J. T., and Enyedi, A. (2007). Plasma membrane Ca^{2+} ATPases as dynamic regulators of cellular calcium handling. *Ann. N.Y. Acad. Sci.* 1099, 226–236. doi: 10.1196/annals.1387.023

Turrens, J. F. (2003). Mitochondrial formation of reactive oxygen species. *J. Physiol.* 552, 335–344. doi: 10.1113/jphysiol.2003.049478

Valko, M., Leibfritz, D., Moncol, J., Cronin, M. T., Mazur, M., and Telser, J. (2007). Free radicals and antioxidants in normal physiological functions and human disease. *Int. J. Biochem. Cell Biol.* 39, 44–84. doi: 10.1016/j.biocel.2006.07.001

Vozza, A., Parisi, G., De Leonardis, F., Lasorsa, F. M., Castegna, A., Amorese, D., et al. (2014). UCP2 transports C4 metabolites out of mitochondria, regulating glucose and glutamine oxidation. *Proc. Natl. Acad. Sci. U.S.A.* 111, 960–965. doi: 10.1073/pnas.1317400111

Weber, A. M., Wong, F. K., Tufford, A. R., Schlichter, L. C., Matveev, V., and Stanley, E. F. (2010). N-type Ca^{2+} channels carry the largest current: implications for nanodomains and transmitter release. *Nat. Neurosci.* 13, 1348–1350. doi: 10.1038/nn.2657

Wilding, J. P., Gilbey, S. G., Bailey, C. J., Batt, R. A., Williams, G., Ghatei, M. A., et al. (1993). Increased neuropeptide-Y messenger ribonucleic acid (mRNA) and decreased neurotensin mRNA in the hypothalamus of the obese (ob/ob) mouse. *Endocrinology* 132, 1939–1944.

Willesen, M. G., Kristensen, P., and Romer, J. (1999). Co-localization of growth hormone secretagogue receptor and NPY mRNA in the arcuate nucleus of the rat. *Neuroendocrinology* 70, 306–316. doi: 10.1159/000054491

Wynne, K., Stanley, S., McGowan, B., and Bloom, S. (2005). Appetite control. *J. Endocrinol.* 184, 291–318. doi: 10.1677/joe.1.05866

Yang, Y., Atasoy, D., Su, H. H., and Sternson, S. M. (2011). Hunger states switch a flip-flop memory circuit via a synaptic AMPK-dependent positive feedback loop. *Cell* 146, 992–1003. doi: 10.1016/j.cell.2011.07.039

Yasuda, T., Masaki, T., Kakuma, T., and Yoshimatsu, H. (2004). Hypothalamic melanocortin system regulates sympathetic nerve activity in brown adipose tissue. *Exp. Biol. Med. (Maywood).* 229, 235–239.

Yoon, Y., Galloway, C. A., Jhun, B. S., and Yu, T. (2011). Mitochondrial dynamics in diabetes. *Antioxid. Redox Signal.* 14, 439–457. doi: 10.1089/ars.2010.3286

York, D. A., Marchington, D., Holt, S. J., and Allars, J. (1985). Regulation of sympathetic activity in lean and obese Zucker (fa/fa) rats. *Am. J. Physiol.* 249, E299–E305.

Yu, X., Shao, X. G., Sun, H., Li, Y. N., Yang, J., Deng, Y. C., et al. (2008). Activation of cerebral peroxisome proliferator-activated receptors gamma exerts neuroprotection by inhibiting oxidative stress following pilocarpine-induced status epilepticus. *Brain Res.* 1200, 146–158. doi: 10.1016/j.brainres.2008.01.047

Zimmerman, M. C., Lazartigues, E., Lang, J. A., Sinnayah, P., Ahmad, I. M., Spitz, D. R., et al. (2002). Superoxide mediates the actions of angiotensin II in the central nervous system. *Circ. Res.* 91, 1038–1045. doi: 10.1161/01.RES.0000043501.47934.FA

17

Effect of treatment modality on the hypothalamic–pituitary function of patients treated with radiation therapy for pituitary adenomas: hypothalamic dose and endocrine outcomes

Andrew Elson[1], Joseph Bovi[1], Kawaljeet Kaur[2], Diana Maas[2], Grant Sinson[3] and Chris Schultz[1]*

[1] *Department of Radiation Oncology, Medical College of Wisconsin, Milwaukee, WI, USA*
[2] *Division of Endocrinology, Metabolism, and Clinical Nutrition, Medical College of Wisconsin, Milwaukee, WI, USA*
[3] *Department of Neurosurgery, Medical College of Wisconsin, Milwaukee, WI, USA*

***Correspondence:**
Chris Schultz, Department of Radiation Oncology, Froedtert Hospital, 3rd Floor East Clinics, 9200 West Wisconsin Avenue, Milwaukee, WI 53226, USA
e-mail: cschultz@mcw.edu

Background: Both fractionated external beam radiotherapy and single fraction radiosurgery for pituitary adenomas are associated with the risk of hypothalamic–pituitary (HP) axis dysfunction.

Objective: To analyze the effect of treatment modality (Linac, TomoTherapy, or gamma knife) on hypothalamic dose and correlate these with HP-axis deficits after radiotherapy.

Methods: Radiation plans of patients treated post-operatively for pituitary adenomas using Linac-based 3D-conformal radiotherapy (CRT) ($n = 11$), TomoTherapy-based intensity modulated radiation therapy (IMRT) ($n = 10$), or gamma knife stereotactic radiosurgery ($n = 12$) were retrospectively reviewed. Dose to the hypothalamus was analyzed and post-radiotherapy hormone function including growth hormone, thyroid stimulating hormone, adrenocorticotropic hormone, prolactin, and gonadotropins (follicle stimulating hormone/luteinizing hormone) were assessed.

Results: Post-radiation, 13 of 27 (48%) patients eligible for analysis developed at least one new hormone deficit, of which 8 of 11 (72%) occurred in the Linac group, 4 of 8 (50%) occurred in the TomoTherapy group, and 1 of 8 (12.5%) occurred in the gamma knife group. Compared with fractionated techniques, gamma knife showed improved hypothalamic sparing for DMax Hypo and V12Gy. For fractionated modalities, TomoTherapy showed improved dosimetric characteristics over Linac-basec treatment with hypothalamic DMean (44.8 vs. 26.8 Gy $p = 0.02$), DMax (49.8 vs. 39.1 Gy $p = 0.04$), and V12Gy (100 vs. 76% $p = 0.004$).

Conclusion: Maximal dosimetric avoidance of the hypothalamus was achieved using gamma knife-based radiosurgery followed by TomoTherapy-based IMRT, and Linac-based 3D conformal radiation therapy, respectively.

Keywords: pituitary adenoma, tomotherapy, gamma knife, hypothalamus, endocrinopathy, IMRT, 3D conformal radiotherapy

INTRODUCTION

Radiotherapy plays an integral role in the management of patients with pituitary adenomas, and this includes both fractionated external beam radiotherapy (EBRT) and stereotactic radiosurgery (SRS). Fractionated EBRT and SRS both afford excellent local control rates for pituitary adenomas, generally on the order of 90% at 10 years (1–3). Both fractionated EBRT and SRS put patients at risk for functional endocrine deficits, which is both a dose and time dependent phenomenon (4). Such abnormalities include deficits in growth hormone (GH), prolactin (PRL), adrenocorticotropic hormone (ACTH), thyroid stimulating hormone (TSH), and gonadotropins follicle stimulating hormone (FSH) and luteinizing hormone (LH), with GH generally being the most radiosensitive endocrine axis (5). In comparison to fractionated EBRT, SRS affords a more convenient option for patients and is becoming a more frequently used modality of treatment (6). However, certain tumor and patient selection criteria may require the use of fractionated radiotherapy. For instance, at the Medical College of Wisconsin (MCW), the use of SRS is generally reserved for patients with pituitary tumors <3 cm in size and with at least 3 mm clearance from the optic chiasm (OC).

The hypothalamus plays a critical role in the functioning of the hypothalamic–pituitary (HP) axis, and radiation-induced injury is believed to effect both the pituitary and the hypothalamus (7). Doses to the hypothalamus as low as 12 Gy may be implicated in increasing the risk of radiotherapy associated endocrinopathies, and doses typically used in the treatment of brain tumors (>50 Gy) commonly result in HP-axis deficiency (8, 9). To better understand the relationship between hypothalamic dose and endocrine dysfunction, we reviewed patients undergoing treatment for pituitary adenomas at our institution. Hypothalamic dose characteristics were analyzed by treatment modality [Linac-based 3D-conformal radiotherapy (CRT), TomoTherapy-based intensity modulated radiation therapy (IMRT), and gamma knife SRS], and endocrine outcomes were assessed accordingly.

MATERIALS AND METHODS

PATIENTS

Between December 2005 and January 2012, 33 patients were identified with pituitary adenomas who underwent gamma knife SRS ($n = 12$), fractionated TomoTherapy-based IMRT ($n = 10$), or fractionated Linac-based 3D-CRT ($n = 11$). All aspects of this retrospective study were approved by the MCW Institutional Review Board. All patients analyzed had routine endocrine follow-up at MCW, and clinical data were obtained from the institutional electronic medical record. Dosimetric information was acquired through restoration of the original treatment plans maintained in the departmental database. Baseline patient characteristics are described in **Table 1**. Pre-radiotherapy endocrine deficits were present in 84.8% of patients, and 45% of patients had functioning adenomas vs. 55% non-functioning. Of all adenomas, 30% were GH secreting, 12% PRL secreting, and 3% ACTH secreting. Four patients were treated with medical therapy to oppose hypersecretory function prior to surgery (two patients treated with a dopamine agonist for PRL secretion in the TomoTherapy group, and two patients treated with octreotide for GH secretion in the gamma knife group). All patients had previously undergone endonasal transsphenoidal surgery. All patients were diagnosed with macroadenomas and underwent a subtotal resection except one patient in the Linac group who underwent a biopsy only. The median study follow-up period was 24 months (range 2–76 months).

Table 1 | Baseline patient characteristics.

	Linac	Tomo Therapy	Gamma knife	Total
N	11	10	12	33
Male (%)	6 (54.5)	6 (60)	5 (41.5)	17 (51.5)
Female (%)	5 (45.5)	4 (40)	7 (58.3)	16 (48.5)
Mean age	43.8	49.2	46	44.4
Transsphenoidal resection (%)	100	100	100	100
Deficit prior to RT (%)	6 (54.5)	10 (100)	12 (100)	28 (84.8)
Non-functioning adenoma (%)	5 (45)	6 (60)	7 (58)	18 (55)
Functioning adenoma (%)	6 (55)	4 (40)	5 (42)	15 (45)
GH secreting (%)	5 (45)	1 (10)	4 (33)	10 (30)
PRL secreting (%)	0 (0)	3 (30)	1 (8)	4 (12)
TSH secreting (%)	0 (0)	0 (0)	0 (0)	0 (0)
ACTH secreting (%)	1 (9)	0 (0)	0 (0)	1 (3)

RADIOTHERAPY

Linac-based 3D-CRT was performed on one of three institutional linear accelerators. Plans were based on a five field non-coplanar design including an anterior "vertex" field requiring a 90° couch rotation. Radiation dose to the target volume ranged from 48.6 to 54 Gy. All 3D-CRT planning was performed using Xio radiation treatment planning software (Elekta/CMS, St Louis, MO, USA).

TomoTherapy-based IMRT was performed on the institutional TomoTherapy unit. IMRT planning was performed using the TomoTherapy radiation planning system (TomoTherapy, Madison, WI, USA). Radiation dose to the target volume ranged from 50 to 54 Gy.

Gamma knife SRS was performed using the Leksell Gamma knife (Elekta AB, Stockholm, Sweden). MRI imaging with a stereotactic head frame was acquired for treatment planning for each case, and planning was performed using Leksell GammaPlan software (Elekta AB, Stockholm, Sweden). Radiation dose to the target volume ranged from 12 to 20 Gy in a single fraction prescribed to the 50% isodose line (IDL).

In this study group at the time of treatment planning and delivery, the hypothalamus was not explicitly contoured, monitored, or identified as an avoidance structure for any of the three treatment techniques.

The determination of eligibility for SRS vs. fractionated EBRT was made primarily based on size of the tumor and distance from the OC, with a requirement of <3 cm tumor with >3 mm clearance from the OC preferred for SRS. The use of 3D-CRT vs. TomoTherapy IMRT was practitioner dependent and partially determined by the year of treatment and the availability of the modality, with a trend toward increased use of TomoTherapy during the later years of the study period. Linac-based IMRT was not performed due to the perceived improved conformality of TomoTherapy over Linac-based IMRT during the study period.

DOSIMETRIC ANALYSIS

In order to analyze hypothalamic dose characteristics of each treatment plan, a hypothalamic contour was retrospectively added in each case. For patients treated with Linac-based 3D-CRT, the treatment plan was restored into the Xio radiation planning system and the hypothalamic contour was added to the structure set, such that dose–volume histogram (DVH) data for the hypothalamus could be acquired. For patients treated with TomoTherapy, plans were restored into both Xio (to allow the hypothalamic contour to be added) and the TomoTherapy planning system (to recover the dose data itself) and fused into Focal (Elekta AB, Stockholm, Sweden) such that dose data from the original plan could be applied to the new hypothalamic contour. For patients treated with gamma knife SRS, the hypothalamic contour was added in Leksell Gamma Plan such that DVH data could be analyzed. Contouring within Gamma Plan was performed directly onto the pre-treatment MRI data set originally acquired using the MRI T1 sequence with contrast. Contouring was performed on pre-radiotherapy MRI T1 weighted images.

After restoration of all plans and construction of the hypothalamic contour was complete, the following parameters were determined: target volume, prescription dose, volume of the hypothalamus, volume of the hypothalamus receiving at least 12 Gy

(V12Gy), Mean hypothalamic dose (DMean Hypo), Maximum hypothalamic dose (DMax Hypo), and the Biologically Equivalent Dose at 2 Gy/Fx for $\alpha/\beta = 3$ (BED2Gy).

HYPOTHALAMIC CONTOURING

The hypothalamic contour was created using MRI-based anatomic landmarks representing surrogate boundaries for the hypothalamus itself. Contouring was performed with the assistance of an MCW neuroradiologist, and contours were reviewed by the senior author (Joseph A. Bovi). Previously published MRI Atlases of the hypothalamus were referenced to identify anatomic landmarks as boundaries for the hypothalamic contour (10, 11). The contouring procedure was also in accordance with a previously published hypothalamic contouring method (8). The hypothalamic contour was a polygonal structure consisting of two separated volumes on each side of the third ventricle or CSF space. The superior most boundary of the contour was set at the axial slice containing the anterior commissure (AC). The inferior most boundary was set at the axial slice containing the OC. Anteriorly, the boundary consisted of the anterior aspect of the third ventricle or the visible edge of the CSF space within the suprasellar cistern. Posteriorly, the contour was drawn to the level of the interpeduncular fossa. The medial border consisted of the third ventricle or the visible CSF space. Laterally, the contour was bounded by the optic white matter tracts or the internal capsule. Representative slices are depicted in **Figure 1**.

ENDOCRINE EVALUATION

Baseline endocrine evaluation was performed on all analyzed patients under the direction of MCW neuroendocrinologists. Each patient had baseline pre-radiotherapy endocrine labs drawn, as well as post-radiotherapy follow-up labs at 6–12 month intervals after treatment indefinitely. Standard endocrine laboratory studies included evaluation of PRL, GH which was evaluated through IGF-1, thyroid studies (TSH and free T4), ACTH which was evaluated with eight AM fasting cortisol, ACTH, and eight AM fasting cosyntropin stimulation test, and gonadotropin function evaluated with estradiol or testosterone, LH and FSH or normal menstrual status in premenopausal women. Reference ranges were as follows: PRL (2.8–23.3 ng/mL female, 4.0–15.2 ng/mL male), IGF-1 (reference range varies with age), TSH (0.45–4.5 μIU/mL), free T4 (0.82–1.77 ng/dL), eight AM cortisol (>10 μg/dL), ACTH (7.2–63.3 pg/mL), FSH (male, 1.5–12.4 mIU/mL, female post menopause 25.8–134.8 mIU/mL, female pre-menopause with normal menstrual cycles considered normal, reference ranges are phase dependent), LH (male, 1.7–8.6 mIU/mL, female post menopause 7.7–58.5 mIU/mL, female pre-menopause with normal menstrual cycles considered normal, reference ranges are phase dependent). Laboratory reference ranges varied slightly during the study period; however, all laboratory values were referenced to the normal ranges listed at the time of lab draw. Pre-radiotherapy deficit was defined as any laboratory values below the reference ranges or any administration of hormone

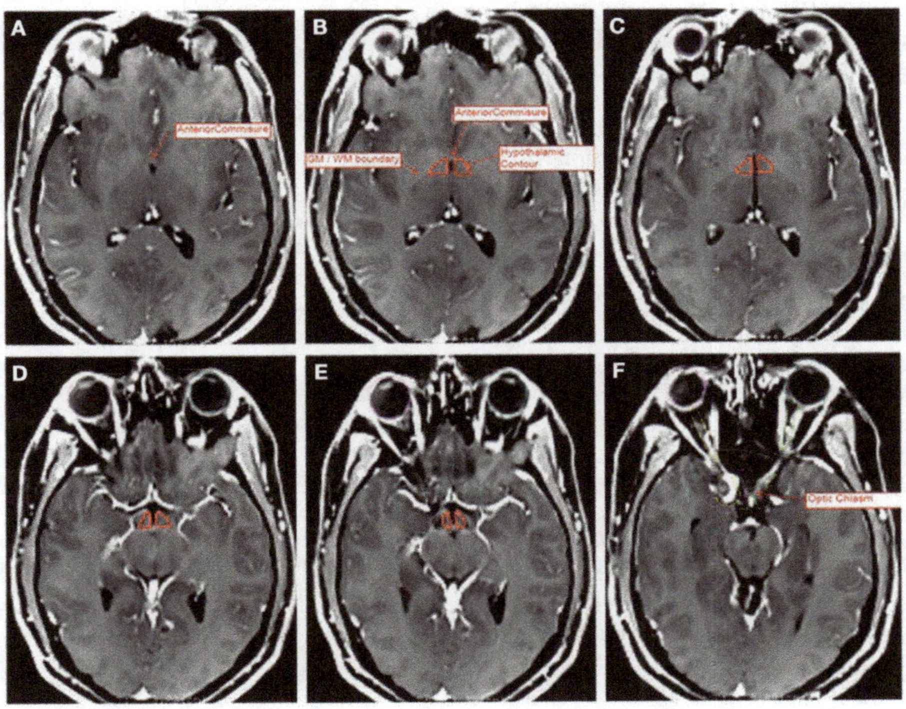

FIGURE 1 | Representative slices of MRI T1 + C images registered to CT data sets for hypothalamic volume contouring. Slices A (superior most) through F (inferior most) depict several anatomic landmarks for the delineation of the hypothalamic contour (red). **(A)** Depicts the superior most slice, at the level of the anterior commissure. **(B–E)** Depict the hypothalamic contour, bounded by the white matter tracts laterally, the third ventricle medially, the CSF space of the suprasellar cistern anteriorly, and the level of the interpeduncular fossa posteriorly. **(F)** Depicts the level of the optic chiasm, at which the contour ends. The contour has been enhanced for ease of visibility.

replacement therapy prior to the start of radiotherapy. Post-radiotherapy endocrinopathy in any axis (PRL, GH, ACTH, TSH, or FSH/LH) was defined as laboratory values on at least two separate lab draws below the reference range identified on a follow-up evaluation, or administration of hormone replacement therapy (such as levothyroxine, hydrocortisone/prednisone, human GH, estrogen/progesterone, or testosterone) as judged necessary by the treating neuroendocrinologist. In addition, PRL elevation post-radiotherapy in a previously non-PRL secreting adenoma was categorized as an endocrine abnormality. Any endocrine laboratory value outside the reference range on a single assessment that subsequently normalized without the administration of hormone therapy was not considered to constitute an endocrinopathy.

STATISTICAL ANALYSIS

With respect to endocrine evaluation, new HP-axis deficits that were not present prior to radiotherapy were considered the primary endpoint. HP-axis event curves using the Kaplan–Meier method were performed, with a new endocrinopathy in any of the five endocrine axes (GH, PRL, ACTH, TSH, or Gonadotropin) constituting an event in the analysis. If multiple endocrinopathies occurred within the same patient, the first endocrinopathy was used for the event curve analysis. Univariate analysis of event free survival by treatment modality was performed using the log-rank test. With respect to dosimetric evaluation, parameters analyzed included hypothalamic mean dose (DMean Hypo), hypothalamic maximum dose (DMax Hypo), and the percentage of hypothalamic volume receiving ≥12 Gy (V12Gy). Dosimetric comparisons by treatment modality for all three groups were performed using one-way ANOVA. TomoTherapy comparison with Linac-based therapy was performed using the Exact Wilcoxon Rank Sum test. Statistics were performed in consultation with the MCW department of Biostatistics using SAS statistics software version 9.3 (The SAS Institute, Cary, NC, USA) and significance was determined by a $p < 0.05$.

RESULTS

DOSIMETRIC COMPARISONS

Dosimetric data are presented in **Table 2**. With respect to the fractionated techniques there was no difference between the Linac-treated group and the TomoTherapy group in terms of target volume (12.7 and 24.5 cc, respectively), prescription dose (50.4 and 50.68 Gy, respectively), volume of the hypothalamus (0.81 and 0.93 cc, respectively), and BED 2 Gy (48.4 and 49.1 Gy, respectively). When comparing the fractionated techniques, there was an improvement in the TomoTherapy group over the Linac group with respect to the hypothalamic V12Gy (76 vs. 100% $p = 0.004$), DMean (44.8 vs. 26.8 Gy $p = 0.02$), and DMax (49.8 vs. 39.1 $p = 0.04$). The gamma knife group was superior to both fractionated techniques in terms of DMax (1.6 Gy) and V12Gy (0%), however DMean for the gamma knife group was not calculated. The hypothalamic volume of the gamma knife group was smaller than that of either of the fractionated groups, likely reflecting differences in the contouring mechanism and the slice thickness of the MRI images available for the Gamma Plan system.

All gamma knife parameters were significantly different than the respective fractionated radiotherapy parameters by the exact Kruskal–Wallis Test. p Values reflect comparison of Linac vs. Tomotherapy by the exact Wilcoxon Rank Sum Test.

PATIENT SURVIVAL, LOCAL CONTROL, AND ENDOCRINE OUTCOMES

All patients were alive and disease free during the study period after completion of fractionated EBRT or gamma knife radiosurgery. No patient exhibited local recurrence as assessed by MRI imaging during follow-up.

Prior to radiotherapy, 28 of 33 (84.8%) of patients had at least one baseline endocrine deficit. Post-radiotherapy for all groups, new endocrine deficits occurred in 13 of 27 (48%) of patients eligible for analysis. A total of 20 new endocrine deficits were identified, with some patients developing more than one endocrinopathy. Deficits by treatment modality were as follows: in the Linac-based 3D-CRT treated group 8 of 11 (72%) patients developed at least one new endocrinopathy, whereas this occurred in 4 of 8 (50%) patients treated with TomoTherapy IMRT and 1 of 8 (12.5%) patients treated with gamma knife SRS. Specific endocrine deficits by treatment modality are displayed in **Table 3**. Of 20 new endocrine deficits identified, 5 (25%) each involved GH, TSH, and PRL, 2 (10%) involved ACTH, and 3 (15%) involved LSH/FSH.

The median event free duration of the functioning pre-radiotherapy hypothalamic–pituitary axes were 18.7 months in the Linac 3D-CRT treatment group, 48.9 months in the TomoTherapy IMRT treatment group, and was not reached in the gamma knife SRS treatment group. The pre-radiotherapy intact endocrine axis event curves for each group are displayed in **Figure 2**. Event

Table 2 | Dosimetric parameters by treatment modality.

Parameter	Linac	Tomo Therapy	Gamma knife	p
Target volume (cc)	12.7	24.5	3.0	0.7
Hypothalamic volume (cc)	0.8	0.9	0.5	0.28
V12Gy Hypo	100%	76%	0%	0.004
DMean Hypo	44.8 Gy	26.8 Gy	NA	0.02
DMax Hypo	49.8 Gy	39.1 Gy	1.6 Gy	0.04
BED2 α/β 3	48.4 Gy	49.1 Gy	60.6 Gy	0.64
Mean prescription dose	50.4 Gy	50.7 Gy	15.8 Gy	0.66

BED2 α/β 3, biologically equivalent dose at 2 Gy per fraction for an α/β ratio of 3.

Table 3 | Specific endocrine deficits by treatment modality.

Hormone abnormality	Linac	Tomo Therapy	Gamma knife	Total (%)
GH	4	1	0	5 (25)
PRL (↓)	1	0	0	1 (5)
PRL (↑)	2	1	1	4 (20)
ACTH	2	0	0	2 (10)
TSH	3	2	0	5 (25)
LSH/FSH	3	0	0	3 (15)
Total	15	4	1	20 (100)

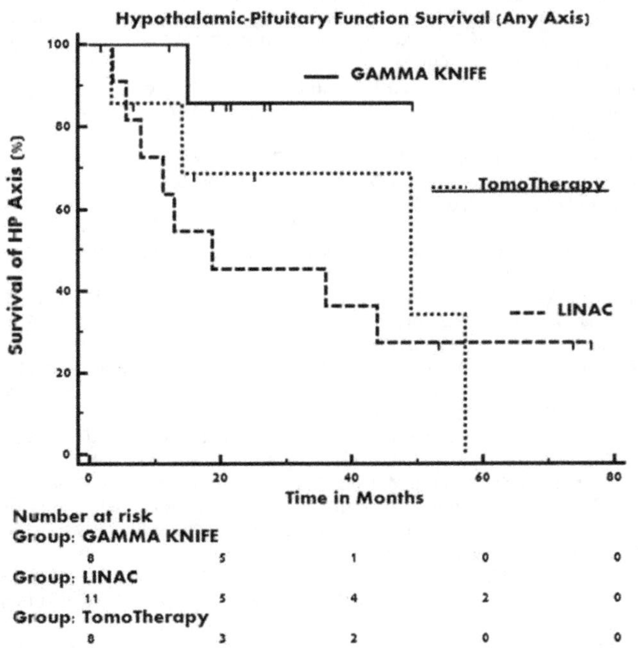

FIGURE 2 | Kaplan–Meier event curves of pre-radiotherapy intact hypothalamic–pituitary axes as a function of time post-radiotherapy. Occurrence of any new endocrinopathy constitutes an event in the plot. Event curve hazard ratios do not differ statistically by the log-rank test.

curve separation was not statistically significant by the log-rank test ($p = 0.36$).

DISCUSSION

One of the most common complications of treatment for pituitary adenomas is endocrine dysfunction, and for this reason long term follow-up is critical to optimize patient outcomes. This risk as it relates to radiotherapy is a phenomenon that depends on dose to the HP-axis, the volume of irradiated tissue, the time interval after irradiation, and underlying HP-axis pathology (12). Patients undergoing both fractionated EBRT and SRS are subject to this risk. Typically endocrinopathies manifest within the first 3 years of treatment, however they can also occur much later (13). Despite the consistent finding that irradiation of pituitary tumors places the patient at risk for hypopituitarism, reports of the actual incidence of treatment-associated endocrine deficits vary widely among both fractionated and radiosurgical series (14, 15). The reason for this heterogeneity is likely multifactorial and involves numerous issues such as the type and extent of surgery prior to radiotherapy, the pre-treatment effect of the tumor itself on the HP-axis, the type of radiotherapy technique, the follow-up interval, and the definition of endocrine dysfunction used. Various definitions of post-treatment endocrine dysfunction have been employed such as the use of strict laboratory cutoff values vs. the administration of hormone replacement therapy, or a combination thereof (16–19).

In this study, the definition of new endocrine deficit included both a consistently abnormal laboratory value as well as the administration of hormone replacement therapy in order to capture these two issues. By doing so, however this study may reflect relatively higher rates of endocrinopathy in comparison to other series. Additionally, it is uncommon to report post-radiotherapy PRL elevation as a new HP-axis endocrinopathy, as this is unlikely to cause symptoms or require intervention. However, this particular abnormality does give insight into the mechanism of dysfunction, as the hypothalamus is known to exert a tonic inhibitory effect on the secretion of PRL by the anterior pituitary through the neurotransmitter dopamine (20, 21). Presumably, a post-radiotherapy rise in PRL would represent damage sustained by the hypothalamus reflected by the inability to maintain this tonic inhibition, and in certain circumstances can be opposed through the use of a dopamine agonist (22).

The exact contribution of the hypothalamus to post-radiotherapy anterior pituitary endocrine deficits is not entirely elucidated, however it is postulated that endocrine changes resulting from hypothalamic damage may occur within a shorter time frame than those associated with damage to the pituitary itself. Agha et al. analyzed HP-axis deficiencies in adults treated with radiotherapy for non-pituitary brain tumors and found that mild to moderate hyperprolactinemia occurred at a shorter median time (33 months) in comparison to GH, ACTH, or gonadotropin deficiency (100 months), possibly reflecting an earlier manifestation of hypothalamic dysfunction in comparison to pituitary dysfunction (18).

Studies of GH deficiency in pediatric patients treated for primary brain tumors as well as total body irradiation (TBI) have revealed that the hypothalamus plays an important role in the pathogenesis of this disorder. Merchant et al. investigated the relationship of the dose to the hypothalamus in the development of GH deficiency and determined that a dose of 16.1 Gy to the hypothalamus would constitute the mean dose required to induce a 50% risk of GH deficiency at 5 years post-radiotherapy (23). GH is known to be the most susceptible endocrine axis to radiotherapy-induced dysfunction, and hypothalamic doses as low as 12 Gy may result in impaired GH release (8). Although susceptibility of the hypothalamus to radiation-induced dysfunction may be more pronounced in children, the same phenomenon has been noted in adult patients as well. Feigl et al. investigated the hypothalamic dose received by 108 patients treated with gamma knife SRS for pituitary adenomas and found that the mean dose was higher in patients with new endocrinopathies than in those without (1.3 vs. 0.8 Gy) (17).

Overall endocrine dysfunction likely reflects the combined effect of damage to both structures (5, 7, 14). In clinical practice, however it is not useful or cost effective to routinely differentiate secondary endocrine deficiencies from tertiary endocrine deficiencies (i.e., anterior pituitary vs. hypothalamic) as this distinction would not typically alter management.

Given the role played by the hypothalamus in the development of radiation-induced hypopituitarism, dose monitoring to this structure with the aim of maximal avoidance is a rational objective. In this study, the parameters DMax Hypo and DMean Hypo were chosen as dose monitoring parameters analogous to those commonly employed for other treatment planning organs at risk (OAR). The parameter V12 Hypo (the volume of the hypothalamus receiving 12 Gy) was chosen as possibly reflective of a "threshold dose" in the fractionated setting, as it has previously been shown through TBI data that dysfunction of the most sensitive HP-axis, GH, is rare with exposure of <12 Gy (9). In addition, in the radiosurgical setting, the volume of brain receiving >12 Gy has been described in QUANTEC as a marker for increased normal tissue complication risk (24).

In this study, dose sparing to the hypothalamus was considerably more favorable in the gamma knife SRS group over the fractionated techniques. This was an expected result, given the highly conformal nature of the gamma knife system and steep dose gradients associated with this technique. It is important to note that to be eligible for this procedure patients must meet certain requirements in terms of tumor size and distance from the optic structures.

With respect to the fractionated techniques, helical TomoTherapy-based IMRT exhibited improved hypothalamic dose sparing in comparison to Linac-based 3D-CRT, likely in part due to the characteristic anterior vertex field of the 3D plans, which projects through the hypothalamus. Improved conformality through IMRT inverse planning is not unique to TomoTherapy, as Linac-based IMRT techniques are capable of producing improved dosimetric profiles in comparison to the Linac-based 3D technique; however this issue was not addressed during the study period as most treating physicians were more comfortable with the use of TomoTherapy IMRT in this setting. The endocrine outcomes of the patients in each of these three groups trended toward improved HP-axis preservation paralleling the hypothalamic sparing properties of the techniques used, however larger patient sample and longer follow-up would likely be required to further clarify the association. Furthermore, routinely incorporating the hypothalamic contour may allow for improved conformal avoidance with either fractionated 3D-CRT or IMRT techniques.

CONCLUSION

In patients treated post-operatively for pituitary adenomas, hypothalamic dose sparing was best achieved using gamma knife-based radiosurgery. With respect to fractionated radiotherapy, TomoTherapy IMRT provides improved hypothalamic dose sparing over Linac-based 3D-CRT. Efforts to minimize hypothalamic dose by monitoring parameters such as DMax Hypo, DMean Hypo, and V12Gy may improve endocrine outcomes post-radiotherapy.

REFERENCES

Brada M, Rajan B, Traish D, Ashley S, Holmes-Sellors PJ, Nussey S, et al. The long-term efficacy of conservative surgery and radiotherapy in the control of pituitary adenomas. *Clin Endocrinol (Oxf)* (1993) **38**(6):571–8. doi:10.1111/j.1365-2265.1993.tb02137.x

Sasaki R, Murakami M, Okamoto Y, Kono K, Yoden E, Nakajima T, et al. The efficacy of conventional radiation therapy in the management of pituitary adenoma. *Int J Radiat Oncol Biol Phys* (2000) **47**(5):1337–45. doi:10.1016/S0360- 3016(00)00503-4

Sheehan JP, Xu Z, Lobo MJ. External beam radiation therapy and stereotactic radiosurgery for pituitary adenomas. *Neurosurg Clin NAm* (2012) **23**(4):571–86. doi:10.1016/j.nec.2012.06.011

Darzy KH, Shalet SM. Hypopituitarism following radiotherapy. *Pituitary* (2009) **12**(1):40–50. doi:10.1007/s11102-008-0088-4

Darzy KH, Shalet SM. Hypopituitarism as a consequence of brain tumours and radiotherapy. *Pituitary* (2005) **8**(3–4):203–11. doi:10.1007/s11102-006-6042-4

Leenstra JL, Tanaka S, Kline RW, Brown PD, Link MJ, Nippoldt TB, et al. Factors associated with endocrine deficits after stereotactic radiosurgery of pituitary adenomas. *Neurosurgery* (2010) **67**(1):27–32. doi:10.1227/01.NEU.0000370978. 31405.A9

Darzy KH. Radiation-induced hypopituitarism after cancer therapy: who, how and when to test. *Nat Clin Pract Endocrinol Metab* (2009) **5**(2):88–99. doi:10.1038/ncpendmet1051

Merchant TE, Goloubeva O, Pritchard DL, Gaber MW, Xiong X, Danish RK, et al. Radiation dose-volume effects on growth hormone secretion. *Int J Radiat Oncol Biol Phys* (2002) **52**(5):1264–70. doi:10.1016/S0360-3016(01)02788-2

Rappaport R, Brauner R. Growth and endocrine disorders secondary to cranial irradiation. *Pediatr Res* (1989) **25**(6):561–7. doi:10.1203/00006450-198906000- 00001

Baroncini M, Jissendi P, Balland E, Besson P, Pruvo JP, Francke JP, et al. MRI atlas of the human hypothalamus. *Neuroimage* (2012) **59**(1):168–80. doi:10.1016/j.neuroimage.2011.07.013

Loes DJ, Barloon TJ, Yuh WT, DeLaPaz RL, Sato Y. MR anatomy and pathology of the hypothalamus. *AJR Am J Roentgenol* (1991) **156**(3):579–85. doi:10.2214/ ajr.156.3.1899763

Toogood AA. Endocrine consequences of brain irradiation. *Growth Horm IGF Res* (2004) **14**(Suppl A):S118–24. doi:10.1016/j.ghir.2004.03.038

Madaschi S, Fiorino C, Losa M, Lanzi R, Mazza E, Motta M, et al. Time course of hypothalamic-pituitary deficiency in adults receiving cranial radiotherapy for primary extrasellar brain tumors. *Radiother Oncol* (2011) **99**(1):23–8. doi:10.1016/j.radonc.2011.02.015

Fernandez A, Brada M, Zabuliene L, Karavitaki N, Wass JA. Radiation-induced hypopituitarism. *Endocr Relat Cancer* (2009) **16**(3):733–72. doi:10.1677/ERC- 08-0231

Sicignano G, Losa M, del Vecchio A, Cattaneo GM, Picozzi P, Bolognesi A, et al. Dosimetric factors associated with pituitary function after gamma knife surgery (GKS) of pituitary adenomas. *Radiother Oncol* (2012) **104**(1):119–24. doi:10.1016/j.radonc.2012.03.021

Kong DS, Lee JI, Lim do H, Kim KW, Shin HJ, Nam DH, et al. The efficacy of fractionated radiotherapy and stereotactic radiosurgery for pituitary adenomas: long-term results of 125 consecutive patients treated in a single institution. *Cancer* (2007) **110**(4):854–60. doi:10.1002/cncr.22860

Feigl GC, Pistracher K, Berghold A, Mokry M. Pituitary insufficiency as a side effect after radiosurgery for pituitary adenomas: the role of the hypothalamus. *J Neurosurg* (2010) **113**(Suppl):153–9. doi:10.3171/2010.8.GKS10959

Agha A, Sherlock M, Brennan S, O'Connor SA, O'Sullivan E, Rogers B, et al. Hypothalamic-pituitary dysfunction after irradiation of nonpituitary brain tumors in adults. *J Clin Endocrinol Metab* (2005) **90**(12):6355–60. doi:10.1210/ jc.2005-1525

Rieken S, Habermehl D, Welzel T, Mohr A, Lindel K, Debus J, et al. Long term toxicity and prognostic factors of radiation therapy for secreting and non-secreting pituitary adenomas. *Radiat Oncol* (2013) **8**:717X–8X. doi:10.1186/1748-717X- 8-18

Platta CS, Mackay C, Welsh JS. Pituitary adenoma: a radiotherapeutic perspective. *Am J Clin Oncol* (2010) **33**(4):408–19. doi:10.1097/COC.0b013e31819d878d

Appelman-Dijkstra NM, Kokshoorn NE, Dekkers OM, Neelis KJ, Biermasz NR, Romijn JA, et al. Pituitary dysfunction in adult patients after cranial radiotherapy: systematic review and meta-analysis. *J Clin Endocrinol Metab* (2011) **96**(8):2330–40. doi:10.1210/jc.2011-0306

Sklar CA, Constine LS. Chronic neuroendocrinological sequelae of radiation therapy. *Int J Radiat Oncol Biol Phys* (1995) **31**(5):1113–21. doi:10.1016/0360-3016(94)00427-M

Merchant TE, Rose SR, Bosley C, Wu S, Xiong X, Lustig RH. Growth hormone secretion after conformal radiation therapy in pediatric patients with localized brain tumors. *J Clin Oncol* (2011) **29**(36):4776–80. doi:10.1200/JCO.2011.37. 9453

Lawrence YR, Li XA, el Naqa I, Hahn CA, Marks LB, Merchant TE, et al. Radiation dose-volume effects in the brain. *Int J Radiat Oncol Biol Phys* (2010) **76**(3 Suppl):S20–7. doi:10.1016/j.ijrobp.2009.02.091

18

The role of the lateral hypothalamus and orexin in ingestive behavior: a model for the translation of past experience and sensed deficits into motivated behaviors

Seth W. Hurley[1] and Alan Kim Johnson[1,2,3,4]*

[1] Department of Psychology, University of Iowa, Iowa City, IA, USA
[2] Department of Pharmacology, University of Iowa, Iowa City, IA, USA
[3] Department of Health and Human Physiology, University of Iowa, Iowa City, IA, USA
[4] François M. Abboud Cardiovascular Center, University of Iowa, Iowa City, IA, USA

***Correspondence:**
Alan Kim Johnson, Department of Psychology, University of Iowa, 11 Seashore Hall E, Iowa City, IA 52242, USA
e-mail: alan-johnson@uiowa.edu

The hypothalamus has been recognized for its involvement in both maintaining homeostasis and mediating motivated behaviors. The present article discusses a region of the hypothalamus known as the lateral hypothalamic area (LHA). It is proposed that brain nuclei within the LHA including the dorsal region of the lateral hypothalamus (LHAd) and perifornical area (PeF) provide a link between neural systems that regulate homeostasis and those that mediate appetitive motivated behaviors. Functional and immunohistochemical data indicate that the LHA promotes many motivated behaviors including food intake, water intake, salt intake, and sexual behavior. Anatomical tracing experiments demonstrate that the LHA is positioned to receive inputs from brain areas involved in regulating body fluid and energy homeostasis. Regions within the LHA send dense projections to the ventral tegmental area (VTA), providing a pathway for the LHA to influence dopaminergic systems generally recognized to be involved in motivated behaviors and their reinforcement. Furthermore, the LHA contains neurons that synthesize orexin/hypocretin, a neuropeptide that promotes many appetitive motivated behaviors. The LHA also receives inputs from brain areas involved in reward-related learning and orexin neuron activation can become conditioned to environmental stimuli that are associated with rewards. Therefore, it is hypothesized that the LHA integrates signaling from areas that regulate body fluid and energy balance and reward-related learning. In turn, this information is "fed into" mesolimbic circuitry to influence the performance of motivated behaviors. This hypothesis may foster experiments that will result in an improved understanding of LHA function. An improved understanding of LHA function may aid in treating disorders that are associated with an excess or impairment in the expression of ingestive behavior including obesity, anorexia, impairments in thirst, salt gluttony, and salt deficiency.

Keywords: motivation, homeostasis, lateral hypothalamus, neural plasticity, salt appetite, thirst, food intake, orexin

INTRODUCTION

In order to survive animals must maintain energy and fluid homeostasis. Calories are continually lost through processes that maintain basic life functions and as a result of behaving. Similarly, terrestrial animals continually lose water and sodium to the environment due to normal physiological and environmental processes including respiration, transpiration, perspiration, urination, and defecation. Some less-common circumstances pose a significant threat to both energy and body fluid homeostasis. For example, sicknesses can evoke states of hypophagia coupled with diarrhea and vomiting that deplete the body of water and sodium. Once the body has become deficient in calories, water, or sodium it is critical for an animal to seek out and ingest substances in the environment to restore homeostasis.

The central nervous system generates motivational states to promote the seeking and ingestion of substances in the environment. The motivational state of hunger, or the seeking and ingestion of food, is necessary for an animal to restore deficits in energy homeostasis. Thirst and sodium appetite (also known as [AKA] salt appetite), or the acquisition and consumption of water and sodium, are necessary to restore fluid balance. These motivated states are accompanied by central nervous system processes that energize behavior (i.e., produce a state of psychological arousal and encourage locomotor behavior) and promote goal directed behavior (Bindra, 1959;

Bolles, 1975). It has been demonstrated that many motivational states are accompanied by a hedonic shift where the pleasurable or aversive responses evoked by specific stimuli are enhanced or inhibited (Garcia et al., 1974; Fanselow and Birk, 1982; Berridge et al., 1984; Mehiel and Bolles, 1988; Berridge and Schulkin, 1989). For example, when sodium-replete rats receive intra-oral infusions of hypertonic saline solutions they exhibit species-specific behavioral responses indicative of aversion (Grill and Norgren, 1978; Berridge et al., 1984) and sodium-replete rats will generally eschew hypertonic saline solutions (Robinson and Berridge, 2013). However, when rats become sodium deficient they exhibit approach behaviors towards saline solutions and will perform responses that are instrumental to obtain sodium (AKA operant responses; Berridge et al., 1984; Clark and Bernstein, 2006; Robinson and Berridge, 2013). Under sodium deficient conditions they even display behavioral responses indicative of pleasure rather than aversion when hypertonic saline solutions are infused intra-orally (Berridge et al., 1984). Similarly, people rate salty foods as more palatable when they are sodium deficient (McCance, 1936; Beauchamp et al., 1990).

The motivated states of hunger, thirst, and salt appetite are strongly influenced by an animal's current state of energy and fluid balance (i.e., homeostatic state). It is reasonable to conceptualize the neural apparatus that monitor energy and fluid homeostasis as sensory systems in their own right. With respect to energy balance, the arcuate nucleus of the hypothalamus (ARH) has received significant attention for its role in sensing peripheral signals related to hunger and satiety (Schwartz et al., 2000). An ensemble of forebrain nuclei lying along the lamina terminalis (LT) are important for detecting signals related to body fluid status (Denton et al., 1996; Johnson and Thunhorst, 1997). The specific structures along the LT are the subfornical organ (SFO), median preoptic area (MnPO), and organum vasculosum of the lamina terminalis (OVLT). To facilitate exposition these structures are collectively referred to as the LT. The SFO and OVLT are sensory circumventricular organs, or brain areas that lack a true blood-brain barrier (Johnson and Gross, 1993) which allows them to monitor substances in the blood that act as indicators of body fluid status (Johnson and Thunhorst, 1997, 2007). It is also worth noting here that there is currently debate as to whether the ARH lacks a blood-brain barrier and is a true circumventricular organ (Mimee et al., 2013). As such, it has been proposed that the LT may also function to detect signals related to energy balance (Mimee et al., 2013; Smith and Ferguson, 2014).

It is important to realize that the ingestion of food, water, and sodium require coordinated activity between neural circuits that sense energy and fluid status and the neural circuitry involved in mobilizing motivated behaviors (Garcia et al., 1974; Roitman et al., 1997; Kelley and Berridge, 2002; Liedtke et al., 2011). Therefore, the brain areas that monitor fluid and energy status must be able to project onto the areas that regulate motivation and reward. One final common pathway that is implicated in the generation of all appetitive motivated behaviors investigated thus far is the dopaminergic projection from the ventral tegmental area (VTA) to the nucleus accumbens (AKA the mesolimbic dopamine system and the A10 dopaminergic cell group; Mogenson et al., 1980; Bozarth, 1994). The ARH and the LT, which are involved in sensing energy and fluid balance, do not appear to directly innervate the VTA (Phillipson, 1979; Geisler and Zahm, 2005; however the ARH does directly project to the nucleus accumbens; Yi et al., 2006; van den Heuvel et al., 2014). As there are no direct projections to the VTA it is likely that areas in the hypothalamus may aid in "bridging the gap" between homeostasis and motivation and reward systems (Mogenson et al., 1980; Swanson and Mogenson, 1981; Swanson and Lind, 1986). For example, retrograde tracing studies have shown that a large region of the hypothalamus contains neurons that project to the VTA (Geisler and Zahm, 2005). This region extends from the dorsomedial hypothalamus (DMH) to the dorsal region of the lateral hypothalamus (LHAd) and appears to be present across the entire anterior-posterior extent of the hypothalamus.

THE EVIDENCE SUPPORTING A ROLE FOR THE LHA IN INTEGRATING HOMEOSTATIC STATE WITH MOTIVATION AND REWARD SYSTEMS

In a classic paper, Stellar (1954) proposed a hypothalamus-centered theory of motivation. Stellar theorized that the hypothalamus contained anatomically dissociable "centers" and each center played a critical role in the promotion of specific motivated behaviors. For example, he posited that the hypothalamus contained centers that specifically control sex, satiety, hunger, and sleep. Stellar's proposal received careful experimental scrutiny and was found to be inadequate to explain emerging data (Miller et al., 1964; Miller, 1965; Hoebel and Teitelbaum, 1966; Booth et al., 1969). Despite the fact that Stellar's theory fell short of elucidating the role of the hypothalamus in specific motivated behaviors, considerable evidence now suggests that areas within the hypothalamus do, in fact, play an important role in promoting appetitive motivated behaviors in general.

Classic experiments that employed short bursts of electrical stimulation directed at the lateral hypothalamic area (LHA) demonstrated that the LHA is involved in motivation and reward processes. Olds and Milner (1954) originally found that rats will perform an operant to obtain acute electrical stimulation of the LHA, an experimental paradigm sometimes referred to as self-stimulation or brain stimulation reward. They interpreted their finding to mean that electrical stimulation of the LHA was rewarding (i.e., LHA stimulation evoked a subjective state of pleasure). If this assessment is correct, it would suggest that some neurons within the LHA are functionally important for coding pleasure from the consumption of rewards. However, others have suggested LHA stimulation may actually produce a subjective state of craving rather than pleasure *per se* (Berridge and Valenstein, 1991). If this interpretation is true it would suggest that a subset of neurons located in the LHAd are involved in the craving that drives animals to seek rewards. It is likely that the motivational and rewarding properties of LHA stimulation are the result of the activation of neurons in the LHA that project to the mesolimbic dopamine system (Phillipson, 1979; Geisler and Zahm, 2005). Recent experiments utilizing anatomical mapping of "hedonic hotspots", or brain areas that appear to code pleasure (Peciña and Berridge, 2000), show that neurons located in the anterior LHA project to a hedonic hotspot in the dorsomedial nucleus accumbens shell (Thompson and Swanson, 2010), and it is possible that LHA stimulation may activate these projection neurons to evoke a sensation of pleasure. Interestingly, if the LHA is stimulated for sufficient intervals (~10–30 s) rats will perform motivated behaviors including drinking, eating, and copulatory behaviors (Wise, 1968). Furthermore, lesions of the LHA abolish food and water intake, copulation, and impair or abolish sodium appetite (Anand and Brobeck, 1951; Montemurro and Stevenson, 1957; Teitelbaum and Epstein, 1962; Wolf, 1964; Wolf and Quartermain, 1967; Cagguila et al., 1973; Grossman et al., 1978; Hansen et al., 1982).

Disruptions in energy or fluid balance alter responding for self-stimulation (Olds, 1958; Morris et al., 2006, 2010). Olds (1958) originally found that food-depriving rats and inducing the motivational state of hunger increased responding for self-stimulation. Furthermore, increased responding for self-stimulation during food deprivation can be prevented by administration of leptin, a hormone that promotes satiety (Fulton et al., 2000). In contrast to food deprivation, sodium depletion reduces responding for self-stimulation (Morris et al., 2010). Reduced responding for self-stimulation is even observed when rats are made salt hungry through administration of an exogenous hormone that promotes salt appetite; despite the fact rats maintain sodium balance during this treatment (Morris et al., 2006). It is unclear as to why the motivational states of hunger and salt appetite produce opposite effects on self-stimulation. However, these studies demonstrate that hunger and salt appetite alter self-stimulation responding and this effect appears to be independent of actual disruptions in energy or fluid homeostasis. For example, leptin normalizes self-stimulation responding without correcting lost calories (Fulton et al., 2000) and self-stimulation responding can be decreased through manipulations that evoke salt hunger without actually inducing a sodium deficit (Morris et al., 2006). Importantly, these experiments support the present hypothesis by showing that the LHA is sensitive to an animal's motivational state.

Some of the strongest evidence supporting a role for the hypothalamus in promoting motivated behavior comes from studies examining orexin (AKA hypocretin). Orexin is a neuropeptide that is expressed primarily in the caudal half of the hypothalamus where it is distributed in an arc that extends from the DMH to the LHAd (**Figure 1**). Orexin appears to be the only known centralized peptide neurotransmitter system as orexin neurons from a relatively circumscribed area send distal projections to diverse brain areas (Peyron et al., 1998). Functionally, orexin neurons have been heavily implicated in a variety of motivated behaviors (Harris et al., 2005; Borgland et al., 2009). Orexin has received significant attention for its capacity to elicit robust food intake (hence the name orexin; Sakurai et al., 1998; Choi et al., 2010) but it is also involved in promoting thirst, salt appetite (Kunii et al., 1999; Hurley et al., 2013a), and reproductive behavior (Muschamp et al., 2007; Di Sebastiano et al., 2010). Orexin neurons can be putatively organized into three cell-clusters in the hypothalamus: a cluster in the DMH, perifornical area (PeF), and the LHAd (**Figure 1**). Both the PeF and LHAd are regions located in the LHA while the DMH lies medially where it abuts the third ventricle. Each orexin cell-cluster contains a subset of orexin neurons that project to the VTA (**Figure 1**; Fadel and Deutch, 2002), and orexin is capable of depolarizing neurons in the VTA (Korotkova et al., 2003). Therefore, orexin neurons provide a mechanism for areas within the LHA to tap into systems traditionally conceived of as being involved in motivation and reward. Evidence also indicates that orexin neurons have direct projections to the nucleus accumbens shell (Peyron et al., 1998; Kampe et al., 2009) where they may act to promote motivated behaviors (Thorpe and Kotz, 2005).

Other major functions of orexin include promoting arousal (Hagan et al., 1999) and sympathetic nervous system responses including the elevation of blood pressure (Samson et al., 1999; Ferguson and Samson, 2003; Kayaba et al., 2003) and the release of stress hormones (Kuru et al., 2000; Spinazzi et al., 2006). It is likely that orexin neurons are activated while an animal is experiencing caloric, hydrational, or sodium deficiency or is in a state of sexual arousal. The subsequent release of orexin throughout the neuraxis encourages the performance of goal-directed behavior by activating brain systems involved in promoting arousal, attention, sympathetic activity, and motivated behavior. Sympathetic activation supports energy mobilization (e.g., increased blood pressure and available glucose levels, and stress hormone release) as well as the redistribution of blood necessary to support increased locomotor activity. Together these central and peripheral responses serve to increase the likelihood that an animal will successfully seek out and consume environmental reinforcers that restore energy and hydrational homeostasis.

Anatomical and immunohistochemical studies support the idea that the LHA aids in integrating signaling from orexigenic peptides with neurocircuitry involved in motivation and reward. Neuropeptide Y (NPY) is expressed in ARH neurons (Hahn et al., 1998) and this neuropeptide induces feeding (Schwartz et al., 2000). Interestingly, NPY neurons send dense projections that are in apposition with orexin neurons located in the LHA (Broberger et al., 1998). Treatments that induce hunger such as hypoglycemia or administration of orexigenic peptides including ghrelin and NPY induce *c-fos* expression in orexin-containing neurons (Moriguchi et al., 1999; Niimi et al., 2001; Toshinai et al., 2003). Additionally, compromising orexin neurotransmission attenuates feeding induced by administration of either NPY or ghrelin. Neurons in the dorsomedial ARH, a region of the ARH that contains a majority of NPY neurons, also project to the PeF and possibly the LHAd (**Figure 2**; Hahn and Swanson, 2010).

In contrast to studies on food intake, relatively little work has been done delineating how the LT may influence motivation and reward neural circuitry. The LT does not appear to directly project to either the VTA (Phillipson, 1979; Geisler and Zahm, 2005) or the nucleus accumbens (Brog et al., 1993), but somehow areas sensing and processing information related to body fluid homeostasis must tap into motivation and reward neurocircuitry. The SFO has been shown to send projections to the DMH, PeF, and LHAd (Swanson and Lind, 1986;

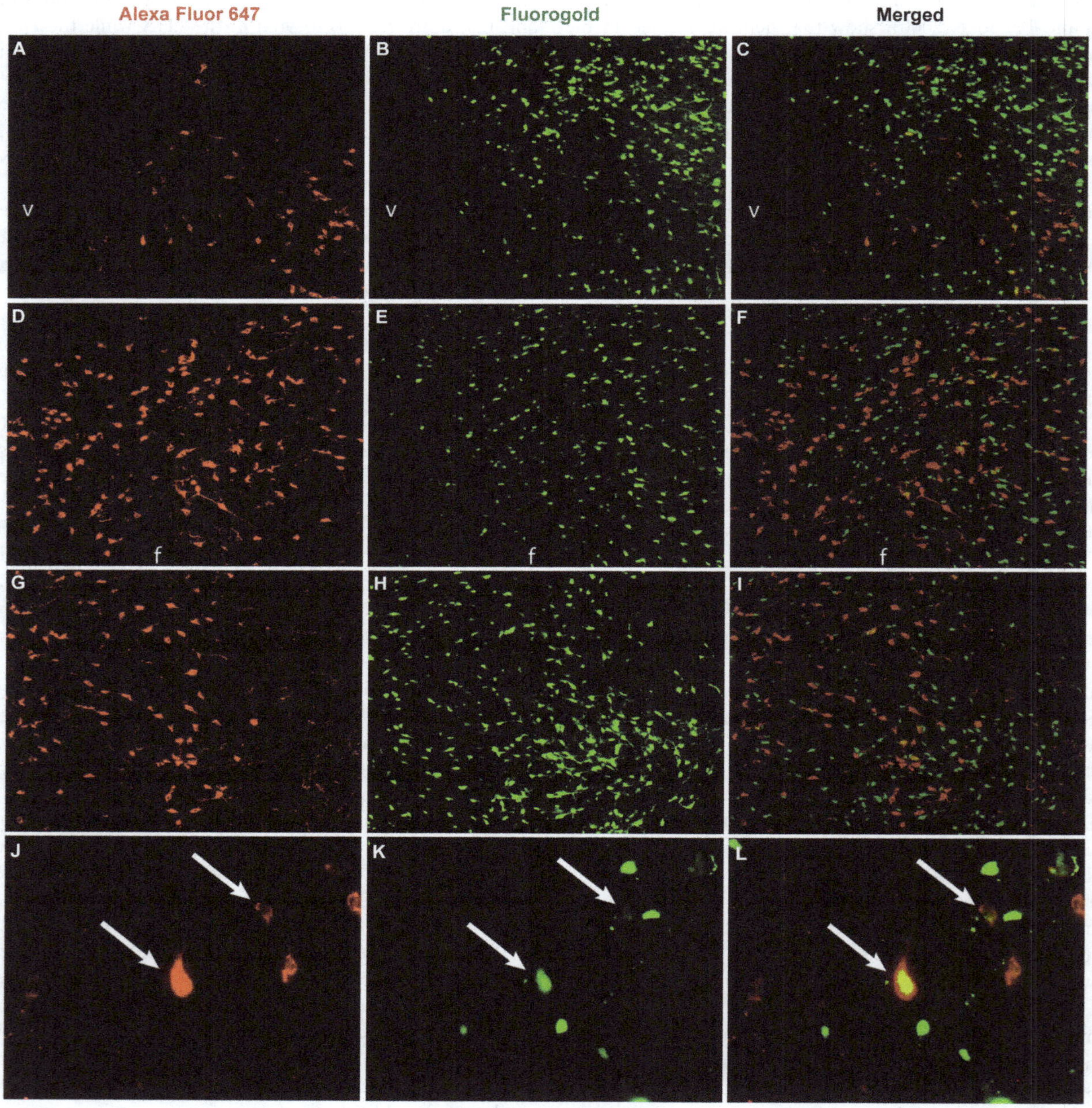

FIGURE 1 | Unpublished data from authors. Co-labeling between orexin and VTA projection neurons in the hypothalamus. The retrograde tracer Fluoro-Gold (Fluorochrome, Denver CO) was microinjected (2% in 250 nl) into the VTA, brains were collected and sliced at 40μm, and then tissue was stained for orexin A immunoreactivity via overnight incubation with an anti-orexin A antibody (1:8000, Phoenix Pharmaceuticals, Burlingame CA) and visualized through incubation with Alexa Fluor 647 (1:200, Jackson ImmunoResearch, West Grove PA) for 1 h. Images **(A–I)** were taken at 10x magnification and images **(J–L)** were taken at 40x. In the DMH **(A–C)**, significant orexin neuron labeling was observed **(A)** in addition to retrogradely labeled neurons from the VTA **(B)**, and some orexin neurons projected to the VTA (**C**, yellow labeling). In the PeF **(D–F)** a subset of orexin neurons **(D)** and retrogradely labeled neurons from the VTA **(E)** co-localized **(F)**. In the LHAd **(G–I)** a subset of orexin neurons **(G)** and retrogradely neurons from the VTA **(H)** colocalized **(I)**. A 40x magnification of labeling observed in the DMH is presented in panels **(J–L)**. Double-labeled neurons are indicated by white arrows. v = ventricle, f = fornix.

Hurley et al., 2013a). Furthermore, recent experiments in our laboratory have shown that iontophoretic application of the retrograde tracer Fluoro-Gold into the posterior portion of the DMH, PeF, and LHAd reveals retrograde labeling across the entirety of the LT (an example of retrograde labeling from an injection that spread from the PeF to the LH is presented in

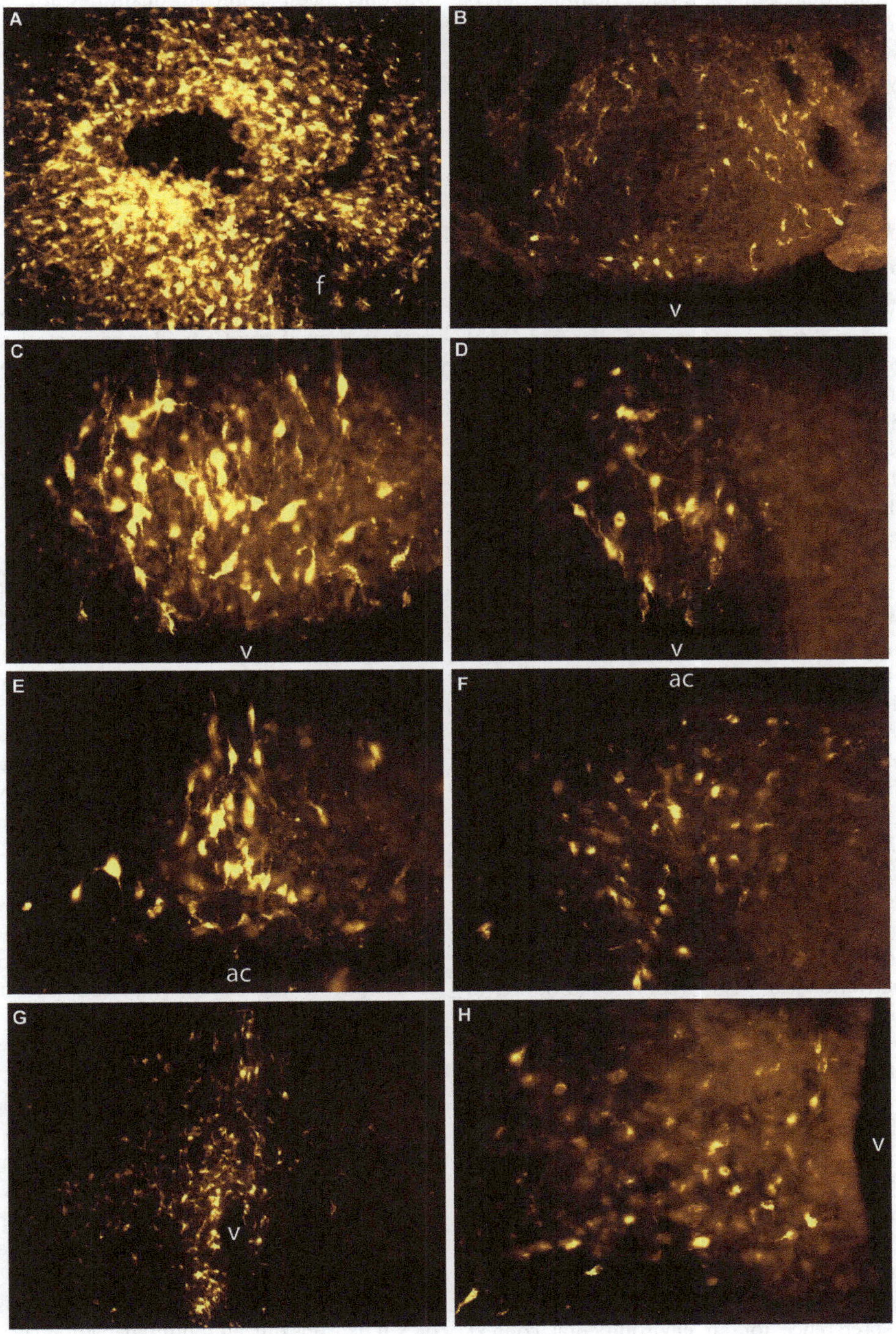

FIGURE 2 | Unpublished data from authors. Retrograde labeling from the LHAd and PeF to the LT and arcuate nucleus of the hypothalamus. 2% Fluoro-Gold in physiological saline was iontophoresed into the PeF and LHAd **(A)**. Retrograde labeling was observed across the LT and in the ARH. Specifically, significant retrograde-labeling was seen in the annulus of the SFO **(B)**, anterior SFO **(C)**, stalk of the SFO **(D)**, dorsal and ventral MnPO **(E, F)**, OVLT **(G)**, and ARH **(H)**. Images were taken at different magnifications to compensate for the size of the brain area. Panels **(A)**, **(B)**, and **(G)** were taken at 10x and **(C)**, **(D)**, **(E)**, **(F)**, and **(H)** were taken at 20x. f = fornix, v = ventricle, ac = anterior commissure.

Figure 2). Others have shown that the PeF receives projections from the entirety of the LT (Hahn and Swanson, 2010). Additionally, we have recently found that orexin neurons are activated when rats depleted of water and sodium are allowed to ingest water and hypertonic saline and that microinjection of an orexin receptor antagonist into the VTA attenuated combined water and sodium intake in depleted rats (Hurley et al., 2013a). Therefore, it is likely that the LT projects to the DMH, PeF and LHAd which, in turn, send orexinergic projections to the VTA. Orexin release in the VTA promotes the ingestion of water and sodium. These experiments provide both anatomical and functional support to the hypothesis that the LHA integrates information about homeostatic state with motivation and reward systems.

THE EVIDENCE SUPPORTING A ROLE FOR THE LHA IN REWARD-RELATED LEARNING

Experiments that examined the effect of sustained LHA stimulation on motivated behaviors provided some of the earliest evidence that the LHA may be involved in reward-related learning. When individual rats receive LHA stimulation they initially exhibit one specific motivated behavior (Valenstein et al., 1970). Some rats will eat, while others will drink or engage in copulatory behaviors. The motivated behavior each rat engages in is referred to as the prepotent behavior. Importantly, the prepotent behavior performed during LHA stimulation can be modified by experience (Valenstein et al., 1970). If the preferred goal object is removed during LHA stimulation, rats will direct their motivated behavior towards another goal object that is present in the environment. For example, if a rat eats during LHA stimulation, food can be removed while a drinking spout remains. In this situation the stimulated rat will now drink from the spout. Importantly, when the LHA is stimulated in future trials when both food and water are present, the rat will essentially split its time between eating and drinking. Therefore, pairing LHA stimulation with the presence of an initially non-preferred goal object causes a rat to direct some of its behavior toward the previously ignored goal object. It appears that LHA stimulation and the subsequent consumption of a goal object results in a form of associative learning that is expressed through changes in prepotent behaviors.

Orexin neuron activation can also become conditioned to stimuli in the environment. In conditioned place preference paradigms a novel environmental context is associated with a reward. After repeated pairings of an environmental context with a reward, rats will exhibit a preference for the context that was paired with reward. The preference that develops in conditioned place preference paradigms appears to be associated with orexin neuron activation. Orexin neurons express *c-fos* in response to environmental contexts that have become associated with drugs of abuse and sex (Harris et al., 2005; Di Sebastiano et al., 2011). Furthermore, lesioning orexin neurons with an orexin conjugated-saporin prevents male rats from exhibiting a conditioned place preference for an environmental context associated with copulation (Di Sebastiano et al., 2011).

Further evidence supporting LHA involvement in associative forms of reward learning comes from the phenomenon of cue-induced feeding. In the cue-induced feeding paradigm, food-deprived rats are allowed to eat in the presence of an environmental cue. This cue essentially becomes a conditioned stimulus (CS+) that is capable of inducing food intake. When the CS+ is presented to rats, even when they are in a satiated state, they will begin eating (Petrovich et al., 2007). Interestingly, rats will only ingest significant quantities of the specific food paired with the CS+, but not novel or familiar foods (Petrovich and Gallagher, 2007). Therefore, it appears that presentation of the CS+ evokes a specific craving for the food paired with the CS+, rather than hunger *per se*. The LHA is one area that is critical for the performance of cue-induced feeding (Petrovich and Gallagher, 2007; Petrovich et al., 2005). The LHA receives inputs from areas involved in associative forms of reward-learning including the amygdala (Krettek and Price, 1978; Everitt et al., 1999) and prefrontal cortex (Gallagher et al., 1999). Neurons that project to the LHA from the basolateral/basomedial amygdala and orbitomedial prefrontal cortex are activated in response to presentation of the CS+ (Petrovich et al., 2005). In addition, contralateral asymmetrical lesions of the basolateral amygdala and LHA prevent cue-induced feeding (Petrovich et al., 2005). Orexin also appears to plays a role in cue-induced feeding as rats exposed to the CS+ express significantly more *c-fos* positive orexin neurons in the PeF (Petrovich et al., 2012).

Finally, the LHA has been implicated in non-associative forms of reward-related learning. When rats are repeatedly depleted of sodium they exhibit an increase in sodium intake (Falk, 1965; Sakai et al., 1987, 1989), a phenomenon termed the sensitization of sodium appetite (Hurley et al., 2013b). Sensitization of sodium appetite is likely to be a form of non-associative learning (Falk, 1966; Frankmann et al., 1986) that is dependent on glutamatergic NMDA receptor-dependent neural plasticity (Hurley and Johnson, 2013). Evidence suggests that sodium appetite sensitization involves neural plasticity in two neural circuits: one circuit governing body fluid homeostasis and another circuit mediating motivation and reward (Roitman et al., 2002; Na et al., 2007). *c-fos* expression induced by sodium depletion is elevated in rats with a history of sodium depletions in the SFO, basolateral amygdala, medial prefrontal cortex, and nucleus accumbens compared to rats with no history of sodium depletions (Na et al., 2007). Furthermore, rats with a history of sodium depletions exhibit enhanced dendritic arborization and length in the nucleus accumbens (Roitman et al., 2002). Many of the areas that appear to undergo sensitization during sodium depletion also send projections to the LHA, including the SFO, prefrontal cortex, and basolateral amygdala. The LHA sends projections to the VTA, which in turn is capable of inducing neural plasticity in nucleus accumbens neurons (Mameli et al., 2009). Finally, additional evidence supports the possibility that orexin neurons undergo neural plasticity from sodium depletion (Liedtke et al., 2011). Activity-regulated cytoskeleton-associated protein, which plays a critical role in neural plasticity (Tzingounis and Nicoll, 2006; Shepherd and Bear, 2011), is upregulated in PeF orexin neurons during sodium depletion (Liedtke et al., 2011).

SYNTHESIS AND CONCLUSIONS

The reviewed experiments support the hypothesis that the LHA contributes to the integration of information related to homeostatic state and past experience with motivation and reward systems. A summary of the anatomical and functional data is presented in **Figure 3**. Nuclei within the LHA, including the PeF and LHAd, receive projections from brain areas that regulate energy and body fluid homeostasis in addition to areas involved

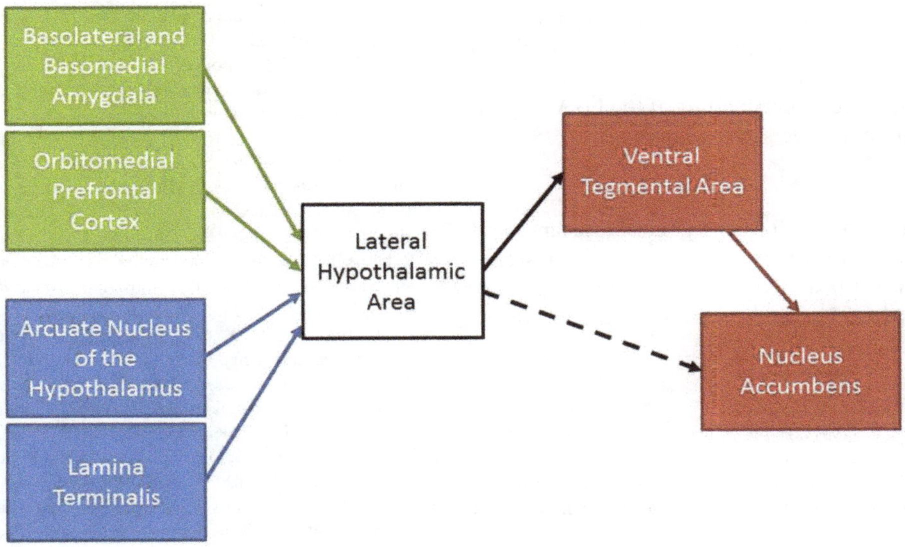

FIGURE 3 | A schematic summary of the reviewed experiments. Areas involved in associative learning (green) and maintaining homeostasis (blue) project to the LHA. The LHA sends projections to motivation and reward areas (red) to initiate motivated behaviors. The LHA also sends projections to the nucleus accumbens that may promote motivated behaviors (dashed line).

in associative learning (Broberger et al., 1998; Petrovich et al., 2005; Hurley et al., 2013a). In turn, these areas of the LHA send projections to the VTA where they promote motivated behaviors, at least partially through the release of orexin in the VTA (Phillipson, 1979; Fadel and Deutch, 2002; Geisler and Zahm, 2005). Although **Figure 3** displays a hierarchical model of LHA functioning dominated by efferent connections to downstream brain areas, it may be the case that this circuitry is actually a neural network which consists of bidirectional inputs between areas involved in learning, homeostasis, and motivation and reward. In this respect, the use of anterograde and retrograde tracer co-injections would provide utility in identifying whether these areas form a neuronal network (for example see Thompson and Swanson, 2010).

As orexin is not exclusively involved in mediating just a single motivated behavior, it is likely that orexin acts to strengthen goal-directed responses associated with several motivated states (Borgland et al., 2009). Cues related to reward presentation and consumption can also induce activation of orexin neurons (Harris et al., 2005; Di Sebastiano et al., 2011; Petrovich et al., 2012), suggesting that past experience influences orexin neuron activity. Therefore, there are at least two conditions that induce orexin neuron activity: (1) the actual seeking and consumption of rewards; and (2) learned associations with rewards. With respect to the second point it is important to point out that orexin can induce neural plasticity in the VTA itself (Borgland et al., 2006). It is unlikely that orexin mediates all of the effects on motivated behaviors observed through manipulations of the LHA, as many projections from the hypothalamus to the VTA are non-orexinergic.

Future work that aims to carefully investigate the role of nuclei located within the LHA will prove fruitful. The LHA actually consists of a collection of heterogeneous brain areas that have unique neuroanatomical connections and cytoarchitecture (Swanson et al., 2005; Hahn and Swanson, 2010). Furthermore, it appears that separate orexin neuron clusters are activated under different experimental conditions (Harris et al., 2005; Harris and Aston-Jones, 2006; Petrovich et al., 2012). Optogenetic manipulations provide a method to test whether these orexin cell clusters have a functionally significant projection to the VTA or nucleus accumbens. Additionally, inactivation of orexin cell clusters should influence the activity of VTA and nucleus accumbens neurons. Finally, it is worth noting that many of the discussed experiments did not dissociate and define the roles of brain nuclei within the LHA and did not discuss the role of the DMH in motivated behaviors. The DMH also receives projections from body fluid homeostasis areas (Swanson and Lind, 1986), sends projections to the VTA (Geisler and Zahm, 2005), and contains orexin neurons (Fadel and Deutch, 2002), all of which are potentially involved in homeostatic behaviors.

HEALTH IMPLICATIONS

From a behavioral perspective, some disorders can be conceived of as problems of ingestion. For example, anorexics fail to ingest sufficient amounts of food while those suffering from obesity ingest too much food. Similarly, some individuals ingest far too much sodium; a phenomenon sometimes referred to as salt gluttony (Schulkin, 1986), while others ingest too little sodium and consequently become sodium deficient causing them to experience autonomic and cardiovascular dysfunction (Bou-Holaigah et al., 1995). Additionally, elderly individuals may exhibit diminished thirst and subsequent dehydration (Rolls and Phillips, 1990; Warren et al., 1994). One approach to understanding these maladies that are marked by a surplus or surfeit in ingestive behavior is to conceive of them as problems of central nervous system functioning related to maintaining homeostasis and appropriately engaging in motivated behavior. As the LHA is critically involved in both maintaining homeostasis and mediating motivated behaviors, an improved understanding of the LHA may aid in diagnosing and treating disorders of ingestion.

ACKNOWLEDGMENTS

The authors thank Young In Kim for her technical assistance and Marilyn Dennis for comments on the manuscript. This research was supported by National Institutes of Health grants HL14388, HL098207, and MH08241. The authors have no disclosures to report.

REFERENCES

Anand, B. K., and Brobeck, J. R. (1951). Hypothalamic control of food intake in rats and cats. *Yale J. Biol. Med.* 24, 123–140.

Beauchamp, G. K., Bertino, M., Burke, D., and Engelman, K. (1990). Experimental sodium depletion and salt taste in normal human volunteers. *Am. J. Clin. Nutr.* 51, 881–889.

Berridge, K. C., Flynn, F. W., Schulkin, J., and Grill, H. J. (1984). Sodium depletion enhances salt palatability in rats. *Behav. Neurosci.* 98, 652–660. doi: 10.1037//0735-7044.98.4.652

Berridge, K. C., and Schulkin, J. (1989). Palatability shift of a salt-associated incentive during sodium depletion. *Q. J. Exp. Psychol. B* 41, 121–138.

Berridge, K. C., and Valenstein, E. S. (1991). What psychological process mediates feeding evoked by electrical stimulation of the lateral hypothalamus? *Behav. Neurosci.* 105, 3–14. doi: 10.1037//0735-7044.105.1.3

Bindra, D. (1959). *Motivation: A Systematic Reinterpretation.* New York, NY: John Wiley and Sons.

Bolles, R. C. (1975). *Theory of Motivation.* 2 Edn., New York: Harper and Row.

Booth, D. A., Coons, E. E., and Miller, N. E. (1969). Blood glucose responses to electrical stimulation of the hypothalamic feeding area. *Physiol. Behav.* 4, 991–1001. doi: 10.1016/0031-9384(69)90055-9

Borgland, S. L., Chang, S. J., Bowers, M. S., Thompson, J. L., Vittoz, N., Floresco, S. B., et al. (2009). Orexin A/hypocretin-1 selectively promotes motivation for positive reinforcers. *J. Neurosci.* 29, 11215–11225. doi: 10.1523/jneurosci.6096-08.2009

Borgland, S. L., Taha, S. A., Sarti, F., Fields, H. L., and Bonci, A. (2006). Orexin A in the VTA is critical for the induction of synaptic plasticity and behavioral sensitization to cocaine. *Neuron* 49, 589–601. doi: 10.1016/j.neuron.2006.01.016

Bou-Holaigah, I., Rowe, P. C., Kan, J., and Calkins, H. (1995). The relationship between neurally mediated hypotension and the chronic fatigue syndrome. *JAMA* 274, 961–967. doi: 10.1001/jama.274.12.961

Bozarth, M. A. (1994). "Pleasure systems in the brain," in *Pleasure: The Politics and the Reality*, ed D. M. Warburton (New York, NY: John Wiley and Sons), 5–14.

Broberger, C., De Lecea, L., Sutcliffe, J., and Hökfelt, T. (1998). Hypocretin/orexin- and melanin-concentrating hormone-expressing cells form distinct populations in the rodent lateral hypothalamus: relationship to the neuropeptide Y and agouti gene-related protein systems. *J. Comp. Neurol.* 402, 460–474. doi: 10.1002/(sici)1096-9861(19981228)402:4<460::aid-cne3>3.3.co;2-j

Brog, J. S., Salyapongse, A., Deutch, A. Y., and Zahm, D. S. (1993). The patterns of afferent innervation of the core and shell in the "Accumbens" part of the rat ventral striatum: immunohistochemical detection of retrogradely transported fluoro gold. *J. Comp. Neurol.* 338, 255–278. doi: 10.1002/cne.903380209

Cagguila, A. R., Antelman, S. M., and Zigmond, M. J. (1973). Disruption of copulation in male rats after hypothalamic lesions: a behavioral, anatomical and neurochemical analysis. *Brain Res.* 59, 273–287. doi: 10.1016/0006-8993(73)90266-7

Choi, D., Davis, J., Fitzgerald, M., and Benoit, S. (2010). The role of orexin-A in food motivation, reward-based feeding behavior and food-induced neuronal activation in rats. *Neuroscience* 167, 11–20. doi: 10.1016/j.neuroscience.2010.02.002

Clark, J. J., and Bernstein, I. L. (2006). Sensitization of salt appetite is associated with increased "wanting" but not "liking" of a salt reward in the sodium-deplete rat. *Behav. Neurosci.* 120, 206–210. doi: 10.1037/0735-7044.120.1.206

Denton, D. A., McKinley, M. J., and Weisinger, R. S. (1996). Hypothalamic integration of body fluid regulation. *Proc. Natl. Acad. Sci. U S A* 93, 7397–7404. doi: 10.1073/pnas.93.14.7397

Di Sebastiano, A. R., Wilson-Pérez, H. E., Lehman, M. N., and Coolen, L. M. (2011). Lesions of orexin neurons block conditioned place preference for sexual behavior in male rats. *Horm. Behav.* 59, 1–8. doi: 10.1016/j.yhbeh.2010.09 006

Di Sebastiano, A. R., Yong-Yow, S., Wagner, L., Lehman, M. N., and Coolen, L. M. (2010). Orexin mediates initiation of sexual behavior in sexually naive male rats, but is not critical for sexual performance. *Horm. Behav.* 58, 397–404. doi: 10.1016/j.yhbeh.2010.06.004

Everitt, B. J., Parkinson, J. A., Olmstead, M. C., Arroyo, M., Robledo, P., and Robbins, T. W. (1999). Associative processes in addiction and reward the role of amygdala-ventral striatal subsystems. *Ann. N Y Acad. Sci.* 877, 412–438. doi: 10.1111/j.1749-6632.1999.tb09280.x

Fadel, J., and Deutch, A. (2002). Anatomical substrates of orexin-dopamine interactions: lateral hypothalamic projections to the ventral tegmental area. *Neuroscience* 111, 379–387. doi: 10.1016/s0306-4522(02)00017-9

Falk, J. L. (1965). Water intake and NaCl appetite in sodium depletion. *Psychol. Rep.* 16, 315–325. doi: 10.2466/pr0.1965.16.1.315

Falk, J. L. (1966). Serial sodium depletion and NaCl solution intake. *Physiol. Behav.* 1, 75–77. doi: 10.1016/0031-9384(66)90044-8

Fanselow, M. S., and Birk, J. (1982). Flavor-flavor associations induce hedonic shifts in taste preference. *Anim. Learn. Behav.* 10, 223–228. doi: 10.3758/bf03212274

Ferguson, A. V., and Samson, W. K. (2003). The orexin/hypocretin system: a critical regulator of neuroendocrine and autonomic function. *Front. Neuroendocrinol.* 24, 141–150. doi: 10.1016/s0091-3022(03)00028-1

Frankmann, S. P., Dorsa, D. M., Sakai, R. R., and Simpson, J. B. (1986). "A single experience with hyperoncotic colloid dialysis persistently alters water and sodium intake," in *The Physiology of Thirst and Sodium Appetite*, eds G. E. de Caro, A. N. Epstein and M. Massi (New York, NY: Plenum Press), 115–121.

Fulton, S., Woodside, B., and Shizgal, P. (2000). Modulation of brain reward circuitry by leptin. *Science* 287, 125–128. doi: 10.1126/science.287.5450.125

Gallagher, M., McMahan, R. W., and Schoenbaum, G. (1999). Orbitofrontal cortex and representation of incentive value in associative learning. *J. Neurosci.* 19, 6610–6614.

Garcia, J., Hankins, W. G., and Rusiniak, K. W. (1974). Behavioral regulation of the milieu interne in man and rat. *Science* 185, 824–831. doi: 10.1126/science.185.4154.824

Geisler, S., and Zahm, D. S. (2005). Afferents of the ventral tegmental area in the rat-anatomical substratum for integrative functions. *J. Comp. Neurol.* 490, 270–294. doi: 10.1002/cne.20668

Grill, H. J., and Norgren, R. (1978). The taste reactivity test. I. Mimetic responses to gustatory stimuli in neurologically normal rats. *Brain Res.* 143, 263–279. doi: 10.1016/0006-8993(78)90568-1

Grossman, S. P., Dacey, D., Halaris, A. E., Collier, T., and Routtenberg, A. (1978). Aphagia and adipsia after preferential destruction of nerve cell bodies in hypothalamus. *Science* 202, 537–539. doi: 10.1126/science.705344

Hagan, J. J., Leslie, R. A., Patel, S., Evans, M. L., Wattam, T. A., Holmes, S., et al. (1999). Orexin A activates locus coeruleus cell firing and increases arousal in the rat. *Proc. Natl. Acad. Sci. U S A* 96, 10911–10916. doi: 10.1073/pnas.96.19.10911

Hahn, T. M., Breininger, J. F., Baskin, D. G., and Schwartz, M. W. (1998). Coexpression of Agrp and NPY in fasting-activated hypothalamic neurons. *Nat. Neurosci.* 1, 271–272.

Hahn, J. D., and Swanson, L. W. (2010). Distinct patterns of neuronal inputs and outputs of the juxtaparaventricular and suprafornical regions of the lateral hypothalamic area in the male rat. *Brain Res. Rev.* 64, 14–103. doi: 10.1016/j.brainresrev.2010.02.002

Hansen, S., Goldstein, M., and Steinbusch, H. (1982). Effects of ibotenic acid-induced neuronal degeneration in the medial preoptic area and the lateral hypothalamic area on sexual behavior in the male rat. *Brain Res.* 239, 213–232. doi: 10.1016/0006-8993(82)90843-5

Harris, G. C., and Aston-Jones, G. (2006). Arousal and reward: a dichotomy in orexin function. *Trends Neurosci.* 29, 571–577. doi: 10.1016/j.tins.2006.08.002

Harris, G. C., Wimmer, M., and Aston-Jones, G. (2005). A role for lateral hypothalamic orexin neurons in reward seeking. *Nature* 437, 556–559. doi: 10.1038/nature04071

Hoebel, B. G., and Teitelbaum, P. (1966). Weight regulation in normal and hypothalamic hyperphagic rats. *J. Comp. Physiol. Psychol.* 61, 189–193. doi: 10.1037/h0023126

Hurley, S. W., Arseth, H. A., and Johnson, A. K. (2013a). "A role for orexin neurons in water and sodium intake," in *Society for Neuroscience* (San Diego, CA).

Hurley, S. W., and Johnson, A. K. (2013). Dissociation of thirst and sodium appetite in the furo/cap model of extracellular dehydration and a role for N-methyl-D-aspartate receptors in the sensitization of sodium appetite. *Behav. Neurosci.* 127, 890–898. doi: 10.1037/a0034948

Hurley, S. W., Thunhorst, R. L., and Johnson, A. K. (2013b). "Sodium appetite sensitization," in *Neurobiology of Body Fluid Homeostasis: Transduction and Integration (Series IV: Frontiers in Neuroscience)*, eds L. A. De Luca, A. K. Johnson and J. V. Menani (Boca Raton, FL: Taylor and Francis), 279–301.

Johnson, A. K., and Gross, P. M. (1993). Sensory circumventricular organs and brain homeostatic pathways. *FASEB J.* 7, 678–686.

Johnson, A. K., and Thunhorst, R. L. (1997). The neuroendocrinology of thirst and salt appetite: visceral sensory signals and mechanisms of central integration. *Front. Neuroendocrinol.* 18, 292–353. doi: 10.1006/frne.1997.0153

Johnson, A., and Thunhorst, R. (2007). The neuroendocrinology, neurochemistry and molecular biology of thirst and salt appetite. *Handb. Neurochem. Mol. Neurobiol. Behav. Neurochem. Neuroendocrinol. Mol. Neurobiol.* 3, 641–687. doi: 10.1007/978-0-387-30405-2_17

Kampe, J., Tschöp, M. H., Hollis, J. H., and Oldfield, B. J. (2009). An anatomic basis for the communication of hypothalamic, cortical and mesolimbic circuitry in the regulation of energy balance. *Eur. J. Neurosci.* 30, 415–430. doi: 10.1111/j.1460-9568.2009.06818.x

Kayaba, Y., Nakamura, A., Kasuya, Y., Ohuchi, T., Yanagisawa, M., Komuro, I., et al. (2003). Attenuated defense response and low basal blood pressure in orexin knockout mice. *Am. J. Physiol. Regul. Integr. Comp. Physiol.* 285, R581–R593. doi: 10.1152/ajpregu.00671.2002

Kelley, A. E., and Berridge, K. C. (2002). The neuroscience of natural rewards: relevance to addictive drugs. *J. Neurosci.* 22, 3306–3311.

Korotkova, T. M., Sergeeva, O. A., Eriksson, K. S., Haas, H. L., and Brown, R. E. (2003). Excitation of ventral tegmental area dopaminergic and nondopaminergic neurons by orexins/hypocretins. *J. Neurosci.* 23, 7–11.

Krettek, J. E., and Price, J. L. (1978). Amygdaloid projections to subcortical structures within the basal forebrain and brainstem in the rat and cat. *J. Comp. Neurol.* 178, 225–253. doi: 10.1002/cne.901780204

Kunii, K., Yamanaka, A., Nambu, T., Matsuzaki, I., Goto, K., and Sakurai, T. (1999). Orexins/hypocretins regulate drinking behaviour. *Brain Res.* 842, 256–261. doi: 10.1016/s0006-8993(99)01884-3

Kuru, M., Ueta, Y., Serino, R., Nakazato, M., Yamamoto, Y., Shibuya, I., et al. (2000). Centrally administered orexin/hypocretin activates HPA axis in rats. *Neuroreport* 11, 1977–1980. doi: 10.1097/00001756-200006260-00034

Liedtke, W. B., McKinley, M. J., Walker, L. L., Zhang, H., Pfenning, A. R., Drago, J., et al. (2011). Relation of addiction genes to hypothalamic gene changes subserving genesis and gratification of a classic instinct, sodium appetite. *Proc. Natl. Acad. Sci. U S A* 108, 12509–12514. doi: 10.1073/pnas.1109199108

Mameli, M., Halbout, B., Creton, C., Engblom, D., Parkitna, J. R., Spanagel, R., et al. (2009). Cocaine-evoked synaptic plasticity: persistence in the VTA triggers adaptations in the NAc. *Nat. Neurosci.* 12, 1036–1041. doi: 10.1038/nn.2367

McCance, R. A. (1936). Experimental sodium chloride deficiency in man. *Proc. R. Soc. Lond. B Biol. Sci.* 119, 245–268. doi: 10.1098/rspb.1936.0009

Mehiel, R., and Bolles, R. C. (1988). Hedonic shift learning based on calories. *Bull. Psychon. Soc.* 26, 459–462. doi: 10.3758/bf03334913

Miller, N. E. (1965). Chemical coding of behavior in the brain. *Science* 148, 328–338. doi: 10.1126/science.148.3668.328

Miller, N. E., Gottesman, K. S., and Emery, N. (1964). Dose response to carbachol and norepinephrine in rat hypothalamus. *Am. J. Physiol.* 206, 1384–1388.

Mimee, A., Smith, P. M., and Ferguson, A. V. (2013). Circumventricular organs: targets for integration of circulating fluid and energy balance signals? *Physiol. Behav.* 121, 96–102. doi: 10.1016/j.physbeh.2013.02.012

Mogenson, G. J., Jones, D. L., and Yim, C. Y. (1980). From motivation to action: functional interface between the limbic system and the motor system. *Prog. Neurobiol.* 14, 69–97. doi: 10.1016/0301-0082(80)90018-0

Montemurro, D., and Stevenson, J. (1957). Adipsia produced by hypothalamic lesions in the rat. *Can. J. Biochem. Physiol.* 35, 31–37. doi: 10.1139/o57-005

Moriguchi, T., Sakurai, T., Nambu, T., Yanagisawa, M., and Goto, K. (1999). Neurons containing orexin in the lateral hypothalamic area of the adult rat brain are activated by insulin-induced acute hypoglycemia. *Neurosci. Lett.* 264, 101–104. doi: 10.1016/s0304-3940(99)00177-9

Morris, M. J., Na, E. S., Grippo, A. J., and Johnson, A. K. (2006). The effects of deoxycorticosterone-induced sodium appetite on hedonic behaviors in the rat. *Behav. Neurosci.* 120, 571–578. doi: 10.1037/0735-7044.120.3.571

Morris, M. J., Na, E. S., and Johnson, A. K. (2010). Mineralocorticoid receptor antagonism prevents hedonic deficits induced by a chronic sodium appetite. *Behav. Neurosci.* 124, 211–224. doi: 10.1037/a0018910

Muschamp, J. W., Dominguez, J. M., Sato, S. M., Shen, R. Y., and Hull, E. M. (2007). A role for hypocretin (orexin) in male sexual behavior. *J. Neurosci.* 27, 2837–2845. doi: 10.1523/jneurosci.4121-06.2007

Na, E. S., Morris, M. J., Johnson, R. F., Beltz, T. G., and Johnson, A. K. (2007). The neural substrates of enhanced salt appetite after repeated sodium depletions. *Brain Res.* 1171, 104–110. doi: 10.1016/j.brainres.2007.07.033

Niimi, M., Sato, M., and Taminato, T. (2001). Neuropeptide Y in central control of feeding and interactions with orexin and leptin. *Endocrine* 14, 269–273. doi: 10.1385/ENDO:14:2:269

Olds, J. (1958). Effects of hunger and male sex hormone on self-stimulation of the brain. *J. Comp. Physiol. Psychol.* 51, 320–324. doi: 10.1037/h0040783

Olds, J., and Milner, P. (1954). Positive reinforcement produced by electrical stimulation of septal area and other regions of rat brain. *J. Comp. Physiol. Psychol.* 47, 419–427. doi: 10.1037/h0058775

Peciña, S., and Berridge, K. C. (2000). Opioid site in nucleus accumbens shell mediates eating and hedonic 'liking' for food: map based on microinjection Fos plumes. *Brain Res.* 863, 71–86. doi: 10.1016/s0006-8993(00)02102-8

Petrovich, G. D., and Gallagher, M. (2007). Control of food consumption by learned cues: a forebrain-hypothalamic network. *Physiol. Behav.* 91, 397–403. doi: 10.1016/j.physbeh.2007.04.014

Petrovich, G., Hobin, M., and Reppucci, C. (2012). Selective Fos induction in hypothalamic orexin/hypocretin, but not melanin-concentrating hormone neurons, by a learned food-cue that stimulates feeding in sated rats. *Neuroscience* 224, 70–80. doi: 10.1016/j.neuroscience.2012.08.036

Petrovich, G. D., Holland, P. C., and Gallagher, M. (2005). Amygdalar and prefrontal pathways to the lateral hypothalamus are activated by a learned cue that stimulates eating. *J. Neurosci.* 25, 8295–8302. doi: 10.1523/jneurosci.2480-05.2005

Petrovich, G. D., Ross, C. A., Gallagher, M., and Holland, P. C. (2007). Learned contextual cue potentiates eating in rats. *Physiol. Behav.* 90, 362–367. doi: 10.1016/j.physbeh.2006.09.031

Peyron, C., Tighe, D. K., van den Pol, A. N., de Lecea, L., Heller, H. C., Sutcliffe, J. G., et al. (1998). Neurons containing hypocretin (orexin) project to multiple neuronal systems. *J. Neurosci.* 18, 9996–10015.

Phillipson, O. (1979). Afferent projections to the ventral tegmental area of Tsai and interfascicular nucleus a horseradish peroxidase study in the rat. *J. Comp. Neurol.* 187, 117–143. doi: 10.1002/cne.901870108

Robinson, M. J., and Berridge, K. C. (2013). Instant transformation of learned repulsion into motivational "wanting". *Curr. Biol.* 23, 282–289. doi: 10.1016/j.cub.2013.01.016

Roitman, M. F., Na, E., Anderson, G., Jones, T. A., and Bernstein, I. L. (2002). Induction of a salt appetite alters dendritic morphology in nucleus accumbens and sensitizes rats to amphetamine. *J. Neurosci.* 22, RC225–RC230.

Roitman, M. F., Schafe, G. E., Thiele, T. E., and Bernstein, I. L. (1997). Dopamine and sodium appetite: antagonists suppress sham drinking of NaCl solutions in the rat. *Behav. Neurosci.* 111, 606–611. doi: 10.1037//0735-7044.111.3.606

Rolls, B. J., and Phillips, P. A. (1990). Aging and disturbances of thirst and fluid balance. *Nutr. Rev.* 48, 137–144. doi: 10.1111/j.1753-4887.1990.tb02915.x

Sakai, R. R., Fine, W. B., Epstein, A. N., and Frankmann, S. P. (1987). Salt appetite is enhanced by one prior episode of sodium depletion in the rat. *Behav. Neurosci.* 101, 724–731. doi: 10.1037//0735-7044.101.5.724

Sakai, R. R., Frankmann, S. P., Fine, W. B., and Epstein, A. N. (1989). Prior episodes of sodium depletion increase the need-free sodium intake of the rat. *Behav. Neurosci.* 103, 186–192. doi: 10.1037//0735-7044.103.1.186

Sakurai, T., Amemiya, A., Ishii, M., Matsuzaki, I., Chemelli, R. M., Tanaka, H., et al. (1998). Orexins and orexin receptors: a family of hypothalamic neuropeptides and G protein-coupled receptors that regulate feeding behavior. *Cell* 92, 573–585. doi: 10.1016/s0092-8674(00)80949-6

Samson, W. K., Gosnell, B., Chang, J., Resch, Z. T., and Murphy, T. C. (1999). Cardiovascular regulatory actions of the hypocretins in brain. *Brain Res.* 831, 248–253. doi: 10.1016/s0006-8993(99)01457-2

Schulkin, J. (1986). "The evolution and expression of salt appetite," in *The Physiology of Thirst and Sodium Appetite*, eds G. De Caro A. N. Epstein and M. Massi (New York: Plenum Press), 491–496).

Schwartz, M. W., Woods, S. C., Porte, D., Seeley, R. J., and Baskin, D. G. (2000). Central nervous system control of food intake. *Nature* 404, 661–671. doi: 10.1038/35007534

Shepherd, J. D., and Bear, M. F. (2011). New views of Arc, a master regulator of synaptic plasticity. *Nat. Neurosci.* 14, 279–284. doi: 10.1038/nn.2708

Smith, P. M., and Ferguson, A. V. (2014). Metabolic signaling to the central nervous system: routes across the blood brain barrier. *Curr. Pharm. Des.* 20, 1392–1399. doi: 10.2174/13816128113199990560

Spinazzi, R., Andreis, P. G., Rossi, G. P., and Nussdorfer, G. G. (2006). Orexins in the regulation of the hypothalamic-pituitary-adrenal axis. *Pharmacol. Rev.* 58, 46–57. doi: 10.1124/pr.58.1.4

Stellar, E. (1954). The physiology of motivation. *Psychol. Rev.* 61, 5–22. doi: 10.1037/h0060347

Swanson, L., and Lind, R. (1986). Neural projections subserving the initiation of a specific motivated behavior in the rat: new projections from the subfornical organ. *Brain Res.* 379, 399–403. doi: 10.1016/0006-8993(86)90799-7

Swanson, L., and Mogenson, G. (1981). Neural mechanisms for the functional coupling of autonomic, endocrine and somatomotor responses in adaptive behavior. *Brain Res.* 3, 1–34. doi: 10.1016/0165-0173(81)90010-2

Swanson, L. W., Sanchez-Watts, G., and Watts, A. G. (2005). Comparison of melanin-concentrating hormone and hypocretin/orexin mRNA expression patterns in a new parceling scheme of the lateral hypothalamic zone. *Neurosci. Lett.* 387, 80–84. doi: 10.1016/j.neulet.2005.06.066

Teitelbaum, P., and Epstein, A. N. (1962). The lateral hypothalamic syndrome: recovery of feeding and drinking after lateral hypothalamic lesions. *Psychol. Rev.* 69, 74–90. doi: 10.1037/h0039285

Thompson, R. H., and Swanson, L. W. (2010). Hypothesis-driven structural connectivity analysis supports network over hierarchical model of brain architecture. *Proc. Natl. Acad. Sci. U S A* 107, 15235–15239. doi: 10.1073/pnas.1009112107

Thorpe, A., and Kotz, C. (2005). Orexin A in the nucleus accumbens stimulates feeding and locomotor activity. *Brain Res.* 1050, 156–162. doi: 10.1016/j.brainres.2005.05.045

Toshinai, K., Date, Y., Murakami, N., Shimada, M., Mondal, M. S., Shimbara, T., et al. (2003). Ghrelin-induced food intake is mediated via the orexin pathway. *Endocrinology* 144, 1506–1512. doi: 10.1210/en.2002-220788

Tzingounis, A. V., and Nicoll, R. A. (2006). Arc/Arg3. 1: linking gene expression to synaptic plasticity and memory. *Neuron* 52, 403–407. doi: 10.1016/j.neuron.2006.10.016

Valenstein, E. S., Cox, V. C., and Kakolewski, J. W. (1970). Reexamination of the role of the hypothalamus in motivation. *Psychol. Rev.* 77, 16–31. doi: 10.1037/h0028581

van den Heuvel, J. K., Furman, K., Gumbs, M. C., Eggels, L., Opland, D. M., Land, B. B., et al. (2014). Neuropeptide Y activity in the nucleus accumbens modulates feeding behavior and neuronal activity. *Biol. Psychiatry* doi: 10.1016/j.biopsych.2014.06.008. [Epub ahead of print].

Warren, J. L., Bacon, W. E., Harris, T., McBean, A. M., Foley, D. J., and Phillips, C. (1994). The burden and outcomes associated with dehydration among US elderly, 1991. *Am. J. Public Health* 84, 1265–1269. doi: 10.2105/ajph.84.8.1265

Wise, R. A. (1968). Hypothalamic motivational systems: fixed or plastic neural circuits? *Science* 162, 377–379. doi: 10.1126/science.162.3851.377

Wolf, G. (1964). Effect of dorsolateral hypothalamic lesions on sodium appetite elicited by desoxycorticosterone and by acute hyponatremia. *J. Comp. Physiol. Psychol.* 58, 396–402. doi: 10.1037/h0048232

Wolf, G., and Quartermain, D. (1967). Sodium chloride intake of adrenalectomized rats with lateral hypothalamic lesions. *Am. J. Physiol.* 212, 113–118.

Yi, C. X., van der Vliet, J., Dai, J., Yin, G., Ru, L., and Buijs, R. M. (2006). Ventromedial arcuate nucleus communicates peripheral metabolic information to the suprachiasmatic nucleus. *Endocrinology* 147, 283–294. doi: 10.1210/en.2005-1051

19

Hypothalamic obesity after craniopharyngioma: mechanisms, diagnosis and treatment

Robert H. Lustig*

Department of Pediatrics, University of California San Francisco, San Francisco, CA, USA

***Correspondence:**
Robert H. Lustig, Division of Pediatric Endocrinology, University of California San Francisco, Box 0434, 500 Parnassus Avenue, San Francisco, CA 94143-0434, USA.
e-mail: rlustig@peds.ucsf.edu

Obesity is a common complication after craniopharyngioma therapy, occurring in up to 75% of survivors. Its weight gain is unlike that of normal obesity, in that it occurs even with caloric restriction, and attempts at lifestyle modification are useless to prevent or treat the obesity. The pathogenesis of this condition involves the inability to transduce afferent hormonal signals of adiposity, in effect mimicking a state of CNS starvation. Efferent sympathetic activity drops, resulting in malaise and reduced energy expenditure, and vagal activity increases, resulting in increased insulin secretion and adipogenesis. Lifestyle intervention is essentially useless in this syndrome, termed "hypothalamic obesity." Pharmacologic treatment is also difficult, consisting of adrenergics to mimic sympathetic activity, or suppression of insulin secretion with octreotide, or both. Recently, bariatric surgery (Roux-en-Y gastric bypass, laparoscopic gastric banding, truncal vagotomy) have also been attempted with variable results. Early and intensive management is required to mitigate the obesity and its negative consequences.

Keywords: craniopharyngioma, hypothalamic obesity, leptin resistance, insulin, octreotide, vagus nerve, sympathetic nervous system, ghrelin

INTRODUCTION

When it comes to brain tumors, the three laws of New York real estate prevail: "Location, location, location." Craniopharyngiomas are problematic less for *what* they are than for *where* they are. The hypothalamus, as is true for most hormonal systems, is the anatomic seat of peripheral energy regulation. When the hypothalamus is damaged, a syndrome of intractable weight gain ensues. This syndrome, termed "hypothalamic obesity," originally described by Babinski (1900) and Frohlich (1901) at the turn of the twentieth century, documents the "organicity" of obesity. Hypothalamic obesity can occur due to the tumor itself, the surgery to extirpate it, or due to subsequent radiation therapy (Bray, 1984; Lustig, 2002). Although this co-morbidity usually manifests in children due to their increased incidence of tumors localized to the posterior fossa (Stahnke et al., 1984; Sorva, 1988; Pinto et al., 2000), adults can also exhibit similar weight gain after completion of therapy (Daousi et al., 2005). Craniopharyngioma accounts for half of the reported cases, with other posterior fossa tumors each contributing smaller numbers. However, the syndrome has also been reported in cases of pseudotumor cerebri, trauma, and infiltrative or inflammatory diseases of the hypothalamus (Bray, 1984).

INCIDENCE AND RISK FACTORS

Hypothalamic obesity can occur in response to any hypothalamic damage. Most studies have been performed in the acute lymphoblastic leukemia (ALL) survivor population (Lustig, 2002; Rogers et al., 2005), in which obesity may be due to several factors, including glucocorticoids and alterations in activity. Nonetheless, the majority of these studies document an abnormal increase in weight for height long after tumor therapy has been discontinued, and many of these studies demonstrate that cranial radiation is an important risk factor (Lustig, 2002).

An extremely high frequency of hypothalamic obesity of 30–77% has been documented after craniopharyngioma treatment (Stahnke et al., 1984; Sorva, 1988; Pinto et al., 2000; Muller, 2008; Vinchon et al., 2009). We analyzed the BMI curves of 148 children with brain tumors who survived longer than 5 years post-therapy, in order to determine risk factors for the development of obesity (Lustig et al., 2003a). We identified four parameters as being predictive. First, those with tumors localized to the hypothalamus or thalamus, along with those originating in the temporal lobe (due to stereoscopic position of the hypothalamus during radiation for this area) gained weight much more rapidly as did those with tumors in the posterior fossa or other hemispheric areas. Secondly, those with tumor histologies prominent in the diencephalon (craniopharyngioma, germinoma, optic glioma, prolactinoma, hypothalamic astrocytoma) also gained weight more rapidly. Third, those with quantitative direct radiation exposure of the hypothalamus of greater than 51 Gy gained excessive weight twice as rapidly after the completion of tumor therapy, even when those with hypothalamic or thalamic locations were removed from the analysis. Lastly, those with some other form of hypothalamic endocrinopathy (i.e., GH deficiency, hypothyroidism, precocious or delayed puberty, ACTH deficiency, diabetes insipidus) exhibited a BMI curve with a steeper upward slope. Thus, each significant risk factor was either linked to hypothalamic location, damage, or dysfunction. Factors not associated with obesity after tumor therapy included hydrocephalus, initial high-dose glucocorticoids, and peripheral or intrathecal chemotherapy.

More recently, Müller et al. (2011) respectively evaluated the long-term outcome data on the Kraniopharyngeom database in

Germany. In this analysis, pre-operative hypothalamic involvement was specifically implicated in the development of post-operative hypothalamic obesity, suggesting again that tumor location is the most important risk factor for obesity.

THE ENERGY BALANCE NEGATIVE FEEDBACK PATHWAY

Animal studies elaborating the negative feedback energy balance pathway have predicted the pathogenesis and symptomatology of hypothalamic obesity. This can best be described as "organic leptin resistance"; that is, a failure in leptin signaling in the afferent arm, due to hypothalamic damage; leading to autonomic dysfunction in the efferent arm, promoting inadequate energy expenditure, and excessive energy storage.

THE AFFERENT ARM

Circulating leptin (derived from peripheral adipocytes) crosses the blood–brain barrier, and synapses on receptors located on neurons within the ventromedial hypothalamus [VMH; which consists of the ventromedial nucleus (VMN) and arcuate nucleus (AN)]. In the energy replete state, both insulin and leptin levels are increased, which acts on a set of "anorexigenic" neurons to increase the synthesis and processing of proopiomelanocortin (POMC) in the VMH to its component peptides, including α-melanocyte stimulating hormone (α-MSH) and its co-localized neuromodulator cocaine–amphetamine regulated transcript (CART), both of which act at the lateral hypothalamic area (LHA) and paraventricular nucleus (PVN) to alter melanocortin receptor-4 (MC_4R) occupancy, which decreases appetite and food intake (Elmquist et al., 1999; Kalra et al., 1999; Schwartz et al., 2000; Balthasar et al., 2005). The stomach hormone ghrelin stimulates, while insulin and leptin inhibit a set of "orexigenic" neurons to inhibit the release of neuropeptide Y (NPY) and agouti-related protein (AgRP), further limiting feeding and providing for unantagonized MC_4R occupancy (Elmquist et al., 1998). Immediately after a meal, ghrelin levels are low, which prevents orexigenic neuronal activation and NPY neurotransmission (Kamegai et al., 2000), keeping hunger at a minimum; furthermore, PYY levels increase after a meal; this hormone binds to the Y_2 receptor on orexigenic neurons, activating gamma-amino butyric acid (GABA), which inhibits signal transduction of NPY to inhibit further food intake (Small and Bloom, 2004).

Conversely, in the fasting state, gastric secretion of ghrelin is increased (Kamegai et al., 2000; Tschöp et al., 2000), while leptin, insulin, and PYY levels are low, which leads to stimulation of the orexigenic pathway (NPY/AgRP), and antagonism of the anorexigenic pathway (α-MSH/CART). The resultant lack of anorexigenic pressure on the MC_4R results in increased feeding behavior and energy efficiency (with reduced fat oxidation), in order to store energy substrate as fat. This is accomplished through signal transduction within the efferent pathway, consisting of the sympathetic nervous system (SNS) and the vagus (see below).

THE EFFERENT ARM

From the PVN and LHA, efferent projections synapse in the locus coeruleus (LC), which controls the SNS; and in the dorsal motor nucleus of the vagus (DMV), which controls the vagus nerve, the chief output of the parasympathetic nervous system.

In the energy replete state, elevated leptin and insulin levels cause the anorexigenic arm to activate the SNS (Muntzel et al., 1994; Vollenweider et al., 1995; Rahmouni et al., 2003). Stimulation of β_2-adrenergic receptors by the SNS (Blaak et al., 1993) increase the expression of numerous genes in skeletal muscle (Viguerie et al., 2004), which promote mitochondrial biogenesis, glycogenolysis, thermogenesis, and increased movement (Boss et al., 1999; Lowell and Spiegelman, 2000), all associated with increased energy expenditure (Collins et al., 1996). The SNS also activates α_{2a}- and α_{2c}-adrenoreceptors on the β-cell, which stimulate G_i and inhibit adenyl cyclase, lower cAMP, and maintain potassium channels in an open configuration with a negative resting membrane potential (Sharp, 1996), in order to reduce pancreatic insulin secretion, and thus reduce energy deposition into adipose tissue. Lastly, SNS activation stimulates the β_3-adrenergic receptor on the adipocyte to promote lipolysis (Susulic et al., 1995). These coordinate sympathetic events serve to reduce adipose tissue leptin expression and secretion; thus this forms a negative feedback loop with the afferent system (**Figure 1**).

Conversely, in the fasting state, leptin and insulin are low, leading to reduced SNS tone, and reduced skeletal muscle thermogenesis, and reduced adipose tissue lipolysis. In addition, the LHA and PVN send efferent projections residing in the medial longitudinal fasciculus to the DMV nerve (Powley and Laughton, 1981). By slowing the heart rate, the vagus reduces myocardial oxygen consumption. Through its effects on the alimentary tract, the vagus promotes peristalsis, and energy substrate absorption. Through its effects on the adipocyte, the vagus promotes increased lipoprotein lipase activity to increase the clearance of energy substrate into adipose tissue (Boden and Hoeldtke, 2003). Lastly, through effects on the β-cell (D'Alessio et al., 2001), the vagus accentuates postprandial insulin hypersecretion in response to a meal, which promotes energy deposition into the adipocyte (Rohner-Jeanrenaud and Jeanrenaud, 1985; Marin et al., 1988; Peles et al., 1995; Lustig, 2003). Overactive vagal neurotransmission increases insulin secretion through three distinct but overlapping mechanisms (Gilon and Henquin, 2001; **Figure 2**):

1. Vagal firing increases acetylcholine availability and binding to the M_3 muscarinic receptor on the β-cell, which is coupled to a sodium channel within the pancreatic β-cell membrane (Miura et al., 1996). As glucose enters the β-cell after ingestion of a meal, the enzyme glucokinase phosphorylates glucose to form glucose-6-phosphate. This increases the generation of intracellular ATP, which induces closure of the β-cell's ATP-dependent potassium channel. Upon channel closure, the β-cell experiences an ATP concentration-dependent β-cell depolarization (Nishi et al., 1987; Zawalich et al., 1989), and the opening of a separate voltage-gated calcium channel within the membrane. Intracellular calcium influx increases acutely, which results in rapid insulin vesicular exocytosis. Concomitant opening of the sodium channel by vagally derived acetylcholine augments the β-cell depolarization, which augments the intracellular calcium influx, and results in insulin hypersecretion (Berthoud and Jeanrenaud, 1979; Komeda et al., 1980; Rohner-Jeanrenaud and Jeanrenaud, 1980).

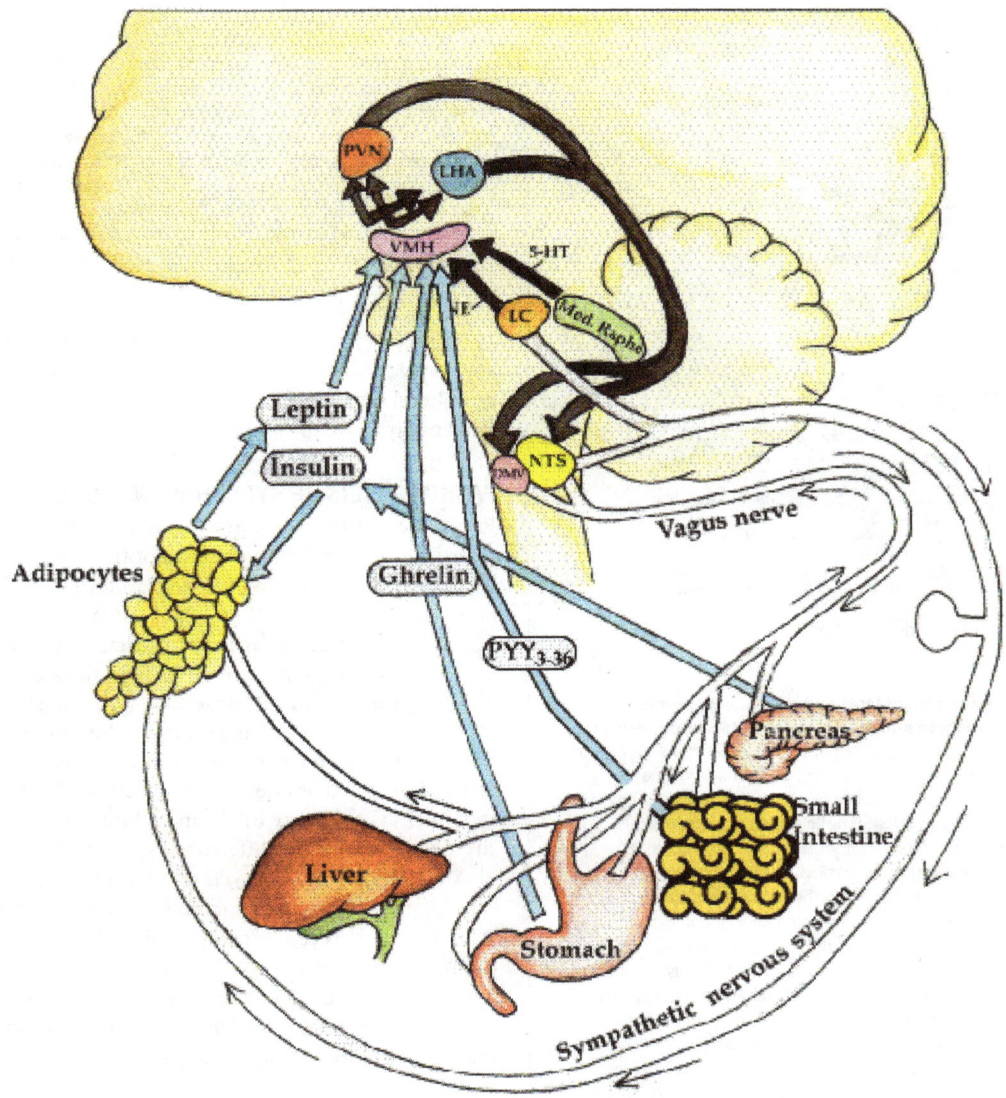

FIGURE 1 | Neuroendocrine regulation of energy balance. *The afferent system*: neural (e.g., vagal) and hormonal (ghrelin, insulin, leptin) signals are generated from the liver, gut, pancreas, and adipose. In addition, norepinephrine from the locus cœruleus and serotonin (5-HT) from the median raphe are elaborated. These signals of satiety vs. hunger, and thinness vs. fatness are interpreted in the ventromedial hypothalamus (VMH). These signals are then integrated in the paraventricular nucleus (PVN) and lateral hypothalamus (LHA). *The efferent system*: efferent signals from these areas in turn stimulate the sympathetic nervous system (SNS) to expend energy by activating β_3-adrenergic receptors and uncoupling proteins in the adipocyte, to release energy the form of lipolysis, heat, or physical activity. Conversely, the parasympathetic nervous system (efferent vagal) increases insulin secretion, with resultant adipogenesis and energy storage, and also increases insulin sensitivity through direct effects on the adipose tissue (Lustig, 2006). From Nature Publishing Group, with permission.

2. Vagally mediated acetylcholine increases phospholipases A_2, C, and D, within the β-cell, which hydrolyze intracellular phosphatidylinositol to diacylglycerol (DAG) and inositol triphosphate (IP_3; Gilon and Henquin, 2001). DAG is a potent stimulator of protein kinase C (PKC; Tian et al., 1996) which phosphorylates myristoylated alanine-rich Protein Kinase C substrate (MARCKS), which then binds actin and calcium–calmodulin, and induces insulin vesicular exocytosis (Arbuzova et al., 1998). IP_3 potentiates release of calcium within β-cells from intracellular stores, which also promotes insulin secretion (Blondel et al., 1994).
3. The vagus also stimulates the release of glucagon-like peptide-1 (GLP-1) from intestinal L-cells, which circulates and binds to the β-cell GLP-1 receptor. Activation of this receptor induces a calcium–calmodulin-sensitive adenyl cyclase, with generation of cAMP, which activates protein kinase A (PKA), stimulating phosphorylation of vesicular proteins, with resultant insulin exocytosis (Kiefer and Habener, 1999).

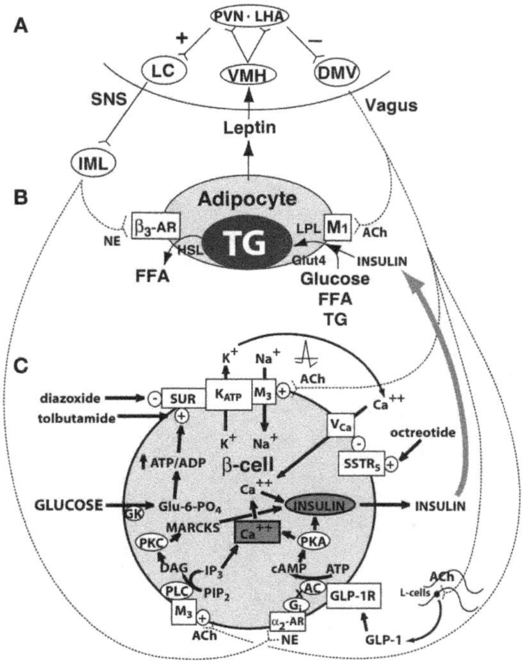

FIGURE 2 | Central regulation of leptin signaling, autonomic innervation of the adipocyte and β-cell, and the starvation response. **(A)** The arcuate nucleus transduces the peripheral leptin signal as one of sufficiency or deficiency. In leptin sufficiency, efferents from the hypothalamus synapse in the locus coeruleus, which stimulates the sympathetic nervous system. In leptin deficiency, efferents from the hypothalamus stimulate the dorsal motor nucleus of the vagus. **(B)** Autonomic innervation and hormonal stimulation of white adipose tissue. In leptin sufficiency, norepinephrine binds to the β_3-adrenergic receptor, which stimulates hormone-sensitive lipase, promoting lipolysis of stored triglyceride into free fatty acids. In leptin deficiency, vagal acetylcholine increases adipose tissue insulin sensitivity (documented only in rats to date), promotes uptake of glucose and free fatty acids for lipogenesis, and promotes triglyceride uptake through activation of lipoprotein lipase. **(C)** Autonomic innervation and hormonal stimulation of the β-cell. Glucose entering the cell is converted to glucose-6-phosphate by the enzyme glucokinase, generating ATP, which closes an ATP-dependent potassium channel, resulting in cell depolarization. A voltage-gated calcium channel opens, allowing for intracellular calcium influx, which activates neurosecretory mechanisms leading to insulin vesicular exocytosis. In leptin sufficiency, norepinephrine binds to α_2-adrenoceptors on the β-cell membrane to stimulate inhibitory G proteins, decrease adenyl cyclase and its product cAMP, and thereby reduce protein kinase A levels and insulin release. In leptin deficiency, the vagus stimulates insulin secretion through three mechanisms. First, acetylcholine binds to a M_3 muscarinic receptor, opening a sodium channel, which augments the ATP-dependent cell depolarization, increasing the calcium influx, and insulin exocytosis. Secondly, acetylcholine activates a pathway that increases protein kinase C, which also promotes insulin secretion. Thirdly, the vagus innervates L-cells of the small intestine, which secrete glucagon-like peptide-1, which activates protein kinase A, contributing to insulin exocytosis. Octreotide binds to a somatostatin receptor on the β-cell, which is coupled to the voltage-gated calcium channel, limiting calcium influx and the amount of insulin released in response to glucose. (Lustig, 2007; reprinted with kind permission of Humana, Totowa, NJ, USA). α_2-AR, α_2-adrenergic receptor; β_3-AR, β_3-adrenergic receptor; AC, adenyl cyclase; ACh, acetylcholine; DAG, diacylglycerol; DMV, dorsal motor nucleus of the vagus; FFA, free fatty acids; G_i, inhibitory G protein; GK, glucokinase; GLP-1, glucagon-like

(Continued)

FIGURE 2 | Continued
peptide-1; GLP-1R, GLP-1 receptor; Glu-6-PO_4, glucose-6-phosphate; Glut4, glucose transporter-4; HSL, hormone-sensitive lipase; IML, intermediolateral cell column; IP_3, inositol triphosphate; LC, locus coeruleus; LHA, lateral hypothalamic area; LPL, lipoprotein lipase; MARCKS, myristoylated alanine-rich protein kinase C substrate; NE, norepinephrine; PIP_2, phosphatidylinositol; PKA, protein kinase A; PKC, protein kinase C; PLC, phospholipase C; PVN, paraventricular nucleus; $SSTR_5$, somatostatin-5 receptor; TG, triglyceride; V_{Ca}, voltage-gated calcium channel; VMH, ventromedial hypothalamus; SUR, sufonylurea receptor (Lustig, 2006). From Nature Publishing Group, with permission.

In this way, the afferent system is entrained with the efferent system by an intricate servo-mechanism to coordinate central and peripheral signals either for appetite and energy storage, or satiety and energy expenditure.

PATHOGENESIS OF HYPOTHALAMIC OBESITY

Rat models of hypothalamic damage, either due to bilateral electrolytic lesions or deafferentation of the VMH, lead to intractable weight gain (Berthoud and Jeanrenaud, 1979; Rohner-Jeanrenaud and Jeanrenaud, 1980; Bray et al., 1981; Jeanrenaud, 1985; Satoh et al., 1997), even upon food restriction (Bray and Nishizawa, 1978). Similarly, children with hypothalamic obesity exhibit weight gain, even in response to forced caloric restriction (Bray and Gallagher, 1975). This seems paradoxical, as one would expect that if hyperphagia were the reason for the obesity, then caloric restriction would be effective in preventing further weight gain. In fact, analysis of energy intake in children with hypothalamic obesity demonstrates no difference vs. control patients with simple obesity (Harz et al., 2003). Instead, both resting energy expenditure (Shaikh et al., 2008) and voluntary energy expenditure (Harz et al., 2003) is severely compromised in these patients. Indeed, the most prominent and concerning complaint in patients with hypothalamic obesity is the persistent fatigue, lack of energy, and lack of physical activity. This generalized malaise is not due to hypopituitarism, as it persists even after full hormonal replacement.

The decrease in energy expenditure is mediated through suppression of SNS activity by the hypothalamic damage. Recent reports demonstrate an impaired ability of such patients to mount an epinephrine response to insulin-induced hypoglycemia (Schofl et al., 2002; Coutant et al., 2003), and document decreased 24-h epinephrine excretion (Coutant et al., 2003), along with decreased urinary homovanillic acid and vanillylmandelic acid (Roth et al., 2007); all pointing to decreased sympathetic tone. It is thought that this malaise and decrease in sympathetic tone may account for decreased rates of lipolysis through the adipocyte β_3-adrenergic receptor (al-Adsani et al., 1997), which results in decreased resting and voluntary energy expenditure.

In addition to "organic leptin resistance," it is possible that such patients also manifest "organic ghrelin resistance," in that ghrelin's suppression of hunger may be attenuated in children with hypothalamic obesity (O'Gorman et al., 2911). This may increase total food intake; although alterations in total food intake in these patients is not different from otherwise healthy obese controls (Harz et al., 2003).

DIAGNOSIS

A retrospective analysis of growth records of children with craniopharyngioma (Muller et al., 2004) indicates that increased weight and BMI gain is evident even before the diagnosis of the tumor. However, after surgery or radiotherapy, the weight gain is immediate, rapid, and highly exaggerated. Evidence of aberrant energy deposition is obvious within the first month. Physicians sometimes confuse this weight gain with glucocorticoid effect, and reduce the dose of maintenance hydrocortisone, which does not impact the obesity, and renders the patient with even more fatigue and malaise.

Children with hypothalamic obesity frequently have normal fasting insulin levels, especially during the rapid weight gain phase. It is important that such metabolic testing be dynamic, as the phenomenon that distinguishes hypothalamic obesity is insulin hypersecretion, not insulin resistance, and so may not be obvious with a fasting insulin level. In addition, stimulation of the alimentary tract so as to activate the vagal efferent component of insulin secretion is required to document the effect. Two sets of studies on insulin dynamics demonstrate insulin hypersecretion (as measured by an increased Corrected Insulin Response, or CIR; Sluiter et al., 1976) on oral glucose tolerance testing (OGTT); and surprisingly these patients also have insulin sensitivity (as measured by an increased Composite Insulin Sensitivity Index (Matsuda and DeFronzo, 1999) within the normal range, and certainly better than BMI-matched healthy obese children (Preeyasombat et al., 2005; Simoneau-Roy et al., 2010; **Figure 3**). However, other studies suggest that some hypothalamic obesity patients may also manifest signs of metabolic syndrome (Tiosano et al., 2003; Srinivasan et al., 2004). These patients may also have an increased incidence of obstructive sleep apnea, which may predispose them to the comorbidities of the metabolic syndrome (O'Gorman et al., 2010). It is not clear whether those patients with both hypothalamic obesity and metabolic syndrome represent a subgroup, or a different pathogenetic phenomenon entirely, or just the late evolution of their morbid obesity. A retrospective evaluation suggests that the degree of hypothalamic involvement of the tumor at its presentation predicts the degree of metabolic disturbance (Müller et al., 2011), though mechanisms for the metabolic alteration are still unclear.

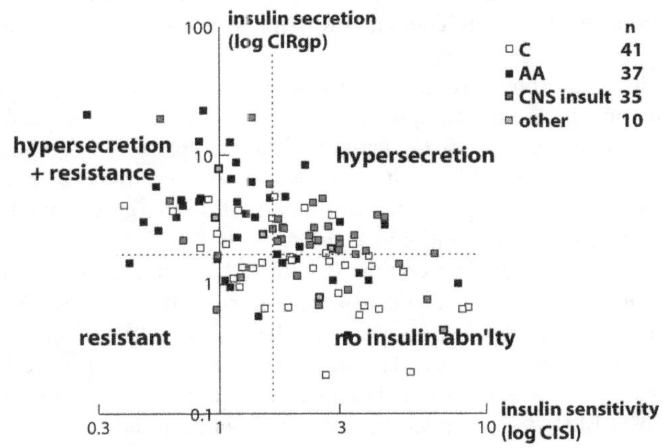

FIGURE 3 | Scatterplot of insulin secretion (Corrected Insulin Response, or CIRgp) vs. sensitivity (Composite Insulin Sensitivity Index, or CISI) plotted logarithmically in 113 obese non-diabetic children. A negative linear correlation was noted ($r = -0.54$, $p < 0.001$). Different racial and etiopathogenic groups tended to plot in different areas. Arbitrary cutoffs (dashed lines) for CIRgp (1.5) and CISI (1.7) divide the plot into four quadrants. The majority of Caucasian children (open squares) plotted in the lower right quadrant, with a CIRgp less than 1.5 and a CISI greater than 1.7, indicating lower insulin secretion and better insulin sensitivity. The preponderance of children with hypothalamic obesity (gray squares) plotted in the upper right quadrant, with a CIRgp of greater than 1.5, and with a CISI of greater than 1.7, indicating insulin hypersecretion with better insulin sensitivity. Finally the majority of African American children (filled squares) plotted in the upper left quadrant, with a CIRgp of greater than 1.5 and a CISI of less than 1.7, indicating both insulin hypersecretion and resistance (Preeyasombat et al., 2005). From Elsevier, with permission.

TREATMENT

The best treatment is prevention. The hypothalamus is extremely sensitive to both surgical intervention and/or external beam radiation (Lustig et al., 2003a). Rather than employing gross total or subtotal resection as a primary therapy for some posterior fossa tumors, newer strategies have been developed which treat them more conservatively, using stereotactic biopsy and conformal irradiation (Karavitaki et al., 2006; Spoudeas et al., 2006). A retrospective single-institutional followup of craniopharyngioma subjected either to gross total resection or stereotactic surgery and conformal radiation demonstrates equal survival and residual rates of hypopituitarism; however those treated with gross total resection exhibit higher incidences of obesity and neurological complications (Merchant et al., 2002).

Bray demonstrated the futility of lifestyle intervention by noting weight gain even with severe caloric restriction (Bray and Gallagher, 1975). Thus, treatment needs to be early and intensive to have any chance at success. A recent report suggests that intensive lifestyle can reduce the rate of BMI gain by half (from 8.4 kg/m^2/year to 4.5 kg/m^2/day), but the rate of increase is still quite unacceptable to rely on (Rakhshani et al., 2010).

PHARMACOTHERAPY

Since the hypothalamus is not amenable to therapy, and aberrant afferent hormonal signal transduction cannot be corrected, pharmacotherapy must instead address the alterations in the efferent pathways. Several attempts to use serotonin or norepinephrine reuptake inhibitors (e.g., phen–fen, fluoxetine, sibutramine) have been met with only salutary efficacy (Molloy et al., 1998). One study assessed the effects of sibutramine 10–15 mg PO qd, with a small but reproducible effect in BMI (Danielsson et al., 2007); however, sibutramine has been withdrawn from the market. These medications work centrally to reduce food intake, but do not work peripherally to stimulate skeletal muscle to increase energy expenditure, and thus have limited value. Mason et al. (2002) used dextroamphetamine 5 mg PO bid, which acts both centrally and peripherally, and achieved weight stability for an interval of 6 months. We have also seen improvement in affect and alertness, which is a major benefit of dextroamphetamine.

In an attempt to reduce hyperinsulinemia, Hamilton have attempted to treat patients with a combination of diazoxide and metformin (Hamilton et al., 2011). Weight gain over 6 months was reduced as compared to pre-treatment; however, side-effects were significant, including edema, and there were some discontinuations.

In an attempt to reduce hyperinsulinemia and simultaneously enhancing insulin action, we examined the effects of the somatostatin analog octreotide (an agonist of the somatostatin-5 receptor on the β-cell, which inhibits the voltage-gated calcium channel; **Figure 2**). A pilot, open-label trial of octreotide 15 μg/kg/day subcutaneously for 6 months in eight subjects (Lustig et al., 1999) demonstrated BMI loss commensurate with the degree of insulin suppression, along with decrease in caloric intake, and subjective improvements in spontaneous physical activity and quality of life. A double-blind, placebo-controlled trial of 20 subjects (Lustig et al., 2003b) resulted in insulin suppression and stabilization of BMI, decreased leptin, decreased caloric intake, increased spontaneous physical activity, and improvement in quality of life commensurate with the degree of insulin suppression. A retrospective analysis demonstrated that octreotide was most effective in those patients who exhibited both insulin hypersecretion with continued insulin sensitivity (Preeyasombat et al., 2005).

SURGERY

The severity and morbidity of obesity in these patients, and the relative lack of alternatives, have led to attempts at bariatric surgery. Inge et al. (2007) reported a 25-kg weight loss after Roux-en-Y gastric bypass in one subject, but whose weight stabilized at an unacceptable level. Recently, Müller et al. (2007) reported in abstract form his experience with four subjects who underwent laparoscopic adjustable gastric banding, with reductions in food intake and slow reductions in BMI. Lastly, vagotomy may be effective in this syndrome (Smith et al., 1983), by reducing the efferent output to both beta-cells and adipocytes. We have recently performed laparoscopic truncal vagotomy in four subjects with hypothalamic obesity, with early results being supportive of this procedure, and with relatively few complications or side-effects (Lustig et al., 2009).

SUMMARY

The hypothalamus interprets afferent signals for energy balance, and transduces them into autonomic efferent signals to either expend or store energy. When this negative feedback system breaks down, as after craniopharyngioma therapy, the phenomenon of hypothalamic obesity ensues. While this disorder is a defect in the afferent pathway, treatment focuses on the efferent pathway, as it is modulable with drugs and surgical techniques that are currently available. Physicians need to explain the risks of this disorder to patients prior to tumor therapy, and must be willing to act quickly and decisively once the intractable weight gain begins, in order to provide intensive management so that the obesity will not get worse.

REFERENCES

al-Adsani, H., Hoffer, L. J., and Silva, J. E. (1997). Resting energy expenditure is sensitive to small dose changes in patients on chronic thyroid hormone replacement. *J. Clin. Endocrinol. Metab.* 82, 1118–1125.

Arbuzova, A., Murray, D., and McLaughlin, S. (1998). MARCKS, membranes, and calmodulin: kinetics of their interaction. *Biochim. Biophys. Acta* 1376, 369–379.

Babinski, M. J. (1900). Tumeur du corps pituitaire san acromegalie et avec arret de developpement des organes genitaux. *Rev. Neurol.* 8, 531–533.

Balthasar, N., Dalgaard, L. T., Lee, C. E., Yu, J., Funahashi, H., Williams, T., Ferreira, M., Tang, V., McGovern, R. A., Kenny, C. D., Christiansen, L. M., Edelstein, E., Choi, B., Boss, O., Aschkenasi, C., Zhang, C. Y., Mountjoy, K., Kishi, T., Elmquist, J. K., and Lowell, B. B. (2005). Divergence of melanocortin pathways in the control of food intake and energy expenditure. *Cell* 123, 493–505.

Berthoud, H. R., and Jeanrenaud, B. (1979). Acute hyperinsulinemia and its reversal by vagotomy following lesions of the ventromedial hypothalamus in anesthetized rats. *Endocrinology* 105, 146–151.

Blaak, E. E., Saris, W. H., and van Baak, M. A. (1993). Adrenoceptor subtypes mediating catecholamine-induced thermogenesis in man. *Int. J. Obes.* 17, S78–S81.

Blondel, O., Bell, G. I., Moody, M., Miller, R. J., and Gibbons, S. J. (1994). Creation of an inositol 1,4,5- triphosphate-sensitive Ca^{2+} store in secretory granules of insulin-producing cells. *J. Biol. Chem.* 269, 27167–27170.

Boden, G., and Hoeldtke, R. D. (2003). Nerves, fat, and insulin resistance. *N. Engl. J. Med.* 349, 1966–1967.

Boss, O., Bachman, E., Vidal-Puig, A., Zhang, C. Y., Peroni, O., and Lowell, B. B. (1999). Role of the β3 -adrenergic receptor and/or a putative β3 -adrenergic receptor on the expression of uncoupling proteins and peroxisome proliferatoractivated receptor-g coactivator-1. *Biochem. Biophys. Res. Commun.* 261, 870–876.

Bray, G. A. (1984). Syndromes of hypothalamic obesity in man. *Pediatr. Ann.* 13, 525–536.

Bray, G. A., and Gallagher, T. F. (1975). Manifestations of hypothalamic obesity in man: a comprehensive investigation of eight patients and a review of the literature. *Medicine (Baltimore)* 54, 301–333.

Bray, G. A., Inoue, S., and Nishizawa, Y. (1981). Hypothalamic obesity. *Diabetologia* 20, 366–377.

Bray, G. A., and Nishizawa, Y. (1978). Ventromedial hypothalamus modulates fat mobilization during fasting. *Nature* 274, 900–902.

Collins, S., Kuhn, C. M., Petro, A. E., Swick, A. G., Chrunyk, B. A., and Surwit, R. S. (1996). Role of leptin in fat regulation. *Nature* 380, 677.

Coutant, R., Maurey, H., Rouleau, S., Mathieu, E., Mercier, P., Limal, J. M., and Le Bouil, A. (2003). Defect in epinephrine production in children with craniopharyngioma: functional or organic origin? *J. Clin. Endocrinol. Metab.* 88, 5969–5975.

D'Alessio, D. A., Kieffer, T. J., Taborsky, G. J., and Havel, P. J. (2001). Activation of the parasympathetic nervous system is necessary for normal meal induced-insulin secretion in rhesus macaques. *J. Clin. Endocrinol. Metab.* 86, 1253–1259.

Danielsson, P., Janson, A., Norgren, S., and Marcus, C. (2007). Impact sibutramine therapy in children with hypothalamic obesity or obesity with aggravating syndromes. *J. Clin. Endocrinol. Metab.* 92, 4101–4106.

Daousi, C., Dunn, A. J., Foy, P. M., MacFarlane, I. A., and Pinkney, J. H. (2005). Endocrine and neuroanatomic predictors of weight gain and obesity in adult patients with hypothalamic damage. *Am. J. Med.* 118, 45–50.

Elmquist, J. K., Ahima, R. S., Elias, C. F., Flier, J. S., and Saper, C. B. (1998). Leptin activates distinct projections from the dorsomedial and ventromedial hypothalamic nuclei. *Proc. Natl. Acad. Sci. U.S.A.* 95, 741–746.

Elmquist, J. K., Elias, C. F., and Saper, C. B. (1999). From lesions to leptin: hypothalamic control of food intake and body weight. *Neuron* 22, 221–232.

Frohlich, A. (1901). Ein fall von tumor der hypophysis cerebri ohne akromegalie. *Weiner Klin. Rundsch.* 15, 883–886.

Gilon, P., and Henquin, J. C. (2001). Mechanisms and physiological significance of the cholinergic control of pancreatic β-cell function. *Endocr. Rev.* 22, 565–604.

Hamilton, J. K., Conwell, L. S., Syme, C., Ahmet, A., Jeffery, A., and Daneman, D. (2011). Hypothalamic obesity following craniopharyngioma surgery: results of a pilot trial of combined diazoxide and metformin therapy. *Int. J. Pediatr. Endocrinol.* 2011, 417949.

Harz, K. J., Muller, H. L., Waldeck, E., Pudel, V., and Roth, C. (2003). Obesity in patients with craniopharyngioma: assessment of food intake and movement counts indicating physical activity. *J. Clin. Endocrinol. Metab.* 88, 5227–5231.

Inge, T. H., Pfluger, P., Zeller, M., Rose, S. R., Burget, L., Sundararajan, S., Daniels, S. R., and Tschöp, M. H. (2007). Gastric bypass surgery for treatment of hypothalamic obesity after craniopharyngioma therapy. *Nat. Clin. Pract. Endocrinol. Metab.* 3, 606–609.

Jeanrenaud, B. (1985). An hypothesis on the aetiology of obesity: dysfunction of the central nervous system as a primary cause. *Diabetologia* 28, 502–513.

Kalra, S. P., Dube, M. G., Pu, S., Xu, B., Horvath, T. L., and Kalra, P. S. (1999). Interacting appetite-regulating pathways in the hypothalamic regulation of body weight. *Endocr. Rev.* 20, 68–100.

Kamegai, J., Tamura, H., Shimizu, T., Ishii, S., Sugihara, H., and Wakabayashi, I. (2000). Central effect of ghrelin, an endogenous growth hormone secretagogue, on hypothalamic peptide gene expression. *Endocrinology* 141, 4797–4800.

Karavitaki, N., Cudlip, S., Adams, C. B., and Wass, J. A. (2006). Craniopharyngiomas. *Endocr. Rev.* 27, 371–397.

Kiefer, T. J., and Habener, J. F. (1999). The glucagon-like peptides. *Endocr. Rev.* 20, 876–913.

Komeda, K., Yokote, M., and Oki, Y. (1980). Diabetic syndrome in the Chinese hamster induced with monosodium glutamate. *Experientia* 36, 232–234.

Lowell, B. B., and Spiegelman, B. M. (2000). Towards a molecular understanding of adaptive thermogenesis. *Nature* 404, 652–660.

Lustig, R. H. (2002). Hypothalamic obesity: the sixth cranial endocrinopathy. *Endocrinologist* 12, 210–217.

Lustig, R. H. (2003). Autonomic dys-function of the (ß-cell and the pathogenesis of obesity. *Rev. Endocr. Metab. Disord.* 4, 23–32.

Lustig, R. H. (2006). Childhood obesity: behavioral aberration or biochemical drive? Reinterpreting the first law of thermodynamics. *Nat. Clin. Pract. Endocrinol. Metab.* 2, 447–458.

Lustig, R. H. (2007). "The efferent arm of the energy balance regulatory pathway: neuroendocrinology and pathology," in *Obesity and Energy Metabolism: Research and Clinical Applications*, ed. P. A. Donahoue (Totowa, NJ: Humana), 69–86.

Lustig, R. H., Post, S. M., Srivannaboon, K., Rose, S. R., Danish, R. K., Burghen, G. A., Xiong, X., Wu, S., and Merchant, T. E. (2003a). Risk factors for the development of obesity in children surviving brain tumors. *J. Clin. Endocrinol. Metab.* 88, 611–616.

Lustig, R. H., Hinds, P. S., Ringwald-Smith, K., Christensen, R. K., Kaste, S. C., Schreiber, R. E., Rai, S. N., Lensing, S. Y., Wu, S., and Xiong, X. (2003b). Octreotide therapy of pediatric hypothalamic obesity: a double-blind, placebo-controlled trial. *J. Clin. Endocrinol. Metab.* 88, 2586–2592.

Lustig, R. H., Rose, S. R., Burghen, G. A., Velasquez-Mieyer, P., Broome, D. C., Smith, K., Li, H., Hudson, M. M., Heideman, R. L., and Kun, L. E. (1999). Hypothalamic obesity in children caused by cranial insult: altered glucose and insulin dynamics, and reversal by a somatostatin agonist. *J. Pediatr.* 135, 162–168.

Lustig, R. H., Tsai, P., Hirose, S., and Farmer, D. L. (2009). "Treatment of hypothalamic obesity by laparoscopic truncal vagotomy: early experience," in *Proceedings of the 8th Lawson Wilkins/European Pediatric Endocrine Society meeting*. New York, NY.

Marin, P., Russeffé-Scrive, A., Smith, J., and Bjorntorp, P. (1988). Glucose uptake in human adipose tissue. *Metab. Clin. Exp.* 36, 1154–1164.

Mason, P. W., Krawiecki, N., and Meacham, L. R. (2002). The use of dextroamphetamine to treat obesity and hyperphagia in children treated for craniopharyngioma. *Arch. Pediatr. Adolesc. Med.* 156, 887–892.

Matsuda, M., and DeFronzo, R. A. (1999). Insulin sensitivity indices obtained from oral glucose tolerance testing: comparison with the euglycemic insulin clamp. *Diabetes Care* 22, 1462–1470.

Merchant, T. E., Kienha, E. N., Sanford, R. A., Mulhern, R. K., Thomp-son, S. J., Wilson, M. W., Lustig, R. H., and Kun, L. E. (2002). Craniopharyngioma: the St. Jude Children's Research Hospital experience 1984–2001. *Int. J. Radiat. Oncol. Biol. Phys.* 53, 533–542.

Miura, Y., Gilon, P., and Henquin, J. C. (1996). Muscarinic stimulation increases Na^+ entry in pancreatic β-cells by a mechanism other than the emptying of intracellular Ca^{2+} pools. *Biochem. Biophys. Res. Commun.* 224, 67–73.

Molloy, P. T., Berkowitz, R., Stallings, V. A., Krell, H., Sutton, L. N., Vaughan, S. N., Loeb, N., and Phillips, P. C. (1998). "Pilot study of evaluation and treatment of tumor-related obesity in pediatric patients with hypothalamic/chiasmatic gliomas and craniopharyngiomas," in *Proceedings of the International Pediatric Oncology Meeting*, Rome, 156.

Müller, H. L., Gebhardt, U., Wessel, V., Schröder, S., Kolb, R., Sörensen, N., Maroske, J., and Hanisch, E. (2007). First experiences with laparoscopic adjustable gastric banding (LAGB) in the treatment of patients with childhood craniopharyngioma and morbid obesity. *Klin. Padiatr.* 219, 323–325.

Muller, H. L. (2008). Childhood craniopharyngioma: recent advances in diagnosis, treatment and follow-up. *Horm. Res.* 69, 193–202.

Muller, H. L., Emser, A., Faldum, A., Bruhnken, G., Etavard-Gorris, N., Gebhardt, U., Oeverink, R., Kolb, R., and Sörensen, N. (2004). Longitudinal study of growth and body mass index before and after diagnosis of childhood craniopharyngioma. *J. Clin. Endocrinol. Metab.* 89, 3298–3305.

Müller, H. L., Gebhardt, U., Teske, C., Faldum, A., Zwiener, I., Warmuth-Metz, M., Pietsch, T., Pohl, F., Sörensen, N., Calaminus, G., and Study Committee of KRANIOPHA-RYNGEOM 2000. (2011). Postoperative hypothalamic lesions and obesity in childhood craniopharyngioma: results of the multinational prospective trial KRANIO-PHARYNGEOM 2000 after 3-year follow-up. *Eur. J. Endocrinol.* 165, 17–24.

Muntzel, M., Morgan, D. A., Mark, A. L., and Johnson, A. K. (1994). Intracerebroventricular insulin produces non-uniform regional increases in sympathetic nerve activity *Am. J. Physiol.* 267, R1350–R1355.

Nishi, S., Seino, Y., Ishida, H., Seno, M., Taminato, T., Sakurai, H., and Imura, H. (1987). Vagal regulation of insulin, glucagon, and somatostatin secretion in vitro in the rat. *J. Clin. Invest.* 79, 1191–1196.

O'Gorman, C. S., Simoneau-Roy, J., Pencharz, P., Adeli, K., and Hamilton, J. (2911). Delayed ghrelin suppression following oral glucose tolerance test in children and adolescents with hypothalamic injury secondary to craniopharyngioma compared with obese controls. *Int. J. Pediatr. Obes.* 6, 285–288.

O'Gorman, C. S., Simoneau-Roy, J., Pencharz, P., MacFarlane, J., MacLusky, I., Narang, I., Adeli, K., Daneman, D., and Hamilton, J. (2010). Sleep-disordered breathing is increased in obese adolescents with craniopharyngioma compared with obese controls. *J. Clin. Endocrinol. Metab.* 95, 2211–2218.

Peles, E., Goldstein, D. S., Akselrod, S., Nitzan, H., Azaria, M., Almog, S., Dolphin, D., Halkin, H., and Modan, M. (1995). Interrelation-ships among measures of autonomic activity and cardiovascular risk factors during orthostasis and the oral glucose tolerance test. *Clin. Auton. Res.* 5, 271–278.

Pinto, G., Bussieres, L., Recasens, C., Souberbielle, J. C., Zerah, M., and Brauner, R. (2000). Hormonal factors influencing weight and growth pattern in craniopharyngioma. *Horm. Res.* 53, 163–169.

Powley, T. L., and Laughton, W. (1981). Neural pathways involved in the hypothalamic integration of autonomic responses. *Diabetologia* 20, 378–387.

Preeyasombat, C., Bacchetti, P., Lazar, A. A., and Lustig, R. H. (2005). Racial and etiopathologic dichotomies in insulin secretion and resistance in obese children. *J. Pediatr.* 146, 474–481.

Rahmouni, K., Haynes, W. G., Morgan, D. A., and Mark, A. L. (2003). Role of melanocortin-4 receptors in mediating renal sympathoactivation to leptin and insulin. *J. Neurosci.* 23, 5998–6004.

Rakhshani, N., Jeffery, A. S., Schulte, F., Barrera, M., Atenafu, E. G., and Hamilton, J. K. (2010). Evaluation of a comprehensive care clinic model for children with brain tumor and risk for hypothalamic obesity. *Obesity (Silver Spring)* 18, 1768–1774.

Rogers, P. C., Meacham, L. R., Oeffinger, K. C., Henry, D. W., and Lange, B. J. (2005). Obesity in pediatric oncology. *Pediatr. Blood Cancer* 45, 881–891.

Rohner-Jeanrenaud, F., and Jeanrenaud, B. (1980). Consequences of ventromedial hypothalamic lesions upon insulin and glucagon secretion by subsequently isolated perfused pancreases in the rat. *J. Clin. Invest.* 65, 902–910.

Rohner-Jeanrenaud, F., and Jeanrenaud, B. (1985). Involvement of the cholinergic system in insulin and glucagon oversecretion of genetic preobesity. *Endocrinology* 116, 830–834.

Roth, C. L., Hunneman, D. H., Gebhardt, U., Stoffel-Wagner, B., Reinehr, T., and Müller, H. L. (2007). Reduced sympathetic metabolites in urine of obese patients with craniopharyngioma. *Pediatr. Res.* 61, 496–501.

Satoh, N., Ogawa, Y., Katsura, G., Tsuji, T., Masuzaki, H., Hiraoka, J., Okazaki, T., Tamaki, M., Hayase, M., Yoshimasa, Y., Nishi, S., Hosoda, K., and Nakao, K. (1997). Pathophysiological significance of the obese gene product, leptin in ventromedial hypothalamus (VMH)-lesioned rats: evidence for loss of its satiety effect in VMH-lesioned rats. *Endocrinology* 138, 947–954.

Schofl, C., Schleth, A., Berger, D., Terkamp, C., Von Zur Muhlen, A., and Brabant, G. (2002). Sympathoadrenal counterregulation in patients with hypothalamic craniopharyngioma. *J. Clin. Endocrinol. Metab.* 87, 624–629.

Schwartz, M. W., Woods, S. C., Porte, D., Seeley, R. J., and Baskin, D. G. (2000). Central nervous system control of food intake. *Nature* 404, 661–671.

Shaikh, M. G., Grundy, R. G., and Kirk, J. M. (2008). Reductions in basal metabolic rate and physical activity contribute to hypothalamic obesity. *J. Clin. Endocrinol. Metab.* 93, 2588–2593.

Sharp, G. W. (1996). Mechanisms of inhibition of insulin release. *Am. J. Physiol.* 271, C1781–C1799.

Simoneau-Roy, J., O'Gorman, C., Pencharz, P., Adeli, K., Daneman, D., and Hamilton, J. (2010). Insulin sensitivity and secretion in children and adolescents with hypothalamic obesity following treatment for craniopharyngioma. *Clin. Endocrinol. (Oxf)* 72, 364–370.

Sluiter, W. J., Erkelens, D. W., Terpstra, P., Reitsma, W. D., and Doorendos, H. (1976). Glucose intolerance and insulin release, a mathematical approach.1. Assay of the beta cell response after glucose loading. *Diabetes* 25, 241–244.

Small, C. J., and Bloom, S. R. (2004). Gut hormones and the control of appetite. *Trends Endocrinol. Metab.* 15, 259–263.

Smith, D. K., Sarfeh, J., and Howard, L. (1983). Truncal vagotomy in hypothalmic obesity. *Lancet* 1, 1330–1331.

Sorva, R. (1988). Children with craniopharyngioma: early growth failure and rapid post-operative weight gain. *Acta Paediatr. Scand.* 77, 587–592.

Spoudeas, H. A., Saran, F., and Pizer, B. (2006). A multimodality approach to the treatment of craniopharyngiomas avoiding hypothalamic morbidity: a UK perspective. *J. Pediatr. Endocrinol. Metab.* 19, 447–451.

Srinivasan, S., Ogle, G. D., Garnett, S. P., Briody, J. N., Lee, J. W., and Cowell, C. T. (2004). Features of the metabolic syndrome after craniopharyngioma. *J. Clin. Endocrinol. Metab.* 89, 81–86.

Stahnke, N., Grubel, G., Lagenstein, I., and Willig, R. P. (1984). Long-term follow-up of children with craniopharyngioma. *Eur. J. Pediatr.* 142, 179–185.

Susulic, V. S., Frederich, R. C., Lawitts, J., Tozzo, E., Kahn, B. B., Harper, M. E., Himms-Hagen, J., Flier, J. S., and Lowell, B. B. (1995). Targeted disruption of the beta 3-adrenergic receptor gene. *J. Biol. Chem.* 270, 29483–29492.

Tian, Y. M., Urquidi, V., and Ashcroft, S. J. H. (1996). Protein kinase C in β-cells: expression of multiple isoforms and involvement in cholinergic stimulation of insulin secretion. *Mol. Cell. Endocrinol.* 119, 185–193. Tiosano, D., Eisenstein, I., Militianu, D., Chrousos, G. P., and Hochberg, Z. (2003). 11β-hydroxysteroid dehydrogenase activity in hypothalamic obesity. *J. Clin. Endocrinol. Metab.* 88, 384.

Tschöp, M., Smiley, D. L., and Heiman, M. L. (2000). Ghrelin induces adiposity in rodents. *Nature* 407, 908–913.

Viguerie, N., Clement, K., Barbe, P., Courtine, M., Benis, A., Larrouy, D., Hanczar, B., Pelloux, V., Poitou, C., Khalfallah, Y., Barsh, G. S., Thalamas, C., Zucker, J. D., and Langin, D. (2004). In vivo epinephrine-mediated regulation of gene express in human skeletal muscle. *J. Clin. Endocrinol. Metab.* 89, 2000–2014.

Vinchon, M., Weill, J., Delestret, I., and Dhellemmes, P. (2009). Craniopharyngioma and hypothalamic obesity in children. *Childs Nerv. Syst.* 25, 347–352.

Vollenweider, L., Tappy, L., Owlya, R., Jequier, E., Nicod, P., and Scherrer, U. (1995). Insulin-induced sympathetic activation and vasodilation in skeletal muscle. Effects of insulin resistance in lean subjects. *Diabetes* 44, 641–645.

Zawalich, W. S., Zawalich, K. C., and Rasmussen, H. (1989). Cholinergic agonists prime the β-cell to glucose stimulation. *Endocrinology* 125, 2400–2406.

20

Sweet taste signaling functions as a hypothalamic glucose sensor

Xueying Ren[1,2], Ligang Zhou[3], Rose Terwilliger[2], Samuel S. Newton[2] and Ivan E. de Araujo[1,2]*

[1] The John B Pierce Laboratory, New Haven, CT, USA
[2] Department of Psychiatry, Yale University School of Medicine, New Haven, CT, USA
[3] Department of Internal Medicine, Yale University School of Medicine, New Haven, CT, USA

***Correspondence:**
Ivan E. de Araujo, The John B Pierce Laboratory, 290 Congress Avenue, New Haven, CT 06519, USA.
e-mail: IAraujo@jbpierce.org

Brain glucosensing is essential for normal body glucose homeostasis and neuronal function. However, the exact signaling mechanisms involved in the neuronal sensing of extracellular glucose levels remain poorly understood. Of particular interest is the identification of candidate membrane molecular sensors that would allow neurons to change firing rates independently of intracellular glucose metabolism. Here we describe for the first time the expression of the taste receptor genes *Tas1r1*, *Tas1r2* and *Tas1r3*, and their associated G-protein genes, in the mammalian brain. Neuronal expression of taste genes was detected in different nutrient-sensing forebrain regions, including the paraventricular and arcuate nuclei of the hypothalamus, the CA fields and dentate gyrus of the hippocampus, the habenula, and cortex. Expression was also observed in the intra-ventricular epithelial cells of the choroid plexus. These same regions were found to express the corresponding gene products that form the heterodimeric T1R2/T1R3 and T1R1/T1R3 sweet and L-amino acid taste G-protein coupled receptors, respectively, along with the taste G-protein α-gustducin. Moreover, in vivo studies in mice demonstrated that the hypothalamic expression of taste-related genes is regulated by the nutritional state of the animal, with food deprivation significantly increasing expression levels of *Tas1r1* and *Tas1r2* in hypothalamus, but not in cortex. Furthermore, exposing mouse hypothalamic cells to a low-glucose medium, while maintaining normal L-amino acid concentrations, specifically resulted in higher expression levels of the sweet-associated gene *Tas1r2*. This latter effect was reversed by adding the non-metabolizable artificial sweetener sucralose to the low-glucose medium, indicating that taste-like signaling in hypothalamic neurons does not require intracellular glucose oxidation. Taken together, our findings suggest that the heterodimeric G-protein coupled sweet receptor T1R2/T1R3 is a candidate membrane-bound brain glucosensor.

Keywords: sweet taste, taste receptor, glucosensing, glucokinase, hypothalamus, hypoglycemia, nutrient chemosensing

INTRODUCTION

Brain glucosensors are specialized neurons that respond to local fluctuations in extracellular glucose levels, modulating their mean firing rate according to changes in glucose concentration (Gonzalez et al., 2008; McCrimmon, 2008). Early electrophysiological studies described the presence of glucosensing neurons in brain regions known to influence glucose homeostasis, including the hypothalamus and the brainstem (Anand et al., 1964; Oomura et al., 1969; Ritter et al., 1981). Later studies have identified the presence of glucosensing neurons in other brain regions including the amygdala (Nakano et al., 1986), septum (Shoji, 1992) and cortex (Lee et al., 1996).

How is glucose sensed by neurons? Glucosensing neurons are generally classified as "glucose-excited" (GE) or "glucose-inhibited" (GI), according to whether their mean firing rate increase or decrease, respectively, in response to local changes in extracellular glucose (Gonzalez et al., 2008; McCrimmon, 2008). In the case of GE neurons, the insulin-secreting β-cells of the pancreas have been adopted as the cellular model of neuronal glucosensing (Matschinsky, 1996; Schuit et al., 2001). In the pancreatic islets, glucose is carried into the cell through facilitated transport via GLUT proteins, resulting in equilibration between extracellular and cytosolic glucose (McCrimmon, 2008). In these cells, intracellular glucose metabolism is controlled by glucokinase (GK), the rate-limiting factor in glycolysis (Matschinsky, 1996; Schuit et al., 2001). The action of GK on glucose results in a series of intracellular events eventually leading to rises in the cytosolic ATP:ADP ratio and subsequent closure of ATP-sensitive potassium (K_{ATP}) channels, which in turn causes cell depolarization (Gonzalez et al., 2008; McCrimmon, 2008). The discovery that both GK and K_{ATP} are expressed in glucosensing regions of the brain then naturally led to the hypothesis that GK and K_{ATP}, like in pancreas, play essential roles in the generation of GE responses to rises in extracellular glucose (Ashford et al., 1990; Kang et al., 2006; Routh, 2002).

However, several lines of evidence strongly suggest that glucosensing neurons might use alternative, GK/K_{ATP}-independent pathways to respond to local fluctuations in glucose levels. For example, rises in glucose concentration at physiological levels fail to elevate cytosolic ATP levels in the hypothalamus (Ainscow et al.,

2002). In addition, K_{ATP} channels are expressed in several regions of the brain, most often in non-glucosensing neurons (Karschin et al., 1997). Another compelling evidence in favor of the existence non-metabolic glucosensing pathways in the brain relates to the lack of expression of pancreatic glucosensor elements in a significant fraction of glucosensing neurons; in fact, over 30% of glucosensing neurons were found to not express GK or SUR1, a subunit of the pancreatic β-cell K_{ATP} channels (Kang et al., 2004). These results have recently led to the hypothesis that the primary role of GK in neurons relates to cellular metabolic support rather than glucosensing *per se* (Gonzalez et al., 2008, 2009). Finally, it is noticeable that GE neurons are present in the hypothalamus of K_{ATP} channel knockout (Kir6.2 null) mice (Fioramonti et al., 2004). Likewise the GE case, GI neurons also seem to make use of GK-independent pathways. In addition to the fact that only a fraction of GI neurons are found to express GK (Kang et al., 2004), stimulating ATP production via lactate infusions did not result in inhibition of hypothalamic GI neurons (Song and Routh, 2005). Moreover, while inhibition of orexin GI neurons by glucose was shown to depend on tandem-pore K_{2P} ion channels (Burdakov et al., 2006), the same study also demonstrates that intracellular applications of glucose did not affect the extracellular action of glucose, suggesting that glucose acts extracellularly on currently undetermined glucose sensors located on the cell membrane (Burdakov et al., 2006). Overall, it must be concluded from the above that at least part of the mechanism regulating neuronal glucosensing involves signaling pathways that do not require intracellular metabolic processing of glucose.

In this study, we propose that one of the metabolism-independent mechanisms that GE and GI neurons might use to respond to local changes in extracellular glucose levels involves a sweet taste-like signaling pathway. Sweet taste signaling is known to be mediated by heterodimeric G-protein coupled receptors and specific downstream signaling elements. More precisely, the transduction of sweet tastants is mediated by the taste genes *Tas1r2* and *Tas1r3* (Bachmanov and Beauchamp, 2007), whose T1R2 and T1R3 products assemble to form the heterodimeric sweet receptor T1R2/T1R3 (Nelson et al., 2001; Zhang et al., 2003; Zhao et al., 2003). A similar mechanism mediates the recognition of L-amino acids via the *Tas1r1* and *Tas1r3* genes (Bachmanov and Beauchamp, 2007; Nelson et al., 2002). T1R2/T1R3 and T1R1/T1R3 receptor signaling are at least in part supported by the taste-specific heterotrimeric G-protein gustducin, formed by α-gustducin (McLaughlin et al., 1992), Gβ3 and Gγ13 (Huang et al., 1999). Because the sweet receptor T1R2/T1R3 is also expressed in the gastrointestinal tract (Bezencon et al., 2007), where it plays important physiological roles by mediating hormonal responses to the presence of tastants in the lumen (Margolskee et al., 2007), we hypothesized that sweet taste-related signaling molecules might also be involved in responses to extracellular levels of brain glucose in a way that is independent from its intracellular metabolic processing.

MATERIALS AND METHODS

AMPLIFICATION AND SEQUENCING OF TASTE GENES FROM MOUSE BRAIN cDNA

Total RNAs were extracted from mouse or rat brain tissue using the TRIzol reagent (Invitrogen), purified by Acid-Phenol:Chloroform (Applied Biosystems) and reverse-transcribed into cDNA using SuperScriptII (Invitrogen) according to the manufacturer's instructions. The cDNA (equivalent to 200 ng RNA) was amplified by real-time (RT)-PCR using an ABIPRISM 7900HT sequence detection system (Applied Biosystems). Taqman primers and probes for the following genes were purchased from Applied Biosystems (Mm99999915_g1 for *GAPDH*, Mm00516381_m1 for *Gnb3*, Mm00458152_ml for *Gng13*. The assay IDs for *Gnat3*, *Tas1r1*, *Tas1r2* and *Tas1r3* are listed in **Table 1**). The cycling conditions were 1 cycle at 50°C for 2 min, 1 cycle at 95°C for 10 min, followed by 50 cycles at 95°C for 15 s and 60°C for 1 min. GAPDH primers were used as internal controls. To confirm the specificity of the products and rule out genomic contamination in the RT-PCR assay, the products of *Gnat3*, and *Tas1r1*, *Tas1r2* and *Tas1r3* from mouse cortex were purified using the QIAquick PCR Purification Kit (Qiagen), ligated into the pDrive cloning vector with the QIAGEN PCR Cloning Kit (Qiagen) and sequenced (the presence of Gnb3 and Gng13 had been shown in brain previously, Huang et al., 1999). Multiple sequence alignment was performed on the sequenced amplified segments using the CLUSTAL W (V. 1.8) software.

RELATIVE QUANTIFICATION OF GENE EXPRESSION LEVELS FROM REAL-TIME PCR DATA

Relative gene expression levels across regions and/or conditions were computed using the $2^{-\Delta\Delta C_T}$ method as described previously (Livak and Schmittgen, 2001). In all experiments, GAPDH was used as an internal reference in order to control for variations in cDNA concentration across samples. Briefly, given a specific sample and a target gene of interest, the quantity $\Delta C_T = (C_{T,\,Target} - C_{T,\,GAPDH})$ was computed, where $C_{T,\,Target}$ and $C_{T,\,GAPDH}$ correspond to the detected threshold cycles for the target gene and GAPDH, respectively, for

Table 1 | Details on taste gene amplification from brain tissue.

Gene	ABI assay ID	Refseq	Amplicon length (bp)	Cloned sequence
Gnat3	Mm01165313_m1	NM_001081143.1	65	TGCACCTCAGCATTTGCTTTCCAGAATATACTGGACCA AACACATTTGAAGATGCAGGGAACTAC
Tas1r1	Mm00473433_m1	NM_031867.1	79	CTGACTGTCTGCAGGTGAGACACAGACCTCTGGTGAC AAGTTGTGACAGGTCTGACAGCTTCAACGGCCATGGCTATCA
Tas1r2	Mm00499716_m1	NM_031873.1	83	CGAGGCTGACCTACATTAGCAATGTGTCCTGGTACACC CCCAACAACACGGTCCCCATATCCATGTGTTCTAAGAGTTGCCAG
Tas1r3	Mm00473459_g1	NM_031872.2	68	AGCTGCAGCAGTCTAAAATGTACTGGCCAGGCAACCA GGTGCCAGTCTCCCAGTGTTCCCGCCAGTGC

this particular sample. To compute the relative expression levels for a target gene across different brain regions, the quantity

$$\Delta\Delta C_T = (C_{T,\text{Target}} - C_{T,\text{GAPDH}})_{R1} - (C_{T,\text{Target}} - C_{T,\text{GAPDH}})_{R2}$$
$$= (\Delta C_T)_{R1} - (\Delta C_T)_{R2}$$

was calculated, where $\mathbf{R}_1$ and $\mathbf{R}_2$ correspond to two different brain regions. Then, the relative levels of expression between regions were computed as $2^{-\Delta\Delta C_T}$. The resulting values were then multiplied by 100 and expressed as percent values, with 100% corresponding to no relative differences in expression levels, by definition, since $2^0 = 1$. By analogy, the relative changes in expression levels of a target gene in a given brain region due to a certain experimental manipulation (e.g., food-deprived vs. fed animals) was computed via the quantity

$$\Delta\Delta C_T = (C_{T,\text{Target}} - C_{T,\text{GAPDH}})_{C1} - (C_{T,\text{Target}} - C_{T,\text{GAPDH}})_{C2}$$
$$= (\Delta C_T)_{C1} - (\Delta C_T)_{C2}$$

where $\mathbf{C}_1$ and $\mathbf{C}_2$ correspond to two different experimental conditions. By analogy, the relative changes in expression levels in a given brain region to specific experimental manipulation were computed as $2^{-\Delta\Delta C_T}$.

One important assumption of the $2^{-\Delta\Delta C_T}$ method concerns the insensitivity of the internal control reference gene to experimental treatment. **Table 2** displays the C_T values for GAPDH for all experimental conditions reported in this study, including GAPDH C_T values associated with the different brain regions analyzed. In each case, appropriate statistical tests were performed to ascertain that GAPDH levels did not vary due to our experimental treatments and/or depend on brain region analyzed.

Finally, the option for $2^{-\Delta\Delta C_T}$, a relative expression method, rather than for an absolute quantification approach is based on the fact that no hypotheses concerning the effects of our experimental treatments on the amount of genes have been formulated *a priori*. While we considered relevant to determine whether gene levels were up- or downregulated according to experimental conditions such as changes in nutritional state, we assumed that such analysis does not require the quantification of absolute gene copy numbers. This is consistent with the principle that absolute quantification should be restricted to situations where it is necessary to determine the absolute transcript copy numbers (Livak and Schmittgen, 2001).

IN SITU HYBRIDIZATION

In situ hybridization (ISH) was performed using radiolabeled riboprobes according to conventional protocols with minor modifications (Newton et al., 2002). The reverse primer included a T7 template sequence (TAATACGACTCACTATAGGGAGA) on the 5'end while the forward primer included a Sp6 template sequence (ATTTAGGTGACACTATAGAA). For *Tas1r2*, PCR product was generated by PCR using gene-specific primers, forward-ccacaccctccacagactcc; reverse-ccacacactcgaagcagcac. For *Gnat3*, primers were forward-cgtgccaaatgagcaagatg; reverse-tctggaaagcaaatgctgagg and for *Tas1r3* primers were forward-acggtgtgacgacatcatgc, reverse-ggtgtagggctctgccacac. Mouse hippocampal cDNA was used as the template for PCR, which was performed in a RT-PCR instrument (SmartCycler; Cepheid, Sunnyvale, CA, USA) using the Quantitect Sybr Green PCR Kit (Qiagen). PCR product was purified by ethanol precipitation and was resuspended in TE buffer. One microgram of each PCR product was used to produce radiolabeled riboprobes using a T7 or Sp6-based *in vitro* transcription kit (Maxiscript, Ambion). Sp6 transcription was used to generate the sense *Tas1r2* probe while T7 transcription was used to produce the sense probe. Specificity of the PCR product was verified by sequencing. Radiolabeled CTP was included in the *in vitro* transcription reaction and 2 million counts were added to each slide. Sections

Table 2 | C_T values for GAPDH under the different experimental conditions.

Experimental condition	GAPDH CTs (mean ± SEM)	Statistical comparison	Does GAPDH vary significantly?
Comparison across brain regions	Hypothalamus = 18.04 ± 0.44 Cortex = 17.02 ± 1.0 Hippocampus = 17.24 ± 0.75	One-way ANOVA across regions	No $p = 0.62$
Fed × hungry	Fed hypothalamus = 17.52 ± 1.32 Fed cortex = 16.28 ± 0.21 Fed hypothalamus = 16.64 ± 0.25 Fed cortex = 16.01 ± 0.18	Two-sample *t*-tests Fed × hungry in hypothalamus and cortex (see "Results")	No $p = 0.16$ $p = 0.37$ df = 4
Obese × lean	Obese hypothalamus = 18.7 ± 0.29 Obese cortex = 17.46 ± 0.17 Lean hypothalamus = 18.87 ± 0.56 Lean cortex = 17.38 ± 0.87	Two-sample *t*-tests Obese × lean in hypothalamus and cortex (see "Results")	No $p = 0.83$ $p = 0.85$ df = 4
Glucose level in cell culture medium	0.1 mM = 15.25 ± 0.22 0.5 mM = 15.23 ± 0.20 1.5 mM = 15.28 ± 0.23 2.5 mM = 15.33 ± 0.24 5.0 mM = 15.38 ± 0.27 10.0 mM = 15.42 ± 0.31	One-way ANOVA across glucose concentrations	No $p = 0.99$
Adding sucralose to cell culture medium	0.5 mM glucose = 17.36 ± 0.18 0.5 mM glucose + 0.5 mM sucralose = 16.86 ± 0.33	Two-sample *t*-test 0.5 mM glucose × 0.5 mM glucose + 0.5 mM sucralose	No $p = 0.26$ df = 4

were opposed to autoradiographic film (Kodak BioMax MR film, Cat# 870 1302) and developed in an automated developer. ISH images were captured using a digital camera (Scion Corporation) and visualized using NIH Image J software. Specificity of probes were tested by verifying that anti-sense probes produced no significant hybridizations to brain tissue (results shown in Figure 1 in Supplementary Material).

IMMUNOHISTOCHEMISTRY

Mice were anesthetized with 5% isoflurane, injected with a lethal dose of Euthasol (0.1 ml i.p.) and cardio-perfused with PBS followed by 4% paraformaldehyde (PFA) in PBS. Brains were removed, postfixed in 4% PFA overnight. All brains were cryoprotected in 30% sucrose in PBS. Thirty micrometer sections were cut using a cryostat. For DAB staining, floating sections were pretreated for 1 h in PBS containing 0.3% H_2O_2 to eliminate endogenous peroxidase activity, incubated overnight with rabbit anti-T1R2, or goat anti-T1R3 (1:50, Santa Cruz Biotechnology and Abcam) in 3% normal donkey serum (NDS) in PBS containing 0.25% Triton X-100 (PBST), and then incubated for 1 h with biotinylated donkey anti-rabbit IgG or anti-goat IgG antibody (1:500, Vector Laboratories) followed by ABC solution (Vectastain ABC elite kit, Vector Laboratories). Signals were visualized in PBS containing 0.02% 3,3′-diaminobenzidine-4HCl, and 0.001% H_2O_2. For immunofluorescent labeling, brain sections were incubated overnight with both rabbit anti-α-gustducin (1:100, Santa Cruz, sc-395) and mouse anti-Neun (1:100, Millipore), and then incubated with Alexa-594 donkey anti-rabbit IgG for 1 h, followed by Alexa-488 donkey anti-mouse IgG for 1 h (Invitrogen), and finally mounted on slides using Vectashield anti-fade (Vector Laboratories, CA, USA). Fluorescence images were obtained using a confocal microscope (Fluoview F1000, Olympus).

IN VIVO STUDIES

Adult male mice with a C57BL/6 background were used. At the time of experiments animals were 3–6 months old. Leptin-deficient *ob/ob* mice and their lean wild-type counterparts were obtained from the Jackson Laboratory (Bar Harbor, ME, USA). For the food-deprivation study, 10 wild-type single-housed animals were either selected to be food-deprived for 24 h (water access only) or to remain under *ad libitum* chow and water access. After this period, animals were anesthetized with an overdose of Euthasol (0.1 ml i.p.) and brains were quickly removed, selected brain areas were dissected and samples were immediately sonicated and treated for total RNA extraction as explained above. For experiments with obese hyperglycemic *ob/ob* animals, procedures were as above, with the exception that all animals in this case were maintained at *ad libitum* conditions. Glucose levels were determined by using a hand-held glucometer (OneTouch) following overnight fasting. All procedures were approved by The J. B. Pierce Laboratory Animal Care and Use Committee.

EMBRYONIC MOUSE HYPOTHALAMIC CELL LINE

Plates containing the Embryonic Mouse Hypothalamic Cell Line N38 (Cellutions Biosystems Inc.) was grown in 1 × DMEM (high glucose, Invitrogen) with 10% fetal bovine serum, and 1% penicillin/streptomycin and maintained at 37°C under 5% CO_2. For the glucose-sensing experiments, the cells were washed with PBS and cultured in a no glucose DMEM medium (Invitrogen), to which was added either one of 0.1, 0.5, 1.5, 2.5, 5 and 10 mM glucose (Sigma-Aldrich) or 0.5 mM glucose + 0.5 mM sucralose (USP), for 45 min before RNA extraction. All the other procedures including amplification and analysis of RT quantitative PCR data were as above. To confirm the specificity of and rule out genomic contamination on the RT-PCR assay, the products of *Gnat3*, and *Tas1r1*, *Tas1r2* and *Tas1r3* from mouse cortex were purified using the QIAquick PCR Purification Kit (Qiagen), ligated into the pDrive cloning vector with the QIAGEN PCR Cloning Kit (Qiagen) and sequenced. Multiple sequence alignment was performed on the sequenced amplified segments using the CLUSTAL W (V. 1.8) software. For immunofluorescence experiments, plated cells were fixed for 20 min with 4% PFA in PBS at room temperature, incubated overnight with goat anti-T1R3 and either rabbit anti-α-gustducin or anti-T1R2. Cultured cells were then incubated with Alexa488 donkey anti-rabbit IgG for 1 h, followed by Alexa-594 donkey anti-goat for 1 h (Invitrogen), and finally mounted on slides using Vectashield anti-fade (Vector Laboratories, CA, USA).

RESULTS

AMPLIFICATION AND CLONING OF TASTE GENES FROM MOUSE BRAIN cDNA

Gene-specific Taqman probes and primers (see "Materials and Methods" section) were used to amplify the following taste-related genes: *Tas1r1*, *Tas1r2*, *Tas1r3*, *Gnat3*, *Gnb3* and *Gng13* from mouse brain cDNA. The first three gene products encode the subunits forming the heterodimeric taste receptors T1R1/T1R3 (L-amino acid, Nelson et al., 2002) and T1R2/T1R3 (sweet, Zhao et al., 2003), and the last three respectively encode the products α-gustducin, Gβ3 and Gγ13 that form the α, β and γ subunits of heterotrimeric taste G-protein gustducin (Huang et al., 1999; McLaughlin et al., 1992). All probes were designed to amplify regions containing exon–exon junctions, and PCR product sizes were verified by gel electrophoresis. To completely exclude the possibility that amplification of taste genes resulted from genomic DNA contamination in the samples, PCR products for *Tas1r1*, *Tas1r2*, *Tas1r3* and *Gnat3* were ligated into pDrive cloning vectors, cloned and sequenced. Sequencing results revealed that the amplified regions corresponded to intronless segments 100% similar to the cDNA published sequences (see **Table 1** for the actual cloned sequences and further details).

TASTE-RELATED GENES ARE HIGHLY EXPRESSED IN HYPOTHALAMUS COMPARED TO CORTEX AND HIPPOCAMPUS

Having established that the taste-related genes above are reliably expressed in the mouse brain, we proceeded to quantify the relative amounts of gene expression across different brain regions. We have used an RT quantitative PCR assay similar to a procedure previously employed to quantify relative amounts of taste-related gene expression in the gastro-intestinal tract (Bezencon et al., 2007). Relative gene expression levels across regions were computed using the $2^{-\Delta\Delta C_T}$ method (see "Materials and Methods" and Livak and Schmittgen, 2001) and were expressed as percent expression levels in hypothalamus relative to either cortex or hippocampus. Values = 100% imply that the hypothalamus displayed no relative differences in expression levels with respect to a given region; values > 100% imply that the hypothalamus displayed relatively higher levels of expression compared to a given region; and values < 100% imply that the hypothalamus displayed relatively lower levels of expression compared to a given region (see "Materials and Methods" for details). Templates were obtained from dissected brains of seven adult male C57B6 mice, and relative quantification was performed using a within-subject design and expressed as mean% levels ± SEM in hypothalamus compared to either cortex or hippocampus.

In the forebrain, we have primarily detected the presence of *Tas1r1*, *Tas1r2*, *Tas1r3*, *Gnat3*, *Gnb3* and *Gng13* in the hypothalamus, hippocampus and cortex. Overall, we found that the hypothalamus displayed the highest levels of taste-related gene expression, followed by cortex and hippocampus. We compared the overall percent levels in hypothalamus (with respect to cortex and hippocampus) against the baseline level of 100%. First, a two-way taste gene × brain region ANOVA revealed significant main effects of taste gene ($F = 10.34$, df = 5, $p < 0.001$) and brain region ($F = 6.92$, df = 1, $p < 0.02$) on expression levels, with no significant interaction effects ($F = 1.04$, df = 5, $p = 0.4$). This result suggests, in particular, a difference in expression levels between cortex and hippocampus when these regions are normalized to hypothalamic expression levels. Next, we analyzed expression levels in cortex and hippocampus, in relation to hypothalamic levels, for each taste gene separately. Most often, taste genes were found to be expressed at significantly higher levels in hypothalamus compared to the hippocampus and, to a lesser extent, the cortex. In fact, *Tas1r1* was found to be significantly more expressed in hypothalamus compared to the hippocampus (250 ± 47% of hypothalamic levels, one-sample *t*-test against 100% baseline $t = 3.15$, df = 6, $p < 0.02$) but only marginally higher in hypothalamus compared to cortex (126 ± 26%, $t = 0.73$, df = 6, $p > 0.3$, **Figure 1A**; red dashed line denotes 100% baseline level). On the other hand, *Tas1r2* was found to be expressed at significantly higher levels in hypothalamus compared to both cortex and hippocampus, with relative expression levels of 121 ± 6% ($t = 3.05$, df = 6, $p < 0.03$) and 156 ± 16% ($t = 3.41$, df = 6, $p < 0.02$), respectively (**Figure 1B**). A pattern similar to *Tas1r2* was observed for *Tas1r3*, with this receptor gene being expressed at significantly higher levels in hypothalamus compared to both cortex and hippocampus, with relative expression levels of 228 ± 45% ($t = 2.8$, df = 6, $p < 0.02$) and 505 ± 207% (one-tailed $t = 1.95$, df = 6, $p < 0.05$), respectively (**Figure 1C**). We have also analyzed the relative expression levels of the taste G-protein genes. For *Gnat3*, although expression levels were on average higher in hypothalamus compared to cortex and hippocampus, such difference did not reach significance (129 ± 31%, $t = 0.94$, df = 6, $p = 0.37$ for cortex and 321 ± 136%, $t = 1.62$, df = 6, $p = 0.15$ for hippocampus, **Figure 1D**). The expression levels of *Gnb3*, on the other hand, were clearly higher in hypothalamus compared to both cortex (735 ± 104%, $t = 6.09$, df = 6, $p < 0.001$) and hippocampus (1413 ± 468%, $t = 2.8$, df = 6, $p < 0.04$, **Figure 1E**). Finally, for *Gng13*, expression levels in hypothalamus were only 85 ± 16% of those observed in cortex, a difference that nevertheless was not significant ($t = -0.84$, df = 6, $p = 0.43$), although levels of this gene were significantly higher in hypothalamus compared to hippocampus (224 ± 49%, $t = 2.5$, df = 6, $p < 0.05$, **Figure 1F**).

Overall, our expression analyses revealed that the taste receptor *Tas1r* genes are highly expressed in the hypothalamus compared to both hippocampus and cortex (with the notable exception of *Tas1r1*). In addition, a similar pattern was observed regarding the associated taste G-protein genes, with the exception of *Gnat3*, the gene encoding for the G-protein α-gustducin, which appears to be more homogenously expressed throughout these three forebrain regions than the other taste genes.

TASTE-RELATED GENES ARE PREFERENTIALLY EXPRESSED IN NEURONS

We were also interested in determining the brain cell types more likely to express the taste-related genes. More specifically, to determine whether taste-related proteins are preferentially expressed in neurons compared to other cell types, we performed double-labeling immunofluorescence experiments using antibodies against taste-related proteins and the neuronal marker NeuN, a neuronal-specific nuclear protein in vertebrates (Mullen et al., 1992). Overall, based on our immunohistochemical (IHC) assay, we found that the expression of taste-related genes in the brain is predominantly neuronal. In **Figures 1G–I** are shown the results of double labeling the hippocampal area with antibodies against α-gustducin and NeuN. Whereas essentially all α-gustducin-expressing cells were also labeled by NeuN, virtually none of the large number of astrocytes in this region reacted to the α-gustducin antibody. The same pattern was found to hold for the hypothalamus; the same IHC procedure applied to the hypothalamus revealed a very consistent overlap between α-gustducin- and NeuN-labeled cells (**Figures 1J–L**). Similar patterns were observed for the other taste gene products including T1R2 and T1R3 (not shown). However, it must be noted that scarce numbers of non-neuronal cells also reacted to taste proteins and their expression in non-neuronal tissue cannot be excluded based on our findings.

ANATOMICAL LOCALIZATION OF TASTE-RELATED GENES AND THEIR PRODUCTS IN THE MOUSE BRAIN

To further explore the anatomical localization of the taste-related genes and their products, we performed both ISH and IHC analyses of taste genes and their associated protein products, respectively. We were especially interested in the expression of the subunits forming the heterodimeric sweet receptor T1R2/T1R3. Overall, the pattern resulting form both analyses were highly consistent. We have detected by *ISH* robust expression of *Tas1r2* and *Tas1r3* in the neurons of the CA fields and dentate gyrus of the hippocampus (**Figures 2A and 3A**, respectively). An equivalent expression pattern was obtaining by IHC using two different antibodies against their products (see "Materials and Methods"), as shown in **Figures 2B and 3B** for T1R2 and T1R3, respectively. In addition, strong expression was found in the hypothalamus, in particular in areas surrounding the ventral part of the third ventricle as pointed in the overall brain section by both ISH (**Figures 2C and 3C**) and IHC (**Figures 2D and 3D**) for T1R2 and T1R3, respectively. Note that IHC allowed us to visualize in particular a population of putative neuroendocrine neurons in the paraventricular nucleus of the hypothalamus reacting to both T1R2 and T1R3 (**Figures 2D and 3D,** respectively). In addition, expression patterns were detected in cortex by both ISH (**Figure 2E**) and IHC (**Figures 2F and 3F**).

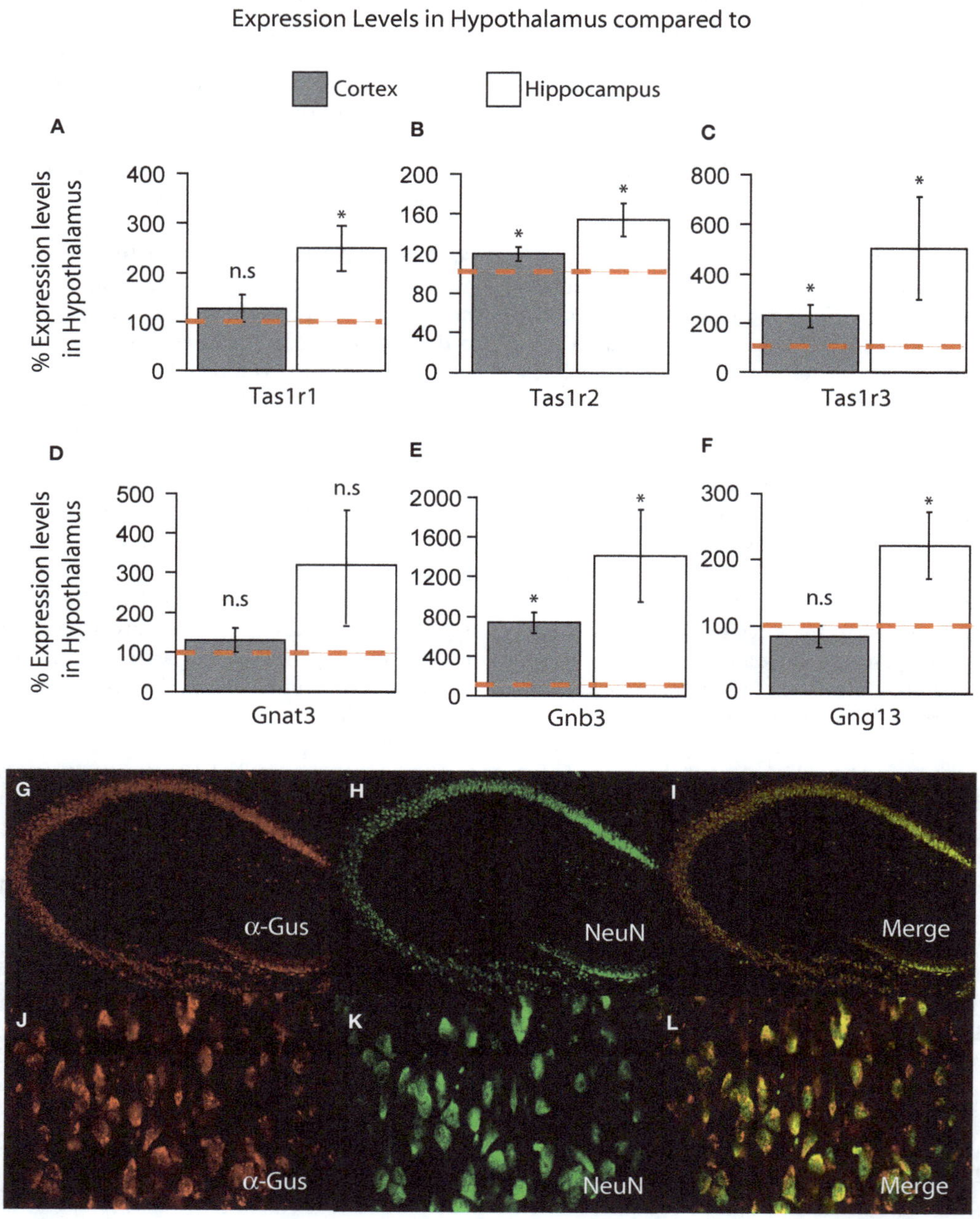

FIGURE 1 | (A–F) Relative levels of expression of taste genes in the mouse hypothalamus compared to cortex and hippocampus. Taste genes were found to be expressed at significantly higher levels in the hypothalamus compared to the other regions found to express these genes, i.e., cortex and hippocampus. The panels depict the results of quantifying the relative levels of expression as obtained by using real-time quantitative PCR methods. Relative gene expression levels across regions were computed using the $2^{-\Delta\Delta C_T}$ method (see "Materials and Methods" and Livak and Schmittgen, 2001) and were expressed as percent expression levels in hypothalamus relative to either cortex or hippocampus. Values = 100% imply that the hypothalamus displayed no relative differences in expression levels with respect to a given region; values > 100% imply that the hypothalamus displayed relatively higher levels of expression compared to a given region; and values < 100% imply that the hypothalamus displayed relatively lower levels of expression compared to a given region (see "Materials and Methods" for details). **(A–C)** Relative levels for taste receptor-related genes *Tas1r1, Tas1r2* and *Tas1r3*, respectively. **(D–F)** Relative levels for taste G-protein-related genes *Gnat3, Gnb3* and *Gng13*, respectively. Note that, overall, the hypothalamus displayed significantly higher levels of expression compared to cortex and hippocampus, with the noted exception of *Tas1r1* in cortex (similar levels in hypothalamus compared to cortex) and the G-protein gene *Gnat3*. See "Results" for details. Dashed red line depicts the 100% baseline levels. (*All $p < 0.05$, one-sample t-test against 100%). n.s.: $p \geq 0.05$. **(G–I)** Co-expression of taste signaling molecules and the nuclear neuronal marker NeuN in the mouse hippocampus as assessed by immunofluorescence methods. Confocal images (×10 magnification) of the mouse hippocampus labeled for α-gustducin **(G)** and NeuN **(H)**. Strong co-expression patterns were observed **(I)**, suggesting that taste-related molecules of the brain are preferentially expressed in neurons. **(J–L)** The same as in **(G–I)**, but for the case of the medial hypothalamus (×60 magnification). Results were qualitatively the same in hypothalamus as in hippocampus.

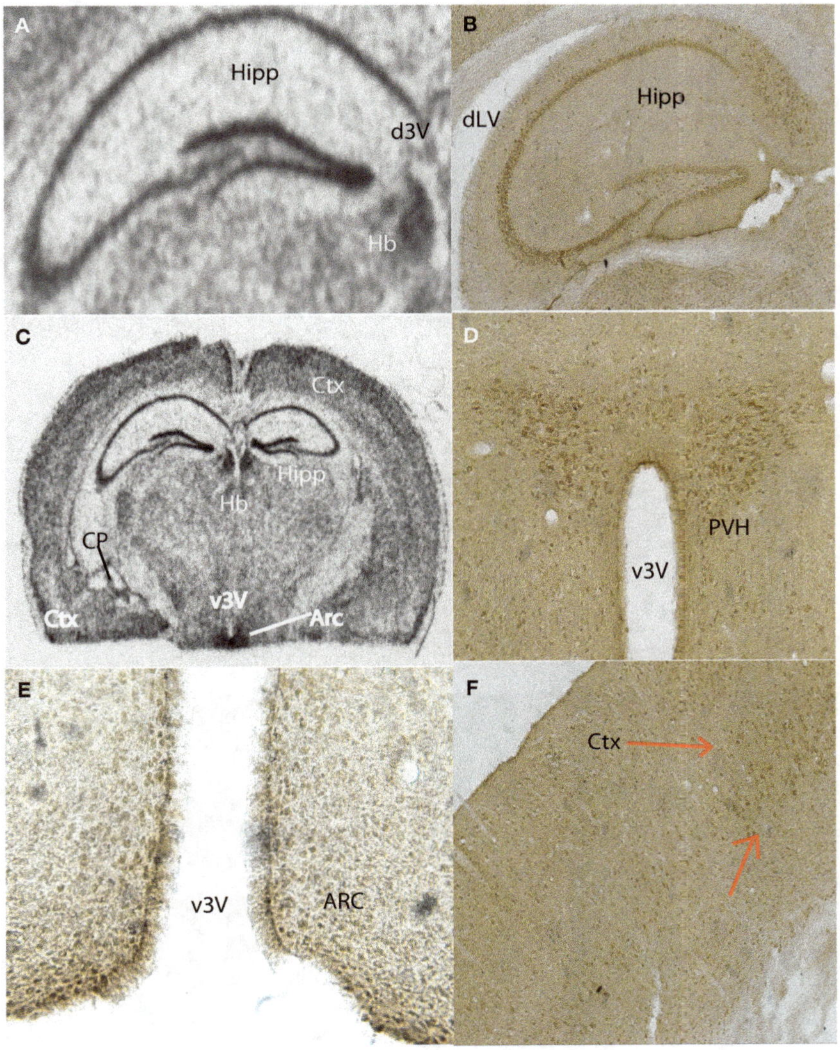

FIGURE 2 | Anatomical distribution of the gene *Tas1r2*, and of its product, the taste receptor subunit T1R2. Images from the mouse hippocampus, hypothalamus and cortex obtained from both in situ hybridization and DAB immunolabeling methods were placed alongside. **(A)** *Tas1r2* and **(B)** T1R2 expression in the hippocampus. Note the strong levels of both gene and protein expression on the CA fields and dentate gyrus, further demonstrating the preferential expression of taste-related elements in neurons. Note also the proximity of the hippocampus to the lateral ventricle. **(C)** Overall view of a brain section hybridized against a *Tas1r2* probe. Note the high levels of expression in hippocampus, periventricular, including arcuate nucleus, of the hypothalamus, cortex and habenula. ISH also identified *Tas1r2* expression in the epithelial cells of the choroid plexus. **(D)** T1R2 expression in the paraventricular nucleus of the hypothalamus. Note the generally higher expression levels of both gene and protein in proximity to the third ventricle. **(E)** T1R2 expression in the arcuate nucleus of the hypothalamus. Note the generally higher expression levels of both gene and protein in proximity to the third ventricle. **(F)** T1R2 expression in the cortex. Note that cortical expression seems to be restricted to layer IV of the cortex for both gene and protein expression. Arc, arcuate nucleus of the hypothalamus; Ctx, cortex; CP, choroid plexus; dLV, dorsal part of the lateral ventricle; d3V, dorsal part of the third ventricle; Hb, habenula; Hipp, hippocampal region; PVH, paraventricular nucleus of the hypothalamus; v3V, ventral part of the third ventricle.

Figures 2E and 3E show the results of immunolabeling against T1R2 and T1R3 antibodies, respectively, in the hypothalamic arcuate nucleus. Finally, it must be noted that additional areas were found to express taste-related genes and proteins, especially areas of the periventricular regions around the dorsal aspect of the third ventricle, including the medial habenula and the epithelial cells of the choroid plexus (shown **Figures 2A–C and 3A–B** for *Tas1r2*/T1R2 and *Tas1r3*/T1R3, respectively) as well as the paraventricular nucleus of the thalamus (not shown).

FOOD DEPRIVATION AND NUTRIENT EXCESS REGULATE EXPRESSION LEVELS OF *Tas1r1* AND *Tas1r2* IN HYPOTHALAMUS BUT NOT CORTEX

To assess the possible functional roles of taste-related signals in the brain, we have performed further RT quantitative PCR analyses on hypothalamic and cortical samples from five mice exposed to 24-h food deprivation and compared the gene expression levels in these animals to those observed in five mice that were fed *ad libitum*. We reasoned that, if taste-related signaling elements play a role in sensing nutrients in the brain, then their levels might be regulated

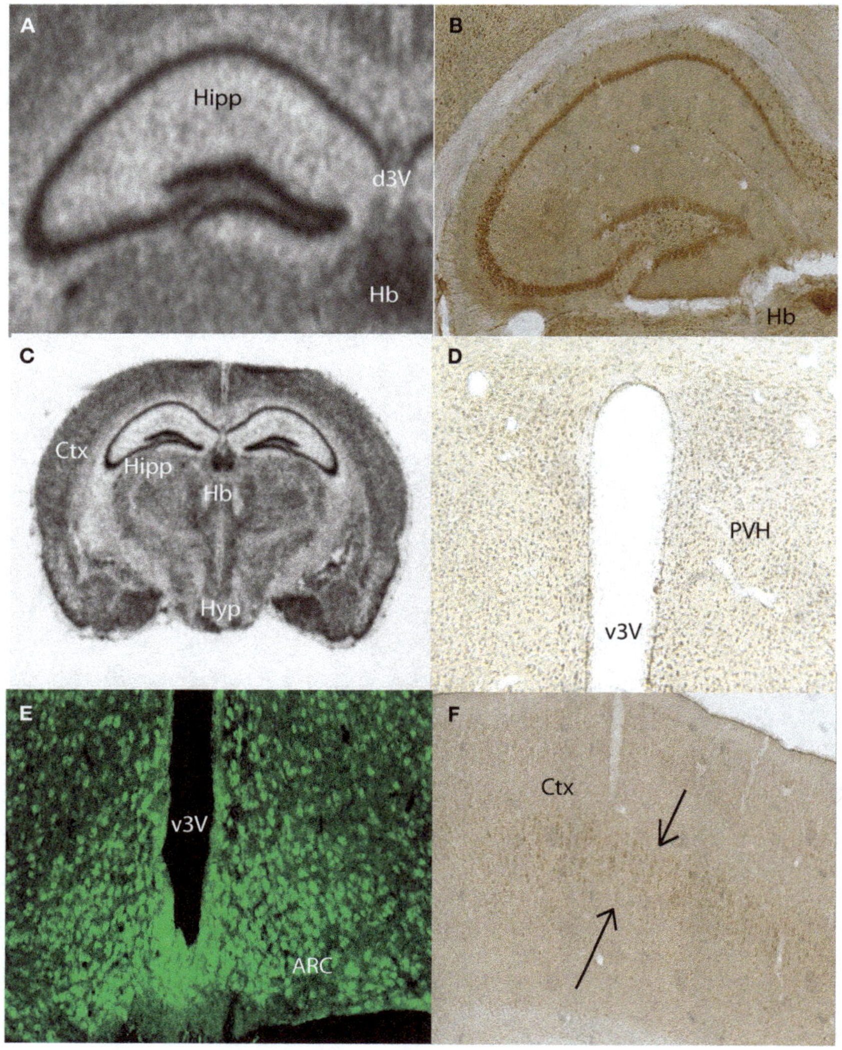

FIGURE 3 | Anatomical distribution of the gene *Tas1r3*, and of its product, the taste receptor subunit T1R3. Images from the mouse hippocampus, hypothalamus and cortex obtained from both in situ hybridization and DAB immunolabeling methods were placed alongside. **(A)** *Tas1r3* and **(B)** T1R3 expression in the hippocampus. Note the strong levels of both gene and protein expression on the CA fields and dentate gyrus, further demonstrating the preferential expression of taste-related elements in neurons. Note also the proximity of the hippocampus to the lateral ventricle. **(C)** Overall view of a brain section hybridized against a *Tas1r3* probe. Note the high levels of expression in hippocampus, hypothalamus, cortex and habenula. ISH also identified *Tas1r3* expression in the epithelial cells of the choroid plexus. **(D)** T1R3 expression in the hypothalamus. In **(D)**, note the generally higher expression levels of both gene and protein in proximity to the third ventricle (PVH). **(E)** T1R3 expression in the arcuate nucleus of the hypothalamus as revealed by immunofluorescence methods. Picture was taken using a confocal microscope. **(F)** T1R3 expression in the cortex. Note that cortical expression seems to be restricted to layer IV of the cortex. ARC, arcuate nucleus of the hypothalamus; Ctx, cortex; CP, choroid plexus; dLV, dorsal part of the lateral ventricle; d3V, dorsal part of the third ventricle; Hb, habenula; Hipp, hippocampal region; Hyp, basal aspect of the hypothalamus; PVH, paraventricular nucleus of the hypothalamus; v3V, ventral part of the third ventricle.

by the nutritional state of the animal, which will determine the concentration and identity of nutrients including glucose and amino acids that actually reach the brain. Overall, we found that the taste receptor genes *Tas1r1* and *Tas1r2* increased their levels of expression following food deprivation in the hypothalamus, but not in cortex, indicating that taste receptor-related genes are sensitive to nutrient levels in the brain regions regulating energy homeostasis. These changes in expression levels seemed to be specific to the taste receptor genes *Tas1r1* and *Tas1r2*. In fact, compared to fed animals, deprived animals showed non-significant decreases in *Gnat3* in both hypothalamus (81 ± 25%, paired within-subject two-sample one-tailed t-test against 100% baseline, df = 4, $t = -0.7$, $p > 0.7$) and cortex (73 ± 26%, $t = -0.1$, $p > 0.8$, see **Figure 4A**); however, *Tas1r1* levels were significantly higher in deprived compared to fed animals in hypothalamus (164 ± 21%, $t = 2.94$, $p < 0.03$) but not in cortex (165 ± 35%, $t = 1.84$, $p = 0.07$, see **Figure 4B**). A similar effect was found for *Tas1r2*: expression levels were significantly higher in deprived, compared to

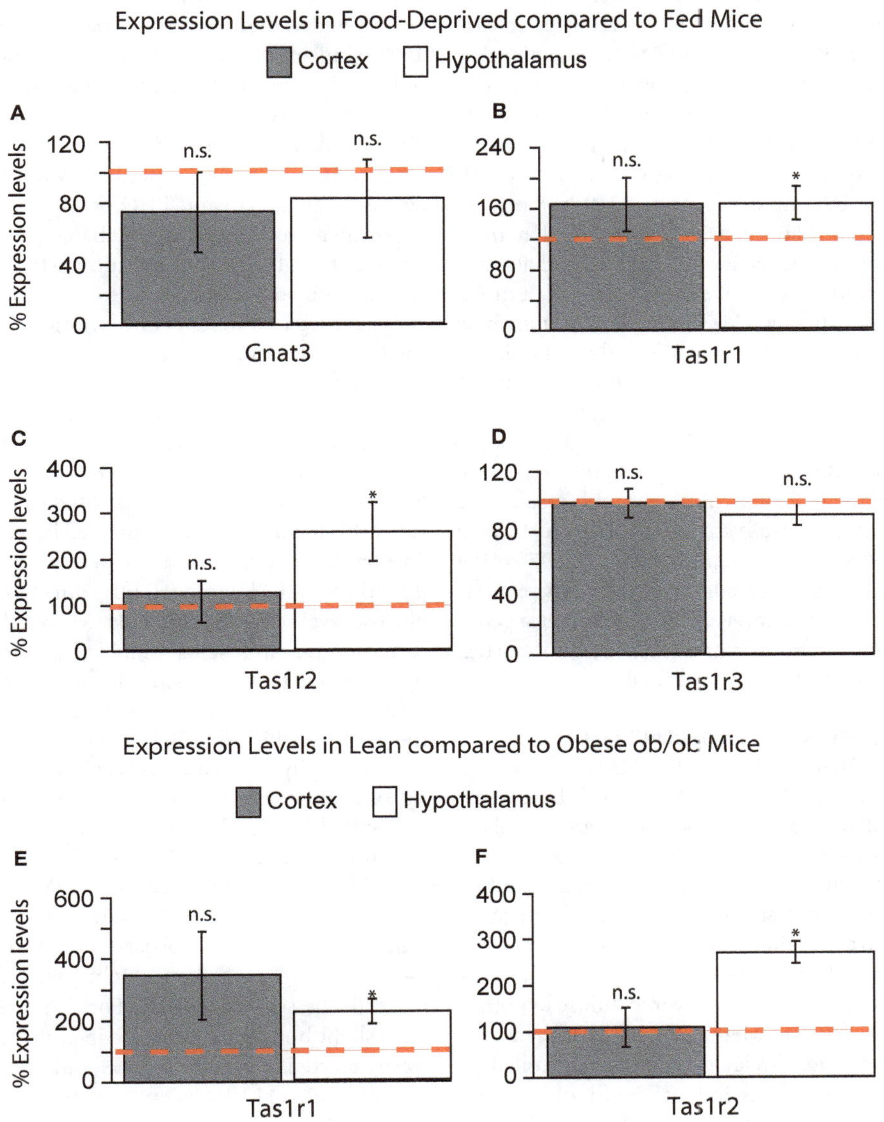

FIGURE 4 | (A–D) Relative levels of expression of taste genes in food-deprived mice compared to fed mice in hypothalamus and cortex. Taste receptor-related genes *Tas1r1* and *Tas1r2* were found to be expressed at significantly higher levels in the hypothalamus, but not cortex, of food-deprived animals when compared to fed animals. The panels depict the results of quantifying the relative levels of expression as obtained by using real-time quantitative PCR methods. Relative gene expression levels across regions were computed using the $2^{-\Delta\Delta C_T}$ method (see "Materials and Methods" and Livak and Schmittgen, 2001) and were expressed as percent expression levels in hypothalamus or cortex observed in deprived compared to fed animals. Values = 100% imply that the brain region displayed no relative differences in expression levels in deprived compared to fed animals; values > 100% imply that the brain region displayed relatively higher levels of expression in deprived compared to fed animals; and values < 100% imply that the brain region displayed relatively lower levels of expression in deprived compared to fed animals (see "Materials and Methods" for details). **(A–D)** Relative levels for taste receptor-related genes *Gnat3, Tas1r1, Tas1r2* and *Tas1r3*, respectively. Note significant changes in *Tas1r1* and *Tas1r2* levels. **(E–F)** Taste receptor-related genes *Tas1r1* and *Tas1r2* were found to be expressed at significantly higher levels the hypothalamus, but not cortex, of lean animals when compared to obese, hyperglycemic *ob/ob* mice. Data are expressed as percent levels of expression in the deprived animals compared to the fed animals, with 100% representing baseline (no relative change) levels. Panels show relative levels for taste receptor-related genes *Tas1r1* **(E)** and *Tas1r2* **(F)**. The other genes did not show significant changes in expression levels. (*All $p < 0.05$, one-sample *t*-test against 100%). Dashed red line depicts the 100% baseline levels.

fed animals in hypothalamus (255 ± 64%, $t = 2.41, p < 0.04$) but not in cortex (124 ± 25%, $t = 0.94, p = 0.2$, see **Figure 4C**). Finally, and rather strikingly given the above, no significant changes were observed for *Tas1r3* in either hypothalamus (90 ± 7%, $t = -1.14, p > 0.8$) or cortex (99 ± 9%, $t = -0.15, p > 0.5$, see **Figure 4D**). These results indicate that the expression levels of the taste receptor genes *Tas1r1* and *Tas1r2* in the hypothalamus are under the control of nutrient availability.

We next asked the question of whether, conversely, abnormally high levels of circulating nutrients could induce a relative decrease in expression levels in hyperglycemic compared to euglycemic mice. We have therefore compared the taste gene expression levels in hypothalamus and cortex between obese hyperglycemic *ob/ob* mice ($n = 5$) and wild-type lean controls ($n = 5$). Hyperglycemia in *ob/ob* was confirmed by measuring blood glucose levels with glucometer (lean: 199 ± 28 mg/dL; obese: 440 ± 58 mg/dL, $p < 0.02$). Based on the results above, we hypothesized that *Tas1r* genes would be expressed at higher levels in the hypothalamus, but not cortex, of lean compared to obese mice. In fact, a direct comparison between *Tas1r* expression levels between lean and obese animals reveal that lean mice displayed significantly higher levels of expression in hypothalamus (205 ± 53%, paired within-subject two-sample one-tailed *t*-test against 100%, $t = 1.94$, $p < 0.04$) but not in cortex (192 ± 54%, $t = 1.69$, $p = 0.056$), although one must note that results from cortex were close to reach significant levels. In any event, once again the main contributors to this result were *Tas1r1* (221 ± 38% in hypothalamus vs. 345 ± 143% in cortex, see **Figure 4E**) and *Tas1r2* (269 ± 58% in hypothalamus vs. 107 ± 41% in cortex, see **Figure 4F**). Overall, the results from our *in vivo* experiments indicate that the expression levels of the taste receptor genes *Tas1r1* and *Tas1r2* in the mouse hypothalamus, but not cortex, reflect the current nutritional state of the animal.

GLUCOSE AND SUCRALOSE SPECIFICALLY MODULATE *Tas1r2* EXPRESSION LEVELS IN A MOUSE HYPOTHALAMIC CELL LINE

It could be argued, however, that the patterns described above result from systemic effects related to prolonged food deprivation or obesity, rather than nutrient sensing *per se*. In fact, one must consider the possibility that systemic factors such as changes in insulin and/or stress hormone levels drive expression levels of taste-related genes in the brain. Therefore, to ascertain that gene levels were primarily under the control of extracellular levels of nutrients, we adopted as an additional experimental model an embryonic mouse hypothalamic cell line (see "Materials and Methods"). We reasoned that, if the levels of expression of taste-related genes are controlled by extracellular availability of nutrients independently of systemic or metabolic factors, then manipulating the levels of nutrients in the medium should suffice to specifically alter taste gene levels in these dissociated cells. In particular, we hypothesized that imposing physiological changes in glucose levels to the medium while maintaining other nutrient levels unaltered should specifically alter expression levels of *Tas1r2*, the sweet-specific gene, while leaving the levels of the other *Tas1rs* unaltered.

Before running the hypothalamic cell culture experiments we ascertained the plausibility of this model by verifying that these cells endogenously express taste-receptor genes. Likewise the case of our fresh brain samples, gene-specific Taqman probes and primers (see "Materials and Methods") were used to amplify the following taste-related genes: *Tas1r1*, *Tas1r2*, *Tas1r3*, *Gnat3*, *Gnb3* and *Gng13* from cultured hypothalamic cells cDNA. As explained above, all probes were designed to amplify regions containing exon–exon junctions, and PCR product sizes were verified by gel electrophoresis. To completely exclude the possibility of genomic DNA contamination in the samples, PCR products for *Tas1r1*, *Tas1r2*, *Tas1r3* and *Gnat3* were ligated into pDrive cloning vectors, cloned and sequenced. Sequencing results revealed that the amplified regions corresponded to intronless segments 100% similar to cDNA, and 100% similar to the sequences cloned from adult mouse brains as described above (see **Table 1** for the actual cloned sequences). These findings were corroborated by probing plated cells with T1R2 and T1R3 antibodies (**Figures 5A,B**) and verifying their co-expression (**Figure 5C**). The same procedure was adopted using antibodies against α-gustducin and T1R2 or T1R3 (not shown).

We then proceeded to assess changes in gene expression levels as a function of glucose concentration in the medium. Specifically, we have quantified the expression levels of taste genes in hypothalamic cells exposed to different concentrations of glucose in the culture medium. We assured that these manipulations in glucose levels were physiologically significant by using concentrations of extracellular glucose close to those found in the rodent hypothalamus during hypo-, eu- and hyperglycemic states (de Vries et al., 2003). More precisely, we have compared the expression levels of taste genes in hypothalamic cells exposed to a severely hypoglycemic (0.1 mM) medium to those observed in cells exposed to higher glucose levels including eu- and hyperglycemic concentrations (from 0.5 up to 10 mM). Importantly, during these experiments only glucose levels were manipulated, whereas levels of other nutrients including L-amino acids remained unaltered. We have therefore hypothesized that increasing glucose levels in the culture medium would produce a significant reduction in the expression levels of the sweet-specific gene *Tas1r2*, but not of the other receptor genes, in cultured hypothalamic cells. Consistent with our hypothesis, hypothalamic cells exposed to a 0.5 mM medium expressed significantly lower levels of *Tas1r2* compared to those exposed to the 0.1 mM medium (157 ± 21% relative decrease in expression with 0.5 mM medium compared to 0.1 mM medium, one-tailed one-sample *t*-test against 100%, $t = 2.68$, df = 4, $p < 0.05$), whereas no significant changes were observed for *Tas1r1* or *Tas1r3* (103 ± 6%, $t = 0.56$, df = 4, $p = 0.3$ and 116 ± 13%, $t = 1.19$, df = 4, $p = 0.14$, respectively, see **Figure 5D**). For G-protein gene levels, except for a slight but robust decrease in *Gnb3* levels, no other changes were detected (for *Gnat3*, *Gnb3* and *Gng13*, 106 ± 4%, $t = 1.46$, df = 4, $p = 0.1$; 113 ± 4%, $t = 2.91$, df = 4, $p < 0.03$ and 113 ± 10%, $t = 1.29$, df = 4, $p = 0.13$, respectively, not shown).

A similar pattern holds for the other glucose concentrations used. In fact, hypothalamic cells exposed to a 1.5 mM medium expressed significantly lower levels of *Tas1r2* compared to those exposed to the 0.1 mM medium (161 ± 23%, $t = 2.61$, df = 4, $p < 0.03$), whereas no significant changes were observed for *Tas1r1* or *Tas1r3* (99 ± 6%, $t = -0.1$, df = 4, $p = 0.54$ and 132 ± 17%, $t = 1.81$, df = 4, $p = 0.07$, respectively, see **Figure 5E**). No changes were associated in this case with the G-protein gene levels (for *Gnat3*, *Gnb3* and *Gng13*, 96 ± 6%, $t = -0.56$, df = 4, $p = 0.69$; 112 ± 12%, $t = 1.0$, df = 4, $p = 0.18$ and 108 ± 8%, $t = 1.03$, df = 4, $p = 0.17$, respectively, not shown). Similarly, hypothalamic cells exposed to a 2.5 mM medium expressed significantly lower levels of *Tas1r2* compared to those exposed to the 0.1 mM medium (162 ± 21%, $t = 2.91$, df = 4, $p < 0.03$), whereas no significant changes were observed for *Tas1r1* or *Tas1r3* (125 ± 18%, $t = 1.39$, df = 4, $p = 0.11$ and 187 ± 54%, $t = 1.59$, df = 4, $p = 0.09$, respectively, see **Figure 5F**). No changes were associated in this case with the G-protein gene levels (for *Gnat3*, *Gnb3* and *Gng13*, 126 ± 19%, $t = 1.32$, df = 4, $p = 0.12$;

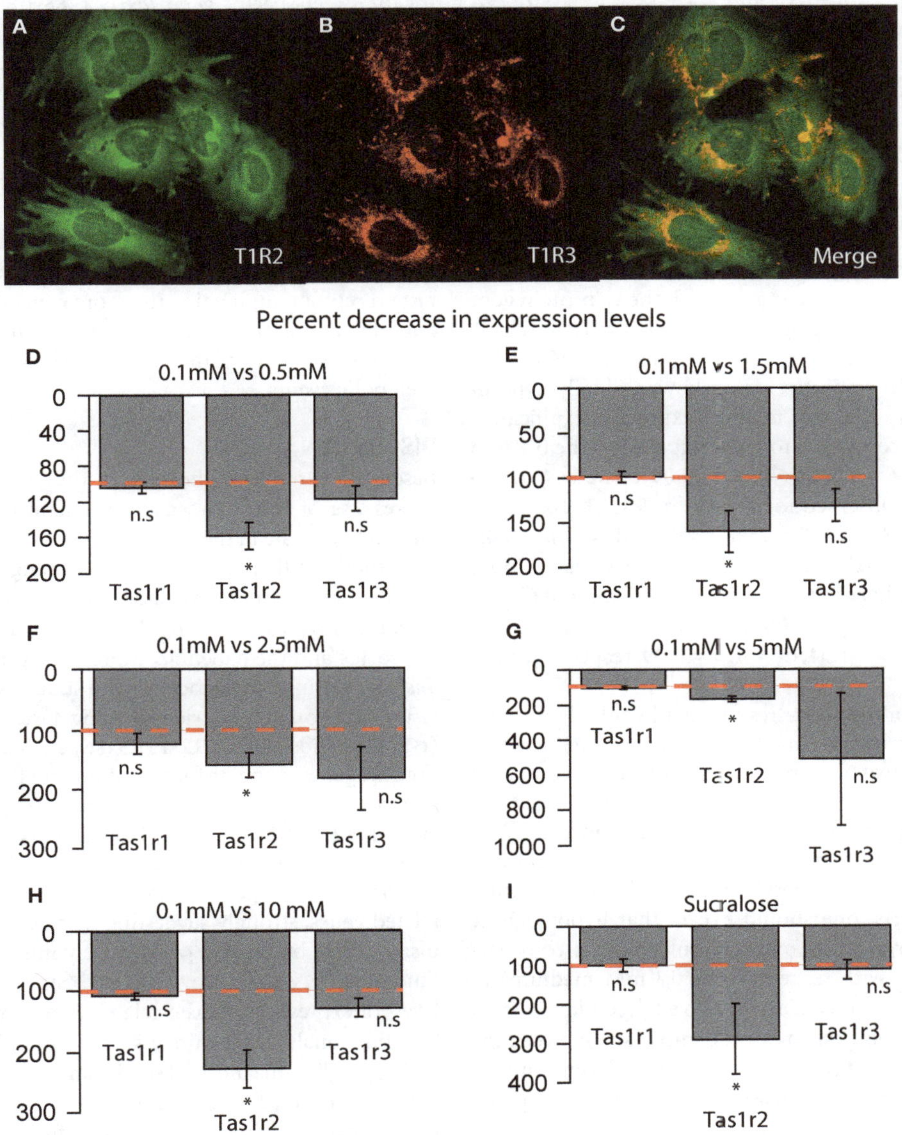

FIGURE 5 | (A–C) Co-expression of taste signaling molecules in the embryonic mouse hypothalamic cell line N38 as assessed by immunofluorescence methods. Confocal images (×10 magnification) of N38 cells that we determine endogenously express taste-related molecules. **(A)** Expression of the receptor subunit T1R2; **(B)** expression of the receptor subunit T1R3; **(C)** merging, showing that these cells express both subunits of the sweet receptor T1R2/T1R3. **(D–E)** Relative decrease in the levels of expression of the sweet-specific receptor gene *Tas1r2* in cultured N38 cells as a function of glucose levels in culture medium. The sweet receptor-specific gene *Tas1r2*, but not others, was found to be expressed at significantly higher levels in N38 cells exposed to a low-glucose medium (0.1 mM) compared to cells exposed to higher glucose levels. The panels depict the results of quantifying the relative levels of expression as obtained by using real-time quantitative PCR methods. Relative gene expression levels across regions were computed using the $2^{-\Delta\Delta C_T}$ method (see "Materials and Methods" and Livak and Schmittgen, 2001) and were expressed as percent decrease in expression levels in cells exposed to a medium containing from 0.5 up to 10 mM glucose compared to cells exposed to a medium containing 0.1 mM glucose. Values = 100% imply that no relative differences in expression levels were detected in cells exposed to a medium containing higher glucose levels (0.5–10 mM) compared to cells exposed to a medium containing 0.1 mM glucose; values < 100% imply that significant decreases in expression levels were detected in cells exposed to a medium containing higher glucose levels compared to cells exposed to a medium containing 0.1 mM glucose. **(D)** Decrease in taste receptor levels produced by increasing glucose medium from 0.1 to 0.5 mM glucose. **(E)** Decrease in taste receptor levels produced by increasing glucose medium from 0.1 to 1.5 mM glucose. **(F)** Decrease in taste receptor levels produced by increasing glucose medium from 0.1 to 2.5 mM glucose. **(G)** Decrease in taste receptor levels produced by increasing glucose medium from 0.1 to 5 mM glucose. **(H)** Decrease in taste receptor levels produced by increasing glucose medium from 0.1 to 10 mM glucose. **(I)** Decrease in *Tas1r2* levels produced by adding 0.5 mM sucralose to 0.5 mM glucose. Values = 100% imply that no relative differences in expression levels were detected in cells exposed to a medium containing 0.5 mM glucose + 0.5 mM sucralose compared to cells exposed to a medium containing 0.5 mM glucose; values < 100% imply that significant decreases in expression levels were detected in cells exposed to a medium containing 0.5-mM glucose + 0.5 mM sucralose compared to cells exposed to a medium containing 0.5 mM glucose. Dashed red line depicts the 100% baseline levels. (*All $p < 0.05$, one-sample *t*-test against 100%). n.s.: $p \geq 0.05$.

151 ± 31%, $t = 1.63$, df = 4, $p = 0.08$ and 124 ± 18%, $t = 1.3$, df = 4, $p = 0.13$, respectively, not shown).

The above was still the case for hypothalamic cells exposed to hyperglycemic media. In fact, hypothalamic cells exposed to a 5.0 mM medium expressed significantly lower levels of *Tas1r2* compared to those exposed to the 0.1 mM medium (167 ± 15%, $t = 4.49$, df = 4, $p < 0.006$), whereas no significant changes were observed for *Tas1r1* or *Tas1r3*, despite the large variance associated with this gene (102 ± 8%, $t = 0.28$, df = 4, $p = 0.39$ and 509 ± 375%, $t = 1.08$, df = 4, $p = 0.16$, respectively, see **Figure 5G**). No changes were associated, once again, with the G-protein gene levels (for *Gnat3*, *Gnb3* and *Gng13*, 103 ± 2%, $t = 1.18$, df = 4, $p = 0.14$; 116 ± 10%, $t = 1.57$, df = 4, $p = 0.09$ and 104 ± 7%, $t = 0.67$, df = 4, $p = 0.26$, respectively, not shown). Finally, hypothalamic cells exposed to a 10.0 mM medium expressed significantly lower levels of *Tas1r2* compared to those exposed to the 0.1 mM medium (227 ± 31%, $t = 4.0$, df = 4, $p < 0.009$), whereas no significant changes were observed for *Tas1r1* or *Tas1r3* (107 ± 4%, $t = 1.64$, df = 4, $p = 0.08$ and 128 ± 15%, $t = 1.88$, df = 4, $p = 0.06$, respectively, see **Figure 5H**). No changes were associated, once more, with the G-protein gene levels (for *Gnat3*, *Gnb3* and *Gng13*, 109 ± 5%, $t = 1.65$, df = 4, $p = 0.08$; 124 ± 18%, $t = 1.29$, df = 4, $p = 0.13$ and 112 ± 7%, $t = 1.54$, df = 4, $p = 0.09$, respectively, not shown).

It is noticeable from the above results that hypothalamic cells exposed to the hyperglycemic media (5 and 10 mM) seem to express considerably greater decreases in *Tas1r2* levels compared to cells exposed to the 1.5 and 2.5 mM euglycemic media (all comparisons with respect to the baseline 0.1 mM medium). In fact, based on the data described in the previous section regarding the comparison between hyperglycemic *ob/ob* mice and their euglycemic counterparts, one should expect that hypothalamic cells exposed to hyperglycemic media should express considerably greater decreases (with respect to the 0.1 mM medium) in *Tas1r2* levels compared to the cells exposed to euglycemic media. In accordance with our hypothesis, a direct comparison between the two conditions revealed that cells exposed to hyperglycemic media expressed significantly greater decreases in *Tas1r2* levels compared to cells exposed to euglycemic media (197 ± 19% vs. 161 ± 14%, respectively, one-tailed two-sample $t = 1.86$, df = 9, $p < 0.05$). Therefore, although the *Tas1r2* levels do not seem to change in strict accordance with fluctuations in extracellular glucose concentrations, this receptor gene does function as a sensor whose expression levels change according to whether glucose levels deviate from euglycemic concentrations, an observation that is consistent with our *in vivo* studies presented above using *ob/ob* mice.

We then reasoned that, if sweet taste-like signaling mechanisms do in fact function as monitors of extracellular levels independently of either systemic or intracellular, GK-mediated mechanisms, then adding the non-metabolizable artificial sweetener sucralose to the medium should produce specific decreases in *Tas1r2*, but not *Tas1r1* or *Tas1r3*, levels. In fact, a one-way ANOVA performed on the percent change data associated with adding sucralose to the 0.5 mM medium revealed a significant main effect of gene ($p < 0.04$) on the relative changes in gene expression level. Conforming to our initial hypothesis, the larger decreases in gene expression levels produced by adding sucralose to the hypoglycemic medium were observed for the sweet-specific gene *Tas1r2* (288 ± 89% of baseline levels), compared to no changes for the L-amino acid specific gene *Tas1r1* (99 ± 16%) or *Tas1r3* (113 ± 25%, **Figure 5I**). No detectable changes in expression were found for taste G-protein-related genes (*Gnat3* 106 ± 18%, *Gng13* 105 ± 12% and *Gnb3* 137 ± 25%, not shown), although the relatively larger although non-statistically significant change in *Gnb3* might indicate a possible specific role of this G-protein in sweet taste.

In conclusion, our experiments with cultured cells provide evidence in favor of a functional role for neuron-expressed sweet taste receptors, supporting the more general proposal that neuronal cells can monitor changes in extracellular levels of glucose via sweet taste signaling pathways that are independent of intracellular metabolic events.

DISCUSSION

Based on the results of the present study, we propose that the brain makes use of nutrient-sensing mechanisms analogous to those known to operate in the periphery, i.e., via G-protein coupled taste receptors and their downstream signaling molecules. More specifically, we have demonstrated that neurons located in different forebrain regions, including the hypothalamus, the hippocampus, the cortex and the habenula, express the genes *Tas1r1*, *Tas1r2* and *Tas1r3*, that in turn encode for the subunits of the heterodimeric G-protein coupled nutrient-sensing taste receptors T1R1/T1R3 (L-amino acids) and T1R2/T1R3 (sweet, Zhao et al., 2003). In addition, the genes encoding for the subunits of the taste-specific heterotrimeric G-protein gustducin, formed by α-gustducin (McLaughlin et al., 1992), Gβ3 and Gγ13 (Huang et al., 1999), were also found to be expressed in these same brain regions. ISH and IHC analyses revealed a high degree of anatomical overlap between these taste-related genes, strongly suggesting that taste-like signaling mechanisms might be capable of effectively influence neuronal activity. Furthermore, we also provide the first supporting evidence that the levels of expression of taste-related genes are under the control of the nutritional state of animal, since we found that food deprivation and hyperglycemia induced significant changes in expression levels of the *Tas1r1* and *Tas1r2* genes in the hypothalamus. Finally, the fact that changes in expression levels as a function of nutritional state were restricted to the hypothalamus in turn suggests that taste-like signaling mechanisms in the brain might be involved in the central regulation of homeostatic processes.

Different lines of evidence support the notion that taste signaling molecules might function as chemosensors in different physiological settings. In fact, seminal work by Hofer, Drenckhahn and colleagues provided the first line of evidence that taste-like signaling mechanisms might be used by the gastrointestinal tract to sense the presence of nutrients in the lumen (e.g., Hofer et al., 1996). They have extended their findings to show that taste mechanisms might also be involved in more general endocrine functions via their expression in the pancreas (Höfer and Drenckhahn, 1998). Early indication that such taste mechanisms play important physiological functions came with the discovery by Rozengurt and colleagues that the taste G-protein α-gustducin is expressed in PYY- and GLP-1-producing L cells of the intestine (Rozengurt and Sternini, 2007; Rozengurt et al., 2006). More recently, it has been shown that taste receptor molecules are richly expressed in the intestinal mucosa, including the sweet receptor T1R2/T1R3 (Bezencon et al., 2007), where it plays important physiological roles by mediating hormonal responses to the presence of tastants in the lumen (Margolskee et al., 2007). Of particular interest to our case is the fact that transcript levels of *Tas1r2* are strongly reduced following jejunal glucose perfusion in mice (Young et al., 2009), a result that closely reflects our own findings in hypothalamus (see below). More generally, we propose that an analogous phenomenon to those observed in the gut takes place with respect to neuronal glucosensing, with similar chemosensory mechanisms acting as glucose receptors in disparate physiological settings.

The principle that taste-like signaling mechanisms might play functional roles in the central nervous system also has its precedents. For example, it has been shown that the tongue-expressed PKD2L1, a polycystic-kidney-disease-like ion channel and candidate mammalian sour taste sensor, is also expressed in specific neurons surrounding the central canal of the spinal cord (Huang et al., 2006). More specifically, it has been demonstrated that the PKD2L1-expressing neurons send terminals to the central canal and trigger action potentials in response to decreases in extracellular pH (Huang et al., 2006).

Among all brain regions, one would expect that nutrient-sensing taste receptors must be found primarily in the hypothalamus, the master brain circuit controlling body homeostasis (Elmquist et al., 1999). In fact, our RT quantitative PCR expression data shows that the hypothalamus expresses significantly higher levels of taste-related genes compared to the cortex or hippocampus. Of particular interest was the expression of taste receptors in hypothalamic regions surrounding the ventral aspect of the third ventricle. This privileged anatomical location allows neurons to have proximal access to the contents of the cerebrospinal fluid and to modulate their responses accordingly. In this regard, it is of interest that T1R2 and T1R3 signals were strongly expressed in the paraventricular nucleus of the hypothalamus, a brain region fundamentally implicated in counter-regulatory responses to hypoglycemia. One interesting topic for future investigation concerns the possibility that paraventricular neurons expressing corticotrophin releasing factor (CRF), a secretagogue factor whose liberation by paraventricular neurons eventually results in adrenal discharge via actions on the anterior pituitary (Porterfield and White, 2007), express sweet taste receptors. CRF release is a fundamental response to deviations from normal glucose levels (McCrimmon, 2008), and the presence of T1R2 and T1R3 in paraventricular regions known to contain CRF-producing neurons is suggestive of chemosensory functions in this region. Of particular interest will be the testing of the hypothesis that T1R2 knockout mice display abnormal counter-regulatory responses to hypoglycemia due to impaired glucosensing abilities in CRF neurons.

The expression of taste sensors in the hippocampus, on the other hand, is seemingly less likely to have been anticipated. However, it must be noted that several molecular studies demonstrated that the hippocampus is a primary target for ligands that reflect body physiology, including ion balance (calcium, magnesium), insulin, immunity response elements, as well as reproductive, satiety and stress hormones (reviewed in Lathe, 2001). This argues that a primary, more fundamental role for the hippocampus refers to sensing soluble molecules present in blood and cerebrospinal fluid (Lathe, 2001). We propose that the currently known list of chemosensory functions of the hippocampus must be expanded to include nutrient sensing. The idea that hippocampal neurons have the ability to sense extracellular levels of nutrients is further corroborated by the fact that, in rats, moderate recurrent hypoglycemia prevented age-related decline in hippocampal-related cognitive functions (McNay et al., 2006), indicating that hippocampal neurons might functionally detect extracellular levels of glucose in this region.

We note that the *Allen Mouse Brain Atlas*[1], a massive ISH project dedicated to map the brain expression of the mouse genome, also displays expression maps for *Tas1r* genes. However, we believe that our expression analyses add considerably to the brain maps reported in the atlas. First, it is not possible to visualize, from the rather weak and diffuse patterns displayed in the atlas, the expression of hypothalamic taste receptors in proximity to the ventral part of the third ventricle. Among these hypothalamic regions, we must mention as of great interest the paraventricular and arcuate nuclei of the hypothalamus. The expression of taste receptor signals in these hypothalamic regions known to be involved in neuroendocrine control strongly suggests a role for these molecules as glucose sensors in the brain (Porterfield and White, 2007). A similar observation holds for structures such as the habenula and the choroid plexus. Another crucial piece of information deriving from our IHC analyses – that cannot be readily obtained from the atlas – refers to the neuronal expression of taste receptor proteins. In fact, our analysis is the first one, to our knowledge, to indicate that nutrient sensing in the brain via taste-like signaling pathways might directly influence electrical neuronal activity. This is particularly relevant for the identification of the chemosensors that have the ability to induce hormone release from neuroendocrine neurons of the paraventricular and arcuate nuclei of the hypothalamus during low glycemic levels (see above).

Finally, the results from our *in vivo* and cell culture experiments indicate that the expression levels of the genes that code for G-protein sweet receptors are under the control of nutritional status. On one hand, our *in vivo* experiments have shown that nutritional deficiency and excess produce opposing effects on the expression levels of *Tas1r1* and *Tas1r2*, with states of nutrient deficiency being associated with upregulation of transcript levels while the opposite effect on gene levels was observed in obese, hyperglycemic mice. However, it could be argued that such effects depended not on neuronal nutrient sensing *per se*, but rather on non-specific systemic effects produced for example by chronic nutrient excess. To resolve the issue of whether nutrient sensing occurs in neuronal cells expressing taste receptors independently of systemic factors or synaptic contact, we have compared the expression levels of taste genes in cultured hypothalamic cells exposed to a severely hypoglycemic (0.1 mM) medium to those observed in cells exposed to higher glucose levels including eu- and hyperglycemic concentrations (from 0.5 up to 10 mM). Consistent with our *in vivo* studies, increasing glucose levels in the culture medium produced a significant reduction in the expression levels of the sweet-specific gene *Tas1r2*, but not of the other receptor genes (since in these experiments only glucose, but not other nutrients including L-amino acids, levels

[1]http://mouse.brain.map.org

were manipulated). Although our experiments with cultured cells showed that *Tas1r2* levels do not seem to change in strict accordance (i.e., linearly) to fluctuations in extracellular glucose, these experiments demonstrate that this membrane receptor gene does function as a sensor whose expression levels change according to whether glucose levels deviate from euglycemic concentrations. In particular, we have shown that hypothalamic cells exposed to hyperglycemic (5 and 10 mM glucose) media express considerably lower levels of *Tas1r2* compared to the cells exposed to euglycemic (1.5 and 2.5 mM) media. This finding might shed further light on the mechanisms underlying deficient central regulation of glucose homeostasis in obese subjects (Elmquist et al., 2005).

The above effects of extracellular glucose concentrations on *Tas1r2* expression levels did not depend on intracellular metabolism of glucose. In fact, the finding that adding the non-metabolizable artificial sweetener sucralose to the cultured cells medium resulted in lower expression levels of *Tas1r2*, the only sweet-specific gene, but not others, suggest that brain glucosensing might be partially mediated by taste-like signaling pathways that do not depend on metabolic actions of GK, the enzyme considered to function as the primary glucosensor in neurons (Karschin et al., 1997). Our findings are consistent with several lines of evidence suggesting that glucosensing neurons might use alternative, GK/K_{ATP}-independent pathways to respond to local fluctuations in glucose levels (reviewed in Gonzalez et al., 2008, 2009). Further studies must determine the extent to which intracellular glucose metabolism might interact with membrane receptors in regulating neuronal responses to extracellular levels of glucose.

Another noticeable aspect of our cell culture experiments relates to the fact that whereas changes in glucose levels or addition of sucralose to the culture medium strongly modulated *Tas1r2* expression levels, no such changes were detected in *Tas1r3* levels. This result is certainly intriguing given the fact that the sweet taste receptor for glucose is the heterodimer T1R2/T1R3. However, some of the characteristics of T1R3 function might provide some explanation for why no significant variations in *Tas1r3* levels were detected as a function of changes in glucose concentrations. It must be noted initially that T1R3 is not a sensory-specific taste gene product; rather, T1R3 has the ability to form dimers with both T1R1 and T1R2, shaping two receptors that, in turn, are sensitive to separate classes of chemicals (Zhao et al., 2003). T1R1 and T1R2, on the other hand, seem to form dimers exclusively with T1R3. In fact, to our knowledge, no functional T1R1/T1R2 dimers have ever been detected in tongue or other tissue (Zhao et al., 2003). One could therefore expect that changes in the levels of a certain nutrient can significantly regulate expression levels of a taste gene only to the extent that the gene is specifically associated with the detection of that nutrient. In the case of our experiments using hypothalamic cells lines, changes in glucose levels were induced while leaving L-amino acid levels unaltered. This might be sufficient to prevent the detection of significant changes in expression levels of *Tas1r3* since quantitative PCR methods can only determine the overall levels of a given transcript. The above could also explain why in these hypothalamic cells experiments *Tas1r2* levels were robustly modulated by glucose while large, although non-significant, variations in *Tas1r3* were observed. This observation is in addition consistent with the fact that *Tas1r1* levels did not respond to changes in glucose levels. Second, T1R3, unlike T1R1 and T1R2, seems to also have the ability to form T1R3/T1R3 homodimers (Zhao et al., 2003). In particular T1R3/T1R3 homodimers display sensitivity to sugars only at relatively high concentrations, e.g., >100 mM (Zhao et al., 2003), which is certainly outside the limits of physiological glucose concentrations in the brain. Although we cannot ascertain, based on transcript levels, that such dimers are expressed in neurons, this is potentially another factor contributing to the insensitivity of *Tas1r3* levels to variations of glucose in the brain at physiological limits. Third, we finally note that T1R3 has been recently implicated in calcium detection by taste cells (Tordoff et al., 2008). Because calcium also acts as a nutritional signal in the brain (Ruat et al., 1995), it is possible that our experimental treatments did not robustly affect *Tas1r3* expression levels because calcium levels have not been explicitly manipulated as an experimental factor. In summary, the lack of specificity of T1R3 to any particular class of nutrients might preclude detection of overall changes in transcript levels of *Tas1r3* in response to the experimental treatments used in our study. We furthermore conjecture that a pervasive change in nutrient concentrations in the brain, involving fluctuations in glucose, L- and D-amino acids, and ionic minerals such as calcium and magnesium, are required to produce sizeable changes in brain *Tas1r3* levels. We conclude with the speculation that changes in *Tas1r2* following variations in brain glucose might enhance the ability of T1R2 to "compete" for dimer formation with T1R3 in detriment of T1R1, although such conjecture has no experimental support at this point.

A similar issue is posed by the lack of significant effects on taste G-protein genes expression levels by changes in nutrient levels. In fact, it appears that all signaling mechanisms downstream to taste G-protein coupled receptors are shared by different classes of chemicals. This holds for the case of both the taste phospholipase PLCβ2 and the non-selective ionic taste channel TRPM5, the deletion of which induces severe impairments in sweet, umami and bitter transduction (Zhang et al., 2003). Similarly, the G-protein gustducin seems to be important not only for sweet taste signaling, but also for umami and bitter detection (Margolskee et al., 2007 Therefore, and likewise the T1R3 case presented above, the fact that taste G-proteins might be part of the transduction pathways of different taste qualities might have precluded us from detecting changes in these molecules based on analyses of transcript levels.

In summary, our study provided the first line of evidence that G-protein coupled taste receptors might operate as membrane-bound chemosensors in brain, and in particular that the sweet T1R2/T1R3 receptor is a candidate to be associated with the elusive brain glucose receptor.

ACKNOWLEDGMENTS

This work has been funded and supported by The John B. Pierce Laboratory. Ligang Zhou is a recipient of a JDRF Research Fellowship. We also thank Jozelia Ferreira for technical assistance with the immunolabeling experiments.

REFERENCES

Ainscow, E. K., Mirshamsi, S., Tang, T., Ashford, M. L., and Rutter, G. A. (2002). Dynamic imaging of free cytosolic ATP concentration during fuel sensing by rat hypothalamic neurones: evidence for ATP-independent control of ATP-sensitive K(+) channels. *J. Physiol.* 544, 429–445.

Anand, B. K., Chhina, G. S., Sharma, K. N., Dua, S., and Singh, B. (1964). Activity of single neurons in the hypothalamic feeding centers: effect of glucose. *Am. J. Physiol.* 207, 1146–1154.

Ashford, M. L., Boden, P. R., and Treherne, J. M. (1990). Glucose-induced excitation of hypothalamic neurones is mediated by ATP-sensitive K+channels. *Pflugers Arch.* 415, 479–483.

Bachmanov, A. A., and Beauchamp, G. K. (2007). Taste receptor genes. *Ann. Rev. Nutr.* 27, 389–414.

Bezencon, C., le Coutre, J., and Damak, S. (2007). Taste-signaling proteins are coexpressed in solitary intestinal epithelial cells. *Chem Senses* 32, 41–49.

Burdakov,D.,Jensen,L.T.,Alexopoulos, H., Williams, R. H., Fearon, I. M., O'Kelly, I.,Gerasimenko,O.,Fugger,L., and Verkhratsky, A. (2006). Tandempore K+channels mediate inhibition of orexin neurons by glucose. *Neuron* 50, 711–722.

de Vries, M. G., Arseneau, L. M., Lawson, M. E., and Beverly, J. L. (2003). Extracellular glucose in rat ventromedial hypothalamus during acute and recurrent hypoglycemia. *Diabetes* 52, 2767–2773.

Elmquist, J. K., Coppari, R., Balthasar, N., Ichinose, M., and Lowell, B. B. (2005). Identifying hypothalamic pathways controlling food intake, body weight, and glucose homeostasis. *J. Comp. Neurol.* 493, 63–71.

Elmquist, J. K., Elias, C. F., and Saper, C. B. (1999). From lesions to leptin: hypothalamic control of food intake and body weight. *Neuron* 22, 221–232.

Fioramonti, X., Lorsignol, A., Taupignon, A., and Penicaud, L. (2004). A new ATP-sensitive K+ channel independent mechanism is involved in glucose-excited neurons of mouse arcuate nucleus. *Diabetes* 53, 2767–2775.

Gonzalez, J.A., Jensen, L. T., Fugger, L., and Burdakov,D.(2008).Metabolism-independent sugar sensing in central orexin neurons. *Diabetes* 57, 2569–2576.

Gonzalez, J. A., Reimann, F., and Burdakov, D. (2009). Dissociation between sensing and metabolism of glucose in sugar sensing neurones. *J. Physiol.* 587, 41–48.

Höfer, D., and Drenckhahn, D. (1998). Identification of the taste cell G-protein, alpha-gustducin, in brush cells of the rat pancreatic duct system. *Histochem. Cell Biol.* 110, 303–309.

Hofer, D., Puschel, B., and Drenckhahn, D. (1996). Taste receptor-like cells in the rat gut identified by expression of alpha-gustducin. *Proc. Natl. Acad. Sci. U. S. A.* 93, 6631–6634.

Huang, A. L., Chen, X., Hoon, M. A., Chandrashekar, J., Guo, W., Trankner, D., Ryba, N. J., and Zuker, C. S. (2006). The cells and logic for mammalian sour taste detection. *Nature* 442, 934–938.

Huang, L., Shanker,Y. G., Dubauskaite, J., Zheng, J. Z., Yan, W., Rosenzweig, S., Spielman, A. I., Max, M., and Margolskee, R. F. (1999). Ggamma13 colocalizes with gustducin in taste receptor cells and mediates IP3 responses to bitter denatonium. *Nat. Neurosci.* 2, 1055–1062.

Kang, L., Dunn-Meynell, A. A., Routh, V. H., Gaspers, L. D., Nagata, Y., Nishimura, T., Eiki, J., Zhang, B. B., and Levin, B. E. (2006). Glucokinase is a critical regulator of ventromedial hypothalamic neuronal glucosensing. *Diabetes* 55, 412–420.

Kang,L.,Routh,V.H.,Kuzhikandathil, E. V., Gaspers, L. D., and Levin, B. E. (2004). Physiological and molecular characteristics of rat hypothalamic ventromedial nucleus glucosensing neurons. *Diabetes* 53, 549–559.

Karschin, C., Ecke, C.,Ashcroft, F. M., and Karschin, A. (1997). Overlapping distribution of K(ATP) channel-forming Kir6.2 subunit and the sulfonylurea receptor SUR1 in rodent brain. *FEBS Lett.* 401, 59–64.

Lathe, R. (2001). Hormones and the hippocampus. *J. Endocrinol.* 169, 205–231.

Lee, K., Dixon, A. K., Rowe, I. C., Ashford, M. L., and Richardson, P. J. (1996). The high-affinity sulphonylurea receptor regulates KATP channels in nerve terminals of the rat motor cortex. *J. Neurochem.* 66, 2562–2571.

Livak, K. J., and Schmittgen, T. D. (2001). Analysis of relative gene expression data using real-time quantitative PCR and the 2-delta/delta (CT) method. *Methods* 25, 402–408.

Margolskee, R. F., Dyer, J., Kokrashvili, Z., Salmon, K. S., Ilegems, E., Daly, K., Maillet, E. L., Ninomiya, Y., Mosinger, B.,and Shirazi-Beechey, S. P. (2007). T1R3 and gustducin in gut sense sugars to regulate expression of Na+-glucose cotransporter 1. *Proc. Natl. Acad. Sci. U. S. A.* 104, 15075–15080.

Matschinsky, F. M. (1996). A lesson in metabolic regulation inspired by the glucokinase glucose sensor paradigm. *Diabetes* 45, 223–241.

McCrimmon, R. (2008). The mechanisms that underlie glucose sensing during hypoglycaemia in diabetes. *Diabet. Med.* 5, 513–522.

McLaughlin, S. K., McKinnon, P. J., and Margolskee, R. F. (1992). Gustducin is a taste-cell specific G protein closely related to transducins. *Nature* 357, 563–569.

McNay, E. C., Williamson, A., McCrimmon, R. J., and Sherwin, R. S. (2006). Cognitive and neural hippocampal effects of long-term moderate recurrent hypoglycemia. *Diabetes* 55, 1088–1095.

Mullen, R. J., Buck, C. R., and Smith, A. M. (1992). NeuN, a neuronal specific nuclear protein in vertebrates. *Development* 116, 201–211.

Nakano, Y., Oomura, Y., Lenard, L., Nishino, H.,Aou, S., andYamamoto, T. (1986). Feeding-related activity of glucose- and morphine-sensitive neurons in the monkey amygdala. *Brain Res.* 399, 167–172.

Nelson,G.,Chandrashekar,J.,Hoon, M. A., Feng, L., Zhao, G., Ryba, N. J. P., and Zucker, C. S. (2002). An amino-acid taste receptor. *Nature* 416, 199–202.

Nelson,G.,Hoon,M.A.,Chandrashekar, J., Ryba, N. J. P., and Zuker, C. S. (2001). Mammalian sweet taste receptors. *Cell* 106, 381–390.

Newton, S. S., Dow, A., Terwilliger, R., and Duman, R. (2002). A simplified method for combined immunohis-tochemistry and in-situ hybridization in fresh-frozen, cryocut mouse brain sections. *Brain Res. Brain Res. Protoc.* 9, 214–219.

Oomura, Y., Ono, T., Ooyama, H., and Wayner, M. J. (1969). Glucose and osmosensitive neurones of the rat hypothalamus. *Nature* 222, 282–284. Porterfield, S. P., and White, B. A. (2007). Endocrine Physiology, 3rd Edn. Philadelphia, PA, Mosby Elsevier.

Ritter, R. C., Slusser, P. G., and Stone, S. (1981). Glucoreceptors controlling feeding and blood glucose: location in the hindbrain. *Science* 213, 451–452.

Routh,V. H. (2002). Glucose-sensing neurons: are they physiologically relevant? *Physiol. Behav.* 76, 403–413.

Rozengurt, E., and Sternini, C. (2007). Taste receptor signaling in the mammalian gut. *Curr. Opin. Pharmacol.* 7, 557–562.

Rozengurt, N., Wu, S. V., Chen, M. C., Huang, C., Sternini, C., and Rozengurt, E. (2006). Colocalization of the alpha-subunit of gustducin with PYY and GLP-1 in L cells of human colon. *Am. J. Physiol. Gastrointest. Liver Physiol.* 291, G792–G802.

Ruat, M., Molliver,M.E.,Snowman, A. M., and Snyder, S. H. (1995). Calcium sensing receptor: molecular cloning in rat and localization to nerve terminals. *Proc. Natl. Acad. Sci. U. S. A.* 92, 3161–3165.

Schuit, F. C., Huypens, P., Heimberg, H., and Pipeleers, D. G. (2001). Glucose sensing in pancreatic beta-cells: a model for the study of other glucose-regulated cells in gut, pancreas, and hypothalamus. *Diabetes* 50, 1–11.

Shoji, S. (1992). Glucose regulation of synaptic transmission in the dorsolateral septal nucleus of the rat. *Synapse* 12, 322–332.

Song, Z., and Routh, V. H. (2005). Differential effects of glucose and lactate on glucosensing neurons in the ventromedial hypothalamic nucleus. *Diabetes* 54, 15–22.

Tordoff, M. G., Shao, H., Alarcón, L. K., Margolskee, R. F., Mosinger, B., Bachmanov, A. A., Reed, D. R., and McCaughey, S. (2008). Involvement of T1R3 in calcium-magnesium taste. *Physiol. Genomics* 34, 338–348.

Young, R. L., Sutherland, K., Pezos, N., Brierley, S. M., Horowitz, M., Rayner, C. K., and Blackshaw, L. A. (2009). Expression of taste molecules in the upper gastrointestinal tract in humans with and without type 2 diabetes. *Gut* 58, 337–346.

Zhang,Y., Hoon, M.A., Chandrashekar, J., Mueller, K. L., Cook, B. W. D., Zucker, C. S., and Ryba, N. J. (2003). Coding of sweet, bitter, and umami tastes: different receptor cells sharing similar signaling pathways. *Cell* 112, 293–301.

Zhao, G. Q., Zhang, Y., Hoon, M. A., Chandrashekar, J., Erienbach, I., Ryba, N. J. P., and Zuker, C. S. (2003). The receptors for mammalian sweet and umami taste. *Cell* 115, 255–266.

Permissions

All chapters in this book were first published by Frontiers; hereby published with permission under the Creative Commons Attribution License or equivalent. Every chapter published in this book has been scrutinized by our experts. Their significance has been extensively debated. The topics covered herein carry significant findings which will fuel the growth of the discipline. They may even be implemented as practical applications or may be referred to as a beginning point for another development.

The contributors of this book come from diverse backgrounds, making this book a truly international effort. This book will bring forth new frontiers with its revolutionizing research information and detailed analysis of the nascent developments around the world.

We would like to thank all the contributing authors for lending their expertise to make the book truly unique. They have played a crucial role in the development of this book. Without their invaluable contributions this book wouldn't have been possible. They have made vital efforts to compile up to date information on the varied aspects of this subject to make this book a valuable addition to the collection of many professionals and students.

This book was conceptualized with the vision of imparting up-to-date information and advanced data in this field. To ensure the same, a matchless editorial board was set up. Every individual on the board went through rigorous rounds of assessment to prove their worth. After which they invested a large part of their time researching and compiling the most relevant data for our readers.

The editorial board has been involved in producing this book since its inception. They have spent rigorous hours researching and exploring the diverse topics which have resulted in the successful publishing of this book. They have passed on their knowledge of decades through this book. To expedite this challenging task, the publisher supported the team at every step. A small team of assistant editors was also appointed to further simplify the editing procedure and attain best results for the readers.

Apart from the editorial board, the designing team has also invested a significant amount of their time in understanding the subject and creating the most relevant covers. They scrutinized every image to scout for the most suitable representation of the subject and create an appropriate cover for the book.

The publishing team has been an ardent support to the editorial, designing and production team. Their endless efforts to recruit the best for this project, has resulted in the accomplishment of this book. They are a veteran in the field of academics and their pool of knowledge is as vast as their experience in printing. Their expertise and guidance has proved useful at every step. Their uncompromising quality standards have made this book an exceptional effort. Their encouragement from time to time has been an inspiration for everyone.

The publisher and the editorial board hope that this book will prove to be a valuable piece of knowledge for researchers, students, practitioners and scholars across the globe.

List of Contributors

Martha Manoli
Developmental Biology, Faculty of Biology, Institute Biology I, University of Freiburg, Freiburg, Germany

Wolfgang Driever
Developmental Biology, Faculty of Biology, Institute Biology I, University of Freiburg, Freiburg, Germany
Centre for Biological Signaling Studies (BIOSS), University of Freiburg, Freiburg, Germany

Ulrich Herget
Developmental Genetics of the Nervous System, Max Planck Institute for Medical Research, Heidelberg, Germany
The Hartmut Hoffmann-Berling International Graduate School of Molecular and Cellular Biology, University of Heidelberg, Heidelberg, Germany

Soojin Ryu
Developmental Genetics of the Nervous System, Max Planck Institute for Medical Research, Heidelberg, Germany

Sophie Croizier, Sandrine Chometton, Dominique Fellmann, Vesna Cvetkovic-Lopes, Christophe Houdayer, Gabrielle Franchi, Amandine Mariot and Pierre-Yves Risold
EA 3922, SFR FED 4234, UFR Sciences Médicales et Pharmaceutiques, Université de Franche-Comté, Besançon, France

Vanessa H. Routh and Zhenyu Sheng
Department of Pharmacology and Physiology, New Jersey Medical School, Rutgers University, Newark, NJ, USA

Lihong Hao, Ammy M. Santiago and Chunxue Zhou
Department of Pharmacology and Physiology, New Jersey Medical School, Rutgers University, Newark, NJ, USA
Department of Pharmacology and Physiology and Graduate School of the Biomedical Sciences, New Jersey Medical School, Rutgers University, Newark, NJ, USA

Valery Grinevich
Schaller Research Group on Neuropeptides, German Cancer Research Center and CellNetwork Cluster of Excellence of the University of Heidelberg, Heidelberg, Germany

Michel G. Desarménien
Institute of Functional Genomics, Centre National de la Recherche Scientifique, Institut National de la Santé et de la Recherche Médicale, Université Montpellier 1, Université Montpellier 2, Montpellier, France

Bice Chini
Consiglio Nazionale delle Ricerche Institute of Neuroscience, Milan. Italy

Maithé Tauber
Reference Centre for Prader-Willi Syndrome – Department of Pediatric Endocrinology, Hôpital des Enfants Centre Hospitalier Universitaire de Toulouse 330, Toulouse, France
Institut National de la Santé et de la Recherche Médicale Unité Mixe de Recherche 1043, Paul Sabatier University Toulouse III, Toulouse, France

Françoise Muscatelli
Institut de Neurobiologie de la Méditerranée Unité Mixe de Recherche U901, Institut National de la Santé et de la Recherche Médicale, Parc Scientifique de Luminy, Marseille, France
Aix-Marseille Université, Institut de Neurobiologie de la Méditerranée Unité Mixe de Recherche 901, Marseille, France

Christin Kosse
Neurophysiology, MRC National Institute for Medical Research, London, UK

Denis Burdakov
Neurophysiology, MRC National Institute for Medical Research, London, UK
MRC Centre for Developmental Neurobiology, King's College London, London, UK

Laura B. Buckman
Department of Molecular Physiology and Biophysics, Vanderbilt University Medical Center, Nashville, TN, USA
Division of Infectious Disease, School of Medicine, University of North Carolina at Chapel Hill, Chapel Hill, NC, USA

Kate L. J. Ellacott
Biomedical Neuroscience Research Group, University of Exeter Medical School, Hatherly Laboratories, Exeter, UK

Michelle Ware, Houda Hamdi-Rozé and Valérie Dupé
Institut de Génétique et Développement de Rennes, Faculté de Médecine, CNRS UMR6290, Université de Rennes 1, Rennes, France

Seth W. Hurley
Department of Psychology, University of Iowa, Iowa City, IA, USA

Priyattam J. Shiromani
Departments of Psychiatry and Behavioral Sciences, Medical University of South Carolina, Charleston, SC, USA
Ralph H. Johnson VA Medical Center, Medical University of South Carolina, Charleston, SC, USA

Anneke Alkemade
Amsterdam Brain and Cognition Center, University of Amsterdam, Amsterdam, Netherlands

Annegret L. Falkner
Neuroscience Institute, New York University School of Medicine, New York, NY, USA

Dayu Lin
Neuroscience Institute, New York University School of Medicine, New York, NY, USA
Department of Psychiatry, New York University School of Medicine, New York, NY, USA

Nathan C. Bingham and Susan R. Rose
Division of Endocrinology, Cincinnati Children's Hospital Medical Center, University of Cincinnati College of Medicine, Cincinnati, OH, USA

Thomas H. Inge
Division of Pediatric General and Thoracic Surgery, Cincinnati Children's Hospital Medical Center, University of Cincinnati College of Medicine, Cincinnati, OH, USA

Sarah M. Burke
Center of Expertise on Gender Dysphoria, Neuroscience Campus Amsterdam, Department of Medical Psychology, VU University Medical Center, Amsterdam, Netherlands
Neuroendocrinology Group, Netherlands Institute for Neuroscience, Amsterdam, Netherlands

Grant Sinson
Department of Neurosurgery, Medical College of Wisconsin, Milwaukee, WI, USA

Peggy T. Cohen-Kettenis
Center of Expertise on Gender Dysphoria, Neuroscience Campus Amsterdam, Department of Medical Psychology, VU University Medical Center, Amsterdam, Netherlands

Dick J. Veltman
Department of Psychiatry, Neuroscience Campus Amsterdam, VU University Medical Center, Amsterdam, Netherlands

Daniel T. Klink
Center of Expertise on Gender Dysphoria, Department of Pediatric Endocrinology, VU University Medical Center, Amsterdam, Netherlands

Julie Bakker
Center of Expertise on Gender Dysphoria, Neuroscience Campus Amsterdam, Department of Medical Psychology, VU University Medical Center, Amsterdam, Netherlands
Neuroendocrinology Group, Netherlands Institute for Neuroscience, Amsterdam, Netherlands
GIGA Neuroscience, University of Liege, Liege, Belgium

Adele Chimento, Rosa Sirianni, Ivan Casaburi and Vincenzo Pezzi
Laboratory of Applied Biology, Department of Pharmacy, Health and Nutrition Sciences, University of Calabria, Cosenza, Italy

Anne Drougard, Audren Fournel, Philippe Valet and Claude Knauf
NeuroMicrobiota, European Associated Laboratory, INSERM/UCL, Institut National de la Santé et de la Recherche Médicale, U1048, Institut des Maladies Métaboliques et Cardiovasculaires (I2MC), CHU Rangueil, Université Paul Sabatier, Toulouse, France

Andrew Elson, Joseph Bovi and Chris Schultz
Department of Radiation Oncology, Medical College of Wisconsin, Milwaukee, WI, USA

Kawaljeet Kaur and Diana Maas
Division of Endocrinology, Metabolism, and Clinical Nutrition, Medical College of Wisconsin, Milwaukee, WI, USA

Roda Rani Konadhode and Dheeraj Pelluru
Departments of Psychiatry and Behavioral Sciences, Medical University of South Carolina, Charleston, SC, USA

Alan Kim Johnson
Department of Psychology, University of Iowa, Iowa City, IA, USA
Department of Pharmacology, University of Iowa, Iowa City, IA, USA
Department of Health and Human Physiology, University of Iowa, Iowa City, IA, USA
François M. Abboud Cardiovascular Center, University of Iowa, Iowa City, IA, USA

Robert H. Lustig
Department of Pediatrics, University of California San Francisco, San Francisco, CA, USA

Xueying Ren and Ivan E. de Araujo
The John B Pierce Laboratory, New Haven, CT, USA
Department of Psychiatry, Yale University School of Medicine, New Haven, CT, USA

Ligang Zhou
Department of Internal Medicine, Yale University School of Medicine, New Haven, CT, USA

Rose Terwilliger and Samuel S. Newton
Department of Psychiatry, Yale University School of Medicine, New Haven, CT, USA

Index

A

Acetylcholine, 78, 101-102, 104, 106, 148, 202-204

Adrenocorticotropic Hormone, 24, 146, 185

Agouti-related Peptide, 41, 44, 78, 140

Androstadienone, 155-157, 159-164

Arcuate Nucleus, 7, 9, 13, 32, 35, 42, 49-52, 84-85, 102, 117, 129, 140, 165, 173, 176, 181-183, 192, 195, 200, 202, 204, 215-216, 223

Arginine Vasopressin, 9, 17, 25-26

Astrocytes, 45, 48, 50, 81-86, 109, 213

Astrogliosis, 82-84, 86

B

Bariatric Surgery, 146, 149-154, 182, 201, 206

C

Cataplexy, 78-79, 100-101, 106

Central Nervous System, 1, 34, 81, 87, 97, 109, 114-115, 144, 146, 154, 171, 174, 183-184, 191, 198, 200, 207-208, 221

Cerebral Cortex, 28-29, 61, 106, 110, 114, 118, 120, 130-131

Cerebrospinal Fluid, 42-43, 65, 100, 183

Chemo-signal, 155, 160-161, 163

Cholecystokinin, 17, 25-26, 102

Circumventricular Organs, 42, 192, 199

Coexpression, 3, 17-25

Corticotropin-releasing Hormone, 14, 17, 25-26, 53

D

Deiodinase, 108-109, 114-116

Diencephalon, 1-3, 6-7, 9, 13, 15, 31-33, 36, 39, 67-68, 91, 97, 130

Dopamine, 25, 33-35, 37-38, 47, 51, 75, 79, 102, 104-105, 130, 140, 142-144, 177, 181, 186, 189, 192, 198-199

E

Early Axon Scaffold, 87-90, 98

Embryogenesis, 2, 60, 62, 87, 91, 95, 97-98, 171

Endocrinopathy, 185, 188-189, 201

Ependymal Cells, 81-82

Estrogen Receptor Alpha, 132-133, 144, 165, 170, 172

F

Functional Magnetic Resonance Imaging, 136, 155

G

Gamma-aminobutyric Acid, 99, 101

Gastrulation, 1

Gender Dysphoria, 155-156, 158-162, 164

Glial Cells, 45, 50, 57, 82, 85, 109-110, 114

H

Histamine, 72-79, 101-102, 107

Homeostasis, 17, 41, 45, 47-50, 52-53, 69, 81-85, 87, 106, 148-149, 173, 175, 177, 179-183, 191-193, 196-199, 209, 216, 221-223

Hyperphagia, 49, 64, 68, 147, 149-150, 153-154, 173, 179-180, 183, 204, 207

Hypoglycemia, 41-42, 44-53, 83, 86, 150-151, 193, 199, 204, 209, 221, 223

Hypomyelination, 82, 110, 115

Hypothalamic Obesity, 146, 150, 153-154, 201-202, 204-207

Hypothalamus, 1-4, 6-7, 9, 11-15, 17-19, 21, 25-26, 28-39, 41-42, 44-52, 54-57, 59, 61, 66-70, 72-75, 78-79, 81-85, 87-95, 97-103, 105-115, 117, 119-120, 122, 127-138, 140-144, 146-148, 150, 155, 157, 159, 164-166, 169-171, 173-183, 185-195, 197-207, 209-218, 220-221, 223

I

Immunohistochemistry, 2, 21, 31, 55, 57, 94, 118-119, 212

Isocortex, 117, 120

L

Lateral Hypothalamic Area, 28, 31, 50-51, 105, 117-118, 181, 191-192, 199, 202, 204

M

Magnocellular Neurons, 17, 55, 57, 65, 68-69

Mammillotegmental Tract, 87, 97

Medial Preoptic Nucleus, 136

Melanin Concentrating Hormone, 28, 44, 78, 99, 101, 105-107, 130

Microglia, 52, 81, 83-84, 86

Mitochondrial Dynamics, 176, 180, 183

Morpholinos, 2, 4, 6, 8, 10

N

Narcolepsy, 35, 39, 72-73, 75, 78-79, 99-101, 105-107, 147, 154

Neonatal Overnutrition, 81-82

Neural Plate, 1, 15, 39-40, 98

Neuroanatomy, 15, 25, 30, 56, 100, 110, 113-114, 117, 130, 181

Neurodegenerative Disorders, 174, 180

Neuroendocrine Neurons, 1, 13, 26, 31, 57, 92, 213, 221

Neuroendocrine System, 17, 41, 47, 69

Neurogenesis, 30-36, 38, 70, 83, 85, 87-88, 90-91, 93-97

Neurohypophysis, 17, 24, 26, 35-37, 57

Neuropeptides, 15, 17-19, 21, 23, 25-26, 49, 54, 65, 69, 79, 86, 107, 129, 131, 147, 199

Neurosecretory Preoptic Area, 17-19

Neurotensin, 17, 25-26, 102, 183

Neurotransmitters, 35, 39, 73, 99, 173

Norepinephrine, 78, 101, 104, 175, 199, 203-205
Notch/proneural Network, 87, 90, 94-95

O
Oligodendrocytes, 81-82, 110
Optogenetic Stimulation, 74, 103-104, 106, 132, 134-136, 142
Orexin, 41, 43, 45-53, 72-80, 99-107, 130, 183, 191, 193-200, 210, 223
Oxytocin, 9, 17, 25-26, 54-55, 62, 65, 67-71

P
Pallidum, 1, 3, 7, 9, 11, 13-15, 29, 31, 36, 61, 98, 117, 120, 128
Paraformaldehyde, 18, 118, 212
Paraventricular Nucleus, 17, 25-26, 44-45, 47-48, 51, 53, 70, 108-109, 113, 115, 117, 174, 203-204, 213, 215-216
Pharmacogenetics, 132
Pituitary Adenoma, 185, 190
Postoptic Commissure, 19, 33, 39, 87-89, 98
Preoptic Region, 1, 3, 6-7, 9, 11, 13, 17, 30
Proneural Network, 87, 90, 94-95

R
Radiotherapy, 146, 185-190, 205

S
Serotonin, 33-35, 73-76, 79, 101-102, 104, 142-143, 203, 205
Sleep-active Neurons, 101, 104-105
Somatostatin, 17-18, 25, 101, 153, 204, 206-207
Sonic Hedgehog, 14, 38-39, 56, 67, 88, 95-98
Subiculum, 61, 102
Substantia Nigra, 34, 36-38, 51, 117-118, 120, 128-130
Suprachiasmatic Nucleus, 31, 105, 110, 112, 200

T
Telencephalon, 1-3, 7, 9, 13-15, 19, 28-39, 88-89, 92, 98, 117-122, 127-128
Thyroid Hormone, 108-109, 114-116, 154, 206
Thyrotropin, 17, 105, 108-109, 114-115, 154
Tomotherapy, 185-186, 188, 190
Tracer Injections, 118
Tractus Postopticus, 28, 30, 34, 36

V
Vasoactive Intestinal Peptide, 17
Ventral Longitudinal Tract, 87-88

www.ingramcontent.com/pod-product-compliance
Lightning Source LLC
LaVergne TN
LVHW082214200926
848484LV00008B/2256